DISEASES OF THE HAIR AND SCALP

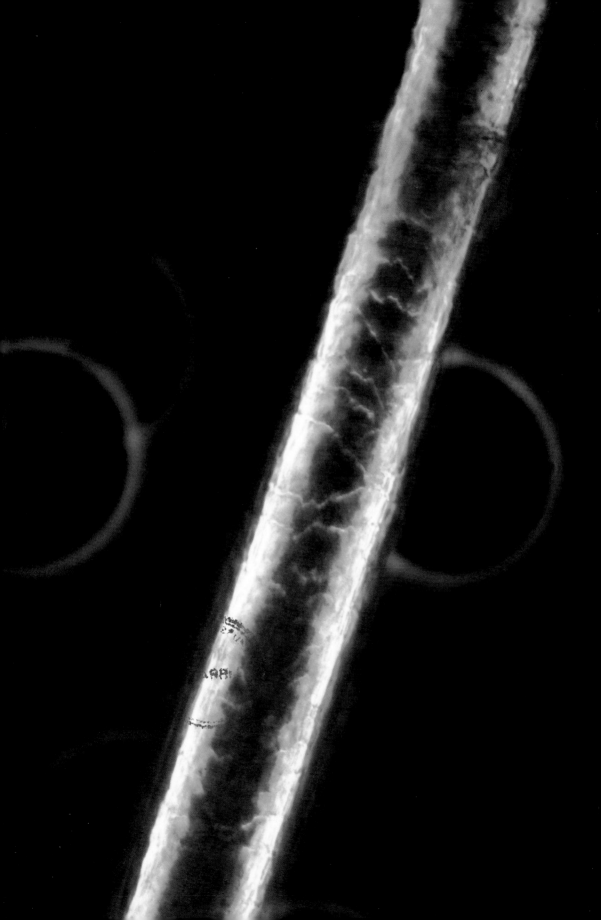

Diseases of the Hair and Scalp

EDITED BY

ARTHUR ROOK
MA, MD, FRCP
Consultant Dermatologist
Cambridge

AND

RODNEY DAWBER
MA, MB, ChB, FRCP
Consultant Dermatologist
John Radcliffe Hospital, Oxford

SECOND EDITION

OXFORD

BLACKWELL SCIENTIFIC PUBLICATIONS

LONDON EDINBURGH BOSTON

MELBOURNE PARIS BERLIN VIENNA

© 1982, 1991 by
Blackwell Scientific Publications
Editorial Offices:
Osney Mead, Oxford OX2 OEL
25 John Street, London WC1N 2BL
23 Ainslie Place, Edinburgh EH3 6AJ
3 Cambridge Center, Cambridge,
  Massachusetts 02142, USA
54 University Street, Carlton
  Victoria 3053, Australia

Other Editorial Offices:
Arnette SA
2, rue Casimir–Delavigne
75006 Paris
France

Blackwell Wissenschaft
Meinekestrasse 4
D-1000 Berlin 15
West Germany

Blackwell MZV
Feldgasse 13
A-1238 Wien
Austria

First published 1982
Second edition 1991

Set by Interprint Ltd, Malta
Printed and bound in Great Britain
by Butler & Tanner Ltd,
Frome and London

DISTRIBUTORS

Marston Book Services Ltd
PO Box 87
Oxford OX2 0DT
(*Orders*: Tel. 0865 791155
         Fax: 0865 791927
         Telex: 837515)

USA
Mosby-Year Book, Inc.
11830 Westline Industrial Drive
St Louis, Missouri 63146
(*Orders*: Tel: (800) 633-6699)

Canada
Mosby-Year Book, Inc.
5240 Finch Avenue East
Scarborough, Ontario
(*Orders*: Tel: (416) 298-1588)

Australia
Blackwell Scientific Publications
(Australia) Pty Ltd
54 University Street
Carlton, Victoria 3053
(*Orders*: Tel: (03) 347-0300)

British Library
Cataloguing in Publication Data

Rook, Arthur
  Diseases of the hair and scalp.—2nd ed.
  1. Man. Hair & scalp. Diseases
  I. Title   II. Dawber, R.P.R. (Rodney PR)
  616.546

  ISBN 0-632-02719-3

Contents

List of Contributors

J.H. BARTH, *Department of Dermatology, Slade Hospital, Oxford OX3 7JH.*

R.P.R. DAWBER, *Department of Dermatology, Slade Hospital, Oxford OX3 7JH.*

D.A. FENTON, *Department of Dermatology, St Thomas's Hospital, Lambeth Palace Road, London SE1 7EH.*

A.R. ROOK, *Department of Dermatology, Addenbrooke's Hospital, Cambridge CB2 2QQ.*

N.B. SIMPSON, *Department of Dermatology, Royal Infirmary, Glasgow G4 0SF.*

F.T. WOJNAROWSKA, *Department of Dermatology, Slade Hospital, Oxford OX3 7JH.*

Preface to the Second Edition

The first edition was aimed mainly at clinicians — dermatologists, physicians and paramedicals who, like us all, find difficulty in handling patients with hair and scalp diseases. It was written at a time when no detailed or comprehensive clinical monograph had been written since Saville and Warren in the 1950s.

As clinicians with a considerable interest in the scientific basis of hair disease we were reassured that the first edition seems to have satisfied a need.

Much has changed during the 1980s in the science and therapeutics within this field — exciting keratin, immunocytochemical, immunological, endocrine and treatment advances, particularly with regard to androgenetic alopecia and alopecia areata. Because of the rapidity of change, we felt it prudent to solicit the considerable expertise of other British authorities to contribute their clinical and scientific skills in writing several chapters — Julian Barth, David Fenton, Nick Simpson and Fenella Wojnarowska have in this way added enormous skill and detail to this second edition.

This book is not meant to be an exhaustive account of everything ever written and thought about regarding the hair and scalp. It inevitably reflects the authors' interests to some degree; but we hope that the detail will prove sufficient to help those working in the field of hair and scalp diseases.

Rodney Dawber
Arthur Rook

Preface to the First Edition

With a few notable exceptions most physicians, including most dermatologists, took little interest in disorders of the hair, apart from ringworm and alopecia areata and certain rare hereditary disorders of the hair shaft, until the development of scientific endocrinology in the present century provided some understanding of the mechanisms underlying certain common disturbances of hair growth. Recent research has greatly increased our knowledge of the complex endocrine influences on the hair, and has also established that a wide range of other metabolic and nutritional disturbances, and some psychiatric states, may first be clinically manifest as, or be accompanied by, changes in the density, pattern, colour or texture of the hair. Apart from those abnormalities of the hair which result from direct external infection, or from chemical or physical trauma, almost all are caused by or are related to systemic processes. The patient who complains of loss of hair, or of the growth of hair which she considers abnormal or excessive, is presenting her physician with a symptom which is as worthy of careful study and investigation as is abdominal pain or cough or any other symptom.

Research by anthropologists and zoologists has thrown much light on the origin and significance of certain common changes in hair pattern, which have in the past wrongly been regarded as abnormal. They have also made it clear that there is no scientific justification for the study of the scalp hair in isolation from the reduced but far from vestigial hair coat in other regions of the body.

This book attempts to present a practical clinical account of the hair and its disorders. It is hoped that it will be of value not only to the dermatologist, but also to other physicians who wish to understand the significance of changes in their patients' hair. The comparative physiology of hair growth is described because it throws light on clinical situations in man. The history of each disorder is discussed briefly, where it explains international inconsistencies in nomenclature, and at greater length where it explains how discredited 'scientific' theories of the past have taken a prominent and sometimes a misleading place in contemporary folk-lore.

Diseases of the scalp are included because they are so often associated with some disturbance of hair growth.

Arthur Rook
Rodney Dawber

Acknowledgements

We would like to express our gratitude to the many colleagues who have supplied us with clinical photographs of their patients. The source of each illustration is acknowledged in the legend which accompanies it.

We greatly appreciate the assistance of Mr C. Gummer, Scientific Officer, Slade Hospital, Oxford, for drawing many figures and for offering constructive criticisms.

Schering Chemicals Limited have kindly paid the cost of the colour frontispiece.

Chapter 1
The Comparative Physiology, Embryology and Physiology of Human Hair

Comparative aspects of the physiology of hair growth
Endocrine influences on follicular activity
The embryology of hair
The growth cycle of the human hair follicle

Comparative aspects of the physiology of hair growth
(References p. 4)

Hair is a characteristic feature of the mammals. The factors which control hair growth and replacement in some mammals other than man have been extensively studied for a variety of motives. Economic pressures have certainly provided a stimulus for research into hair growth in the sheep and in other species which directly or indirectly serve man's needs. In addition, very numerous experimental investigations have been carried out on the common laboratory mammals.

These studies in mammals other than man are of great importance to the physician in clinical practice for they throw much light on the origin and significance of the complex mechanisms by which the growth and replacement of human hair are regulated.

Although a striking feature of hair in man is its relative sparcity, where it is present it is often long and plentiful and by no means vestigial (Goodhart 1960). Man has largely lost the general covering of body hair which protects the skin of other primates. Ashley Montagu (1964) suggests that this reduction in body hair may have followed the adoption of a hunting way of life which necessitated the development of a mechanism for the rapid loss of body heat. The eccrine sweat glands were evolved and selection pressures then favoured the partial loss of the covering of hair which impaired their function.

The head hair and the beard are adornments directly concerned with sexual display (Patzer 1985); many authors writing in the fields of ethnology, anthropology, sociology and psychology have suggested more profound functions for adult body hair—even mystical and magical significance (Leach 1958). Pubic hair is in general much better developed in man than in other species and axillary hair is an almost exclusively human characteristic. It is probable that the hair in both sites is concerned with the wider dissemination of the odour of the apocrine glands, which become functional at the age at which this hair develops.

The general covering of body hair in many mammals has an important function in conserving heat, and in some the colour or pattern of colours serves as

1

camouflage. In mammals living in geographical regions in which there are marked seasonal changes in temperature, a heavy coat which made survival possible throughout the cold winter could well be a handicap in warmer weather. Moulting evolved under such climatic conditions to allow the necessary seasonal adjustments of the weight (and in some species also of the colour) of the coat. However, moulting is not necessarily seasonal; it may correlate with age or with reproductive cycles (Ebling 1965).

Wave moulting
The pattern of moulting varies greatly from species to species and even in successive cycles in a single species (Ebling 1965). Moulting may be related to age, the texture, density and colour of successive coats adapting the young animal to the changed circumstances of each stage of development. Synchronous shedding of hair is a pathological event except in the very young. In many species, spontaneous moults start in one region and progress in a wave across the body. Age related moulting in rats and mice starts on the belly and moves over the flanks to the back. In the adult rabbit these waves of hair shedding and replacement start in the anterior dorsal region and move posteriorly and ventrally.

Seasonal moulting occurs in many species in the spring and autumn; in others there are three moults each year. For example, in the stoat, *Mustela erminea* (Rothschild 1942, 1944), moults occur in the autumn, winter and spring. The winter moult starts on the belly and moves towards the back. In the spring, the wave passes in the opposite direction. Aquatic rodents such as the beaver and the muskrat undergo almost continuous coat replacement but suspend moulting at the peak of the breeding season (Ling 1972). Aquatic mammals such as seals moult usually after the breeding season.

Many other mammals have seasonal moults. Ebling (1965) makes the important point that all the follicles in any particular region of the body do not necessarily behave in the same fashion. For example, in a wild sheep, the moufflon, the moult is complete only in the outer coat; the shorter wool fibres continue to grow (Ryder 1960).

Mosaic moulting
In the species so far mentioned, with the exception of the mouflon, with the two distinct populations of follicles, the follicles in each region of the body are synchronized in more or less the same stage of the moulting cycle. In the human scalp, however, postnatally the activity of each follicle appears to be independent of that of its neighbours (Ebling 1986). This so-called mosaic pattern of moulting has been said to occur in the guinea-pig which, on this account, has been regarded as a particularly valuable species for laboratory studies on hair growth (Bosse 1965). Subsequent studies in the guinea-pig (Jackson & Ebling 1970, 1971, 1972) on the effects of oestradiol on the hair cycles suggest that there is a wave pattern of follicular activity in this animal, which is partially obscured by the lack of

synchrony between different types of follicle, although there is a marked degree of synchrony within each type. Waves of hair growth appear to move from anterior to posterior (Tejima *et al.* 1968). A number of observations (reviewed by Jackson 1972) suggest that moulting in the human scalp too, may not be strictly of the mosaic pattern, because more than one type of follicle may be concerned.

The significance of moulting
Moulting is in general a mechanism of adaptation to changing environmental temperatures and conditions, but in some species it shows also some correlation with the sexual cycle. In the rabbit (Farooq *et al.* 1963) hair loosening occurs towards the end of pregnancy and the doe plucks the loosened hair to line her nest. Postpartum shedding of hair occurs also in women, but its practical significance is questionable.

The regulation of moulting
The photoperiod—the duration of daylight—has been shown to have a strong influence on the moulting cycle as well as on the sexual cycle in a number of animals (Ebling 1965). Temperature itself appears to have little direct influence on the cycles. It is postulated that the increase in the photoperiod in the spring and its decrease in the autumn influence the moulting cycle through the eyes, the hypothalamus and the hypophysis, which then directly modifies follicular activity through the thyroid and adrenal, and indirectly through the gonads.

Both the sexual cycle and the hair cycle are intrinsic rhythms, which may in some species be adjusted by environmental factors acting through the endocrine system. In man, the sexual cycle and the hair cycle have become largely disengaged from environmental influences, but the hormones of environmental adaptation and the sex hormones still influence follicular activity under physiological as well as pathological conditions. Hormonal influences on the hair follicle in species other than man can throw much light on the phenomena observed in man, and will therefore be reviewed in some detail.

Endocrine influences on follicular activity (see also Chapter 4)

The investigations of the mechanisms by which follicular activity is regulated has been greatly advanced by grafting experiments carried out in rats (Johnson 1965, 1977). The transplantation of dorsal and ventral skin flaps in rats, in a two stage operation to avoid interference with the blood supply of the flaps, showed that the wave of hair replacement developed in each graft at the same time as on the donor and several grafts showed the direction of passage of the wave in the graft to be the opposite to that in the surrounding skin. If grafts are exchanged between rats of different ages so that the waves of hair replacement are out of phase, the timing of the waves on the graft is that of the donor for at least two cycles when the donor is the younger rat. If the donor is the older rat the timing of the first and subsequent cycles is that of the host. The implication of these studies, and of others in rats joined in parabiosis, is that each follicle has an inherent rhythm of cyclical activity, but that the timing of the events of that cycle can be influenced by systemic factors.

The donor dominance in grafted skin is of great practical importance in plastic surgery, and provides the basis for the treatment of common baldness by grafting from the occipital to the frontovertical regions of the scalp.

The influence of the nervous system on hair growth is uncertain. Hair follicles have a well-developed nerve supply mediating their sensory function (Heyden 1969; Giacometti & Montagna 1969; Hashimoto 1979; Lynn 1988). It has been claimed that after denervation of the skin in mice, the hair grew more slowly after plucking and remained shorter (Omard 1970). Other work in various species showed increased hair growth after sympathectomy, but this seems likely to be a result of increased blood flow. Moreover, in the normal hair cycle the cyclical increase in blood flow in anagen is a consequence of increased metabolic activity and not its cause.

The effects of hormones on the hair cycles in laboratory rodents have been extensively studied (Houssay *et al.* 1965; Ebling 1986). Cortisol inhibits the initiation of anagen in the resting follicle, and gonadectomy and adrenalectomy accelerate it. Oestradiol in the albino rat also delays the initiation of follicular activity and reduces the rate of hair growth and the loss of club hairs. Thyroid stimulates follicular activity. Thyroidectomy in rats and mice slightly reduces the rate of growth of hair and the shaft diameter of the wool fibres (Rougeot 1965).

In the rat the covering of hair in adult life is probably brought about by prolactin. Thyroxin increases hair length in female rats (Rensels & Callahan 1959).

References

Bosse, K. (1965) Growth and replacement of hair in the guinea-pig. In *Comparative Physiology and Pathology of the Skin*, p. 151, eds. A.J. Rook & G.S. Walton. Blackwell Scientific Publications, Oxford.

Ebling, F.J. (1965) Comparative and evolutionary aspects of hair replacement. In *Comparative Physiology and Pathology of the Skin*, p. 87, eds. A.J. Rook & G.S. Walton. Blackwell Scientific Publications, Oxford.

Ebling, F.J. (1986) Biology of hair follicles. In *Dermatology in General Medicine*, 3rd edn, p. 213, eds. T.B. Fitzpatrick, A.Z. Eisen, K. Wolff, I.M. Freedberg & K.F. Austin. McGraw-Hill, New York.

Farooq, A., Denenberg, V.H., Ross, S., Savin, P.B. & Zarrow, M.X. (1963) Maternal behaviour in the rabbit: endocrine factors involved in hair loosening. *American Journal of Physiology*, **204**, 271.

Giacometti, L. & Montagna, W. (1969) The innervation of human hair follicles. In *Advances in Biology of the Skin*, vol. IX, *Hair Growth*, p. 393, eds. W. Montagna & R.L. Dobson. Pergamon Press, Oxford.

Goodhart, C.B. (1960) The evolutionary significance of human hair patterns and skin colouring. *Advances in Science*, **17**, 53.

Hashimoto, K. (1979) Nerven und Blutversorgung des Haarfollikels. In *Haar und Haarkrankheiten*, p. 95, ed. C.E. Orfanos. Fischer, Stuttgart.

Heyden, B. (1969) Über die Innervation des behaarten Haut des Menschen. *Acta Anatomica*, **74**, 20.

Houssay, A.B., Epper, C.E. & Pazo, J.H. (1965) Neurohormonal regulation of the hair cycles in rats and mice. In *Biology of the Skin and Hair Growth*, p. 641, eds. A.G. Lyne & B.F. Short. Angus & Robertson, Sydney.

Jackson, D. (1972) Hair replacement in the guinea-pig and in man. *British Journal of Dermatology*, **87**, 509.

Jackson, D. & Ebling, F.J. (1970) The effect of oestradiol on moulting in the guinea-pig, *Cavia porcellus*, L. *Journal of Clinical Endocrinology*, **48**, 4.

Jackson, D. & Ebling, F.J. (1971) The guinea-pig hair follicle as an object for experimental observation. *Journal of the Society of Cosmetic Chemists*, **22**, 701.

Jackson, D. & Ebling, F.J. (1972) The activity of hair follicles and their response to oestradiol in the guinea-pig, *Cavia porcellus*, L. *Journal of Anatomy*, **111**, 303.

Johnson, E. (1965) Growth and replacement of hair in rodents. In *Comparative Physiology and Pathology of the Skin*, p. 137, eds. A.J. Rook & G.S. Walton. Blackwell Scientific Publications, Oxford.

Johnson, E. (1977) The control of hair growth. In *The Physiology and Pathophysiology of the Skin*, vol. 4, p. 1351, ed. A. Jarrett. Academic Press, London.

Leach, E.R. (1958) Magical hair. *Anthropological Institute of Great Britain and Ireland*, **88**, 147.

Ling, T.K. (1972) Adaptive function of vertebrate molting cycles. *American Zoologist*, **12**, 77.

Lynn, B. (1988) Structure, function and control: afferent nerve endings in the skin. In *Pharmacology of the Skin*, vol. I, p. 175, eds. M.W. Greaves & S. Shuster. Springer-Verlag, Berlin.

Montagu, A. (1964) Natural selection and man's relative hairlessness. *Journal of the American Academy of Dermatology*, **187**, 357.

Omard, E. (1970) Regeneration of hair: a neural effect. *American Zoologist*, **10**, 323.

Patzer, G.L. (1985) *The Physical Attractiveness Phenomena*. Plenum Publications, New York.

Rensels, E.G. & Callahan, W.P. (1952) The hormonal basis for pubertal maturation of hair in the albino rat. *Anatomical Record*, **135**, 21.

Rothschild, M. (1942) Change of pelage in the stoat, *Mustela erminea*, L. *Nature*, **149**, 78.

Rothschild, M. (1944) Pelage change of the stoat, *Mustela erminea*, L. *Nature*, **154**, 180.

Rougeot, J. (1965) Thyroid hormones and the wool cuticle. In *Biology of the Skin and Hair Growth*, p. 625, eds. A.G. Lyne & B.F. Short. Angus & Robertson, Sydney.

Ryder, M.L. (1960) A study of the coat of the moufflon, *Ovis musimon*, with special reference to seasonal change. *Proceedings of the Zoological Society of London*, **135**, 387.

Tejima, Y., Okada, Y., Kanno, F., Kikuchi, K. & Isobe, G. (1968) Studies on hair cycle in the guinea-pig (Abstract). *5th Congress of the International Federation of Societies of Cosmetic Chemists*, Tokyo, p. 40.

The embryology of hair
(References p. 8)

A knowledge of the embryology of the hair follicle is essential for the dermatologist, not only because it may eventually lead to an understanding of many of the structural defects of the hair shaft, but also because the sequence of events by which the hair follicle is formed in foetal life is partly recapitulated in each cycle of follicular activity. It is surprising therefore that, as Pinkus (1958) has pointed out, the subject attracted until relatively recently little interest among either clinicians or anatomists except in Germany. Albert von Kölliker (1817–1905), Swiss by birth, became Professor of Anatomy in Wurzburg in 1847, and was a pioneer in the application of the cell theory in comparative anatomy and embryology. In 1850 he published an important article on the embryology of the skin in the journal of which he was co-founder (Kölliker 1850). P.G. Unna (1850–1929) of Hamburg was the first dermatologist to give serious attention to this subject (Unna 1876). The few English-language texts that did not ignore completely the embryology of the hair quoted *Stohr's Histology*, which also appeared in English translation in 1896. The German work became still more widely known with the publication in 1910 of the *Manual of Human Embryology*, edited by Keith and Moll to which F. Pinkus contributed an important chapter.

The scientific approach in the United States to diseases of the hair, based on studies of the embryology and physiology of the hair follicle, was given great impetus by Martin Engman, Professor of Dermatology, Washington University, St Louis, who had worked for a year in Unna's clinic. Engman initiated a long-term research programme, in which C.H. Danforth, Mildred Trotter, L.D. Cady and others took part. The publications of this group (Danforth 1925) laid the foundations for much subsequent work on the hair.

This account of the embryology of the hair follicle is based largely on the writings of Pinkus (1958), Sengel (1976) and Spearman (1977); also the work on local interactions in mammalian hair growth (Oliver 1980) has suggested that possibly more significance should be given to dermal papillary cell precursors in initiating hair follicle growth embryologically.

The primitive hair germs, seen as focal crowding of the nuclei of basal cells in foetal epidermis, form at the end of the second or the beginning of the third month, in the eyebrow region and on the upper lip and the chin. These are the sites in which vibrissae are present in mammals other than man. Electron microscopic studies (Breathnach & Smith 1968) showed that the initial crowding of the cells in the primitive or pregerm stage is not at first associated with the other significant changes in the cells concerned. The factors determining the sites of individual hair formations are unknown. During the fourth month primary hair germs form between the existing ones, and secondary germs develop in relation to the primary germs, so that the follicles are in groups of three.

It is often stated that no new hair follicles can be formed *in utero* (or postnatally) after the initial population is complete by 20–22 weeks of foetal development. This is certainly true in health but in conditions such as dermal tumours overlying follicular neogenesis may be seen (Dalziel & Marks 1986).

As the hair germ enlarges it becomes asymmetrical and grows obliquely downwards (Fig. 1.1). This solid column of cells, now known as the hair peg, the broad tip of which becomes slightly concave, carries before it the aggregation of mesodermal cells which will form the papilla.

As the follicle elongates, its lower end becomes bulbous, and the concavity at the tip deepens to enclose the dermal papilla. Two swellings appear at the posterior edge of the follicle; the upper swelling is the germ of the sebaceous gland (Fig. 1.2).

The layer of cells immediately surrounding the enclosed papilla constitutes the matrix. Between the epithelial cells melanocytes can be seen, and at first these are scattered throughout the lower part of the bulb and in the outer root sheath. The mesodermal cells surrounding the bulb begin to form the connective tissue sheath (Fig. 1.3).

Above the bulb a cone of cells differentiates from the matrix; these will form the hair. A second concentric cone of cells surrounding the first is the future inner root

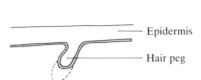

Fig. 1.1 Formation of the epidermal hair peg.

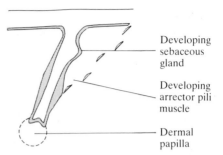

Fig. 1.2 Oblique growth of the peg. The tip of the peg has become concave and encloses the dermal papilla. The upper bulge represents the future sebaceous gland; the lower bulge, the site of attachment of the arrector muscles.

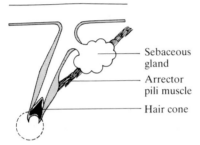

Fig. 1.3 The sebaceous gland has formed. The cone of the internal root sheath is evident.

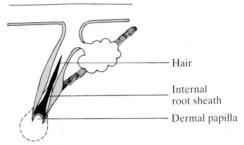

Fig. 1.4 The tip of the hair emerges from the protection of the internal root sheath.

sheath. The outer of the three components of the inner root sheath differentiates first as Henle's layer which keratinizes slightly higher in the follicle, and inside this again is the cuticle of the internal root sheath, the overlapping tile-like cells of which project downwards towards the base of the follicle. The differentiation of Henle's and Huxley's layers reaches an advanced stage before presumptive cuticular or corneal cells can be detected (Robins & Breathnach 1970). The inner cone gives rise to the cortex and the hair cuticle; there is no medulla in foetal hair. The cone of the internal root sheath pushes upwards and protects the tip of the hair as it grows up into the hair canal (Fig. 1.4). In subsequent hair cycles the internal root sheath disintegrates below the level of the sebaceous duct. The first hair coat of long fine lanugo is shed *in utero* about 1 month before birth at full term (Kligman 1961). The second coat of shorter lanugo, in all areas except the scalp where the hair may be both longer and of larger calibre, is shed during the first 3 or 4 months of life, almost imperceptibly, or as a wave terminating in almost complete alopecia; these first and second coats are synchronized in growth and in the sequence of shedding. The more or less unsynchronized mosaic pattern of hair growth then becomes established.

References

Breathnach, A.S. & Smith, J. (1968) Fine structure of the early hair germ and dermal papilla in the human foetus. *Journal of Anatomy*, **102**, 511.

Dalziel, K. & Marks, R. (1986) Hair follicle-like change over histiocytomas. *American Journal of Dermatopathology*, **8**(6), 462.

Danforth, C.H. (1925) Hair with special reference to hypertrichosis. *A.M.A. Archives of Dermatology*, **11**, 494.

Kligman, A.M. (1961) Pathologic dynamics of human hair loss. *Archives of Dermatology*, **83**, 175.

Kölliker, A. (1850) Zur Entwicklungsgeschichte der äussern Haut. *Zeitschrift für wissenschaftlicher Zoologie*, **2**, 67.

Oliver, R.F. (1980) Local interactions in mammalian hair growth. In *The Skin of Vertebrates*, p. 199, eds. R.I.C. Spearman & P.A. Riley. Linnean Society Symposium Series, No. 9.

Pinkus, F. (1910) The development of the integument. In *Manual of Human Embryology*, vol. 1, p. 243, eds. H. Kubel & F. Mall. Lippincott, Philadelphia.

Pinkus, H. (1958) Embryology of hair. In *The Biology of the Skin*, vol. IX, *Hair Growth*, p. 1, eds. W. Montagna & R.A. Ellis. Academic Press, London.

Robins, E.J. & Breathnach, A.S. (1970) Fine structure of bulbar end of human foetal hair follicle at stage of differentiation of inner root sheath. *Journal of Anatomy*, **107**, 131.

Sengel, P. (1976) *Morphogenesis of Skin*. Cambridge University Press, Cambridge.

Spearman, R.I.C. (1977) Hair follicle development, cyclical changes and hair form. In *The Hair Follicle*, p. 1268, ed. A. Jarrett. Academic Press, London.

Unna, P.G. (1876) Beiträge zur Histologie und Entwicklungsgeschichte der menschlichen Oberhaut und ihrer Anhangsgebilde. *Archiv für microscopisch Anatomie und Entwicklungsmach*, **12**, 665.

Unna P.G. (1896) *The Histopathology of the Diseases of the Skin*. William F. Clay, Edinburgh.

The growth cycle of the human hair follicle
(References p. 16)

From the time it is first formed each hair follicle undergoes repeated cycles of active growth and of rest. What controls the cyclical events remains unknown but it is probable that the dermal papilla produces potent proliferative and morphogenic stimuli. The relative duration of phases of the cycle varies with the age of the individual and the region of the body, and can be modified by a variety of factors, both physiological and pathological (Jarrett 1977; Ebling 1986).

The events of the follicular cycle (Kligman 1959) are most readily understood if a follicle is first examined in the final stage of its full development and active growth—metanagen (Fig. 1.5).

Catagen

Mitosis in the matrix decreases and then stops and the follicle enters catagen (Parakkal 1970) which is complete within a few days. The melanocytes in the tip of the papilla resorb their dendrites and as keratinization of hair and inner root sheath

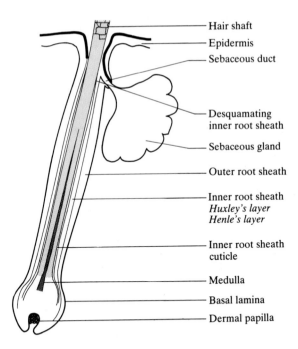

Hair shaft
Epidermis
Sebaceous duct

Desquamating
inner root sheath

Sebaceous gland

Outer root sheath

Inner root sheath
Huxley's layer
Henle's layer

Inner root sheath
cuticle

Medulla

Basal lamina

Dermal papilla

Fig. 1.5 A follicle in metanagen (anagen 6).

continues, the terminal portion of the hair which has become club-shaped lacks pigment, and keratinized fibres extend from it to between epithelial cells. Since mitosis has ceased the lower part of the follicle becomes shortened and the connective tissue sheath, particularly the vitreous membrane, becomes thickened and corrugated. The inner root sheath disintegrates and disappears. The cells of the external root sheath form a sac in the base of which are the germ cells of the follicle. Beneath the sac lies the dermal papilla, which moves upwards as the follicle shortens. The club is surrounded by a capsule of partially keratinized cells and becomes bound to the unkeratinized cells in the base of the sac. The follicle is now in telogen. It is still not clear what initiates spontaneous catagen; the reduction in blood supply is not a primary change; the destruction of the lower two-thirds of the follicle is already underway before the capillary loops are affected (Ellis & Moretti 1957) (Fig. 1.6).

Telogen

Telogen is the resting phase of the hair cycle. The club hair with its relatively unpigmented bulb is held in the sac by the intercellular junctions and may be retained in the follicle until metanagen is well-established in the next cycle or for more than one subsequent hair generation (Fig. 1.7). The follicle re-enters anagen spontaneously at the end of telogen, or may be induced to do so prematurely if the resting club hair is plucked.

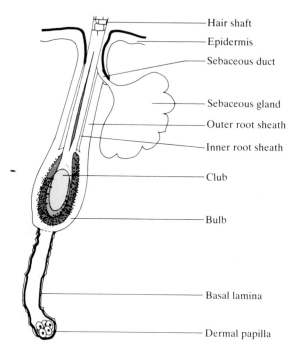

— Hair shaft
— Epidermis
— Sebaceous duct

— Sebaceous gland
— Outer root sheath
— Inner root sheath

— Club

— Bulb

— Basal lamina

— Dermal papilla

Fig. 1.6 Catagen.

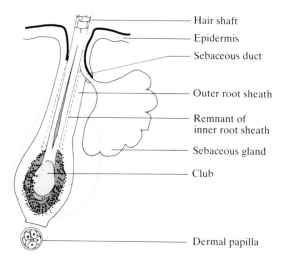

— Hair shaft
— Epidermis
— Sebaceous duct

— Outer root sheath

— Remnant of
inner root sheath

— Sebaceous gland

— Club

— Dermal papilla

Fig. 1.7 A club hair in a
telogen follicle.

Anagen (Chase 1954)

The sequence of events in anagen to some extent recapitulates those of the original morphogenesis of the follicle in foetal skin (Spearman 1977). In stage I of anagen the cells of the dermal papilla increase in size and show increased RNA synthesis;

simultaneously the germinal cells at the base of the sac show vigorous mitotic activity. In stage II, the lower part of the follicle grows down, enclosing the dermal papilla. As the follicle reaches its maximum length the proliferation of the matrix cells gives rise to the cone of the internal root sheath, a distinctive feature of stage III. In stage IV, the melanocytes lining the papilla develop dendrites and begin to form melanin; the hair has formed but is still within the cone of the internal root sheath. The keratogenous zone becomes established just below the level of the sebaceous duct. In stage V, the tip of the hair has emerged from the cone of the internal root sheath (Fig. 1.8). Stage VI, also known as metanagen, begins as soon as the hair emerges at the skin surface and it continues until the onset of catagen. Stages I–V of anagen are known collectively as proanagen.

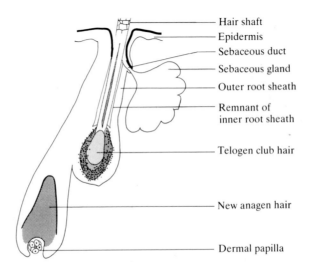

Hair shaft
Epidermis
Sebaceous duct
Sebaceous gland
Outer root sheath
Remnant of inner root sheath
Telogen club hair
New anagen hair
Dermal papilla

Fig. 1.8 Early anagen. The new hair will grow up beside the club hair.

The dynamics of the follicular cycle in the human scalp
The normal duration of anagen in any individual scalp follicle is genetically determined and ranges from 2 to over 5 years. The approximate average duration of anagen is easily remembered as 1000 days (Orentreich 1969). Telogen lasts approximately 100 days. The ratio of anagen to telogen hairs is therefore approximately 90:10 since, under normal conditions, the percentage of hairs in catagen at any given moment is small. The population of follicles in the human scalp is approximately 100,000—blondes have more and redheads fewer. The average number of hairs shed daily is therefore 100. The nature of 'biological variability' means that all the above figures are approximate; they are comparatively of use in representing the dynamics of follicular activity.

The average density of hair follicles in the newborn is $1135/cm^2$. Dilution by growth in surface area has reduced this to 795 towards the end of the first year and to 615 by the third decade. Between the ages of 30 and 50 the destruction of some follicles has reduced the number to 485, after which there is only slight further reduction in old age. In a clinically bald scalp many follicles are reduced in size but the total count is less drastically reduced. Average figures for bald scalp (age 45–70 years) were 330 and (70–85) 280 (Giacometti 1965).

The role of the photoperiod in adjusting moulting cycles in some species of mammal has suggested that similar effects might occur in man. Most observers have failed to record any consistent relation between moulting in man and the seasons. However, Orentreich (1969) recorded short-term variations superimposed on a long-term seasonal variation with maximum loss in November in the northern temperate regions.

The trichogram
Studies of the dynamics of the follicular cycle depend largely on the trichogram, the ratio of anagen to telogen hairs (A/T ratio), as established by the microscopic examination of plucked hairs (Fig. 1.9) (Braun-Falco 1966; Meiers 1967). This technique gives reliable results provided that certain precautions are taken; over 50 hairs must be plucked as the standard deviation is unacceptably high if the sample is too small (Bosse 1967); the hair should not have been washed during the week before the examination, as washing the hair extracts hairs nearing the end of telogen and thus artificially reduces the percentage in this phase recorded in the trichogram (Braun-Falco & Fischer 1966). The hair root is less damaged by a sharp

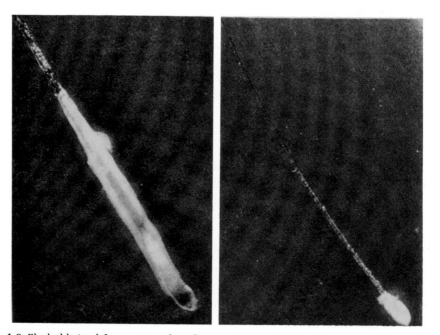

Fig. 1.9 Plucked hairs: left, anagen; right, telogen.

quick pluck than by slow traction. The studies of Headington (1984) suggest that transverse (horizontal) sections of cylindrical scalp biopsies provide further useful details of the cyclical events of the hair follicle and with less potential for observer and 'experimental' errors.

Important differences in the trichogram are recorded with age and with the region of the scalp. The highest A/T ratio—over 90%—is found in children. In adult men, even in those not clinically bald, the proportion of hairs in telogen is highest in the frontovertical region. No marked regional variations were found in non-bald women (Braun-Falco 1966), but differences are present in women with androgenetic alopecia. Witzwl and Braun-Falco (1963) examined scalp hairs from 146 clinically normal subjects; they found an average in all sites in women of 85% in anagen and 11% in telogen, and in men 83 and 15% respectively. Catagen hairs accounted for 2.1% of the total in women and 3.2% in men but were demonstrable in only 48% of women and 46% of men.

Racial variation in follicular density is well-illustrated by studies of the predominantly dark-haired population of the Argentine (Barman *et al.* 1965). The follicular density in adults ranged from 175–300/cm^2 (average of 223; the density of follicles decreased with age in all regions and the hair became finer) but the diameter was not related to the total population. The proportion of telogen hairs increased with age and was greatest in the frontovertical region in both sexes.

In regions of the body other than the scalp anagen is relatively short and telogen relatively long. There is some disagreement between the figures given by different authors, most of whom reported wide variations in each site. Saitoh *et al.* (1970) made their observations by time-lapse photography and also reviewed the findings of some earlier observers.

	Anagen	Telogen
Moustache	16	6
Finger	12	9
Arms	13	13
Leg	21	19

Pinkus (1947) observed a single follicle on the dorsum of one hand daily for 6 years, during which time 12 hairs were formed. The average lifespan of each hair was 180 days (107–195). The hairless intervals lasted, in six instances, 27–52 days, and in the other six 76–92 days.

The rate of hair growth
Several different techniques have been employed to measure the rate of hair growth in man (Barth 1986, 1987). Myers and Hamilton (1951) observed the length of time required for the regrowth of the hair in 90% of follicles after plucking. The time interval ranged from 129 days on the vertex of the scalp and 117 days on the temples, to 92 days on the chin. Plucking the hair damaged the follicle, and

observations based on regrowth after plucking are not necessarily applicable to spontaneous regrowth (Silver *et al.* 1969). Observations of individual uninjured follicles (Saitoh *et al.* 1970) showed that new hairs took 3 weeks to reach the scalp surface. By direct measurement of the regenerated hairs, Myers and Hamilton (1951) found the daily growth rate to be 0.35 mm/day on the vertex and on the temple, and slightly greater in these sites in women than in men. Barman *et al.* (1964) measured daily shavings and obtained essentially similar figures. Using the intradermal injection of [^{35}S] cystine to measure linear growth of scalp hair gave a daily average of 0.37 mm (range 0.31–0.41) (Munro 1966). Saitoh and his colleagues in Japan (Saitoh *et al.* 1969) used a capillary tube technique for measuring the rate of hair growth. They recorded an average growth rate of 0.44 mm on the vertex and on the chest, 0.29 mm at the temples and 0.27 mm in the beard. Time-lapse photography showed a constant growth rate in each follicle and no significant diurnal variation.

Pecoraro *et al.* (1970) studied in 126 subjects aged 10–74, the density and rate of growth of axillary hair. The axilla was divided into three subregions, central, brachial, and thoracic. There were no significant sex differences in hair density. Hair density and growth rate were highest in the central area. The hairs in the three subregions showed different quantitative responses to pregnancy. In all three subregions the hair density decreased with age. In contrast the pubic hair (Astore *et al.* 1979) showed a trichogram little influenced by ageing or by pregnancy.

The mitotic activity at a given level of the germinative matrix of a follicle is inversely proportional to the distance from the base of the dermal papilla (Van Scott *et al.* 1963). There is a consistent proportional relationship between the volume of the hair matrix and the size of the papilla, the latter depending on the size of the population of germinative cells and hence the size of the hair (Epstein & Maibach 1969).

The length of the hair
The length of each hair is genetically determined. It depends obviously on the duration of anagen and the rate of growth (Fig. 1.10); also if hair is intrinsically weak, for example cystine/sulphur deficiency syndromes, or weakened due to hair cosmetic abuse, then premature breakage and weathering may occur giving shorter length.

Systemic influences on the hair cycle
Androgens increase the growth rate as well as the calibre of the shaft in androgen-dependent sites such as the beard. Androgen-blocking agents reduce the growth rate in such sites. In the scalp genetically predisposed to androgenetic alopecia, however, androgen reduces the shaft diameter and the rate of growth and the duration of anagen.

Oestrogen retards the rate of growth during anagen but prolongs the duration of anagen. Thyroxine advances the onset of anagen in resting follicles and cortisone retards it.

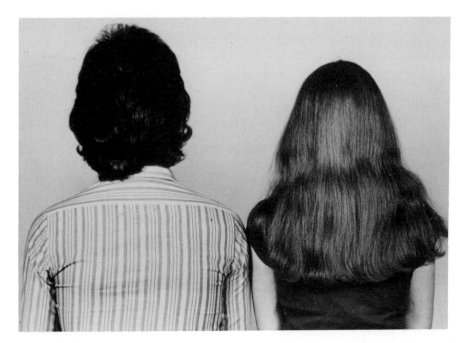

Fig. 1.10 Differences in hair length depend on the duration of anagen, a genetically determined characteristic. Neither of these subjects had had a haircut for over 18 months; length was initially the same.

Local influences on hair growth

Anything causing epithelial hyperplasia initiates a new anagen in resting follicles, for example wounds cause hair growth beyond the edges of the wound (Chase 1969). Telogen skin contains an inhibitor of hair growth (Paus *et al.* 1990).

Inflammatory changes, as in ringworm infections, cause telogen to synchronize in the area of scalp surrounding the lesions, thus limiting the extension of the lesion (Bosse 1967).

The widespread belief that shaving increases the rate of growth and shaft diameter of hair is difficult to destroy. Trotter (1923) showed that neither shaving nor exposure to sunlight had any effect on hair growth. In a further paper in 1928 she repeated that shaving did not have any effect on the growth of the beard. Over 40 years later, Lynfield and MacWilliams (1970) reported that five young men had shaved one leg only for several months, leaving the other leg as a control. There was no difference between the two sides in the weight of hair produced or in the shaft diameter or in the rate of growth.

Whether nerve supply directly affects hair growth and the hair cycle remains unknown though in many neurological abnormalities hair changes have been described. These are discussed by Soria *et al.* (1989)—shorter hair growth was noted on the right side of the scalp in syringomyelia with impaired pain and temperature sensation in this area. Some denervated areas show less abundant hair growth whilst in others hypertrichosis is a feature. In causalgia there is usually obvious hair loss in the affected area. After trigeminal nerve surgery a wedge-shaped temporal area of hair loss may develop; increased greying may be seen under similar surgical conditions.

References

Astore, I.P., Pecoraro, V. & Pecoraro, E.G. (1979) The normal trichogram of pubic hair. *British Journal of Dermatology*, **101**, 441.

Barman, J.M., Pecoraro, V. & Astore, I. (1964) Method, technique and computations in the study of the trophic state of human scalp hair. *Journal of Investigative Dermatology*, **42**, 421.

Barman, J.M., Astore, I. & Pecoraro, V. (1965) The normal trichogram of the adult. *Journal of Investigative Dermatology*, **44**, 233.

Barth, J.H. (1986) Measurement of hair growth. *Clinical and Experimental Dermatology*, **11**, 127.

Barth, J.H. (1987) Normal hair growth in children. *Pediatric Dermatology*, **4**, 173.

Bosse, K. (1967) Der Einfluss der Entzündigung auf das Haarwachstum. *Hautarzt*, **18**, 218.

Bosse, K. (1967) Vergleichende Untersuchungen zur Physiologie und Pathologie des Haarwechsels unter besonderer Berücksichtigung seiner Synchronisation. II. Methodische Untersuchungen zur Haarwechselstatusbestimmung und ihre Anwendung an Mensch und Meerschweinchen. *Hautarzt*, **18**, 35.

Braun-Falco, O. (1966) Dynamik des normalen und pathologischen Haarwachstum. *Archiv für klinische und experimentelle Dermatologie*, **227**, 419.

Braun-Falco, O. & Fischer, C. (1966) Über den Einfluss des Haarwaschens auf das Haarwurzelmuster. *Archiv für klinische und experimentelle Dermatologie*, **226**, 136.

Chase, H.B. (1954) Growth of the hair. *Physiological Review*, **34**, 113.

Chase, H.B. (1969) Physical factors which influence the growth of hair. In *Advances in Biology of the Skin*, vol. IX, *Hair Growth*, p. 435, eds. W. Montagna & R.L. Dobson. Pergamon Press, Oxford.

Ebling, F.J. (1986) Biology of hair follicles. In *Dermatology in General Medicine*, 3rd edn, p. 213, eds. T.B. Fitzpatrick, A.Z. Eisen, K. Wolff, I.M. Freedberg & K.F. Austin. McGraw-Hill, New York.

Ellis, R.A. & Moretti, G. (1957) Vascular pattern associated with catagen hair follicles in the human scalp. *Annals of the New York Academy of Science*, **53**, 448.

Epstein, E.L. & Maibach, H.I. (1969) Cell proliferation and movement in human hair bulbs. In *Advances in Biology of the Skin*, vol. IX, *Hair Growth*, p. 83, eds. W. Montagna & R.L. Dobson. Pergamon Press, Oxford.

Giacometti, L. (1965) The anatomy of the human scalp. In *Advances in Biology of the Skin*, vol. IX, *Hair Growth*, p. 97, eds. W. Montagna & R.L. Dobson. Pergamon Press, Oxford.

Headington, J.T. (1984) Transverse microscopic anatomy of the human scalp: a basis for a morphometric approach to disorders of the hair follicle. *Archives of Dermatology*, **120**, 449.

Jarrett, A. (1977) *The Hair Follicle*. Academic Press, London.

Kligman, A.M. (1959) The human hair cycle. *Journal of Investigative Dermatology*, **33**, 307.

Lynfield, Y.L. & MacWilliams, P. (1970) Shaving and hair growth. *Journal of Investigative Dermatology*, **55**, 170.

Meiers, H.G. (1967) Die Methode des Trichogrammes. *Arztliche Kosmetologie*, **6**, 22.

Munro, D.D. (1966) Hair growth measurement using intradermal sulphur-35 L-cystine. *Archives of Dermatology*, **93**, 119.

Myers, R.J. & Hamilton, J.B. (1951) Regeneration and rate of growth of hair in man. *Annals of the New York Academy of Science*, **53**, 862.

Orentreich, N. (1969) Scalp hair regeneration in man. In *Advances in Biology of the Skin*, vol. IX, *Hair Growth*, p. 99, eds. by W. Montagna & R.L. Dobson. Pergamon Press, Oxford.

Parakkal, P.F. (1970) Morphogenesis of the hair follicle during catagen. *Zeitschrift für Zellforschung*, **104**, 174.

Paus, R., Stenn, K.S. & Link, R.E. (1990) Telogen skin contains an inhibitor of hair growth. *British Journal of Dermatology*, **122**, 777.

Pecoraro, V., Astore, I. & Barman, J.N. (1970) Growth rate and hair density of the human axillae. *Journal of Investigative Dermatology*, **56**, 362.

Pinkus, F. (1947) The story of a hair root. *Journal of Investigative Dermatology*, **9**, 91.

Saitoh, M., Uzuka, M., Sakamoto, M. & Kobori, M. (1969) Rate of hair growth. In *Advances in Biology of the Skin*, vol. IX, *Hair Growth*, p. 183, eds. W. Montagna & R.L. Dobson. Pergamon Press, Oxford.

Saitoh, M., Uzaka, M. & Sakamoto, M. (1970) Human hair cycle. *Journal of Investigative Dermatology*, **54**, 65.

Silver, A.F., Chase, H.B. & Arsenault, C.T. (1969) Early anagen initiated by plucking compared with early spontaneous anagen. In *Advances in Biology of the Skin*, vol. IX, *Hair Growth*, p. 265, eds. W. Montagna & R.L. Dobson. Pergamon Press, Oxford.

Soria, E., Fine, E. & Paroski, M. (1989) Asymmetrical growth of scalp hair in syringomyelia. *Cutis*, **43**, 33.

Spearman, R.I.C. (1977) Hair follicle development, cyclical changes and hair form. In *The Hair Follicle*, p. 1268, ed. A. Jarrett. Academic Press, London.

Trotter, M. (1923) The resistance of hair to certain supposed growth stimulants. *Archives of Dermatology and Syphilology*, **7**, 93.

Trotter, M. (1928) Hair growth and shaving. *Anatomical Record*, **37**, 373.

Van Scott, E.J., Ekel, T.M. & Auerbach, R. (1963) Determinants of rate and kinetics of cell division in scalp hair. *Journal of Investigative Dermatology*, **41**, 269.

Witzel, M. & Braun-Falco, O. (1963) Über den Haarwurzelstatus am menschlichen Capillitium unter physiologischen Bedingungen. *Archiv für klinische und experimentelle Dermatologie*, **216**, 221.

Chapter 2
Hair Follicle Structure, Keratinization and the Physical Properties of Hair

Physiology and biochemistry
(References p. 30)

All the cell layers within the outer root sheath are products of the hair matrix in the bulb (Figs 2.1a and b). The area of active cell division is in the lower bulb and in the upper bulb adjacent to the dermal papilla. From the upper bulb to the zone of complete keratinization cells stream upwards and undergo successively the phases of orientation into layers, hardening and keratinization.

The outer root sheath is not a product of the hair matrix but consists of a sleeve of cells continuous with, and similar in structure to, the surface epidermis. It is, however, an intimate part of the hair follicle which possesses many 'subsections' which are anatomically and functionally separate (Hashimoto & Ito 1989).

Hair bulb

The hair matrix is made up of rapidly dividing cells in the lower bulb and the upper bulb surrounding the dermal papilla. These cells are several layers deep and have a very rapid turnover; it has been suggested that each matrix cell divides every 23–72 hours (Van Scott et al. 1963). Unlike the epidermal basal layer, there appears to be no diurnal variation in mitotic rate or chalone inhibition in the matrix (Bullough & Lawrence 1958; Kligman 1959; Epstein & Maibach 1969); these cells appear to be working 'full-out' during metanagen (Wright & Alison 1984), this being the suggested reason for psoriatic hair bulb matrix cell kinetics being normal (Shahrad & Marks 1976). At the end of the anagen phase of the follicular cycle continuous cell division slows down and finally ceases in catagen.

Matrix cells possess a characteristic ultrastructure (Fig. 2.2). Most of the cell is occupied by the large spherical nucleus; within the scanty cytoplasm are many

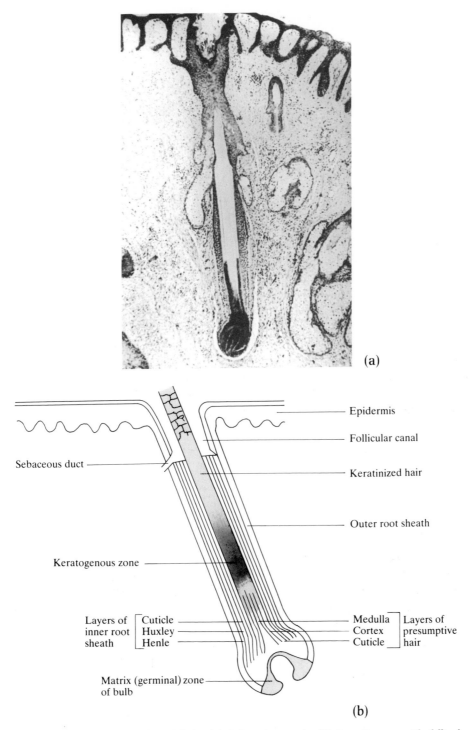

Fig. 2.1 A mature anagen hair follicle: (a) light micrograph, (b) line diagram with follicular components labelled.

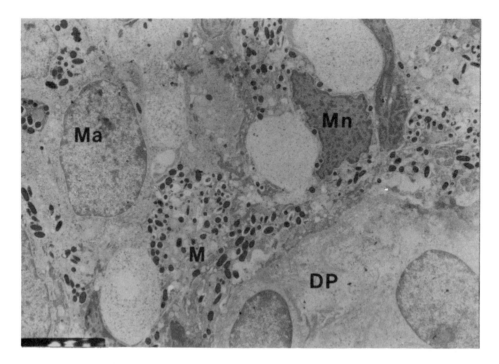

Fig. 2.2 Electron micrograph at the junction of the dermal papilla (DP) and hair bulb. A melanocyte (Mn) containing mature melanosomes (M) is seen adjacent to a hair bulb matrix cell (Ma).

ribosomes and some mitochondria. Rough surface endoplasmic reticulum, a compact Golgi zone adjacent to the nucleus and arrays of cisternae and vesicles compose the rest of the cytoplasm. The cells are rich in RNA (Fraser *et al.* 1972). Desmosomal attachments and gap junctions are present between adjacent cells and, as in epidermal keratinocytes, filaments extend from the desmosomes into the cell cytoplasm. There are considerably fewer attachment sites between matrix cells than are found in the epidermal basal layer; this may facilitate easier movement of cells from the matrix to the upper bulb and suprabulbar area. The cells surrounding the dermal papilla are precursors of the hair fibre and the more peripheral matrix cells give rise to the inner root sheath. In the suprabulbar part of the follicle these cells become relatively long and thin, with distinct cell boundaries (Auber 1952). The overall size of the cells and the relative amount of cytoplasm noticeably increase (Montagna & Van Scott 1958). These changes may relate to greater water content and protein synthesis. Ribosomes are mostly strung together as polysomes and a few bound ribosomes are evident. Golgi bodies are poorly developed in this region and consist of a few vesicles adjacent to the nucleus; the endoplasmic reticulum is poorly developed (Parakkal & Maltoltsy 1964). Both nuclei and nucleoli remain prominent in suprabasal cells.

The various layers ascending the follicle first become noticeable as cells of different shapes. Medullary cells remain relatively large and spherical whilst presumptive hair cortex cells become spindle-shaped. The structure of each layer will be considered separately, from its development from the appropriate bulbar matrix cells, through differentiation and cell death associated with keratinization higher up the follicle.

Medullary cells

These differentiate from matrix cells adjacent to the apex of the dermal papilla. Distinctive microscopic changes can be observed before other cell layers are distinguishable. Irregular dense granules develop from the Golgi apparatus (Auber 1952) and these enlarge by coalescing. By cytological and histochemical methods the granules can be differentiated from epidermal keratohyalin, though as will be seen later, the granules have some biochemical similarities to the inner root sheath protein (Harding & Rogers 1971). Medullary cells do not produce these proteins in significant amounts and harden by a different biochemical process than the keratin-forming cells of the cortex and cuticle (Powell & Rogers 1986). The function of medullary granules in man is not known. Medullary cells produce some filaments which are aggregated into bundles and are randomly distributed in the cytoplasm.

As differentiation proceeds glycogen granules become evident, particularly near the nucleus and other cytoplasmic organelles begin to disintegrate. Mitochondria begin to swell, the cristae lose orientation and the density of the matrix decreases. Finally the mitochondria become vacuolated like empty vessels. Fully formed medullary cells are wedged between projections of cortical cells and in the fully developed hair, mature cells are arranged along the core of the hair with spaces between them.

In vellus and lanugo hair, no medullary cells form and even terminal hair follicles may reveal complete absence or only infrequent medullary cells (Fig. 2.3a).

Cortical cells

These become visible microscopically, at a higher level in the follicle than presumptive medullary cells, as spindle-shaped cells which produce increasing amounts of cytoplasmic filaments parallel both to the long axis of the cell and the hair follicle (Figs 2.4 and 2.5). The filaments grade into dense α-keratin fibrils but have no clear connection with tonofibrils. This zone of keratinization shows evidence of intense protein synthesis (Parakkal 1969), many polysomes being seen together with strong nucleolar and cytoplasmic staining for RNA. The higher keratogenous zone shows increasing evidence of cytolysis; hydrolases are released from lysosomes (acid phosphatase stain) and the phospholipid reaction increases (Braun-Falco 1958a). At the same stage, nuclear degradation occurs. Ribosomes are the final organelle to disappear. Stable sulphydryl groups (cysteine reaction) are increasingly found towards the upper keratogenous zone. The fully keratinized

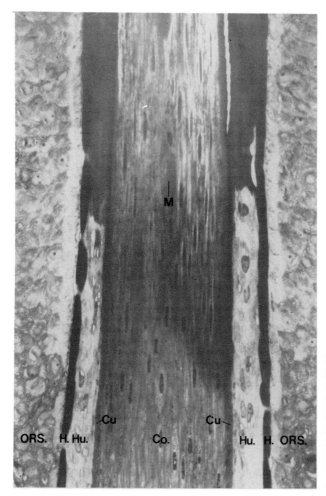

Fig. 2.3 (a) Concentric layers of the hair follicle (resin embedded section). Within the cortex (Co) only occasional medullary cells are present (M). Within the outer root sheath (ORS), all layers show keratinization, which in the Huxley layer (Hu) is only evident in the upper area.

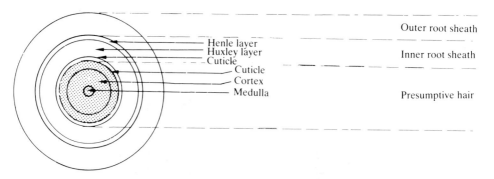

(b) Concentric cell layers of suprabulbar portion of an anagen hair follicle

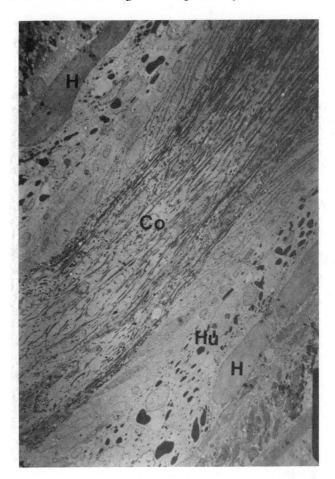

Fig. 2.4 Hair follicle (longitudinal section), showing the central cortex (Co) surrounded by the root sheaths. The Henle layer (at H) is keratinized.

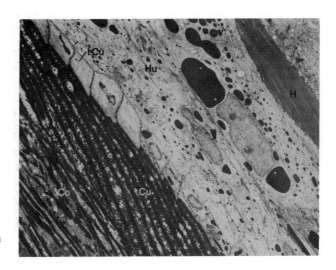

Fig. 2.5 Hair follicle (electron micrograph). The inner root sheath cuticle (I.Cu) is visible adjacent to the hair cuticle (Cu). The Huxley layer (Hu) shows numerous (black) trichohyalin granules.

'dead' cortical cells retain a membranous nuclear outline (nuclear 'ghost') which persists into the hair shaft.

Cuticle cells

Presumptive cuticular cells elongate in the suprabulbar region and become flattened; during differentiation the cells increasingly overlap (Fig. 2.5). Tonofibrils and desmosomes are present but no α-keratin fibrils are produced. Increasing protein synthesis occurs during hardening and keratinization and dense cytoplasmic granules are visible. Reactive phospholipids and cysteine sulphydryl groups are detectable, contributing to the formation of a matrix rather than fibrillar, protein structure (Birkbeck & Mercer 1957).

Hardening (keratin bonding) zone (Fig. 2.1b)

During this phase before complete cell death and keratinization, the hair first acquires its strength and flexibility in the cuticle and cortex (Auber 1952). The hair fibre decreases in diameter by about 25%, probably due to a combination of water loss due to plasma membrane permeability changes, and contraction of keratin complexes from cytoplasmic water loss. In the final stages of keratin bonding, bound sulphydryl is oxidized to cystine and the cysteine reaction of the keratinized area decreases to negligible amounts.

Inner root sheath (Figs 2.3b and 2.5)

The inner root sheath consists of three layers, from within outwards, the cuticle, Huxley's and Henle's layers; the cuticle is one cell thick whilst Huxley's layer is several cells deep. The cuticle interlocks with the cells of the hair cuticle and is intimately associated with it. All three layers are formed from the peripheral mass of matrix cells in the hair bulb. There is no evidence in man to support the idea that the basal cells of the outer root sheath cells overlying the hair bulb contribute to the formation of the Henle layer.

All three layers undergo differentiation in the same sequence but at different rates; firstly, the Henle layer, then the Huxley layer and finally, the cuticle. The late stages of hardening and cell death further up the follicle begin in the Henle layer (Fig. 2.4), then the cuticle and finally, Huxley's layer. It is important to note that complete hardening and differentiation of the inner root sheath occurs before the layers of the developing hair within it. Keratinization proceeds by the secretion of increasing amounts of trichohyalin and flattening of the cells. The trichohyalin granules (Fig. 2.5) are mostly attached to tonofilaments. The final stage of differentiation involves the disintegration of the nucleus, other organelles and the trichohyalin which becomes diffusely visible as electron-dense material between keratin filaments. This is particularly evident in the inner root sheath cuticle. In the lower follicle the junction between the outer root sheath and the Henle layer is maintained by desmosomes and gap junctions; higher up the follicle, after inner root sheath differentiation is complete, the relation with the outer root sheath is maintained by intercellular cement and by interdigitation between cells. The Huxley and Henle layers possess similar intimate methods of contact. With maturation, inner root sheath cells demonstrate thickening of plasma membranes and the deposition of amorphous intercellular material; cells shrink during keratinization, the mature inner root sheath thus becoming a rigid cylindrical tube surrounding the softer ascending hair structures within it (Fig. 2.3a). The fully formed inner root sheath shows detectable amounts of cystine, RNA and phospholipid, probably released from the degradation of hydrolysed organelle membranes and trichohyalin (Jarrett 1958). At the level of the follicular canal, desmosomal contacts between adjacent cells begin to be broken down and the cells, singly or in groups, are shed into the follicular canal. This desquamation is probably facilitated by hydrolases of lysosomal origin. The exact source of these enzymes is not known but they may be from the inner or outer root sheath (Straile 1962) or from sebaceous secretion.

The prime function of the inner root sheath is probably to mould the hair within it. It effects this by hardening in advance of the hair; since the cuticles of the hair and inner root sheath are closely apposed, in health, the fully keratinized fibre takes the shape of the root sheath (Straile 1962; Swift 1977).

Outer root sheath (Figs 2.3a and 2.6)
This layer surrounds the hair follicle as a sleeve of cells several layers thick that is continuous with the epidermis (Hashimoto & Ito 1989). It is divisible into two parts: a short lower part surrounding the outer part of the bulb, and the upper part from the neck of the bulb to the level of the sebaceous duct. The area surrounding the follicular opening has the same structure and biochemical characteristics as the surface epidermis and will not be considered further.

The part surrounding the hair bulb is one or two cells thick, the outer layer being elongated and the inner layer markedly flattened. In the suprabulbar area it is

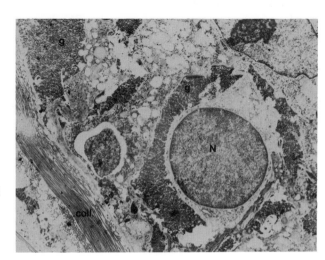

Fig. 2.6 Outer root sheath. The nucleus (N) is surrounded by cytoplasmic glycogen (g). Adjacent to the cell is the perifollicular connective tissue membrane (coll.).

usually three cells thick and only becomes multilayered approximately half way along the follicle. The outer cell layer is the germinative layer continuous with the epidermal basal cells (Parakkal 1969); differentiation occurs in a centripetal direction towards the inner root sheath, the cells enlarging, flattening and becoming vacuolated. The exact fate of the cells adjacent to the Henle layer is not known though it seems likely that movement towards the surface occurs; this certainly occurs in some sheep and mice in which keratinized cells from the upper part of the outer root sheath are shed into the follicular canal along with the inner root sheath. It is possible that some keratinization occurs in the differentiating cells next to the inner root sheath (Jarrett 1958).

The outer root sheath differs from the follicular canal in containing prominent Golgi vesicles associated with well-developed rough endoplasmic reticulum; the amorphous cytoplasmic granules produced during differentiation probably develop from this organelle. The granules are not membrane bound. Membrane-limited vesicles are also present together with glycogen particles (Parakkal 1969). The outer root sheath does not produce keratohyalin. The epidermis of the follicular canal differs from the surface epidermis only in degree. Ribosomes are arranged as polysomes lying free in the cytoplasm with only small Golgi vesicles and very little endoplasmic reticulum. The keratohyalin granules are smaller and rounder and more membrane-coating granules are seen than in the surface epidermis. Towards the sebaceous duct the membrane-coating granules decrease both in size and number. The exact function of the outer root sheath is not known. During the early stages of the anagen phase of the hair cycle it elongates rapidly because of a high rate of mitotic activity which ceases when the follicle reaches its full length; subsequent mitotic activity only continues at a rate equal to cell death or cytoplasmic obliteration (Bullough & Lawrence 1958; Montagna & Van Scott 1958) though some investigators have detected higher rates than this (Straile 1962). In general, the outer root sheath is considered a relatively static region displaying little indication of cell movement. However, the observation that partial keratinization occurs in the innermost cells adjacent to the Henle layer suggests that the moving cylinder of inner root sheath plus hair may pull along the inner cells of the outer root sheath; these cells may also have a role in the differentiation and breakdown of the Henle layer. The outward migration of outer root sheath cells in facilitating the movement of the cell layers within it during metanagen (anagen 6), may account for the final outward movement of the terminal part of the hair during the last half of catagen after hair growth has ceased (Straile *et al.* 1961).

Histochemistry (Swift 1977)

Knowledge of the chemical nature of the various morphological components of the hair follicle has accumulated by three major methods: histochemistry and electron histochemistry, autoradiography and analysis of material extracted from different parts of the follicle (Gillespie 1983).

As in the epidermis and nail plate, the major protein structures are keratins in nature—filamentous or matrix types in different sites. Keratins are highly differentiated, insoluble and resistant proteins in the horny cells of vertebrate animals; but of course most constituents of the keratin filaments already exist in the keratinocytes giving rise to the horny cells in the epidermis, hair and nail (Ogawa and Yoshike 1984). In hair follicle terms, keratinization, the differentiation of keratinocytes, is very complex since there are several specific concentric rings of keratinocytes with differing keratinization characteristics; the major zone of keratinization takes place in mid-follicle and is particularly obvious in the cells, giving rise to the hair cortex above this zone.

Other, more detailed texts, describe the probable *in vivo* chemical processes of keratinization in the different cell layers (Gillespie 1983; Ogawa & Yoshike 1984; Baden 1988; Goldsmith 1986; Moll *et al.* 1988). It is of general interest that much of the 'hardening' and keratinization within differentiating matrix keratino-cytes ascending the follicle involves transglutaminase mediated cross-linkages as well as the more well-known —S$=$S— (Cu^{2+} dependent) type. This is particularly well seen in the internal root sheath and hair medulla.

Cystine and cysteine

In the hair follicle the presumptive cuticle and cortex contain cysteine sulphydryl groups followed by cystine disulphide cross-links (hard keratin) in the fully keratinized hair; only small amounts are to be found in root sheaths, particularly the Henle layer. Stabilization and hardening in the follicle are accompanied by an increase in birefringence of the cortical zone. An α-keratin pattern without orientation has been found in the lower bulb using X-ray diffraction studies; keratinization is associated with the development of orientated α-keratin as seen in the hair cortex. This α-pattern precedes the formation of disulphide-rich proteins and corresponds to the development of fibrillar bundles in the cortical zone which subsequently acquire cystine-rich proteins (Rudall 1964). Autoradiographic studies have suggested that α-keratin-like, low sulphur fibrils (microfibrils) are formed first, and at a later stage an amorphous sulphur-rich matrix protein (interfibrillar) is deposited.

Nucleic acids

The dividing cells of the hair follicle matrix stain densely for DNA; through the suprabulbar region the intensity fades and the nuclei lose this stain during keratinization. Dermal papillary cell nuclei are strongly positive for DNA. The basal cells of the follicle show the greatest concentration of RNA. Differentiating cortical cells also contain large amounts of RNA associated with great numbers of ribosomes between cytoplasmic fibrillar bundles. As the cortical cells keratinize, RNA staining stops abruptly.

Carbohydrates

Glycogen is the main carbohydrate reserve store. Dermal papillary vascular endothelial cells contain glycogen but this is absent from follicular matrix cells; all the differentiated cell layers in the follicle contain glycogen but as cells harden, the amount decreases progressively. Glycogen staining disappears as catagen succeeds the various phases of anagen.

Acid mucopolysaccharides are detectable in the follicle connective tissue sheath and the dermal papilla; metachromatic stains are also positive in the peripheral layers of the outer root sheath. Very little acid mucopolysaccharide is detectable in the presumptive hair. Using electron, histochemical methods a polysaccharide-rich layer is detectable around matrix cells of the hair bulb, particularly near desmosomes; this coat vanishes from differentiating hair cells but is retained in the inner root sheath—the retention of this coat may be important in the breakdown of the inner root sheath higher up in the follicle.

Lipids
Very little histochemical work has been carried out to detect lipids in hair follicles. Typically only undifferentiated matrix cells show lipid staining and only in small amounts. Prior to trichohyalin deposition early inner root sheath cells contain lipid granules. Phospholipid is evident in matrix cells and in the inner root sheath; these decrease as hardening proceeds.

Arginine and citrulline
Intensive staining for arginine is found in association with trichohyalin droplets in the developing medulla and inner root sheath. This decreases as cells undergo hardening. The structure of trichohyalin has been investigated extensively (Rogers 1964a, b; Fraser *et al.* 1972). Both the inner root sheath and medullary proteins are rich in acidic and basic amino acids, contain citrulline and are virtually devoid of cystine. Rogers (1964a, b) proposes that the medullary and inner root sheath trichohyalin globules contain arginine-rich protein (arginine trichohyalin) which by desimidation of the arginine is transferred into citrulline. In biological terms, it seems likely that this method of inner root sheath and medullary hardening has evolved to limit the use of disulphide bond keratinization, which requires considerable amounts of sulphur-containing amino acids, to the cuticle and cortex. This is of great importance in coat formation in animals but whether it is of significance in man is not known.

Enzymes (Braun-Falco 1958b)
Optical histochemical techniques have demonstrated the presence of many enzymes within the hair follicle, in particular phosphorylase, aldolase, succinic dehydrogenase, cytochrome oxidase, alkaline phosphatase, acid phosphatase, glucose-6-phosphatase, esterases, carbonic anhydrase, aminopeptidase, β-glucuronidase and arginase. Alkaline phosphatase activity is present along the basement membrane and around the periphery of dermal papillary cells. Acid phosphatase activity is associated with premelanosomes, Golgi apparatus and endoplasmic reticulum of melanocytes.

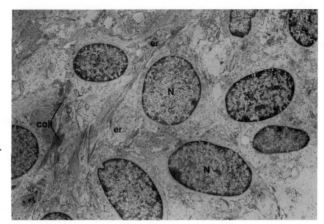

Fig. 2.7 Dermal papillary cells. The cytoplasm shows endoplasmic reticulum (er). Collagen fibres (coll) are present between the cells.

Dermal papilla (Fig. 2.7)

The connective tissue contained within the hair bulb is the dermal papilla. The size of the papilla and surrounding bulb are directly related to the size of the hair produced (Durward & Rudall 1958; Schinckel 1961). In anagen follicles the dermal papilla is attached to a basal plate of connective tissue by a narrow stalk. In small follicles there may be no visible vasculature but terminal hair follicles show variable numbers of papillary blood vessels. Papillary cells in the anagen follicle (Fig. 2.7) have prominent Golgi complexes and rough endoplasmic reticulum with bound ribosomes; even in the telogen phase appreciable cytoplasmic volume is still evident. At the beginning of anagen papillary cells show a marked increase in RNA content (Roth 1965). There is a close relationship between the mitotic activity of dermal papillary cells and hair bulb matrix cells (Straile 1965). The fact that papillary cell activity does not predate that in matrix cells is against the idea of the papilla initiating the anagen phase, but it seems probable that the dermal papilla determines the cyclical rhythm of the follicle (Cohen 1965). In rat vibrissae follicles, dermal–epidermal recombination and transplantation techniques have suggested a crucial role for the dermal papilla in follicle development, the maintenance of follicles and the control of hair growth (Young & Oliver 1976; Oliver 1980). Early *in vitro* studies on cultured human dermal papillae cells suggest similar properties to rat vibrissae but shorter survival time (Messenger *et al.* 1986). Papillary capillary endothelial cells undergo mitotic activity during anagen (Helwig 1958) but these changes occur secondary to those in bulb matrix cells. In human anagen follicles the ratio of papillary cells to matrix cells is approximately 1:9.

Perifollicular structures

A hyaline membrane surrounds the follicle; it is thin in the upper part and thick in the lower third. Two layers of collagen fibres surround the lower part, the inner one orientated parallel to the long axis and the outer one perpendicular. These layers are in continuity with the areolar tissue around the sebaceous gland and the papillary layer of the dermis; they also connect to the dermal papilla via the stalk.

The blood supply to the follicle arises from the subdermal arterial plexus supplying the capillary tuft in the dermal papilla; connected to this are numerous shunts forming a rich plexus around the lower third of the follicle. No cross-shunts are detectable in the parallel vessels that run from about this zone to the higher region at the level of the sebaceous gland where a plexus is again present. Above this, the parallel longitudinal vessels terminate in capillaries surrounding the follicular opening.

The whole length of the follicle is surrounded by many sensory nerves (Lynn 1988; Winkelmann 1988); many of these end in blunt terminals. This rich nerve supply reflects the clinical fact that hair fibres act as subtle organs of touch; this is clearly obvious to those subjects who lose all their body hair from disease or drugs. As well as the sensory follicular nerve supply efferent autonomic fibres supply the arrector pilorum muscle. All follicles appear to be innervated, usually by several myelinated fibres. The responses evoked by hair movement are mainly rapidly adapting. Ultrastructural studies have revealed a unique association between nerve terminals and pairs of Schwann cell processes in some hair follicles (Winkelmann 1988). In the hairy skin of many mammals, including man, small elevated areas are found often associated with large Tylotrich hairs. These contain the terminals of a single large myelinated axon located in close contact with Merkel cells deep in the epidermis. These are called Pinkus corpuscles (Haarscheibe); they react to light pressure (Sinclair 1981). A considerable amount of work has been carried out in recent years on a variety of peptides in cutaneous and hair follicle nerves; their exact physiological and pathological significance is yet to be clarified (Weihe & Hartschuh 1988).

References

Auber, L. (1952) The anatomy of follicles producing wool fibres with special reference to keratinisation. *Transactions of the Royal Society of Edinburgh*, **62**, 191.

Baden, H.P. (1988) Keratin. In *Pharmacology of the Skin*, vol. I, p. 31, eds. M.W. Greaves & S. Shuster. Springer-Verlag, Berlin.

Birkbeck, M.S.C. & Mercer, E.H. (1957) The electron microscopy of the human hair follicle. II. The hair cuticle. *Journal of Biophysical and Biochemical Cytology*, **3**, 215.

Braun-Falco, O. (1958a) The fine structure of the anagen hair follicle of the mouse. In *Advances in the Biology of the Skin*, vol. IX, *Hair Growth*, ch. 29, eds. W. Montagna & R.L. Dobson. Pergamon Press, Oxford.

Braun-Falco, O. (1958b) Histochemistry of the hair follicle. In *The Biology of Hair Growth*, ch. 4, eds. W. Montagna & R.A. Ellis. Academic Press, New York.

Bullough, W.S. & Lawrence, E.B. (1958) The mitotic activity of the follicles. In *The Biology of Hair Growth*, p. 171, eds. W. Montagna & R.A. Ellis. Academic Press, New York.

Cohen, J. (1965) The dermal papilla. In *Biology of the Skin and Hair Growth*, ch. 12, eds. A.G. Lyne & B.F. Short. Angus and Robertson, Sydney.

Durward, A. & Rudall, K.M. (1958) The vascularity and patterns of growth of hair follicles. In *The Biology of Hair Growth*, p. 189, eds. W. Montagna & R.A. Ellis. Academic Press, New York.

Epstein, W.L. & Maibach, H.I. (1969) Cell proliferation and movement in human hair bulbs. In *Advances in Biology of the Skin*, vol. IX, *Hair Growth*, p. 83, eds. W. Montagna & R.L. Dobson. Pergamon Press, Oxford.

Fraser, R.D.B., MacRae, T.P. & Rogers, G.E. (1972) *Keratins: Their Composition, Structure and Biosynthesis*. Thomas, Springfield.

Gillespie, J.M. (1983) The structural proteins of hair: isolation, characterization and regulation of biosynthesis. In *Biochemistry and Physiology of the Skin*, vol. I, p. 475, ed. L.A. Goldsmith. Oxford University Press, Oxford.

Goldsmith, L.A. (1986) Cytokeratins—promiscuous molecules. *Archives of Dermatology*, **122**, 594.

Harding, H.W.J. & Rogers, G.E. (1971) The E-lysine cross-linkage in citrulline-containing protein fractions from hair. *Biochemistry*, **10**, 624.

Hashimoto, K. & Ito, M. (1989) Keratinization of outer root sheath of human hair. In *Acne and Related Disorders*, 1st edn, p.3, eds. R. Marks & G. Plewig. Martin Dunitz, London.

Helwig, E.B. (1958) Pathology of psoriasis. *Annals of the New York Academy of Science*, **73**, 924.

Jarrett, A. (1958) The chemistry of inner root sheath and keratins. *British Journal of Dermatology*, **70**, 271.

Kligman, A.M. (1959) The human hair cycle. *Journal of Investigative Dermatology*, **33**, 307.

Lynn, B. (1988) Structure, function, and control: afferent nerve endings in the skin. In *Pharmacology of the Skin*, vol. I, p. 175, eds. M.W. Greaves & S. Shuster. Springer-Verlag, Berlin.

Messenger, A.G., Senior, H.J. & Bleehen, S.S. (1986) The *in vitro* properties of dermal papilla cell lines established from human hair follicles. *British Journal of Dermatology*, **114**, 425.

Moll, I., Heid, H.W., Franke, W.W. & Moll, R. (1988) Patterns of expression of trichocytic and epithelial cytokeratins in mammalian tissue. *Differentiation*, **39**, 167.

Montagna, W. & Van Scott, E.J. (1958) The anatomy of the hair follicle. In *The Biology of Hair Growth*, p. 11, eds. W. Montagna & R.A. Ellis. Academic Press, New York.

Ogawa, H. & Yoshike, T. (1984) Keratin, keratinisation and biochemical aspects of dyskeratosis. *International Journal of Dermatology*, **23**, 507.

Oliver, R.F. (1980) Local interactions in mammalian hair growth. In *The Skin of Vertebrates*, p. 199, eds R.I.C. Spearman & P.A. Riley. Linnean Society Symposium Series, No. 9.

Parakkal, P.F. (1969) The fine structure of the anagen hair follicle of the mouse. In *Advances in Biology of the Skin*, vol. IX, *Hair Growth*, ch. 29, eds. W. Montagna & R.L. Dobson. Pergamon Press, Oxford.

Parakkal, P.F. & Maltoltsy, A.G. (1964) A study of the differentiating products of the hair follicle. *Journal of Investigative Dermatology*, **43**, 23.

Powell, B.C. & Rogers, G.E. (1986) Hair keratins:composition, structure and biogenesis. In *Biology of the Integument*, p. 696, eds. J. Bereiter-Hahn, A.G. Maltoltsy & K.S. Richards. Springer-Verlag, Berlin.

Rogers, G.E. (1964a) Structural and biochemical features of the hair follicle. In *The Epidermis*, p. 202, eds. W. Montagna & W.C. Lobitz. Academic Press, New York.

Rogers, G.E. (1964b) Isolation and property of inner root sheath cells of the hair follicle. *Experimental Cell Research*, **33**, 264.

Roth, S.I. (1965) The cytology of the murine resting (telogen) hair follicle. In *Biology of the Skin and Hair Growth*, p. 1, eds. A.G. Lyne & B.F. Short. Angus and Robertson, Sydney.

Rudall, K.M. (1964) The biomolecular structure of hair keratins. In *Progress in the Biological Sciences in Relation to Dermatology*, vol. 2, p. 355, eds. A. Rook & R.H. Champion. Cambridge University Press, London.

Schinckel, P.G. (1961) Mitotic activity in wool fibre follicle bulbs. *Australian Journal of Biological Sciences*, **14**, 659.

Shahrad, P. & Marks, R. (1976) Hair follicle kinetics in psoriasis. *Journal of Investigative Dermatology*, **94**, 7.

Sinclair, D. (1981) *Mechanisms of Cutaneous Sensation*. Oxford University Press, Oxford.

Straile, W.E. (1962) Possible functions of the external root sheath during growth of the hair follicle. *Journal of Experimental Zoology*, **150**, 207.

Straile, W.E. (1965) Root sheath dermal papilla relationships and the control of hair growth. In *Biology of the Skin and Hair Growth*, ch. 3, eds. A.G. Lyne & B.F. Short. Angus and Robertson, Sydney.

Straile, W.E., Chase, H.B. & Arsenault, C. (1961) Growth and differentiation of hair follicles between periods of activity and quiescence. *Journal of Experimental Zoology,* **148,** 205.

Swift, J.A. (1977) The histology of keratin fibres. In *The Chemistry of Natural Protein Fibres,* ch. 3, ed. R.S. Asquith. Wiley, London.

Van Scott, E.J., Ekel, T.M. & Auerbach, R. (1963) Determinants of rate and kinetics of cell division in scalp hair. *Journal of Investigative Dermatology,* **41,** 269.

Weihe, E. & Hartschuh, W. (1988) Multiple Peptides in Cutaneous Nerves. In *Seminars in Dermatology,* vol. 7 (4), p. 284, eds. A.J. Rook & H.I. Maibach. Grune and Stratton, Philadelphia.

Winkelmann, R.K. (1988) Cutaneous sensory nerves. In *Seminars in Dermatology,* vol. 7, p. 236, eds. A.J. Rook & H.I. Maibach. Grune & Stratton, Philadelphia.

Wright, N.A. & Alison, M. (1984) *Biology of Epithelial Cell Populations,* vol. 1. Oxford University Press, Oxford.

Young, R.D. & Oliver, R.F. (1976) Morphological changes associated with the growth cycle of vibrissal follicles in the rat. *Journal of Embryology and Experimental Morphology,* **36,** 597.

Hair structure
(References p. 41)

The main part of the fully keratinized hair fibre in the cortex, which is made up of closely packed interdigitating spindle-shaped cells whose axis is parallel to the hair axis. Covering this is the cuticle, composed of six to eight layers of flattened cells which overlap each other from root to tip (Figs 2.8a and b). In man, a third component may be present in terminal hairs, the central medulla (Fig. 2.9). It consists of specialized cells which contain air spaces (Fig. 2.10).

It is of great interest to paleantologists that hair structure is very stable and resists breakdown even for thousands of years after death, for example, bog bodies (Stead *et al.* 1986).

Surface structure
Mammalian hairs are covered with a thin layer termed the epicuticle (Fraser *et al.* 1972) which is approximately 2.5 nm thick. It has been suggested in the past that the epicuticle covers the entire surface of the hair but more recently it has been localized as part of the cell membrane complex (Robbins 1979), perhaps chemically associated with the intercellular binding material. The epicuticle is not morphologically evident on microscopy. It is probably best to consider the epicuticle to be a lipid-containing surface membrane made up of the cytoplasmic membrane and/or the A-layer to which remnants of protein from the exocuticle are attached (Swift & Holmes 1965; Swift 1977).

Cuticle (Wolfram & Lindemann 1971) (Fig. 2.11)
Human hair is surrounded by six to ten layers of cuticle cells, each being approximately 0.2–0.5 µm thick; at the proximal end the hair is therefore encased by a 1-µm thick layer of cuticular material. The number of layers varies but little from coarse to fine hairs and thus, in the latter, the cuticle may account for up to 10% of the fibre by weight. Cuticular cells overlap and on surface examination of the fibre they are seen to be imbricated (like roof tiles). The free margin of the cells

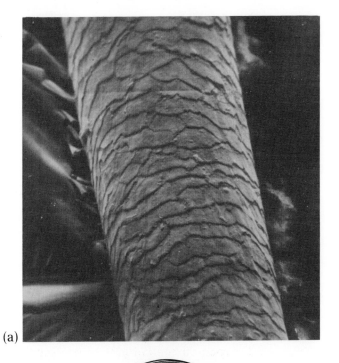

(a)

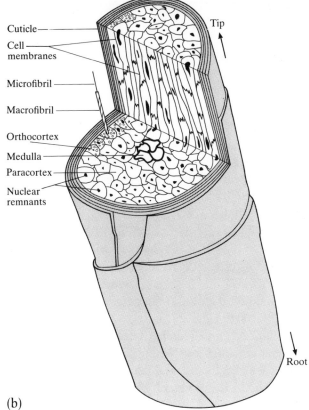

Cuticle

Cell membranes

Microfibril

Macrofibril

Orthocortex

Medulla

Paracortex

Nuclear remnants

Tip

Root

Fig. 2.8 (a) Surface structure of scalp hair at root end, showing overlapping cuticular cells closely apposed to underlying cells. The lower margin points towards the tip (scanning electron micrograph). (b) Diagram to show component parts of the hair shaft at the root end.

(b)

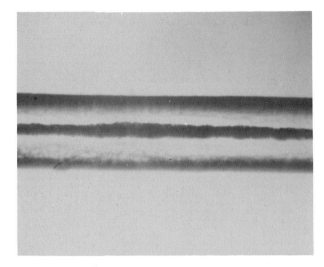

Fig. 2.9 Medullated terminal hair showing continuous (dark) central medulla. Many terminal hairs show only intermittent medullation.

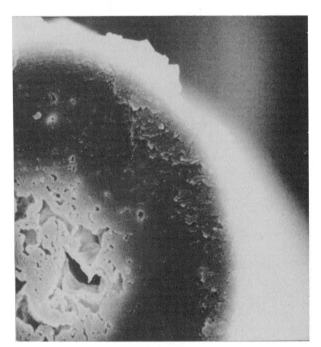

Fig. 2.10 Normal medullated terminal scalp hair (transverse section). Scanning electron micrograph showing air spaces in the medulla (lower left) and darker compact surrounding cortex.

points towards the tip. The free length of each fibre visible at the surface is mainly dependent on the overall diameter of the hair, i.e. in vellus hair three-quarters of the surface cuticle cell is visible with a relatively large distance between the free margin of successive scales of terminal hair in which scale margins appear closer. The cell junctions between adjacent cuticle cells and the cuticle and underlying cortex are usually flat, and folds are infrequently, but regularly, seen, which may contribute to the mechanical strength of the cuticle.

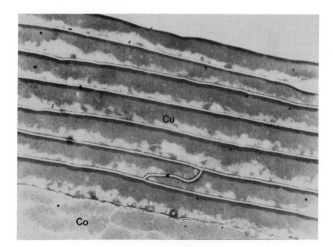

Fig. 2.11 Hair cuticle layers (Cu) surrounding the central cortex (Co) (electron micrograph).

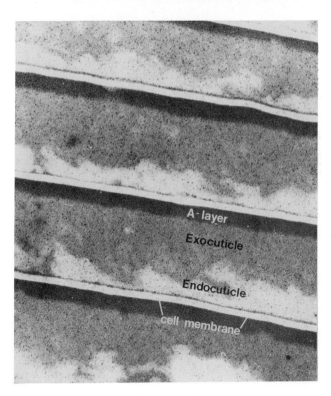

Fig. 2.12 Hair cuticle (electron micrograph — silver methenamine stain).

Each cuticle cell is composed of lamellar components (Fig. 2.12). The outer cell membrane complex is from 5 to 25 nm thick. Within each cell are three major layers—the cystine-rich A-layer, the exocuticle and the endocuticle. The cuticle cell contents generally lack fine structure, though Orfanos & Ruska (1968a) have observed fine structure in the exocuticle made up from interwoven thread-like osmophilic units approximately 3 nm in diameter; other authors have interpreted these results cautiously (Swift 1977) suggesting that the units could be the product of the high magnification methods used.

The outer exocuticle is approximately 0.2 μm thick and the inner endocuticle 0.1 μm thick in human scalp hair; the junction between the two layers is generally irregular. The A-layer is of constant thickness in each cell and approximately 40 nm thick. The endocuticle has an irregular substructure of membrane-like elements which are probably the remnants of cytoplasmic structures. The mechanism controlling the migration of 'strong' high sulphur protein (exocuticle) to the outer part of each cuticular cell requires careful genetic control. This control may be lost in diseases such as trichothiodystrophy.

Cortex (Orfanos & Ruska 1968b)
This component constitutes the main bulk of the hair and is the part contributing most to the mechanical properties of the fibres. Cortical cells are closely packed and orientated to the axis of the hair; they are approximately 3–6 μm in diameter and up to 100 μm long. Each cell contains a nuclear remnant (nuclear 'ghost') which is stellate in transverse section. The major structures within cortical cells are the closely packed macrofibrils (Fig. 2.13).

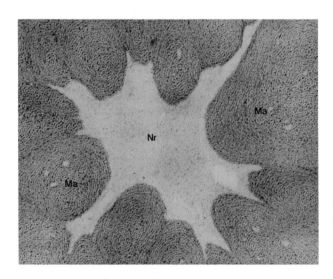

Fig. 2.13 Hair cortex. The central nuclear remnant (Nr) is surrounded by macrofibrils (Ma) (electron micrograph — silver methenamine stain).

Each macrofibril is a solid cylindrical unit 0.1–0.4 μm in diameter and of variable length, but often the whole cell length. Between the macrofibrils is a variable amount of intermacrofibrillar matrix and melanin granules; this matrix is analogous in structure to the cuticular endocuticle and contains the remnants of cytoplasmic organelles. In some cells macrofibrils are so densely packed that individual units are difficult to see by electron microscopy (paracortical cells), whilst others are less densely aggregated (orthocortical cells). Human hair cortex is generally considered to be of the paracortical cell type throughout the cortical thickness, though Swift (1977) has described Monogolian (straight) hair as paracortical, Caucasian (curly) as mainly paracortical and Negro (woolly) as segmented into two zones—the other side of the crimp curl being ortho- and the inner paracortical.

Macrofibrils are composed of rod-like microfibrils approximately 7 nm in diameter, arranged in whorls (pseudo-hexagons), and embedded in a structureless intermicrofibrillar matrix (Fig. 2.14). Routine transmission electron microscopic studies suggest that these microfibrils are parallel and are longitudinally orientated within the macrofibril, but Johnson & Sikorski (1965) have described a spiral arrangement of macrofibrils.

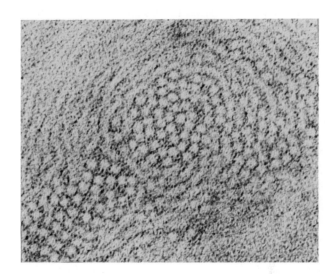

Fig. 2.14 Details of the structure of a hair cortex macrofibril. The dark staining matrix protein surrounds densely packed circular microfibrils (silver methenamine stain).

Medulla (Marhle & Orfanos 1971)

In many lower animals, for example the porcupine quill, the medulla constitutes a continuous central part of the fibre. However, in human hair the medulla is typically only found in terminal hair and may be continuous (Fig. 2.9), discontinuous or even absent. Wildman (1954) has subdivided medullary types into 'latticed' and 'simple' patterns for continuous medulla, and 'fragmented' and 'ladder' patterns for discontinuous medulla.

The medulla in all keratin fibres consists of a cortex-like framework of spongy keratin supporting thin shells of amorphous material bounding air spaces of variable size.

Chemical composition of hair (Montagna & Parakkal 1974; Robbins 1979)

Human hair is a very complex fibre made up of various morphological components and several different chemical species. For convenience and simplicity the different chemical components are described separately in most texts and in relating the chemical basis of hair function and physical properties. However, it is very important to note that human hair is an integrated system with the chemical components acting together. The chemical composition of hair varies somewhat with its water content. The main component is protein which is 65–95% of the hair weight; the protein is keratinous and is a condensation polymer of amino acids. Other constituents include water, lipids, pigment and trace elements.

Protein (Gillespie 1983; Powell and Rogers 1986)
Most of the extractable keratinous protein is contained within cortical cells, but significant and important fractions are present within the cuticle; medullary proteins are probably of little physico-chemical significance in human hair. It is characteristically insoluble and resistant to proteolytic enzymes. Because of solubility problems, it is difficult to compare quantitative results from different laboratories. Solubility may vary from 10 to 70%. Solubilization involves breaking disulphide bonds by either reduction or oxidation. The proteins produced by reduction are keratins; those from oxidation are keratoses, S-carboxymethyl keratins (SCMK proteins). SCMK proteins produced by reduction separate into a low sulphur group (SCMKA proteins, mol. wt. 45,000) and a high sulphur group (SCMKB proteins, mol. wt. 20,000)—these compose 60 and 30% respectively of the total protein of hair (Fraser *et al.* 1972). After oxidation, the keratoses can be separated into α-keratose and γ-keratose; in relation to sulphur content and amino acid content α- and γ-keratoses are similar to SCMKA and SCMKB proteins respectively. As well as these two protein groups, 2–3% of the protein consists of low-sulphur heterogeneous protein that is rich in glycine and tyrosine (Zahn & Biela 1968).

Much recent work on the detail of keratins produced normally has suggested differences between individuals—possibly of forensic significance (Lee *et al.* 1978); also further refinement of the techniques may at last lead to a logical classification of hereditary hair shaft defects (Hordinsky *et al.* 1987).

To summarize, human hair contains a large number of proteins extracted by a variety of methods but it is quite likely that these are the technical products of much fewer proteins present *in vivo*. It has been shown by electron histochemical methods that in the cortex hair, the high-sulphur proteins are predominantly in the matrix and the low-sulphur in the filamentous protein.

During the last 20 years many investigators have analysed the constituent amino acids of whole hair specimens; such analysis is often quoted for genetically diseased hair. The results are of limited use since they only provide average values for the amino acid contents of average proteinaceous substances of the hair; also some amino acids undergo hydrolytic decomposition. Hydrochloric acid (5–6 N) is most commonly used for keratin fibre analysis and using this method the following amino acids have been shown to undergo partial decomposition: cystine, threonine, tyrosine, phenylalanine, arginine and tryptophan.

Table 2.1 Amino acid composition of normal hair (residues per 100 residues extracted)

Amino acid	Amount	Amino acid	Amount
Lysine	2.8	Alanine	4.8
Histidine	0.8	Cystine	17.5
Arginine	5.6	Valine	5.9
Aspartic acid	5.0	Methionine	0.5
Threonine	6.9	Isoleucine	2.7
Serine	11.7	Leucine	6.1
Glutamic acid	11.1	Tyrosine	1.9
Proline	3.6	Phenylalanine	1.4
Glycine	6.5		

The amino acids isolated from normal hair are shown in Table 2.1 together with average relative amounts found by quantitative analysis (Dawber 1985). The figures are gross and in health and disease cannot be compared unless a large number of varying factors are taken into consideration; these include genetic variation, weathering, diet, cosmetic treatment and the extraction and analytical methods used. In general, male scalp hair contains more cystine than female hair, whilst dark hair is said to contain more cystine than light shades. The tip of scalp hair contains significantly less cystine and cysteine than the root end; the converse applies for cysteic acid. For details of these and other studies of factors varying amino acid composition, the reader is referred to more comprehensive texts (Asquith 1977; Robbins 1979; Baden 1988).

Human hair cuticle is said to contain more cystine, cysteic acid, proline, threonine, isoleucine, methionine, leucine, tyrosine, phenylalanine and arginine than whole hair (Bradbury 1973); using different methods other workers obtained broadly similar results (Blout *et al.* 1960). In general, cuticular cells contain a higher proportion of amino acids not usually found in α-helical polypeptides than whole hair. The chemical composition of the A-layer and exocuticle are considerably different from the endocuticle in that they are highly cross-linked by cystine, giving a tough and resilient layer. The endocuticle contains very little cystine.

Since both by weight and volume the cortex makes up the main part of the hair fibre, whole fibre analytical studies relate closely to cortical chemistry. The greatest error will be in those amino acids present in smallest quantities

Medullary protein is notoriously insoluble and difficult to isolate; consequently, complete analytic studies have not so far been possible. Much of the known information has come from analysis of porcupine quill proteins (Rogers 1964a). Medulla has a very low cystine and sulphur content and contains relatively large quantities of acidic and basic amino acids and hydroxyamino acids.

Water content

Water content is important in relation to its physical and cosmetic properties. The density of dry hair is 1.09 on the basis of geometrical weight measurements and 1.37 from pycnometric measurements. Consequently, the porosity is about 20% and hence it is hygroscopic. When impregnated with water its weight increases by 12–18%. The process of absorption is very rapid; 75% of the maximum possible amount of water is absorbed within 4 minutes (Ryabukhin 1980). The water binding of amino and guanidino groups is responsible for the large percentage of water absorption capacity of keratin, particularly at low humidities; peptide bonds are preferential sites for hydration. It is thought that at low relative humidities ($<25\%$), water molecules are bonded to hydrophilic sites by hydrogen bonds. With increasing humidity more water is absorbed producing a decrease in the energy binding of water already associated with the protein. At greater than 80% relative humidity water on water absorption becomes more and more important.

Hair lipids

Much of our knowledge of hair lipids comes from 'fat solvent' studies. Depending on the solvent used, different results are obtainable; ethanol removes more lipid from hair than do solvents such as benzene, ether or chloroform. The values obtained represent mainly sebum and the chromographic fractions obtained consist primarily of free fatty acids and neutral fats: esters, glyceryl, wax, hydrocarbons and alcohols.

The lipids of human hair are often thought of as of minor importance. It has been shown that hair lipid increases after puberty in both sexes. This declines with age in women but not to the same extent in men. Negroid hair produces more lipid than Caucasian hair. Squalene content in children is approximately one-quarter that of adults, whilst cholesterol exists in similar proportions. In relation to age or sex, there is no difference with regard to fatty alcohol content of human hair lipid.

Trace elements (Brown & Crounse 1980; Dormany 1986; Fenton *et al.* 1988; Valkovic 1988)

It is not known to which chemical group in hair structure trace elements are attached; however, the principal metal content of human hair probably exists as an integral part of fibre structure, i.e. as salt linkages or coordinated complexes with the side chains of pigment or proteins.

Trace elements may be incorporated into hair from several sources, both exogenous and endogenous (Hopps 1971). Of endogenous sources, the matrix, connective tissue papilla, the sebaceous, eccrine and apocrine glands and the surface epidermis are important. The environment also contributes greatly, particularly by pollution, for example from industry and hair cosmetics; scalp hair has been used in many studies as a sensitive index of environmental pollution. Until recently, the most frequently investigated elements in hair have been As,

Cd, Cr, Cu, Hg, Pb and Zn (Chatt *et al.* 1980). Techniques such as nuclear activation, X-ray fluorescence and emission, and atomic absorption and emission have enabled submicrogram quantities to be determined. An international coordinated programme on activation analysis of trace element pollutants in human hair has been set up by the International Atomic Energy Agency based in Vienna (Ryabukhin 1980). It is hoped to standardize methods used so that different studies around the world can be coordinated and correlated. With standardization of methods it is possible that the method of photon activation analysis may prove to be as unique for each individual as fingerprints. This method enables elements such as C, N, O, F, Cr, Y, Zn, Mo, Cd, Sn, I, Sr, Pb, Tl and Bi to be analysed that are difficult by other methods.

The total ash content of human hair varies from 0.26 to 0.94% of dry weight. The number of elements reported in human hair depends on the method used but the following have been detected: Ca, Mg, Sr, B, Al, Si, Na, K, Zn, Cu, Mn, Fe, Ag, Au, Hg, As, Pb, Sb, Ti, W, Mo, I, P and Se. The vast majority are from extraneous sources but substances such as As and Tl used as poisons are sensitively localized in hair after ingestion.

Hair shape

The shape of the hair varies with body site and with race (Swift 1977; Lindelöf *et al.* 1988).

Mongoloid hair is typically straight and of round bore, whilst Caucasoid hair is curly and tends to be oval in cross-section; Negroid hair is woolly and distinctly oval. Caucasoid and Negroid hair tend to have a smaller diameter than Mongoloid hair.

Pubic, beard and eyelash hairs are generally oval in all racial types. There is no detectable difference in hair shape between men and women with respect to race or body site.

References

Asquith, R.S. (1977) *The Chemistry of Natural Protein Fibres.* Wiley, London.

Baden, H.P. (1988) Keratin. In *Pharmacology of the Skin*, vol. 1, p. 31, eds. M.W. Greaves & S. Shuster. Springer-Verlag, Berlin.

Blout, E.R., de Loye, D., Bloom, S.M. & Forman, G.D. (1960) *Journal of the American Chemical Society*, **82**, 3787.

Bradbury, J.H. (1973) The structure and chemistry of keratin fibres. *Advances in Protein Chemistry*, **27**, 111.

Brown, A.C. & Crounse, R.G. (1980) *Hair, Trace, Elements and Human Illness.* Praeger, New York.

Chatt, A., Secord, C.A., Tiefenbach, B. & Jervis, R.E. (1980) Scalp hair as a monitor of community exposure to environmental pollutants. In *Hair, Trace Elements and Human Illness*, ch. 3, eds. A.C. Brown & R.G. Crounse. Praeger, New York.

Dormany, T.L. (1986) Trace element analysis of hair. *British Medical Journal*, **293**, 975.

Fenton, D.A., Morris, I.W. & Kendall, M.D. (1988) Energy-dispersive X-ray microanalysis (EDX): a method to assess the elemental composition of hair. *British Journal of Dermatology*, **119**, 46.

Fraser, R.D.B., MacRae, T.P. & Rogers, G.E. (1972) *Keratins: Their Composition, Structure and Biosynthesis.* Thomas, Springfield.

Gillespie, J.M. (1983) The structural proteins of hair: isolation, characterization and regulation of biosynthesis. In *Biochemistry and Physiology of the Skin*, vol. I, p. 475, ed. L.A. Goldsmith. Oxford.

Hopps, H.C. (1971) The biological basis of using hair and nail for analysis of trace elements. In *Proceedings of the Symposium on Trace Substances in Environmental Health*, 8th edn, p. 1, ed. D.D. Hemphill. University of Missouri, Columbia.

Hordinsky, M., Berry, S. & Sundby, S. (1987) Hair protein patterns in a new autosomal dominant ectodermal dysplasia. *Archives of Dermatology*, **123**, 715.

Johnson, D.J. & Sikorski, J. (1965) *Proceedings of the 3rd International Wool Textile Research Conference*, Paris, p. 53.

Lee, L.D., Ludwig, K. & Baden, H.P. (1978) Matrix proteins of human hair as a tool for identification of individuals. *Forensic Science*, **11**, 115.

Lindelöf, B., Forslind, B., Hedblad, M-A. & Kaveus, U. (1988) Human hair form. *Archives of Dermatology*, **124**, 1359.

Marhle, G. & Orfanos, G.E. (1971) The spongious keratin and the medullary substance of human scalp hair. *Archiv für dermatologische Forschung*, **241**, 305.

Montagna, W. & Parakkal, P.K. (1974) *The Structure and Function of Skin*, p. 232. Academic Press, New York.

Orfanos, C. & Ruska, H. (1968a) The fine structure of human hair. I. Cuticle. *Archiv für klinische und experimentelle Dermatologie*, **231**, 97.

Orfanos, C. & Ruska, H. (1968b) The fine structure of human hair. II. The hair cortex. *Archiv für klinische und experimentelle Dermatologie*, **231**, 264.

Powell, B.C. & Rogers, G.E. (1986) Hair keratins:composition, structure and biogenesis. In *Biology of the Integument*, p. 696, eds. J. Bereiter-Hahn, A.G. Maltoltsy & K.S. Richards. Springer-Verlag, Berlin.

Robbins, C.R. (1979) *Chemical and Physical Behaviour of Human Hair*, p. 7. Van Nostrand–Reinhold, New York.

Rogers, G.E. (1964a) Structural and biochemical features of the hair follicle. In *The Epidermis*, p. 202, eds. W. Montagna & W.C. Lobitz. Academic Press, New York.

Ryabukhin, Y.S. (1980) International coordinated program of trace element pollutants on human hair. In *Hair, Trace Elements and Human Illness*, p. 5, eds. A.C. Brown & R.G. Crounse. Praeger, New York.

Stead, I.M. & Bourke, J.B. (1986) *The Lindow Man: The Man in the Bog*. British Museum Publications, London.

Swift, J.A. (1977) The histology of keratin fibres. In *The Chemistry of Natural Protein Fibres*, p. 1, ed. R.S. Asquith. Wiley, London.

Swift, J.A. & Holmes, A.W. (1965) Degradation of human hair by papain. *Textile Research Journal*, **35**, 1014.

Valkovic, V. (1988) *Fundamentals and Methods of Measurement of Elemental Composition*, vol. 2. CRC Press, London.

Wildman, A.B. (1954) *The Microscopy of Animal Textile Fibres*. Wool Industries Research Association, Leeds.

Wolfram, L.J. & Lindemann, M.K.O. (1971) Some observations on the hair cuticle. *Journal of the Society of Cosmetic Chemists*, **22**, 839.

Zahn, H. & Biela, M. (1968) Tyrosin reiche Proteine in Ameisensäureextrakt von reduzierter Welle. *European Journal of Biochemistry*, **5**, 567.

Physical properties of hair (Dawber 1985)
(References p. 49)

The physical properties of biological materials are a function of their geometric shape and of the intrinsic properties of the individual constituent materials. Hair keratin is the only human protein that is able to have its exact physical properties analysed. Most of the early work on keratin fibres was carried out on wool (Chapman 1969) and much of the equipment now used for assessing human hair characteristics has evolved from prototypes used in earlier wool research (Robbins 1979). A considerable amount of work has been carried out in applying basic laws of physics and engineering to hair tensile properties, but it is important to state that such laws cannot exactly apply in the field of biomechanics. The 'strength' of human hair resides in the cortex which has a composite structure in which discontinuous fibres—keratin fibrils within longitudinal orientated cell envelopes—are embedded in a sulphur-rich matrix. In engineering terms, fibre/matrix composites are structures in which two or more components are combined to make best use of the favourable properties of the components whilst at the same time mitigating against some of their less desirable characteristics. Natural composites can sustain loads and resist loads far more efficiently than man-made composites, and hair is no exception (Fraser & Macrae 1980; Harris 1980). The cortical matrix is easily deformed by mechanical stress and energy is transmitted evenly into the fibrils, possibly by shearing forces at the fibre/matrix interface. Whatever the efficiency of the hair cortex as a composite, without an intact overlying cuticle, human hair resists external mechanical stresses poorly, as in excessive weathering due to cosmetic abuse. Therefore in assessing hair for biochemical efficiency, it is important to consider the cuticle, epicuticle, intercellular cement substance and the plasma membranes of both the cortex and cuticle (Spearman 1977). Since the medulla is absent from vellus hair and is frequently absent or discontinuous in terminal hair, it is not generally considered important in this context, though in lower animals this is certainly not the case.

The physical properties of hair can be divided into elastic deformations including stretching, bending, stiffness, torsion, cross-sectional area and shape, density, friction and static charge.

Elastic properties

Probably the most important mechanical property of hair is elasticity by which it resists forces tending to change its shape, volume and length and also enables it to recover its original form when the force is removed. Every deforming force of an elastic substance is balanced by a force tending to return it to its normal condition. The commonest types of strain are stretching (the ratio of increase in length to the original length), compression (the ratio of decrease in length to the original length), shear, bending and torsion (Mitchell & Feughelman 1960). Each type of stress and strain has a modulus (the ratio of stress to strain). The modulus that has received the greatest amount of attention in hair studies has been Young's modulus, a measure of elasticity to stretching. Young's modulus is defined by the equation:

$$\frac{FL}{al} \text{ dynes per unit area (cm}^2),$$

where F = force (dynes) applied per unit area of cross-section, a = unit area of cross-section, L=length of fibre before stretching, l=increase in length on stretching.

In considering the response of hair to stretching, another law of physics must be considered, Hooke's Law. This states that in elastic substances, strains are proportional to the stresses producing them. Thus, when an elastic fibre is pulled, the change in length is proportional to the force applied. A typical load–elongation curve for human hair is shown in Fig. 2.15; Hooke's Law only applies up to point 1 on the curve. Up to this point, the fibre is able to return to its original state.

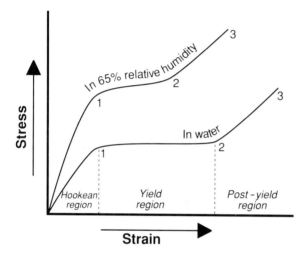

Fig. 2.15 Load/extension curves for human hair.

Irreversible changes occur in the hair in the yield region even if the fibre returns to its normal length. In the post-yield region, resistance to stress increases greatly until the breaking point is reached. When hair is stretched up to 30% of its original length in water and allowed to return to its former length, the curve of relaxation is separated from the elongation curve (Fig. 2.16). Under these circumstances, the work of elongation is greater than the work of recovery; the ratio of these two work values is known as the hysteresis curve. When normal hairs are stretched to between 30 and 70% more than their original length above the hysteresis region, the relaxation curve is the same as for extension (Alexander, Hudson & Earland 1963). Normal scalp hair fibres break if stretched to approximately 80% of the initial length.

The effects of many different factors on the tensile properties of hair have been studied in great detail.

The moisture content of hair increases with increasing relative humidity (RH). The effect of 65% RH and 100% RH on the load–extension curve can be seen in Fig. 2.15. In general, Young's modulus falls as RH rises, whilst hair extensibility prior to breaking is directly proportional to RH (Robbins 1979).

Both the wet and dry elastic properties of hair are directly proportional to shaft

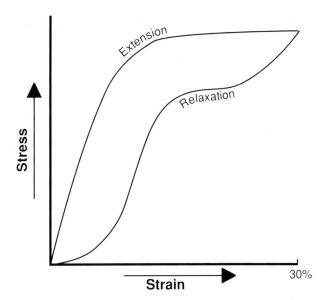

Fig. 2.16 Load/extension and recovery curves for human hair.

diameter as assessed by investigations at fixed RH. The breaking stress decreases with increasing hair diameter.

The elastic modulus of human hair decreases with increasing temperature as do the post-yield modulus and fibre strength. Hair extensibility prior to breaking point increases directly with temperature.

Bleaching and permanent waving markedly alter the elastic properties of hair, the latter particularly so. Bleaching decreases tensile properties by up to 25% (Alexander *et al.* 1963; Robbins 1979). Permanent waving reduces disulphide cross-links and causes molecular 'shifting' on reoxidation. Both the reduction and reoxidation phases alter tensile properties; stress to breaking point is up to 15% less, and stress to 20% extension up to 18% less than for untreated hair. Stretching hairs in aqueous reduction solutions results in lower stresses to achieve a particular strain; reoxidation improves this towards normal.

Dyeing from a light to a darker shade produces negligible change in elastic properties, whilst any impairment on lightening hair colour depends on the extent of disulphide bond oxidation (bleaching).

Sunlight and artificial ultraviolet β-radiation cause photochemical degradation of cystine to cysteic acid and thus impair elastic properties in a similar way to bleaching, but to a small degree since disulphide bond disruption is less following ultraviolet radiation (UVR) exposure.

Elastic properties of hair in disease (Goldsmith & Baden 1971)
Dawber (1972) found that hair from a family with pili annulati, though not clinically fragile, always breaks through the abnormal bands; breaking stress analysis, however, showed only a 2% reduction compared to normal controls.

Swanbeck *et al.* (1970) studied tensile strength, strain at breaking point and elastic modulus in male pattern baldness, alopecia areata and defluvium capillorum; no significant abnormalities were found. However, in congenital ectodermal dysplasia both tensile strength and elastic modulus were reduced whilst in congenital ichthyosiform erythroderma only elastic modulus was decreased.

Both hypothyroidism and acromegaly cause an alteration in the yield region of the stress/strain curve at low levels of RH (Korostoff *et al.* 1970).

In view of the importance of the disulphide bond with regard to tensile strength of hair, it is likely that all sulphur, cystine and high-sulphur, protein-deficient hairs will have abnormal tensile properties (Clarke & Buhrke 1954), though only occasional reports have appeared to substantiate this. Brown *et al.* (1970) studied a congenital defect of hair showing trichoschisis, alternate birefringence and low sulphur content and found that dry hair had a lower degree of extension at a lower stress than normal. Stress–strain testing of low sulphur hair in water (Baden *et al.* 1976) showed that the fibres extended more at lower tensions before breaking; these results were similar to those from hairs with chemically reduced disulphide bonds.

Most of the studies described above, investigating elastic properties of hair, are carried out at fixed rates of extension with the hair held at each end. For other methods of evaluating stretching properties of hair the reader is referred to the description by Robbins (1979); the use of techniques such as the oscillating beam method, stress relaxation, stretch rotation and the set and supercontraction method has largely been limited to the hair cosmetic and wool industries.

Hair structure following stretching
The fusiform cortical cells increase in length during stretching; this change occurs during the Hookean phase of extension (Fig. 2.15). It seems unlikely that any slip occurs between adjacent cells in view of the firm adhesion present due to plasma membrane interdigitations and strong cement substance. X-ray diffraction studies have shown that further stretching modifies intracellular keratin structure. There is an increase in the meridional spacings in the alpha helix (Fraser *et al.* 1972) which are like stretched spiral springs. This action is possible because of the weak hydrogen bonds between the keratin fibrils and the matrix protein. As strain increases in the yield and post-yield zones (Fig. 2.16) matrix disulphide bonds are disrupted and cell membranes may fracture in advance of the breaking point (Rudall 1964). Following elastic recoil, disulphide bonds probably reform at different points in the keratin molecule as in permanent waving.

It is important to note that many of the properties of hair fibres described above may not be relevant under normal circumstances since the force required to pull hair out of its follicle (Tsuda 1957), even in the anagen phase of the hair cycle, may frequently be less than that needed to construct load–extension curves (Figs 2.15 and 2.16). Certainly the majority of hairs plucked for anagen–telogen analysis possess roots, i.e. they are released from the scalp before the breakage point is reached.

Hair bending and stiffness

When a hair fibre is bent the arc that is formed contains three longitudinal zones within it—the outer layers of the arc are stretched, the inner layers compressed and a central zone undergoes neither stretching nor compression. Stiffness of hair implies a resistance to bending. This property of hair has received very little attention from clinicians though several authors have shown that bending forces damage cuticular structure in the outer part of the bending arc in normal (Swift & Brown 1972) and knotted hair (Dawber 1974). Also the transverse fracture and breakage of monilethrix internodes is probably due to the inability of the narrowed hair to withstand bending forces (Dawber 1980).

Several methods have been described in an attempt to quantitate bending forces (Robbins 1979) but none of the techniques can specifically measure the extension and compression forces within the bent section. It has been suggested that hair stiffness parallels the linear stretching properties and is varied by similar factors.

Density of human hair (Morton & Hearle 1962)

The absolute density of keratin fibres is difficult to measure. At RH of 60% the density is approximately 1.32, the same as wool fibres. No studies of hair density in disease have been carried out; bleaching and permanent waving have no significant effect on hair density.

Variations in hair fibre dimensions

The measurements which are most commonly used for comparative studies are length and diameter. If the hair is taken to be cylindrical, then volume, cross-sectional area, radius and surface area can easily be calculated. These measurements need to be made to enable fundamental elastic properties to be studied. Single hair cross-sectional dimensions can be measured by various methods, including linear density, light microscopy, vibrascopy, calipers and laser beam diffraction. Centrifugation can be used for multiple hair determinations (Robbins 1979).

Much of the work carried out in this field has been by physical anthropologists, anatomists, forensic scientists and cosmetic scientists. Hayashi *et al.* (1975) studied differences in hair diameter, the hair index—the ratio of the least diameter to the greatest diameter—and the area of the cuticle expressed as a percentage of the area of cross-section in 55 subjects of 18 races in Europe, Asia and America. The diameter measurements showed that hair from white races and their hybrids— German, Italian and English—are finer than hair from Latin Mongoloid races. Scalp hair diameter varies from 40 to 120 μm; Caucasoid scalp hair varies from 50 to 90 μm whilst Mongoloid scalp hair is the coarsest with a mean diameter of approximately 120 μm.

Hair length increases slightly as RH rises, whilst hair diameter increases to a much greater degree. Swelling of this type is much less than in unstretched hair when the hair is under tension below 60% RH; at greater than 60% RH swelling of hair is greater than that of unstretched fibres.

Mechanical properties of hair cuticle

Linear stretching of hair fibres alters cortical structure before any cuticular damage occurs. Cuticular cells are able to move over each other, since the flat overlapping cells do not normally interdigitate like cortical cells. These overlapping scales give a rough surface to hair fibres which are thus susceptible to frictional damage.

Friction is defined as the force tending to resist motion when one body slides over another. The force (F) necessary to slide one object over another is proportional to the normal load pressing the surfaces together (W):

$$F = \mu W.$$

The constant μ is the coefficient of friction; the force to start movement governs the coefficient of static friction (μ_s) and that force necessary to maintain force determines the coefficient of kinetic friction (μ_k). μ_k is usually less than μ_s. The methods used to measure friction in keratin fibres have been well described (Meredith & Hearle 1959).

Hair exhibits a directional frictional effect in that it is easier to move a surface in a root to tip direction than in a tip to root direction. Wet friction is higher than dry friction for both human hair and wool fibres; friction is not dependent on hair shaft diameter or temperature. Bleaching and permanent waving increase the coefficient of kinetic friction, whilst high conditioning shampoos and cream rinses decrease μ_k.

Electrical (static) charge of hair

Dry hairs are poor conductors of electricity, whilst wet hairs are very good. When dry hair is rubbed and pressed during combing and brushing, under suitable conditions, static electricity is produced. This is associated with 'flyaway' hair and is due to electrons or ions that are not moving. Frictional electricity is called tribo-electricity; it is more likely to develop in fibres with a high electrical resistance, for example hair or wool, than those with a lower resistance such as cotton and rayon (Morton & Hearle 1962). Decreasing levels of RH decrease electric resistance and lessen the propensity for tribo-electricity production. Most women know that combing and brushing in hot conditions causes greater flyaway than in cool conditions; experimental combing has confirmed this observation in showing that electrical resistance decreases as the temperature rises. Semi-quantitative experiments have shown that a useful way to minimize static build up is to reduce the effort of combing by making the hair comb easier.

The sign of the charge that develops when hairs are rubbed against each other is related to the direction of rubbing. If a single fibre in a group of hairs all orientated in the same direction is pulled out root first it becomes positively charged; if it is pulled out tip first, a negative charge is produced. Hair is thus dielectrically anisotropic at its surface.

Cream rinses and certain shampoos (high cleansing or high conditioning) decrease flyaway by reducing static charge as a result of lower kinetic frictional force during combing or brushing. They also lower the electrical resistance of fibres by increasing hair moisture.

References

Alexander, P., Hudson, P.F. & Earland, C. (1963) *Wool: Its Chemistry and Physics*, 2nd edn. Chapman & Hall, London.

Baden, H.P., Jackson, C.E., Weiss, I., Jumbow, K., Lee, I., Kubilus, J. & Gold, R.J.M. (1976) The physicochemical properties of hair in the BIDS syndrome. *American Journal of Human Genetics*, **28**, 514.

Brown, A.C., Belser, R.B., Crounse, R.G. & Wehr, R.F. (1970) A congenital hair defect, trichoschisis with alternating birefringence and low sulphur content. *Journal of Investigative Dermatology*, **34**, 496.

Chapman, B.M. (1969) A review of the mechanical properties of keratin fibres. *Journal of the Textile Institute*, **60**, 181.

Clarke, G.L. & Buhrke, V.E. (1954) Effects of elemental sulphur in the diet on the load extension hysteresis in single wool fibres. *Science (New York)*, **120**, 40.

Dawber, R.P.R. (1972) Investigations of a family with pili annulati associated with blue naevi. *Transactions of St. John's Hospital Dermatological Society*, **58**, 51.

Dawber, R.P.R. (1974) Knotting of hair. *British Journal of Dermatology*, **91**, 169.

Dawber, R.P.R. (1980) Weathering of hair in some genetic hair dystrophies. In *Hair, Trace Elements and Human Illness*, eds. A.C. Brown & R.G. Crounse. Praeger, New York.

Dawber, R.P.R. (1985) Physical properties of hair and nails. *Bioengineering and the Skin*, **2**, 39.

Fraser, R.D.B., MacRae, T.P. & Rogers, G.E. (1972) *Keratins: Their Composition, Structure and Biosynthesis*. Thomas, Springfield.

Fraser, R.D. & MacRae, T.P. (1980) Molecular structure and mechanical properties of keratins. In *The Mechanical Properties of Biological Materials*, p. 9, eds. J.F. Vincent & J.D. Currey. Proceedings of Society for Experimental Biology Symposium, No. 34. Cambridge University Press, Cambridge.

Goldsmith, L.A. & Baden, H.P. (1971) The mechanical properties of hair. Chemical modifications and pathological hairs. *Journal of Investigative Dermatology*, **56**, 200.

Harris, B. (1980) The mechanical behaviour of composite materials. In *The Mechanical Properties of Biological Materials*, p. 37, eds. J.F. Vincent & J.D. Currey. Proceedings of Society for Experimental Biology, No. 34. Cambridge University Press, Cambridge.

Hayashi, A., Taneda, D. & Ogawa, K. (1975) Trichogram. *Journal of Investigative Dermatology*, **60**, 70.

Korostoff, E., Rawnsley, H.M. & Shelley, W.B. (1970) Normalised stress–strain relationships of human hair perturbations by hypothyroidism. *British Journal of Dermatology*, **83**, 27.

Meredith, R. & Hearle, J. (1959) *Physical Methods of Investigating Textiles*. Interscience, New York.

Mitchell, T.W. & Feughelman, M. (1960) The torsional properties of single wool fibres. I. Torque–twist relationships and torsional relaxation in wet and dry fibres. *Textile Research Journal*, **30**, 662.

Morton, W. & Hearle, J. (1962) *Physical Properties of Textile Fibres*. Butterworth Scientific Publications, London.

Robbins, C.R. (1979) *Chemical and Physical Behaviour of Human Hair*. Van Nostrand–Reinhold, New York.

Rudall, K.M. (1964) The biomolecular structure of hair keratins. In *Progress in the Biological Sciences in Relation to Dermatology*, Vol. 2, eds. A. Rook & R.H. Champion. Cambridge University Press, London.

Spearman, R.O.C. (1977) The physical properties of hair. In *The Physiology and Pathophysiology of the Skin*, Vol. 4, ch. 44, ed. A. Jarrett. Academic Press, London.

Swanbeck, G., Nyren, J. & Juhlin, L. (1970) Mechanical properties of hairs from patients with different types of hair diseases. *Journal of Investigative Dermatology*, **54**, 248.

Swift, J.A. & Brown, A.C. (1972) The critical determination of the changes in the surface architecture of human hair due to cosmetic treatment. *Journal of Society of Cosmetic Chemists*, **23**, 695.

Tsuda, K. (1957) Study on the extractive strength of human head hairs. *Journal of Kyoto Prefecture Medical University*, **61**, 936.

Chapter 3
The Hair in Infancy and Childhood

Physiological aspects
(References p. 52)

The entire body of the foetus is covered by lanugo hair which is fine, soft, poorly pigmented and has no central medulla. There are two growths of lanugo hair, the first of which is normally shed at 7–8 months *in utero*, and the second is shed, often unnoticed, soon after birth. Significant lanugo is only seen after birth on a premature infant. The postnatal loss of lanugo hair is followed by the growth of vellus hair which is medullated, fine and poorly pigmented. It is often best seen on the face and forearms. Terminal hair is thicker, often pigmented and typically grows on the scalp, eyebrows and eyelashes before puberty and subsequently at the characteristic secondary sexual sites. Vellus hair continues to grow throughout life, even in the areas usually considered to have only terminal hairs such as the scalp where vellus hair may constitute 6–25% of the hair population (Danforth 1925; Trotter & Duggins 1948). A single follicle is probably capable of producing lanugo, vellus and terminal hairs.

There is an intermediate form of hair on the scalp which appears rapidly at 3–7 months and lasts until 2 years of age. It is coarser than lanugo hair, is sparsely pigmented and has a clearly formed but fragmented medulla compared with terminal hair which has greater pigmentation but a less well-defined medulla at this age (Duggins & Trotter 1950) (see Fig. 3.1).

At birth there is a total (histological) follicle density on the scalp of $1135/cm^2$; however, as the head enlarges the density falls to $795/cm^2$ at 3–12 months and $615/cm^2$ by the third decade (Giacometti 1964). The density of emergent hair shafts is lower than the histological density of follicles as there is only one terminal hair per follicular unit. The prepubertal child (3–9 years) has a density on the

51

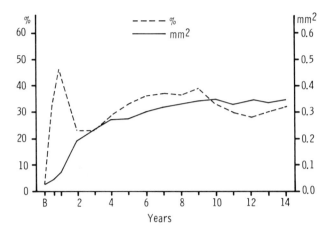

Fig. 3.1 Comparison of the cross-sectional area and the incidence of a medulla in hairs and their change with age. Intermediate hair is demonstrated by the peak of medullated hairs occurring in the first 2 years (adapted from Duggins & Trotter 1950).

crown of the scalp of 250 shafts/cm² and 170–205 on the surrounding scalp; boys have a slightly greater density of scalp hairs than girls (Pecoraro *et al.* 1964). There may be a variation in hair density which is dependent upon hair colour (Pinkus 1927).

References

Danforth, C.H. (1925) Studies on hair: with special reference to hypertrichosis. *AMA Archives of Dermatology and Syphilology*, **12**, 76.

Duggins, O.H. & Trotter, M. (1950) Age changes in head hair from birth to maturity. II. Medullation in hair of children. *American Journal of Physical Anthropology*, **8**, 399.

Giacometti, L. (1964) The anatomy of the human scalp. In *Advances in Biology of the Skin*, vol. VI, *Aging*, p. 97, ed. W. Montagna. Pergamon Press, Oxford.

Pecoraro, V., Astore, I., Barman, J.M. & Araujo, C.I. (1964) The normal trichogram in the child before puberty. *Journal of Investigative Dermatology*, **42**, 427.

Pinkus, F. (1927) Die normale Anatomie der Haut. In *Handbuch der Haut und Geschlechtskrankheiten*, vol. I, *Anatomie der Haut*, p. 116, ed. J. Jadassohn. Verlag von Julius Springer, Berlin.

Trotter, M. & Duggins, O.H. (1948) Age changes in head hair from birth to maturity. I. Index and size of hair of children. *American Journal of Physical Anthropology*, **6**, 489.

Hair growth
(References p. 56)

Well-formed follicles containing hair roots in the anagen growth phase can be seen over the entire scalp at 20 weeks gestation (Barman *et al.* 1967; Smith & Gong 1974; Findlay & Harris 1977). During the 26th to 28th week, the scalp hair roots change to catagen and then telogen in a progressive wave from the frontal to the parietal regions over a period of 7–10 days (Barman *et al.* 1967). Many of these telogen hairs are shed *in utero* (Kligman 1961). The roots in the occipital region remain in anagen until a time near birth when they too abruptly enter telogen (Barman *et al.* 1967; Saadat *et al.* 1976). After the telogen hair in the frontal and parietal regions has been shed, the roots re-enter anagen in a wave similar to the conversion to telogen and form the second pelage (Pecoraro *et al.* 1964b; Kostanecki *et al.* 1965; Barman *et al.* 1967).

At birth there are two consecutive waves of hair, each of which is growing over the scalp from the forehead to the nape of the neck (see Fig. 3.2). These waves can be identified by hair root studies. While the newer wave consists only of anagen

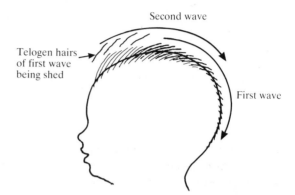

Fig. 3.2 The direction of the first two postnatal hair waves before the development of the 'mosaic' pattern — see text.

roots, the previous wave is converting to telogen prior to being shed and is represented by a gradient of telogen roots which is maximal frontally; this suggests that the earlier wave is being shed in the same direction (Pecoraro *et al.* 1964a). From the frontal to parietal regions there is, therefore, a gradual overlap of predominantly second growth over first growth hairs (due to the delay in shedding after conversion to telogen), and at the occipital region there are predominantly first growth hairs, few of which have entered telogen. This progression to a second pelage is delayed in infants with dark complexion who therefore have more abundant hair at birth (Pecoraro *et al.* 1964b; Barman *et al.* 1967). Careful observation of the primary hair will show that hair from the vertex is lost in a caudal fashion until the last hair is lost from a fringe above the nape of the neck (Trotter & Duggins 1948).

There is an area over the occiput in which the primary hairs do not enter telogen until after birth. These hairs remain in the scalp for 8–12 weeks and then fall. As the telogen hairs predominate on the occiput (Sadaat *et al.* 1976), their fall commonly produces an area of alopecia. This area typically has clearly defined borders on the lower and lateral margins and has been described as 'occipital alopecia of the newborn' (see Fig. 3.3). Often the parietal region will also have a considerable proportion of hairs in telogen at birth and this hair will also be shed after 8–12 weeks leaving only hair on the vertex. It has been suggested that immediately after birth there is loss of hair over the frontoparietal area analogous to adult male-pattern alopecia (see Fig. 3.4) (Hamilton 1951; Von Steigleder & Schultka 1963).

During foetal life and at least the first 4 postnatal months, all the scalp hair

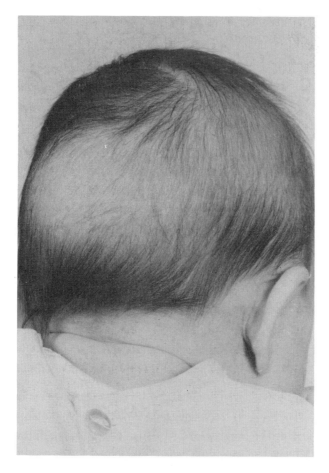

Fig. 3.3 Occipital alopecia due to the loss of synchronized telogen hairs in a child aged 14 weeks.

follicles are synchronized in the same phase of the growth cycle so that the waves of growth described above occur. Towards the end of the first year there is a change in the relationship of the growth cycle of adjacent hairs; there is a loss of synchronization and a random, or mosaic, pattern emerges. Once this conversion has occurred there will be a uniform distribution of hairs at all stages of the growth cycle. However, there is considerable variation in the age at which the mosaic pattern develops (Bosse & Rubisz-Brzezinska 1965) and it is not uncommon for children to have little hair for many months after the initial postnatal telogen fall. Once the mosaic pattern has developed it is maintained unless modified by disease, i.e. telogen effluvium (Kligman 1961).

There is a gradual transition during the years prior to puberty of scalp hair from vellus through intermediate to terminal hairs (Duggins & Trotter 1950). During this time there is a change in the shape and size of the hair shaft which may be related to the different hair forms. At birth the shaft is round and during the first 2 years it assumes an oval cross-section which is maintained throughout life. The cross-sectional area rapidly rises to 0.25 mm² at 3 years but thereafter more

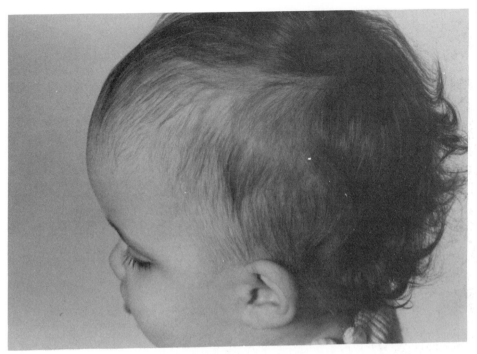

Fig. 3.4 Child aged 7 months demonstrating wave of hair fall which is progressing over the frontoparietal regions.

gradually to 0.40 mm² at 17 years (Trotter & Duggins 1948). Dark hair has a thicker cross-section than light-coloured hair. There is probably no significant sex difference in shaft calibre (Pecoraro *et al.* 1964b; Trotter & Duggins 1948; Trotter 1930). The hair of girls aged less than 20 years has a more variable and elliptical cross-section than boys (Steggerda & Seibert 1941) and this is particularly marked in the first 4 years of life (Trotter 1930).

The proportion of medullated scalp hairs rises steeply from 0 to 60% from 3–7 months, falls to 23% at 2 years and then gradually rises in proportion to shaft cross-sectional area (see Fig. 3.1). The pattern of medullation after 2 years is consistent with the change to terminal hairs. The medullated, thin hair at 6–18 months is an intermediate form which suddenly replaces vellus and is separate from the succeeding terminal hair (Duggins & Trotter 1950).

Overall hair density is slightly greater in boys than in girls (199 vs. 185/cm²) with a gradation from the vertex to occipital and parietal regions. Root estimations reveal low overall telogen counts (< 10%) but with a slightly higher telogen count over the frontoparietal region than the occiput (8–12% vs. 1–5%) suggesting a shorter anagen phase in these areas (Pecoraro *et al.* 1964b).

Linear growth has been poorly studied in children. The daily growth rate is marginally faster (0.05 mm) on the vertex of the scalp in comparison with the surrounding scalp (0.30–0.35 mm/day) (Pecoraro *et al.* 1964b; Myers & Hamilton

1951; Flesch 1954). It is likely that there are racial differences, the daily rate in Zulus being only 0.23 mm (Sims 1967). Linear growth is 5–15% faster in boys aged 3–9 years than in girls (Pecoraro *et al.* 1964b). Thigh hair grows at 0.13–0.20 mm/day (Myers & Hamilton 1951; Trotter 1924); the faster rate of scalp than body hair growth is maintained into adulthood. These measurements may not be comparable as they are not controlled for such factors as race or hair curl.

Overall hair length is variable and specific for an individual. It is proportional to the duration of anagen and the daily growth rate. The duration of anagen is probably the limiting factor and may be genetically determined.

References

Barman, J.M., Pecoraro, V., Astore, I. & Ferrer, J. (1967) The first stage in the natural history of the human scalp hair cycle. *Journal of Investigative Dermatology,* **48**, 138.

Bosse, K. & Rubisz-Brzezinska, J. (1965) Der Haarwechsel des Säuglings. *Archiv für klinische und experimentelle Dermatologie,* **221**, 166.

Duggins, O.H. & Trotter, M. (1950) Age changes in head hair from birth to maturity. II. Medullation in hair of children. *American Journal of Physical Anthropology,* **8**, 399.

Findlay, G.H. & Harris, W.F. (1977) The topology of hair streams and whorls in man with an observation on their relationship to epidermal ridge patterns. *American Journal of Physical Anthropology,* **46**, 427.

Flesch, P. (1954) Hair growth. In *Physiology and Biochemistry of the Skin,* p. 601, ed. S. Rothman. University of Chicago Press, Chicago.

Hamilton, J.B. (1951) Patterned loss of hair in man: types and incidences. *Annals of the New York Academy of Sciences,* **53**, 708.

Kligman, A.M. (1961) Pathologic dynamics of human hair loss. *Archives of Dermatology,* **83**, 175.

Kostanecki, W., Pawlowski, A. & Lozinska, D. (1965) Der Haarwurzelstatus bei Neugeborenen. *Archiv für klinische und experimentelle Dermatologie,* **221**, 162.

Myers, R.J. & Hamilton, J.B. (1951) Regeneration and rate of growth of hairs in man. *Annals of the New York Academy of Sciences,* **53**, 562.

Pecoraro, V., Astore, I. & Barman, J.M. (1964a) Cycle of the scalp hair of the newborn child. *Journal of Investigative Dermatology,* **43**, 145.

Pecoraro, V., Astore, I., Barman, J.M. & Araujo, C.I. (1964b) The normal trichogram in the child before puberty. *Journal of Investigative Dermatology,* **42**, 427.

Saadat, M., Khan, M.A., Gutberlet, R.L. & Heald, F.P. (1976) Measurement of hair in normal newborns. *Pediatrics,* **57**, 960.

Sims, R.T. (1967) Hair growth in kwashiorkor. *Archives of Disease in Childhood,* **42**, 397.

Smith, D.W. & Gong, B.T. (1974) Scalp hair patterning: its origin and significance relative to early brain and upper facial development. *Teratology,* **9**, 17.

Steggerda, M. & Seibert, H.C. (1941) Size and shape of head hair from six racial groups. *Journal of Heredity,* **32**, 315.

Trotter, M. (1924) The life cycles of hair in selected regions of the body. *American Journal of Physical Anthropology,* **7**, 427.

Trotter, M. (1930) The form, size and color of head hair of American whites. *American Journal of Physical Anthropology,* **14**, 433.

Trotter, M. & Duggins, O.H. (1948) Age changes in head hair from birth to maturity. I. Index and size of hair of children. *American Journal of Physical Anthropology,* **6**, 489.

Von Steigleder, G.K. & Schultka, O. (1963) Wechsel des Kopfhaares bei Kindern im ersten Lebensjahr. *Zeitschrift für Haut und Geschlechtskrankheiten,* **34**, xi.

Trichoglyphics: hair-slope patterns
(References p. 62)

Hair patterns are determined by the direction of hair streams. Although vellus and terminal hairs are present at all sites, vellus hairs being short, fine and poorly pigmented are apparent only on close observation; consequently terminal hairs tend to dominate the overall impression of patterning.

Hair does not grow vertically but leaves the skin at an angle; this angulation is precisely determined so that streams or patterns are formed. The patterns form spiralling or non-spiralling sprays emanating from central foci or whorls (Samlaska *et al.* 1989). It is impossible to cover a three-dimensional surface with parallel streams without a point from which the streams originate. Whorls and streams are probably formed as early as 10–12 weeks, and certainly by 18 weeks (Smith & Gong 1974).

The central point of a whorl is characterized by the divergent growth of a small group of hairs. The apparent orderliness of the spiral does not conform to any mathematical pattern and is not reflected by the histological root pattern in the foetus. The individual follicles are curved away from the axis of the emergent shaft (Findlay & Harris 1977) unlike other follicles which are in line with their shaft.

Whorls can be seen on the parietal region of the scalp, at the inner canthi of the eyes and often at other sites of depressions and projections such as the axillae, the olecranon of the elbow, the umbilicus, and the anus (Smith & Gong 1974; Findlay & Harris 1977), although they may develop at any site (Pinkus 1927). The back and the posterior aspect of the thigh are common sites for whorls although there are no topographical points to centre the whorls (see Fig. 3.5). When two streams converge, they split and fuse into lateral streams forming a cross, for example, the axillary whorls merge on the upper arm and join over the upper sternum to form a cross (see Fig. 3.6).

There is a single parietal scalp whorl in at least 95% of infants (Lauterbach & Knight 1927; Smith & Gong 1973, 1974; Wunderlich & Heereman 1974; Tirosh *et al.* 1987) which does not change throughout life. Most whorls (80%) are clockwise. Their position on the scalp is inconsistent and is not related to handedness (Lauterbach & Knight 1927). A frontal upsweep ('cowlick') due to a counterstream of hair from the forehead is present in 7% (Smith & Gong 1974) (see Fig. 3.7); it may affect a portion or the complete length of the anterior hair line.

Several hypotheses have been proposed to explain the generating force behind the evolution of hair slopes and streams: physical and local chemical factors.

Scalp hair patterns on the heads of children with abnormal brain development, for example, microcephaly and turrencephaly, are grossly abnormal with frontal upsweep and aberrant or absent parietal whorls (see Table 3.1). Smith (Smith & Gong 1973, 1974; Smith & Greely 1978) believes that this pattern is the result of differential shearing forces within the skin during foetal development. The

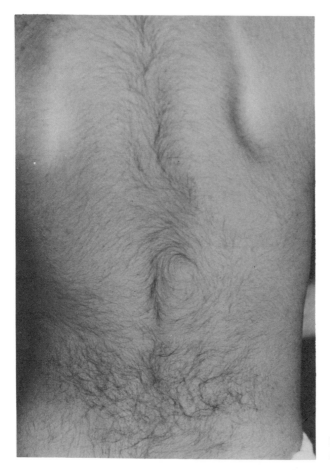

Fig. 3.5 Hair whorl on the back of an Indian child aged 3 years.

outgrowth of the foetal brain produces a shearing force on the lower dermis against the epidermis. The hair roots are, therefore, angled to the epidermis with the deepest part pointed towards the site of greatest cerebral outgrowth, the apex of which forms the whorl. When there is minimal cerebral growth there is no stretch and no whorl develops; the face then becomes the dominant growth area with the hair shafts angled from the forehead over the crown of the head.

There is some support for this hypothesis from animal experiments. If skin flaps of mature animals are raised and rotated by 180°, the hair continues to grow in its original direction (Trotter & Dawson 1931; Durward & Rudall 1949). However, if the flap is rotated before the hair follicles are fully developed in an immature animal, the hair may grow in a similar direction to the surrounding non-transposed hair. This may be due to the effects of stretch as the animal grows but the effect of scar tissue around the graft cannot be entirely discounted (Trotter & Dawson 1932).

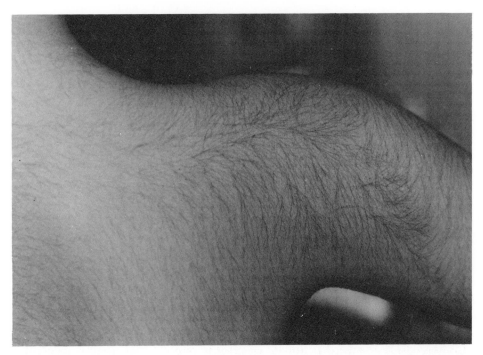

Fig. 3.6 Hair streams flowing from the axilla around the arm and fusing into a single stream over the shoulder.

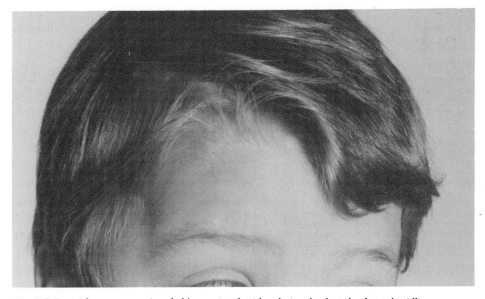

Fig. 3.7 Frontal upsweep or 'cowlick' associated with a hair whorl at the frontal midline.

Table 3.1 Abnormalities of scalp hair whorls (Smith & Gong 1974)

Disorder	Scalp whorl location
Malformations	
Turrencephaly	Whorl near top of projection
Dicephaly	Widely spaced biparietal whorls with midline confluence of hair streams
Microcephaly	Absent or poorly developed parietal whorl. Midline whorl over posterior fontanel. Anterior whorl
Trigonocephaly	Widely spaced biparietal whorls with midline confluence
Dysmorphic syndromes	
Down's syndrome	Midline whorl over posterior fontanel
13-trisomy	Areas of scalp aplasia with outflaring hair patterns. Anterior upsweep with anterior scalp whorl
Prader–Willi	Anterior upsweep with anterior whorl
Rubinstein–Taybi	Anterior whorl

This hypothesis of physical forces is not endorsed by the pattern of follicles at the centre of the whorl. As only the 'follicle neck' is in line with the shaft (Findlay & Harris 1977; Durward & Rudall 1949) it is possible that there is differential bidirectional growth between the superficial and deep parts of the dermis. Hair whorls have been seen lying in dermatoglyphic patterns on the arms and may reflect the three-dimensional development of the skin (Findlay & Harris 1977).

Computer-aided mathematical models suggest that the morphology of the hair shaft, the relationship both between individual follicles and between follicles and their associated sebaceous gland can be explained by the local production, diffusion and response of surrounding tissue to an active substance or 'morphogen' (Nagorka 1984; Mooney & Nagorka 1985). However, no such substance has been isolated.

Negroes with short curly hair do not usually develop a scalp pattern with hair streams, and only 10% have a parietal whorl (Wunderlich & Heereman 1974).

Abnormalities of scalp hair whorls
(References p. 62)

The association between congenital dysmorphic features has already been mentioned and the patterns described by Smith & Gong (1974) are summarized in Table 3.1. A comparative study of 348 mentally retarded children demonstrated an increased incidence of multiple scalp hair whorls (Fig. 3.8) and other dysmorphic features (Fig. 3.9) compared with 1399 normal children. The authors suggested that multiple whorls might be considered to be a dysmorphic sign (Tirosh *et al.* 1987; Samlaska *et al.* 1989).

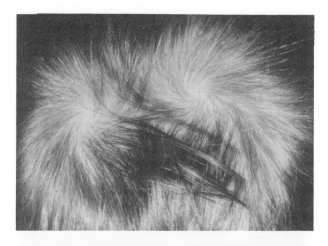

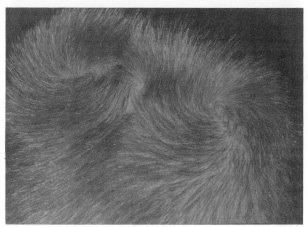

Fig. 3.8 Double and triple parietal whorls in developmentally normal 2- and 3-year-olds (courtesy of C.P. Samlaska M.D., Washington, USA).

Abnormalities of the scalp hair line

Displacement of the hair line occurs in a number of syndromes:
low anterior hair line—Cornelia de Lange syndrome, lipoatrophic diabetes, foetal hydantoin syndrome, Rubinstein–Taybi syndrome;
low posterior line—multiple pterygium syndrome, Turner's syndrome, Noonan's syndrome.

Unruly hair (Mortimer 1985)
(References p. 62)

Unruly hair in children may be due to hair shaft abnormalities, abnormalities of scalp hair patterning (see above) or a physiological phenomenon.

Hair shaft abnormalities may be classified into those associated with increased

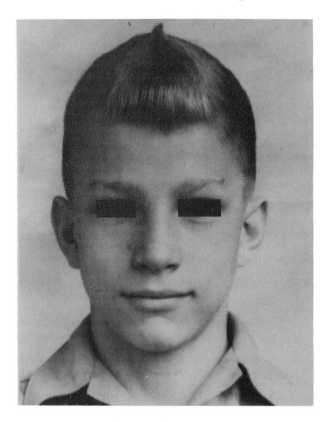

Fig. 3.9 Ridgeback anomaly. The hair waves are growing towards the vertex from all around the scalp instead of the normal spiralling pattern away from the crown. This pattern does not fit any of the theories propounded in the text and may represent intrinsic factors of the hair follicles (courtesy of C.P. Samlaska M.D., Washington, USA and Samlaska *et al.* (1989), *Archives of Dermatology*).

shaft fragility (pili torti) or without shaft fragility (woolly hair, cheveux incoif-fables).

Smith & Greely (1978) noted that many normal infants had hair that stood up and could not be combed flat. This phenomenon occurs to a mild degree over the vertex in 12% of normal infants and more completely in 2%.

References

Durward, A. & Rudall, K.M. (1949) Studies on hair growth in the rat. *Journal of Anatomy*, **83**, 325.

Findlay, G.H. & Harris W.F. (1977) The topology of hair streams and whorls in man with an observation on their relationship to epidermal ridge patterns. *American Journal of Physical Anthropology*, **46**, 427.

Lauterbach, C.E. & Knight, J.B. (1927) Variations in whorl of head hair. *Journal of Heredity*, **18**, 107.

Mooney, J.R. & Nagorka, B.N. (1985) Spatial patterns produced by a reaction–diffusion system in primary hair follicles. *Journal of Theoretical Biology*, **115**, 299.

Mortimer, P.S. (1985) Unruly hair. *British Journal of Dermatology*, **113**, 467.

Nagorka, B.N. (1984) Evidence for a reaction–diffusion system as a mechanism controlling mammalian hair growth. *Biosystems*, **16**, 323.

Pinkus, F. (1927) Die normale Anatomie der Haut. In *Handbuch der Haut und Geschlechtskrankheiten*, vol. 1, *Anatomie der Haut*, p. 116, ed. J. Jadassohn. Verlag von Julius Springer, Berlin.

Samlaska, C.P., Benson, P.M. & James, W.D. (1989) The ridgeback anomaly: a new follicular pattern of the scalp. *Archives of Dermatology*, **125**, 98.

Smith, D.W. & Gong, B.T. (1973) Scalp hair patterning as a clue to early fetal brain development. *Journal of Pediatrics*, **83**, 374.

Smith, D.W. & Gong, B.T. (1974) Scalp hair patterning: its origin and significance relative to early brain and upper facial development. *Teratology*, **9**, 17.

Smith, D.W. & Greely, M.J. (1978) Unruly scalp hair in infancy: its nature and relevance to problems of brain morphogenesis. *Pediatrics*, **61**, 783.

Tirosh, E., Jaffe, M. & Dar, H. (1987) The clinical significance of multiple hair whorls and their association with unusual dermatoglyphics and dysmorphic features in mentally retarded Israeli children. *European Journal of Pediatrics*, **146**, 568.

Trotter, M. & Dawson, H.L. (1931) The direction of hair after rotation of skin in the guinea pig: an experiment on hair slope. *Anatomical Record*, **50**, 193.

Trotter, M. & Dawson, H.L. (1932) The direction of hair after rotation of skin in the newborn albino rat: a second experiment on hair slope. *Anatomical Record*, **53**, 19.

Wunderlich, R.C. & Heereman, N.A. (1974) Hair crown patterns of human newborns: studies on parietal whorl locations and their direction. *Clinical Pediatrics*, **14**, 1045.

Circumscribed alopecia in infancy
(References p. 67)

The differential diagnosis of circumscribed alopecia in infancy present at or soon after birth depends upon an accurate history and careful examination.

Obstetric trauma at birth may be followed by scarring or temporary shedding of hair over a contusion or haematoma. Pressure from the uterine cervix may produce an annular pattern of hair loss which may be temporary or permanent with scarring (Neal *et al.* 1984; Prendiville & Esterley 1987). Trauma is often wrongly incriminated in cases of aplasia cutis congenita but the shape and situation of these raw areas or paper thin scars should establish the true diagnosis.

Naevi are the commonest cause of circumscribed congenital alopecias. Epidermal naevi in infancy are flat or only slightly thickened and totally or partially devoid of hair. The slightly warty texture of the surface should suggest the diagnosis, which becomes obvious as the child grows older.

Cicatricial alopecia not preceded by inflammatory changes is rarely present at birth but may develop during childhood in association with a number of hereditary syndromes, for example incontinentia pigmenti.

The most distinctive form of follicular aplasia is triangular alopecia of the temples (Tosti 1987) but more common, though often discovered in the course of a routine examination of the scalp, is a small circumscribed, but not sharply defined, area of alopecia in which follicles are absent or are few and of vellus type (Barth & Dawber 1987).

Sutural alopecia is an inconstant feature of the Hallermann–Streiff syndrome but is not present in early infancy.

Alopecia areata has occurred in infancy, but the diagnosis should be made with caution.

Three infants with subdural meningocoeles developed alopecia (Bitz & Donalies 1970); in one it developed over the lesion. The hair re-grew after surgical treatment.

Aplasia cutis congenita

Aplasia cutis congenita (ACC) occurs in a heterogeneous group of disorders in which localized or widespread areas of skin are absent at birth. The incidence of congenital skin defects affecting the scalp is 0.03% of all births in Holland (Van Dijke *et al.* 1987; Leung *et al.* 1988). Neuroectodermal defects may mimic this entity (Commens *et al.* 1989).

Pathogenesis
Several hypotheses have been forwarded; most have emphasized mechanical factors such as vascular events, amniotic bands, trauma, uterine compression and intra-uterine herpes simplex infection (Freiden 1986). Reports of maternal ingestion of methimazole causing ACC have not been supported by epidemiological evidence (Van Dijke *et al.* 1987). Other reports have emphasized that ACC may be due to a primary failure of embryonic differentiation (Anderson & Novy 1942).

As scalp ACC most commonly involves the parietal whorl, Smith has invoked his hypothesis of mechanical forces (Stephen *et al.* 1982). He suggests that the whorl acts as the central point of outgrowth of the foetal brain and is stretched from all around; he further suggests that in ACC this stretching compromises the vasculature and results in cutaneous rupture. This concept of skin tension is supported by the thinning out of the dermal appendages adjacent to the lesion (see below).

Most cases of isolated scalp ACC are sporadic but there have been many pedigrees demonstrating autosomal dominant inheritance and involvement in identical twins (Sybert 1985; Freiden 1986).

Histopathology
Ulcers extend to a variable depth. Healed areas show a flattened epidermis, dermal fibrosis and a complete absence of dermal structures. The skin bordering the lesions reveals a gradual transition from normal skin to an area deficient in elastic fibres. In the intermediate zone, the dermal appendages are found to be absent, rudimentary or malformed; they decrease in numbers centripetally in proportion to the decrease in elastic fibres (Gross *et al.* 1957; Croce *et al.* 1973).

Clinical features
Aplasia cutis congenita may be present at birth as a sharply circumscribed ulcer with a raw red base simulating a wound or it may be completely scarred. Isolated lesions are seen on the scalp in 85% of cases and it is usually placed close to the site of the parietal scalp whorl (Demmel 1975; Stephen *et al.* 1982). Scalp lesions are single in 70–75% of cases, double in 20% and triple in 8% (Ingalls 1933) (see Fig. 3.10). They are often round but may be oval, linear, rhomboidal or stellate (Demmel 1975). They are usually 1–2 cm in diameter but may involve more extensive areas of skin.

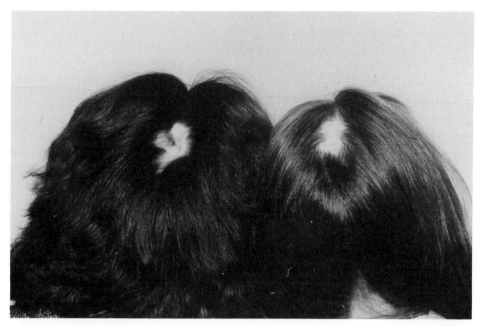

Fig. 3.10 Aplasia cutis congenita, here seen in mother and daughter; no other member of this family tree was affected.

The defects may heal rapidly to leave an atrophic, or more rarely, a keloidal scar (Moschella 1962; Lassman & Sims 1975). Even extensive defects may heal if they are not too deep, but may result in considerable cosmetic disfigurement; 20–30% may have associated involvement of the calvaria directly beneath the lesions. The mortality from scalp defects due to meningitis or haemorrhage has been reported to be 20% (Anderson & Novy 1942; Demmel 1975); although infection is now more often controllable there is still an appreciable risk of thrombosis, haematoma or erosion of the sagittal sinus (Croce *et al.* 1973; Lavine *et al.* 1978; Schneider *et al.* 1980).

Aplasia cutis congenita occurs in a wide spectrum of disorders:
1 isolated scalp ACC;
2 scalp ACC with limb abnormalities;
3 scalp ACC with associated epidermal and organoid naevi;
4 ACC overlying embryonal defects;
5 ACC with foetus papyraceus or placental infarcts;
6 ACC with epidermolysis bullosa;
7 ACC localized to the extremities;
8 ACC caused by specific teratogens;
9 ACC with specific syndromes.
It has been reported with a diversity of associated features. The latter include cleft lip and palate (Kosnik & Sayers 1975), tracheo-oesophageal fistula (Kosnik

& Sayers 1975; Deeken & Caplan 1970), double uterus (Cutlip *et al.* 1967). patent ductus arteriosus (Deeken & Caplan 1970), polycystic kidneys (O'Brien & Drake 1960), mental retardation (Lassman & Sims 1975), cutis marmorata (South & Jacobs 1978) and ocular abnormalities (Leung *et al.* 1988).

Treatment
Small lesions are best left to heal spontaneously and control of infection is the principal aim. For these lesions any decision about surgical removal of the bald area may be left until the child is older. However, for larger lesions, the risks of haemorrhage or meningitis have led to the recommendation for early skin grafting (Croce *et al.* 1973; Lavine *et al.* 1978).

Congenital triangular alopecia

The first description and illustration of this distinctive congenital defect were given by Sabouraud (1905) in his *Manual of Topographical Dermatology* under the name 'aire alopécique temporale congénital'. Although there have only been 36 published cases, the condition cannot be uncommon as 14 were seen in a single department over a period of only 3 years (Bargman 1984; Tosti 1987).

Pathology
The affected area demonstrates a normal epidermis and vellus hair follicles (Tosti 1987).

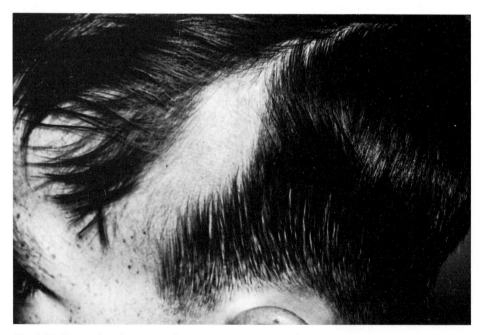

Fig. 3.11 Triangular alopecia. In this patient it was bilaterally symmetrical.

Clinical features

The practically bald triangular areas are present at birth but are not usually noticed by the parents until the third to sixth years (Tosti 1987), possibly because infants' hair is generally fine and sparse. It is possible that in some cases the first hair coat is normal as in some other forms of congenital circumscribed alopecia. The base of each triangle impinges on, and may or may not involve, the temporal hair line. The triangle overlies the frontotemporal suture and measures 3–5 cm from base to apex. It is usually unilateral, but may be bilateral (Fig. 3.11). It remains unchanged throughout life and, as far as is known, is of no more than cosmetic significance.

Treatment

No therapy is usually indicated. Hair replacement with grafting has been used with cosmetic success (Bargman 1984).

References

Anderson, N.P. & Novy, F.G. (1942) Congenital defects of the scalp. *AMA Archives of Dermatology and Syphilology*, **46**, 257.

Bargman, H. (1984) Congenital temporal triangular alopecia. *Canadian Medical Association Journal*, **131**, 1253.

Barth, J.H. & Dawber, R.P.R. (1987) Focal naevoid hypotrichosis. *Acta Dermato-Venereologica*, **67**, 187.

Bitz, D. & Donalies, C. (1970) Alopecia partialis beim klinische progradiunten chronischen subduralen Hydrom des Säuglings. *Padiatrie und Grenzgebiete*, **9**, 101.

Commens, C., Rogers, M. & Kan, A. (1989) Heterotropic brain tissue presenting as bald cyst with a collar of hypertrophic hair. *Archives of Dermatology*, **125**, 1253.

Croce, E.J., Purohit, R.C. & Janovski, N.A. (1973) Congenital absence of skin (aplasia cutis congenita). *Archives of Surgery*, **106**, 732.

Cutlip, D.B. Jr., Cryan, D.M. & Vineyard, W.R. (1967) Congenital scalp defects in a mother and child. *American Journal of Diseases of Children*, **113**, 597.

Deeken, J.H. & Caplan, R.M. (1970) Aplasia cutis congenita. *Archives of Dermatology*, **102**, 386.

Demmel, U. (1975) Clinical aspects of congenital skin defects. *European Journal of Pediatrics*, **121**, 21.

Freiden, I.J. (1986) Aplasia cutis congenita: a clinical review and proposed classification. *Journal of the American Academy of Dermatology*, **14**, 6446.

Gross, H., Lindemayr, W. & Pospisil, G. (1957) Zur Kenntnis der Aplasia cutis. *Neue Österreiche Zeitschrift für Kinderheilkunde*, **2**, 94.

Ingalls, N.W. (1933) Congenital defects of scalp; studies in pathology of development. *American Journal of Obstetrics and Gynecology*, **25**, 861.

Kosnik, E.J. & Sayers, M.P. (1975) Congenital scalp defects: aplasia cutis congenita. *Journal of Neurosurgery*, **42**, 32.

Lassman, L.P. & Sims, D.G. (1975) Congenital midline scalp and skull defect. *Archives of Disease in Childhood*, **50**, 958

Lavine, D., Lehman, J.A. Jr. & Thomas, R. (1978) Congenital scalp defect with thrombosis of the sagittal sinus. *Plastic and Reconstructive Surgery*, **61**, 599.

Leung, R.S.C., Beer, W.E. & Mehta, H.K. (1988) Aplasia cutis congenita presenting as a familial triad of atrophic alopecia, ocular defects and a peculiar scarring tendency of the skin. *British Journal of Dermatology*, **118**, 715.

Moschella, S.L. (1962) Congenital defects of scalp with keloid formation. *Archives of Dermatology*, **86**, 63.

Neal, P.R., Merk, P.F. & Norins, A.L. (1984) Halo scalp ring: a form of localized scalp injury associated with caput succedaneum. *Pediatric Dermatology*, **2**, 52.

O'Brien, B.McC. & Drake, J.E. (1960) Congenital defects of the skull and scalp. *British Journal of Plastic Surgery*, **13**, 102.

Prendiville, J.S. & Esterley, N.B. (1987) Halo scalp ring: a cause of scarring alopecia. *Archives of Dermatology*, **123**, 992.

Schneider, B.M., Berg, R.A. & Kaplan, A.M. (1980) Aplasia cutis congenita complicated by sagittal sinus hemorrhage. *Pediatrics*, **66**, 948.

South, D.A. & Jacobs, A.H. (1978) Cutis marmorata telangiectasia congenita (congenital generalized phlebectasia). *Journal of Pediatrics*, **93**, 944.

Stephen, M.J., Smith, D.W., Ponzi, J.W. & Alden, E.R. (1982) Orgin of scalp vertex aplasia cutis. *Journal of Pediatrics*, **101**, 850.

Sybert, V.P. (1985) Aplasia cutis congenita: a report of 12 new families and review of the literature. *Pediatric Dermatology*, **3**, 1.

Tosti, A. (1987) Congenital triangular alopecia. *Journal of the American Academy of Dermatology*, **16**, 991.

Van Dijke, C.P., Heydendael, R.J. de Kleine, M.J. (1987) Methimazole, carbimazole and congenital skin defects. *Annals of Internal Medicine*, **106**, 60.

The scalp in infancy
(References p. 69)

Many naevi may be present on the scalp at birth or may develop during the first few weeks of life.

Greasy scaling and crusting, particularly in the frontovertical regions, is characteristic of seborrhoeic dermatitis.

Cephalhaematoma

Birth trauma resulting in subperiosteal haemorrhage is the cause of this uncommon scalp lesion which, in about 25% of cases, may be associated with an underlying fracture of the skull (Kendall & Woloshin 1952). It presents as a firm but compressible swelling, often with a palpable rim of periosteum. Most of these lesions resolve during the first 6 weeks of life, but they may calcify and persist for months or years (Soloman & Esterly 1973).

Gonococcal scalp abscess

The slight injury to the scalp which may be inflicted by the electrode for foetal heart monitoring may provide a portal of entry for infection. Two infants with such a gonococcal infection have been described (Reveri & Krishnamurhy 1979).

Pubertal hair growth
(References p. 69)

Before puberty terminal hairs only occur on the scalp, eyebrows and eyelashes. At puberty there is a conversion of vellus to terminal hairs at other sites of the body. The pubic area is the first to appear and is followed by the axillae after an interval of about 2 years. In boys facial hair appears at the same time as axillary hair. Terminal hairs start at the corners of the lips and spread over the upper lip

Table 3.2 Presence (%) of body hair in American boys (Reynolds 1951)

Area	14 years	16 years	18 years
Pubic	97	100	100
Axillary	40	97	100
Anterior leg	46	90	100
Anterior thigh	30	67	95
Forearm	14	37	80
Abdomen	14	37	75
Buttocks	14	33	50
Chest	3	7	40
Lower back	3	7	20
Upper arms	0	0	10
Shoulders	0	0	0

before appearing on the chin and then cheeks. An orderly sequence of hair conversion follows on the body—the lower legs, thighs, forearms, abdomen, buttocks, chest, back, upper arms and shoulders (Reynolds 1951) (see Table 3.2). The development of pubic hair does not correlate well with genital development (Tanner 1975).

There is a standardized assessment and grading of the evolution of pubic hair. Girls enter puberty earlier and, therefore, develop and complete an adult pattern of hair earlier than boys (Marshall & Tanner 1969, 1970). The difference in the age of onset of puberty probably explains the variation between racial groups (Tanner 1975; Reynolds & Wines 1951; Neyzi *et al.* 1975). There is also a variation of 1–2 years within each racial group (Tanner 1975).

Hirsuties in childhood

The pathophysiology of hirsuties is discussed in depth in Chapter 4. The differential diagnosis in children includes congenital adrenal hyperplasia, polycystic ovary syndrome (Yen 1980) and hormone secreting tumours of the adrenal gland. The development of sexual characteristics in girls under 8 years and boys under 9 years may be due to precocious puberty or to precocious adrenarche. Precocious puberty is the development of the usual secondary characteristics and demands detailed endocrine investigation. Precocious adrenarche is characterised by the development of pubic and axillary hair *without* any features of sexual development or virilism (particularly cliteromegaly in girls) and is due to premature activation of adrenal androgen production (Savage & Evans 1984).

References

Kendall, N. & Woloshin, H. (1952) Cephalhaematoma associated with fracture of the skull. *Journal of Pediatrics*, **41**, 125.

Marshall, W.A. & Tanner, J.M. (1969) Variations in pattern of pubertal changes in girls. *Archives of Disease in Childhood,* **44**, 291.

Marshall, W.A. & Tanner, J.M. (1970) Variations in pattern of pubertal changes in boys. *Archives of Disease in Childhood,* **45**, 13.

Neyzi, O., Alp, H., Yalcindag, A., Yakacikli, S. & Orphon, A. (1975) Sexual maturation in Turkish boys. *Annals of Human Biology,* **2**, 251.

Reveri, M. & Krishnamurthy, C. (1979) Gonococcal scalp abscess. *Journal of Pediatrics,* **94**, 819.

Reynolds, E.L. (1951) The appearance of adult patterns of body hair in man. *Annals of the New York Academy of Sciences,* **53**, 576.

Reynolds, E.L. & Wines, J.V. (1951) Physical changes associated with adolescence in boys. *American Journal of Diseases of Children,* **82**, 529.

Savage, D.C.L & Evans, J. (1984) Puberty and adolescence. In *Textbook of Paediatrics,* 3rd edn, p. 372, eds. J.O. Forfar & G.C. Arneil. Churchill Livingstone, Edinburgh.

Soloman, L.M. & Esterly, N.B. (1973) Major problems in clinical pediatrics. In *Neonatal Dermatology,* vol. IX, p. 47. Saunders, Philadelphia.

Tanner, J.M. (1975) Growth and endocrinology of the adolescent. In *Endocrine and Genetic Diseases of Childhood and Adolescence,* 2nd edn, p. 14, ed. L.I. Gardner. Saunders, Philadelphia.

Yen, S.S.C. (1980) The polycystic ovary syndrome. *Clinical Endocrinology,* **12**, 177.

Chapter 4
Hair Patterns: Hirsuties and Baldness

Introduction

This chapter concerns the problem of hair patterning with particular reference to hirsuties in the female and common baldness in both sexes. The text is based on the (philosophical) premise that both situations represent a continuum of hairiness in men and women. However, the degree of pattern change may be determined by age, sex and hormonal status, as will be discussed in the following pages. The concepts of 'normal' and 'pathological' are, therefore, invalid for most of the population.

The extent to which these patterns are considered abnormal depends on social pressures; for example, the loss of head hair as common baldness in males is equated with senility and hence loss of sexual potency in some races while in others the myth of baldness and increased sexuality prevails. Men from the former culture consider common baldness to be abnormal while those from the latter are more content with their bodily habitus. A similar situation occurs in women with respect to loss of scalp hair and increase in body hair.

This chapter considers regional variations in hair type and distribution and progresses to the problems of hirsuties and common baldness.

Regional variations in hair patterns
(References p. 76)

The variations in hair pattern related to age, genetic constitution and endocrine status have been studied thoroughly in only a few regions of the body, and in a very limited number of races. The available information is summarized below, largely as an inducement to further, more detailed, investigations. Few investigators, however, attempt to correlate the hair patterns in different regions with different races. Danforth & Trotter (1922), who examined soldiers on demobilization, noted that dark-haired individuals tended to have more body hair than fair-haired individuals, but that there were racial differences unrelated to pigmentation, in that fair-haired men of Italian descent had more body hair than did fair-haired Scandinavians.

The pinna

Hairiness of the pinna—the external ear—is a conspicuous racial character which has aroused much interest among geneticists and anthropologists, but has received little attention from clinicians (Kamalam & Thambiah 1990).

The development of coarse hairs on the pinna occurs most frequently, and with the longest and densest hairs, in Indians. Normally only males are affected. The incidence and severity of the hairiness increase from the age of about 20 to over 50. By the 7th decade about 70% of men in Madras and about 30% in West Bengal are affected (Stern *et al.* 1964). In Indians the sulcus at the side of the ear bears most hairs, but the top of the ear and other sites may also be involved. The degree of hairiness ranges from a few hairs to large bushy tufts. In the Maltese (Gates & Vella 1962) and in Israeli populations (Slatis & Apelbaum 1963) the total incidence is lower than in Indians, and the top of the ear is the site most extensively affected. Hypertrichosis of the pinna has been regarded as a classical example of a sex-linked recessive trait (Dronamraju & Haldane 1962). However, many pedigrees are not compatible with inheritance by a γ-linked fully penetrant gene (Sarkar *et al.* 1961). Dronamraju (1963) favoured multifactorial inheritance. However, vellus hairs are present on the female pinna and until studies have been made on the pinnae of virilized females, sex-influenced autosomal inheritance remains a possibility (Sarkar & Ghosh 1963; Stern *et al.* 1964). There is evidence that the growth of coarse hairs on the pinna is androgen dependent. In Caucasoid males they begin to appear after the 24th year and increase in number until about the 58th year (Hamilton 1947).

A detailed investigation of the ear hair patterns in American Caucasoid and Negro males was carried out (Setty 1969). There were wide variations in the pattern and in the extent of hypertrichosis, both tending to increase with age. Over 45% of the Negroes but only 15% of the Caucasoids had no terminal hairs on their pinnae. The patterns on the two ears were not necessarily identical. The patterns in other races also have been studied. There are marked differences in the relative frequency of different patterns, but in all the hypertrichosis becomes significant, if it does so at all, by middle life.

The presence of marked hypertrichosis of the margin of the pinna in the majority of infants born to diabetic mothers (Eklund *et al.* 1960) has not been explained. Wallis (1897) found such hair in some normal infants.

Chest

The growth of terminal hair on the chest begins in the normal male soon after puberty, but the hair does not attain its greatest extent and density until the 6th decade. The pattern most frequently encountered in mature Caucasoid American males covered the sternum, with lateral extensions below the clavicles and below the nipples (Setty 1961a). This same author described and defined other patterns.

Quantitative studies of coarse sternal hairs (Hamilton *et al.* 1969) provided data which are applicable also to other androgen-dependent sites. The number of sternal hairs, their mean length and shaft diameter rose slowly from puberty to reach a peak in the 5th or 6th decade. Thereafter the number of hairs slowly declined, but there was little reduction in their size.

In some individuals with an extensive chest hair pattern, circular bare areas form above and medial to the nipples (Setty 1961b). The prevalence of this so-called 'pectoral alopecia' is not well documented. In a hospital population in the United States such bare areas were found in 46% of Negroes and 16% of Caucasoids (Gompertz 1960).

Back

The patterns of terminal hair growth on the backs of American Caucasoid males have been defined and classified (Setty 1962). Extensive covering of the back tends to accompany extensive chest hairs, but the genetic significance of striking variations in pattern is not clear.

Axillae

Terminal hair in the axillae usually appears about 2 years after the first pubic hair, but there is much individual variation and axillary hair may occasionally appear first (Tanner 1964). Coarse hairs appear at an earlier age than in the beard. In old age the follicles tend to atrophy (Hamilton & Terada 1963).

Axillary hair growth in Caucasoids and Japanese has been compared (Hamilton & Terada 1963). In both sexes axillary hair was much sparser in the Japanese than in the Caucasoids. Not only were there fewer hairs but in a larger proportion of older subjects there were no hairs at all.

Abdominal wall and pubes

This region has been particularly well studied on account of the obvious relationship of its hair patterns to other pubertal developments (Pryor 1956; Thomas & Ferriman 1957).

Using the distribution of hair at and above the upper border of the pubic triangle as a criterion, Dupertuis *et al.* (1945) proposed the terms horizontal, acuminate and disperse to describe the grosser variations in pattern. They studied 1060 American Caucasoid men and 309 women. The horizontal pattern was found in 90% of women and in 38% of 18-year-old males; this pattern persisted in 17% of fully adult males. The remaining 10% of women showed an acuminate pattern, which was found also in 50% of males. Extensive—'disperse'—abdominal hair in men aged 30–40 tended to be associated with much terminal hair on chest and thighs.

Of 3858 fit British men examined by McGregor (1961) 4.05% showed a horizontal pattern, 85.2% an acuminate or disperse pattern and 10.2% an intermediate pattern. The differences between this series and that reported by Dupertuis *et al.* (1945) can largely be explained by differences in the age composition of the two groups of subjects.

The development of pubic hair was studied in 557 Caucasoid American girls (Reynolds & Wines 1948). Sparse pigmented hair first appeared on average at the age of 11 years and the full pubic triangle was complete by 13.9.

Pubic hair becomes thinned after the menopause and in those women in whom the pattern has been acuminate it becomes horizontal (Beek 1950). Large doses of oestrogen, such as are prescribed in some patients with carcinoma of the prostate, may lead to the development of a horizontal abdominal hair pattern in men (Fig. 4.1).

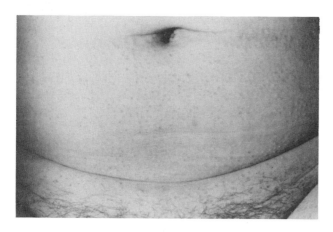

Fig. 4.1 Female pattern of abdominal hair in a male receiving oestrogen treatment.

Penis and scrotum
Penile hair patterns of four types all occur over a wide age range (Setty 1969) as do the three scrotal hair patterns (Setty 1970) which are essentially similar in American Negroes and Caucasoids.

Arms
On the arms four well-defined patterns of hair growth have been differentiated. Fairly full cover of the upper limbs, sparing only the flexor aspect of the upper arms,

was found in some 70% of Caucasoid American men (Setty 1964). In another 25% there was no terminal hair on the upper arms. In 3% only the forearms bore terminal hair. Other patterns were exceptional.

In familial hypertrichosis cubiti—the hairy elbows syndrome (Beighton 1970; Andreev & Stransky 1979)—hypertrichosis of the lower third of the upper arms and the upper third of the forearms is present from early infancy, becomes worse in the next year or two and then partially regresses. The mode of inheritance is uncertain (Fig. 4.2).

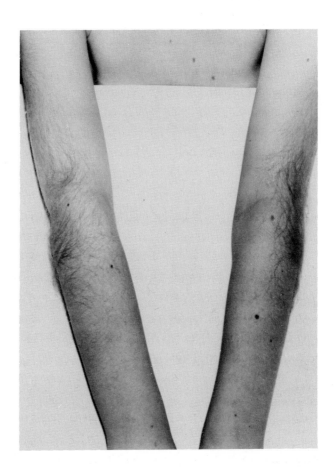

Fig. 4.2 'Hairy elbows' in a girl aged 11.

The fingers

There have been many anthropological studies of the incidence and patterns of hair on the backs of the fingers. Hair is present on the proximal phalanx of the index, middle, ring and little fingers of most individuals of most races, and in most the dorsum of the middle phalanx of the index finger is hairless (Ikoma 1972). Hair on the proximal phalanx of the thumb, and on the middle phalanx of the middle and ring fingers shows individual and racial variation. It was less common in a North American Indian tribe than in Japanese, and was more common still in Canadians of European descent. Genetic studies in Japan (Ikoma 1973) and Germany

(Sommer 1971) showed that the trait is transmitted dominantly and is controlled by multiple alleles. In identical twins there was concordance in the numbers of hairy phalanges, and in the shape, position, size and density of the hairy patches (Sommer 1971).

Thigh and leg

In adult male American Caucasoids and Negroes four patterns of terminal hair could be differentiated (Setty 1968). The thigh is completely covered with the exception of an area of variable extent on the lateral aspect of the upper thigh. The lower leg, too, may be completely covered, but far more frequently the anterolateral aspect of the lower leg, or the entire lower two-thirds of the lower leg is bare. The incidence of such bare areas, sometimes referred to as peroneal alopecia, has been found to be in the region of 35% in the US and in England (Ronchese & Chace 1939). The differences in the relative frequency of the various thigh and leg patterns were fully analysed by Setty (1968). Similar studies in other races would be helpful; the findings of Shah (1957) in women in the Bombay area of India suggest possible racial differences in the sensitivity of thigh follicles to androgen.

References

Andreev, V.C. & Stransky, L. (1979) Hairy elbows. *Archives of Dermatology*, **115**, 761.
Beek, C.H. (1950) A study on extension and distribution of the human body-hair *Dermatologica*, **101**, 317.
Beighton, P. (1970) Familial hypertrichosis cubiti: hairy elbows syndrome. *Journal of Medical Studies*, **7**, 158.
Danforth, C.H. & Trotter, M. (1922) The distribution of body hair in white subjects. *American Journal of Physical Anthropology*, **5**, 259.
Dronamraju, K.R. (1963) A note on the age of onset of hypertrichosis pinnae auris in Orissa, West Bengal and Ceylon. *Journal of Geriatrics*, **58**, 324.
Dronamraju, K.R. & Haldane, J.B.S. (1962) Inheritance of hairy pinnae. *American Journal of Human Genetics*, **14**, 102.
Dupertuis, C.W., Atkinson, W.B. & Elftman, H. (1945) Sex differences in pubic hair distribution. *Human Biology*, **17**, 137.
Eklund, J., Hjelt, L. & Lumme, T. (1960) Hirsutism in the children of diabetic mothers. *Annales Paediatricae Fenniae*, **6**, 232.
Gates, R.R. & Vella, F. (1962) Hairy pinnae in Malta. *Lancet*, **ii**, 357.
Gompertz, M.L. (1960) A note on the incidence of pectoral alopecia *American Journal of Digestive Disorders*, **5**, 437.
Hamilton, J.B. (1947) A secondary sexual character that develops in an organ common to both sexes but normally only in men. With a discussion of the relation of this character to endocrine stimulation. *Journal of Clinical Endocrinology*, **7**, 465.
Hamilton, J.B. & Terada, H. (1963) Interdependence of genetic ageing and endocrine factors in hirsutism. In *The Hirsute Female*. p. 20, ed. R.B. Greenblatt. Thomas, Springfield.
Hamilton, J.B., Terada, H., Mestler, G.E. & Tinman, W. (1969) I. Coarse sternal hairs; a male secondary sexual character that can be measured quantitatively: the influence of sex, age and genetic factors. II. Other sex-differing characters: relationship to age, to one another and to values for coarse sternal hairs. In *Hair Growth*. p. 129, eds. W. Montagna & R.L. Dobson. Pergamon Press, Oxford.
Ikoma, E. (1972) An anthropological study on digital hair. *Journal of the Anthropological Society (Nippon)*, **80**, 283.

Ikoma, E. (1973) A genetic study of human hair. *Japanese Journal of Human Genetics*, **18**, 259.

Kamalam, A. & Thambiah, A.S. (1990) Genetics of hairy ears in south Indians. *Clinical and Experimental Dermatology*, **15**, 192.

McGregor, D. (1961) Distribution of pubic hair in a sample of fit men. *British Journal of Dermatology*, **73**, 61.

Pryor, H.B. (1956) Certain physical and physiological aspects of adolescent development in girls. *Journal of Pediatrics*, **8**, 52.

Reynolds, E.L. & Wines, J.V. (1948) Individual differences in physical changes associated with adolescence in girls. *American Journal of Diseases of Children*, **75**, 329.

Ronchese, F. & Chace, R.R. (1939) Patterned alopecia about the calves and its apparent lack of significance. *Archives of Dermatology and Syphilology*, **40**, 416.

Sarkar, S.S. & Ghosh, R.R. (1963) Hairy pinnae in the Bengalee female. *Lancet*, i, 1432.

Sarkar, S.S., Banerjee, A.R., Bhattacharjee, P. & Stern, C. (1961) A contribution to the genetics of hypertrichosis of the ear rims. *American Journal of Human Genetics*, **13**, 214.

Setty, L.R. (1961a) The distribution of chest hair in Caucasoid males. *American Journal of Physical Anthropology*, **19**, 285.

Setty, L.R. (1961b) Bare areas in regions of pilosity of the chest and abdomen. *Journal of the National Medical Association*, **53**, 394.

Setty, L.R. (1962) Hair patterns on the back of white males. *American Journal of Physical Anthropology*, **20**, 365.

Setty, L.R. (1964) The distribution of hair of the upper limb in Caucasoid males. *American Journal of Physical Anthropology*, **22**, 143.

Setty, L.R. (1968) The distribution of hair of the lower limb in white and Negro males. *American Journal of Physical Anthropology*, **29**, 51.

Setty, L.R. (1969) Hair patterns of the pinnae of white and Negro males. *American Journal of Physical Anthropology*, **31**, 153.

Setty, L.R. (1969) Penile hair patterns of whites and Negroes. *Journal of the National Medical Association*, **61**, 67.

Setty, L.R. (1970) Scrotal hair patterns of whites and Negroes. *Journal of the National Medical Association*, **62**, 156.

Shah, P.N. (1957) Human body hair—a quantitative study. *American Journal of Obstetrics and Gynecology*, **73**, 1255.

Slatis, H.M. & Apelbaum, A. (1963) Hairy pinna of the ear in Israeli populations. *American Journal of Human Genetics*, **15**, 74.

Sommer, K. (1971) Untersuchungen zur Genetik des Merkmals 'Fingerbehaarung'. *Humangenetik*, **11**, 155.

Stern, C., Centerwell, W.R. & Sarkar, S.S. (1964) New data on the problem of γ-linkage of hairy pinnae. *American Journal of Human Genetics*, **16**, 455.

Tanner, J.M. (1964) The adolescent growth spurt and development age. In *Human Biology*, p. 325, eds. G.A. Harrison, J.S. Wiseman, J.M. Tanner & N.A. Barnicot. Clarendon Press, Oxford.

Thomas, P.K. & Ferriman, D.G. (1957) Variation in familial pubic hair growth in white women. *American Journal of Physical Anthropology*, **15**, 171.

Wallis, H.M. (1897) On the growth of hair upon the human ear and its testimony to the shape, size and position of the ancestral organ. *Proceedings of the Zoological Society of London*, **11**, 298.

Hirsuties

History (References p. 78)

The first historical descriptions of female virilism are ascribed to Hippocrates (Medvei 1982). His writings contain descriptions of two women who became generally hairy with beards and whose bodies 'assumed a masculine appearance'.

They both became amenorrhoeic and died soon afterwards. Amboise Pare (1510–1590) described women who 'degenerate into a male type and are called masculine women . . . because they are robust, aggressive and arrogant, and have a man's voice and become hairy and develop beards'. He attributed these features to the retention of menstrual blood flow.

Henry Sampson described a girl in 1698 who was a sickly infant but recovered at 3 years to become hale, hearty and strong, and grew axillary and pubic hair and a beard. She died quite suddenly at 6 years. The autopsy revealed an enlarged kidney and large smooth 'testes' (Medvei 1982). Three separate accounts of a similar story in the late 19th century describe a 3-year-old whose skin was 'covered with a remarkable growth of black hair' and who had thick bushy eyebrows, a moustache and enlarged genitals. Pathological specimens were re-examined in 1898 and described as a cortical carcinoma (Medvei 1982).

The prognosis for bearded women is not always so grave. A report in the *Lancet* (Chowne 1852) describes a Swiss woman who, when 5 months pregnant, presented for certification of her gender in order to satisfy the 'scruples in the mind of persons who would . . . perform the marriage ceremony'. In due course, she gave birth to a healthy fair baby.

This early medical literature has been complemented by the works of early medical artists. The most famous paintings are 'The Woman with Two Beards' painted by Willem Keys (1520–1550), which has unfortunately been stolen from the museum in Aachen, and 'La Mujer Barbuda' commissioned by the Duke of Alcala and painted, albeit reluctantly, in 1631 by José de Ribera (1591–1652). The latter work records a 52-year-old women who, despite being bald and bearded, succeeded in suckling her own child. A different story is told by the statue of the bearded St Wilgefort who stands in Westminster Abbey; she is alleged to have grown a beard to repel an unwanted suitor (Cooper 1971).

Despite these elegant and graphic descriptions, the first scientific descriptions of the underlying diseases have been made quite recently. De Crecchio described adrenal hyperplasia in 1865 and Bullock and Sequiera (1905) associated it with hirsutism. Polycystic ovaries were described by Stein and Leventhal in 1935.

References

Bullock, W. & Sequiera, J.H. (1905) The relation of the suprarenal capsules to the sexual organs. *Transactions of the Pathological Society of London*, **56**, 189.
Chowne, W.D. (1852) Remarkable case of hirsute growth in a female. *Lancet*, **i**, 421 & 514; **ii**, 51.
Cooper, W. (1971) *Hair: Sex, Society, Symbolism*. Aldus Books, London.
Medvei, V.C. (1982) *A History of Endocrinology*, p. 237. MTP Press, Lancaster.
Stein, I.F. & Leventhal, M.C. (1935) Amenorrhoea associated with bilateral polycystic ovaries. *American Journal of Obstetrics and Gynecology*, **29**, 181.

Hirsuties (References p. 83)

Definition

Hirsuties may be defined as the growth of terminal hair on the body of a woman in the same pattern and sequence as that which develops in the normal post-pubertal male.

There is an orderly pattern in the appearance of terminal body hair in males after puberty. The first site affected is the upper lip which is followed by the chin and cheeks and then, the lower legs, thighs, forearms, abdomen, buttocks, chest, back, upper arms and shoulders (Reynolds, 1951). There is, however, a considerable variation in the degree of body hair that an individual man may grow. It is best to consider that the quantity of body hair possessed by an individual male lies on a spectrum which is determined by individual variation and race. Mongolian males, for example, have little or no facial and body hair, whereas Mediterranean males are covered with an exuberant pelage.

A similar situation exists in females. The identical pattern of hair growth may be seen in women as in men; however, the female growth is quantitatively inferior (Beek 1950). It is, therefore, spurious to suggest that there are female and male patterns of hair growth—there are simply different degrees on a single scale.

The main problem lies in the separation of hirsuties from normality. The development of body hair growth in the female should not be considered a disease process *per se*; it is a spectrum of biological variation of which the hairy extreme is frequently, but not always, associated with a recognized endocrinopathy which produces a state of hyperandrogenism, for example, polycystic ovarian disease. The exact point at which an individual woman is to be considered hirsute is blurred.

Perception of hirsuties is by definition subjective and women present with a wide variation in severity. Both the severity of the hirsuties and the degree of acceptance are dependent on racial, cultural and social factors. Even the criteria for the definition of hirsuties used by physicians vary widely (Shah 1957; Ferriman & Gallwey 1961; McKnight 1964; Lunde & Grottum 1984). Should a woman be considered hirsute if she, or her physician, feels that she is too hairy?

In order to solve this issue different groups have evolved different grading schemes for hair growth. The study by Ferriman & Gallwey (1961), which has become the standard grading system, has defined hirsuties purely on quantitative grounds. The consequence of the use of total hair scores to define hirsuties means that the definition of hirsuties lies only with the observing physician's assessment.

Other physicians have examined women complaining of hirsuties and compared them with controls. Their studies are not strictly comparable due to variations in subjective assessments; however, they have demonstrated that there is a considerable overlap in the grades of hirsuties between those women who consider themselves to be hirsute and control women, and that this overlap area may contain as many as 16% of each group (Lunde & Grottum 1984). This overlap has occurred irrespective of whether the women themselves have initiated the assessment or whether they have been referred by a physician (Shah 1957; Lunde & Grottum 1984). Hair on the face, chest or upper back is a good discriminating factor between hirsute women and controls with similar hair growth scores. Involvement of these sites is more likely to ensure early presentation for therapy than hair growth on more covered sites such as the limbs and buttocks.

Hirsuties or hypertrichosis?
The difference between hirsuties and hypertrichosis is not entirely semantic. Hirsuties is defined as androgen-dependent hair and is characterized by a specific pattern of hair growth, as described above, in which the individual hair shafts are coarse and curly. Generalized hypertrichosis differs in that the density of hair growth is uniform over the hairless body and the hair shafts tend to be fine and uniform (see Fig. 4.3). The importance of differentiation is that hirsuties is due to androgenic stimulation whereas hypertrichosis is due to other underlying factors which are usually unidentified (see Chapter 8).

Prevalence and racial factors
Hair is second only to the skin as a feature of racial difference. Facial and body hair is less commonly seen on the Mongolian (Hamilton 1958), Negroid and American Indian races than on the Caucasians (Fig. 4.3). Even amongst Caucasians there are differences; hair growth is heavier on those of Mediterranean than Nordic ancestry

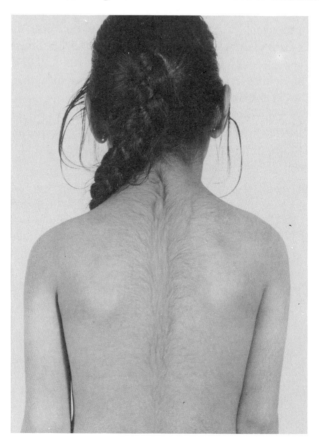

Fig. 4.3 Racial hypertrichosis. A normal Iranian girl aged 8.

(Greenblatt 1983). Indeed, 'the noble features'of Provençal women were described by the travel writer Max Nordau (1849–1923) as 'cruelly distorted by an entirely virile hair growth . . . which needs the razor'.

The pattern of hair growth in hirsuties within different racial groups is identical (Shah 1957; Ferriman & Gallwey 1961; McKnight 1964; Lunde & Grottum 1984); however, different criteria have made the determination of the comparative incidence and severity within these groups difficult to assess. Only one study of a random population states how many women considered themselves to be hirsute. McKnight (1964) examined 400 unselected students, 60% of whom were Welsh; 9% were considered by both the women and investigator to be hirsute and 4% were considered to be disfigured by their facial hair growth.

The patterns of hair growth for normal women have been compared with those complaining of hirsuties in India (Shah 1957) and in Norway (Lunde & Grottum 1984). Both studies have stressed the importance of hair on the lip, chin, chest and upper back as sites which differentiate between those women who consider themselves to be hirsute from those who do not.

These investigators have also studied hair growth in women who were not complaining of hirsuties and the patterns are tabulated in Table 4.1. These studies have been rigorously performed and confirm ethnic variations in density of hair growth. It is important to the definition of hirsuties that a sizeable proportion of normal women have some terminal hairs on their faces, breasts or lower abdomen (Fig. 4.4).

Table 4.1 Presence (%) of terminal hair at different body sites in women

Site	Country and age range surveyed				
	England[1] (15–44)	India[2] (15–48)	Norway[3] (16–44)	Wales[4] (?18)	USA[5] (18–24)
Lip	41	0	8	26	—
Chin	10	0	4	—	—
Upper arm	18	3	55	—	—
Lower arm	78	50	88	—	—
Chest	16	0	54	17	
Upper abdomen	0	} 3	4	—	} 35
Lower abdomen	25		29	35	
Upper back	0	0	6	3	
Lower back	13	5	24	16	
Thigh	34	30	46	—	—
Leg	94	66	96	—	—

Hair growth is defined as the presence of terminal hairs greater than 0.5 mm in length. Number of women in each group: England 257, India 100, Norway 100, Wales 400, USA 350. [1]Ferriman & Gallwey (1961); [2]Shah (1957); [3]Lunde & Grottum (1984); [4]McKnight (1964); [5]Danforth & Trotter (1922).

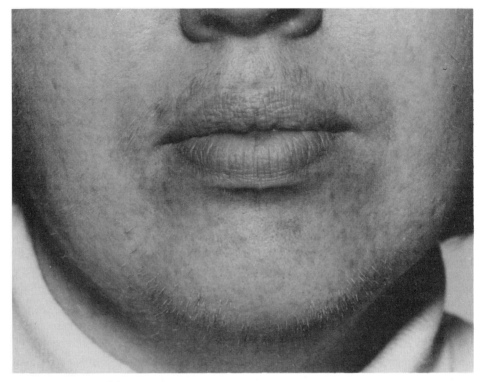

Fig. 4.4 Hirsutism of the upper lip and chin in a woman aged 35. She also has acne.

Familial factors

There have been few accounts of the familial relationship in hirsuties. Lorenzo (1970) studied 90 hirsute women and found an increased incidence of hirsutism in their female relatives compared with control populations. McKnight (1964) reported that 14% of hirsute Welsh women gave a positive family history. This tendency to familial clustering in hirsutism might have been anticipated as some of the underlying disorders which result in hyperandrogenism may have a familial basis; for example, congenital adrenal hyperplasia is linked to the major histocompatibility complex (Gordon *et al.* 1985) and a very strong family relationship has been reported in the polycystic ovary syndrome (Hague *et al.* 1988).

Social factors

The role of society in hirsuties is to determine the threshold level for normality and this is now determined by the media. Women receive a barrage of advertisements for cosmetics which are based on the premise that only a woman with a hairless body can be both normal and healthy. A woman who comes to this society and who might previously have accepted her 'hairy body' will be persuaded that she is unacceptable in her new culture until she becomes devoid of hair.

Psychological factors

Hirsute women are generally considered to be subject to social and psychological pressures due to their excess hair (Editorial 1975), or why would they seek medical help?

There have, however, been few studies on the psychological status of hirsute women. Meyer and Zerssen (1960) concluded on the basis of a small sample of patients studied within a psychoanalytic framework that many patients suffered reactive psychic disturbances. These were mostly neurotic disorders but included sexual difficulties and avoidance of sexual contact. A small controlled study by Rabinowitz *et al.* (1983) revealed increased levels of anxiety but no relationship between the degree of hirsuties and the level of anxiety was found. In contrast, Callan *et al.* (1980), using a more rigorous methodology to assess psychological profiles, were unable to detect significant differences in comparison with normative data.

Another approach to the psychological aspect of hirsuties has been to implicate 'stress' as an aetiological factor for, rather than as a result of, hirsuties. Segre states, in his monograph on the *Hirsute Female* (Segre 1967), that: 'Lack of peace of mind appears at the core of the problem. We believe it to be both a cause and result of hirsutism.' This view has been endorsed (Rook 1980) but has little substantiation in the literature other than in anecdotal reports. The onset of hirsutism in 4 of 10 hirsute women was noted to coincide with a period of emotional stress (Merivale 1951). Bush and Mahesh (1959) reported stress-induced hirsutism in a young woman whose unstressed twin was not hirsute.

References

Beek, C.H. (1950) A study on extension and distribution of the human body-hair. *Dermatologica*, **101**, 317.

Bush, I.E. & Mahesh, V.B. (1959) Adrenocortical hyperfunction with sudden onset of hirsutism. *Journal of Endocrinology*, **18**, 1.

Callan, A., Dennerstein, L., Burrows, G.D. & Hyman, G.J. (1980) The psychoendocrinology of hirsutism. In *Obstetrics, Gynaecology and Psychiatry 1980*, p. 43, eds. L. Dennerstein & G.D. Burrows. University of Melbourne, Melbourne.

Danforth, C.H. & Trotter, M. (1922) The distribution of body hair in white subjects. *American Journal of Physical Anthropology*, **5**, 259.

Editorial. (1975) Endocrine treatment in hirsutism. *British Medical Journal*, **ii**, 461.

Ferriman, D. & Gallwey, J.D. (1961) Clinical assessment of body hair growth in women. *Journal of Clinical Endocrinology*, **21**, 1440.

Gordon, M.T., Conway, D.I., Anderson, D.C. & Harris, R. (1985) Genetics and biochemical variability of variants of 21 hydroxylase deficiency. *Journal of Medical Genetics*, **22**, 354.

Greenblatt, R.B. (1983) Hirsutism—ancestral curse or endocrinopathy. In *Hirsutism and Virilism*, p. 1, eds. V.B. Mahesh & R.B. Greenblatt. John Wright PSG, Boston.

Hague, W.M., Adams, J., Reeders, S.T., Peto, T.E.A. & Jacobs, H.S. (1988) Familial polycystic ovaries: a genetic disease? *Clinical Endocrinology*, **29**, 593.

Hamilton, J.B. (1958) Age, sex and genetic factors in the regulation of hair growth in men: a comparison of Caucasian and Japanese populations. In *The Biology of Hair Growth*, p. 399, eds. W. Montagna & R.A. Ellis. Academic Press, New York.

Lorenzo, E.M. (1970) Familial study of hirsutism. *Journal of Clinical Endocrinology and Metabolism*, **31**, 556.

Lunde, O. & Grottum, P. (1984) Body hair growth in women: normal or hirsute. *American Journal of Physical Anthropology*, **64**, 307.

McKnight, E. (1964) The prevalence of 'hirsutism' in young women. *Lancet*, **i**, 410.

Merivale. W.H. (1951) The excretion of pregnanediol and 17-ketosteroids during the menstrual cycle in benign hirsutism. *Journal of Clinical Pathology*, **4**, 78.

Meyer, A.E. & Zerssen, D.V. (1960) Frauen mit sogenanntem idiopathischem Hirsutismus. *Journal of Psychosomatic Research*, **4**, 206.

Nordau, M. quoted by Medvei, V.C. (1982) *A History of Endocrinology*, p. 243. MTP Press, Lancaster.

Rabinowitz, S., Cohen, R. & Le Roith, D. (1983) Anxiety and hirsutism. *Psychology Reports*, **53**, 827.

Reynolds, E.L. (1951) The appearance of adult patterns of body hair in man. *Annals of the New York Academy of Sciences*, **53**, 576.

Rook, A.J. (1980) Aspects of cutaneous androgen-dependent syndromes. *International Journal of Dermatology*, **19**, 357.

Segre, E.J. (1967) *Androgens, Virilization and the Hirsute Female*, p. 92. Thomas, Springfield.

Shah, P.N. (1957) Human body hair—a quantitative study. *American Journal of Obstetrics and Gynecology*, **73**, 1255.

Pilosebaceous physiology in relation to hirsuties (References p. 86)

There are three types of hair. *Lanugo* hair is the form which only occurs *in utero* and may be seen on preterm babies born before 36 weeks gestation. There are two forms of postnatal hair: vellus and terminal. *Vellus* hair is fine, short and poorly pigmented; it grows all over the body except on the palms, soles, parts of the genitalia and peri-ungual tissue. *Terminal* hair is thicker, longer, has a central medulla and is often strongly pigmented; it is seen after birth on the scalp, eyebrows and eyelashes.

At puberty the production of androgens in both sexes stimulates the conversion of vellus to terminal hair in the axillary and pubic regions. In the male, terminal hair growth further develops in an orderly sequence on the upper lip, chin and cheeks, lower legs, thighs, forearms, abdomen, buttocks, chest, back, upper arms and shoulders (Reynolds 1951). The full development of hair growth does not occur in all men. There is a complete range of body hair growth in men and there are as many men with only a sparse beard and no body hair as there are with a complete pelage. There has been no study of hair growth through puberty to adulthood in women who become hirsute; it is assumed that the sequence is identical.

Terminal hair growth on the lower arms and legs occurs in both sexes (Shah 1957; McKnight 1964) and is conventionally considered to be unrelated to sex hormones (Ferriman & Gallwey 1961; Rook 1965); however, there are reasons to question this belief. Firstly, men have hairier arms and legs than women. Similarly, hirsute women have hairier arms and legs than non-hirsute women (Shah 1957; McKnight 1964; Lunde & Grottum 1984). Indeed, only 40% of women not complaining of hirsuties have no terminal hair on their arms and legs (Pedersen 1943). Secondly, treatment of hirsute women with the anti-androgen spironolactone results in a reduction in hair growth on the forearm (Barth *et al.* 1989).

Hair follicles can alter their morphology into different sizes and hair types. Vellus hairs can transform into terminal hairs and vice versa (Montagna & Parakkal 1974). This is the mode of terminal hair formation at secondary sexual sites on the body after puberty, and the reverse process on the scalp for vertical balding (Uno *et al.* 1985). The process of transformation between hair types is unknown but the process is believed to be mediated by androgens.

The relationship between androgens and hair growth

The first systematic correlation of hair growth and androgens was made as recently as 1942 by the American anatomist, James Hamilton (Hamilton 1942). He observed that men castrated before or during puberty did not become bald, that eunuchs treated with testosterone became bald and that the progression of this process ceased when therapy was withheld. These observations have been crucial in our understanding as there is no clear relationship in men between serum androgens and the process of balding (Burton *et al.* 1979).

Early studies on body hair growth in men similarly found no relationship with serum androgens (Ewing & Rouse 1978) but any relationship may have been obscured by the relative insensitivity of clinical grading scales. The exact relationship between androgens and hair growth has been clarified by the elucidation of the two main forms of androgen insensitivity: 5α-reductase deficiency and androgen receptor defects (Griffin & Wilson 1980).

Males born with androgen receptor deficiency (complete testicular feminization) express no peripheral androgen effects and appear as phenotypic women with abdominal testes but do not develop axillary, pubic or body hair at puberty (Kuttenn *et al.* 1979). However, in 5α-reductase deficiency which is characterized by an inability to convert testosterone to dihydrotestosterone (DHT), there is systemic virilization of genotypic males at puberty; they grow axillary and pubic hair but little or no hair at other body sites (Fisher *et al.* 1978). The role of DHT has been further highlighted by a study which reported that linear growth of facial hair in men was related to serum DHT whereas hair density was related to testosterone (Farthing *et al.* 1982). This might suggest that although testosterone is necessary for expression of terminal hair, DHT is required for regulation of its growth.

There have been several attempts to correlate hair growth in women with plasma androgen levels but these reports have yielded conflicting results. Reingold & Rosenfield (1987) noted a considerable variability between hair growth scores and free testosterone but no significant relationship. Ruutiainen *et al.* (1985) have calculated a complex formula for multiple plasma androgen levels (testosterone/ sex hormone-binding globulin + androstenedione/100 + dehydroepiandrosterone sulphate/100); this correlates with hair growth only in women with idiopathic hirsuties. In a further study, the same group, Ruutiainen *et al.* (1987) found a relationship between hair growth and salivary testosterone levels, but in this study no selection of patients was required. A different ratio has been determined for female baldness (De Villez & Dunn 1986) (3-α androstanediol glucuronide/sex hormone-binding globulin). These relationships are clearly unsatisfactory because they cannot explain the differential response to androgens by hair follicles at different sites on the body. The development of hair follicle and dermal papilla models *in vitro* may help to answer these questions.

References

Barth, J.H., Cherry, C.A., Wojnarowska, F. & Dawber, R.P.R. (1989) Spironolactone is an effective and well tolerated systemic anti-androgen therapy for hirsute women. *Journal of Clinical Endocrinology and Metabolism*, **68**, 966.

Burton, J.L., Ben Halim, M.M., Meyrick, G., Jeans, W.D. & Murphy, D. (1979) Male pattern alopecia and masculinity. *British Journal of Dermatology*, **100**, 567.

De Villez, R.L. & Dunn, J. (1986) Female androgenic alopecia: the 3-alpha,17-beta-androstanediol glucuronide/sex hormone binding globulin ratio as a possible marker for female pattern baldness. *Archives of Dermatology*, **122**, 1011.

Ewing, J.A. & Rouse, B.A. (1978) Hirsutism, race and testosterone levels: comparison of east asians and euroamericans. *Human Biology*, **50**, 209.

Farthing, M.J.G., Mattei, A.M., Edwards, C.R.W. & Dawson, A.M. (1982) Relationship between plasma testosterone and dihydrotestosterone concentrations and male facial hair growth. *British Journal of Dermatology*, **107**, 559.

Ferriman, D. & Gallwey, J.D. (1961) Clinical assessment of body hair growth in women. *Journal of Clinical Endocrinology*, **21**, 1440.

Fisher, L.K., Kogut, M.D., Moore, R.J., Goebelsmann, U., Weitzman, J.J., Isaacs, H.Jr., Griffin, J.E. & Wilson, J.D. (1978) Clinical, endocrinological, and enzymatic characterisation of two patients with 5-alpha-reductase deficiency: evidence that a single enzyme is responsible for the 5-alpha-reduction of cortisol and testosterone. *Journal of Clinical Endocrinology and Metabolism*, **37**, 653.

Griffin, J.E. & Wilson, J.D. (1980) The syndromes of androgen resistance. *New England Journal of Medicine*, **302**, 198.

Hamilton, J.B. (1942) Male hormone stimulation is prerequisite and an incitant in common baldness. *American Journal of Anatomy*, **71**, 451.

Kuttenn, F., Mowszowicz, I., Wright, F., Baudot, N., Jaffiol, C., Robin, M. & Mauvais-Jarvis, P. (1979) Male pseudohermaphroditism: a comparative study of one patient with 5-alpha-reductase deficiency and three patients with the complete form of testicular feminisation. *Journal of Clinical Endocrinology and Metabolism*, **49**, 861.

Lunde, O. & Grottum, P. (1984) Body hair growth in women: normal or hirsute. *American Journal of Physical Anthropology*, **64**, 307.

McKnight, E. (1964) The prevalence of 'hirsutism' in young women. *Lancet*, **i**, 1410.

Montagna, W. & Parakkal, P.F. (1974) *The Structure and Function of Skin*, 3rd edn, p. 172. Academic Press, New York.

Pedersen, J. (1943) Hypertrichosis in women. *Acta Dermato-Venereologica*, **23**, 1.

Reingold, S.B. & Rosenfield, R.L. (1987) The relationship of mild hirsutism or acne in women to androgens. *Archives of Dermatology*, **123**, 209.

Reynolds, E.L. (1951) The appearance of adult patterns of body hair in man. *Annals of the New York Academy of Science*, **53**, 576.

Rook, A. (1965) Endocrine influences on hair growth. *British Medical Journal*, **i**, 609.

Ruutiainen, K., Erkkola, R., Kaihola, H-L., Santti, R. & Irjala, K. (1985) The grade of hirsutism correlated to serum androgen levels and hormonal indices. *Acta Obstetricia et Gynecologica Scandinavica*, **64**, 629.

Ruutiainen, K., Sannika, E., Santti, R., Erkkola, R. & Adlercreutz, H. (1987) Salivary testosterone in hirsutism: correlations with serum testosterone and the degree of hair growth. *Journal of Clinical Endocrinology and Metabolism*, **64**, 1015.

Shah, P.N. (1957) Human body hair—a quantitative study. *American Journal of Obstetrics and Gynecology,* **73**, 1255.

Uno, H., Cappas, A. & Schlagel, C. (1985) Cyclic dynamics of hair follicles and the effect of minoxidil on the bald scalps of stumptailed macaques. *American Journal of Dermatopathology,* **7**, 283.

Androgen physiology in normal women (References p. 91)

The physiological mechanism for androgenic activity may be considered in three stages: (i) production of androgens by the adrenals and ovaries; (ii) their transport in the blood on carrier proteins [principally sex hormone-binding globulin (SHBG)]; and (iii) their intra-cellular modification and binding to the androgen receptor.

Adrenal and ovarian androgen production

The first sign of androgen production in women occurs 2–3 years before the menarche, is due to adrenal secretion and is known as the adrenarche (Reiter *et al.* 1977; Sklar *et al.* 1980). The signal for this development is unknown, but Rosenfield *et al.* (1971) have postulated that stimulation of the adrenals by adrenocorticotrophic hormone (ACTH) may result in increased dehydroepiandrosterone (DHA) production as a result of either of two mechanisms. There may be increased activity of C_{17-20}-lyase which redirects glucocorticoid precursors towards the androgen pathway or there may be a reduced forward metabolism of DHA as a result of reduced activity of Δ^5-3β-hydroxysteroid dehydrogenase: this process represents a maturation of the adrenal zona reticularis. The major androgens secreted by the adrenals are androstenedione, DHA and DHA sulphate (DHAS). Their control during post-pubertal life is unknown but it is thought that androstenedione and DHA may be controlled by ACTH as their serum levels mirror those of cortisol (Rosenfield *et al.* 1975; James *et al.* 1978). It is difficult to ascertain the control mechanism for DHAS as it has a prolonged plasma half-life of 10–20 hours (Rosenfeld *et al.* 1975).

Ovarian androgen production begins under the influence of the pubertal secretion of luteinizing hormone (LH) and takes place in the theca cells. Androstenedione is the predominant androgen secreted by the ovaries during the reproductive years, and testosterone after the menopause. Androgen secretion continues throughout the cycle but peaks at the middle of an ovulatory cycle (Vermeulen & Verdonck 1976). Androstenedione secretion is greater from the ovary containing the dominant follicle (Baird *et al.* 1974).

In normal women the majority of testosterone production (50–70%) is derived from peripheral conversion of androstenedione in skin and other extra-splanchnic sites (Horton & Tait 1966; Kirschner & Bardin 1972). The remaining proportion is secreted directly by the adrenals and ovaries. The relative proportion estimated from each gland varies between reported studies from 5 to 20% from the ovary and 0 to 30% from the adrenal (Kirschner & Bardin 1972; Moltz *et al.* 1984). DHA is the source of less than 10% of circulating androstenedione and 1% of circulating testosterone (Horton & Tait 1967; Kirschner *et al.* 1973).

Androgen transport proteins

In non-pregnant women the majority of circulating androgens are bound to a high-affinity β-globulin, called sex hormone-binding globulin (SHBG). A further 20–25% is transported loosely bound to albumin and about 1% circulates freely. The free steroid is believed to be active and the binding protein is therefore of paramount importance. The affinity of the androgens for SHBG is proportional to their biological activity.

The function of SHBG is unknown. It is probable that its main role is to buffer acute changes in unbound androgen levels and to protect androgens from degradation. Burke and Anderson (1972) have suggested that it also acts as a biological amplifier. High oestrogen levels increase SHBG and therefore reduce available androgen; high androgen levels reduce SHBG and increase available free androgen.

Androgen metabolism in the skin

Androgen action in the skin depends first upon the conversion of relatively inactive 'pre-hormones' to more potent forms, and then their binding to nuclear receptor proteins. The existence of these mechanisms was first established in the prostate and subsequently there have been a series of studies delineating the ability of the skin to interconvert androgens *in vitro* (see review by Beazley *et al.* 1982). These findings are summarized in Fig. 4.5.

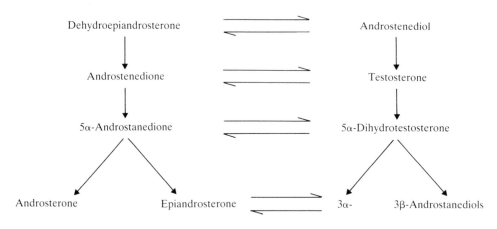

Fig. 4.5 Metabolic pathways for androgen hormones in human skin.

There are regional variations in cutaneous androgen metabolism; for example, whole skin biopsies from genital skin predominantly convert testosterone to DHT whereas abdominal and dorsal skin convert testosterone to androstenedione (Kim & Herrmann 1968; Flamigni *et al.* 1971). These variations reflect the sensitivity of genital tissue to androgenic stimulation. Variations between the face and axilla are probably due to the different activities within the epidermal appendages (Dijkstra *et al.* 1987); the face contains sebaceous glands and favours androstenedione production from testosterone whereas the axilla contains apocrine glands and favours DHT production (Hay & Hodgins 1973).

The importance of testosterone and DHT lies in their ability to bind to the androgen receptor (AR) and therefore to mediate the androgen effect. The AR can be detected both in the cytosol and the nucleus. The receptor binds to either testosterone or DHT in the cytosol and is translocated to the nucleus for the androgen message to take effect (see Fig. 4.6). DHT binds to the receptor more readily and securely than does testosterone (Wilson & French 1976) and may be more important in securing a cellular effect.

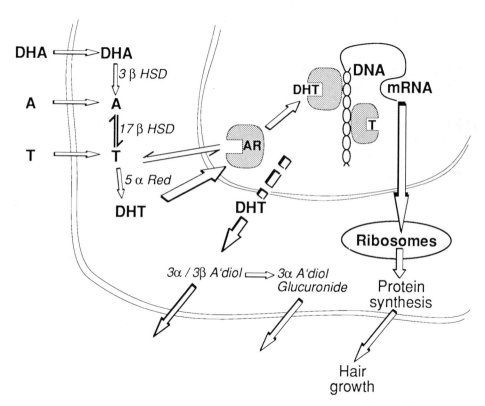

Fig. 4.6 Molecular mechanism of action of androgens on skin. DHA: dehydroepiandrosterone. A: androstenedione. T: testosterone. DHT: dihydrotestosterone. A'diol: androstanediol. AR: androgen receptor. 3β and 17β HSD: 3β- and 17β- hydroxysteroid dehydrogenase. 5α red: 5α- reductase.

Most investigations of the AR in skin have, for technical reasons, been performed on cultures of skin fibroblasts. Fibroblasts derived from genital skin contain more AR binding capacity than do cells from pubic skin and much more than cells from non-sexual sites (neck, abdomen and wrist) (Keenan *et al.* 1975). Interestingly, AR in pubic skin fibroblasts do not demonstrate any difference between men and women (Eil *et al.* 1985). Studies on whole skin have only examined the cytosolic AR (Mowszowicz *et al.* 1981). These results are difficult to interpret as AR is predominantly a nuclear protein, even in the relative absence of androgens (Husmann *et al.* 1990).

Androgen dependence of 5α-reductase. There appear to be two types of 5α-reductase involved in sexual differentiation. In genital skin 5α-reductase is androgen independent, whereas 5α-reductase in the terminal hair bearing pubic skin is regulated by androgens both *in vivo* (Mauvais-Jarvis *et al.* 1971; Wilson *et al.* 1988) and *in vitro* (Mowszowicz *et al.* 1983). This induction is dependent upon the presence of androgen receptors.

Androstanediol glucuronide. 3α- and 3β-Androstanediol are the reduction products of DHT and are subsequently conjugated to glucuronides. There has been considerable interest in this product as a marker of cutaneous androgen metabolism. Firstly, 3α-A'diol is synthesized extra-splanchnically (Morimoto *et al.* 1981). Secondly, it is only detectable at low levels in subjects with 5α-reductase deficiency (Horton 1984). Thirdly, it is synthesized by genital skin (Lobo *et al.* 1987) and fourthly, it correlates with the presence of body hair and acne (Lookingbill *et al.* 1988). However, its value as a marker of cutaneous androgen metabolism is now in question as its presence in serum is entirely dependent upon ovarian/adrenal androgen production (Rittmaster 1988) and 3α-A'diol correlates well with body mass independently of hirsutism (Scanlon *et al.* 1988).

Androgen metabolism in isolated hair follicles
Plucked hair follicles possess the same metabolic pathways that exist in whole skin (see Fig. 4.5). DHA is metabolized to androstenedione and androstanedione (Fazekas & Sandor 1973) and is hydroxylated to 7α-hydroxy-DHA (Vermorken *et al.* 1979). The interconversion of androstenedione and testosterone physiologically favours androstenedione formation (Sansone-Bazzono *et al.* 1972; Schweikert & Wilson 1974 a,b; Vermorken *et al.* 1979; Goos *et al.* 1982) except in homogenized follicles in the presence of NADPH (Takayasu & Adachi 1972). The predominant 5α-reduced product is therefore the relatively inactive androgen androstanedione (Sansone-Bazzono *et al.* 1972; Vermorken *et al.* 1979). Hair follicles also contain aromatase and can convert androstenedione to oestrone (Schweikert *et al.* 1975). The hair follicle would, therefore, appear to protect itself from androgenic stimulation by metabolizing androgens away from the effector pathway of testosterone and DHT.

The act of plucking damages the hair follicle as part of the germinative matrix and the dermal papillae are left in the skin. As the papilla is thought to exert a controlling influence over hair growth, cultured papilla cells have been been examined and found to contain AR and metabolizing enzymes (Murad *et al.* 1985; Messenger *et al.* 1988; Sawaya *et al.* 1988); these studies have not been performed in hirsuties.

References

Baird, D.T., Burger, P.E., Heavon-Jones, G.D. & Scaramuzzi, R.J. (1974) The site of secretion of androstenedione in non-pregnant women. *Journal of Endocrinology*, **63**, 201.

Beazley, J.M., Wade, A.P., Hipkin, L.J. & Davis, J.C. (1982) Skin metabolism of androgens and the control of hair growth. In *Androgens and Anti-androgen Therapy*, p. 41, ed. S.L. Jeffcoate. John Wiley, Chichester.

Burke, C.W. & Anderson, D.C. (1972) Sex-hormone-binding globulin is an oestrogen amplifier. *Nature*, **240**, 38.

Dijkstra, A.C., Goos, C.M.A.A., Cunliffe, W.J., Sultan, C. & Vermorken, A.J.M. (1987) Is increased 5α-reductase activity a primary phenomenon in androgen-dependent skin disorders? *Journal of Investigative Dermatology*, **89**, 87.

Eil, C., Cutler, G.B. Jr. & Loriaux, D.L. (1985) Androgen receptor characteristics in skin fibroblasts from hirsute women. *Journal of Investigative Dermatology*, **84**, 62.

Fazekas, A.G. & Sandor, T. (1973) The metabolism of dehydroepiandrosterone by human scalp hair follicles. *Journal of Clinical Endocrinology and Metabolism*, **36**, 582.

Flamigni, C., Collins, W.P., Koullapis, E.N., Craft, I., Dewhurst, C.J. & Sommerville, I.F. (1971) Androgen metabolism in human skin. *Journal of Clinical Endocrinology*, **32**, 737.

Goos, C.M.A.A., Wirtz, P., Vermorken, A.J.M. & Mauvais-Jarvis, P. (1982) Androgenic effect of testosterone and some of its metabolites in relation to their biotransformation in the skin. *British Journal of Dermatology*, **107**, 549.

Hay, J.B. & Hodgins, M.B. (1973) Metabolism of androgens *in vitro* by human facial and axillary skin. *Journal of Endocrinology*, **59**, 475.

Horton, R. (1984) Markers of peripheral androgen production. In *Sexual Differentiation: Basic and Clinical Aspects*, p. 261, eds. M. Serio, M. Motta, M. Zanisi & L. Martini. Raven Press, New York.

Horton, R. & Tait, J.F. (1966) Androstenedione production and interconversion rates measured in peripheral blood and studies on the possible site of its conversion to testosterone. *Journal of Clinical Investigation*, **45**, 301.

Horton, R. & Tait, J.F. (1967) *In vivo* conversion of dehydroisoandrosterone to plasma androstenedione and testosterone in man. *Journal of Clinical Endocrinology and Metabolism*, **27**, 79.

Husmann, D.A., Wilson, C.M., McPhaul, M.J., Tilley, W.D. & Wilson, J.D. (1990) Antipeptide antibodies to two distinct regions of the androgen receptor localise the receptor protein to the nuclei of target cells in the rat and human prostate. *Endocrinology*, **126**, 2359.

James, V.H.T., Tunbridge, D., Wilson, G.A., Hutton, J.D., Jacobs, H.S., Goodall, A.B., Murray, M.A.F. & Rippon, A.E. (1978) Central control of steroid hormone secretion. *Journal of Steroid Biochemistry*, **9**, 429.

Keenan, B.S., Meyer, W.J. III, Hadjian, A.J. & Migeon, C.J. (1975) Androgen receptor in human skin fibroblasts: characterisation of a specific 17β-hydroxy-5α-androstan-3-one protein complex in cell sonicates and nuclei. *Steroids*, **25**, 535.

Kim, M.H. & Herrmann, W.L. (1968) *In vitro* metabolism of dehydroepiandrosterone sulphate in foreskin, abdominal skin and vaginal mucosa. *Journal of Clinical Endocrinology and Metabolism*, **28**, 187.

Kirschner, M.A. & Bardin, C.W. (1972) Androgen production and metabolism in normal and virilised women. *Metabolism*, **21**, 667.

Kirschner, M.A., Sinhamahapatra, S., Zucker, I.R., Loriaux, L. & Nieschlag, E. (1973) The production, origin and role of dehydro-epiandrosterone and 5-androstenediol as androgen prehormones in hirsute women. *Journal of Clinical Endocrinology and Metabolism*, **37**, 183.

Lobo, R.A., Paul, W.L., Gentzschein, E., Serafini, P.C., Catalino, J.A., Paulson, R.J. & Horton, R. (1987) Production of 3α-androstanediol glucuronide in human genital skin. *Journal of Clinical Endocrinology and Metabolism*, **65**, 711.

Lookingbill, D.P., Egan, N., Santen, R.J. & Demers, L.M. (1988) Correlation of serum 3α-androstanediol glucuronide with acne and chest hair density in men. *Journal of Clinical Endocrinology and Metabolism*, **67**, 986.

Mauvais-Jarvis, P., Crepy, O. & Bercovici, J.P. (1971) Further studies on the pathophysiology of testicular feminisation syndrome. *Journal of Clinical Endocrinology and Metabolism*, **32**, 568.

Messenger, A.G., Thornton, M.J., Elliot, K. & Randall, V.A. (1988) Androgen responses in cultured human hair papilla cells (Abstract). *Journal of Investigative Dermatology*, **91**,382.

Moltz, L., Sorensen, R., Schwartz, U. & Hammerstein, J. (1984) Ovarian and adrenal vein steroids in healthy women with ovulatory cycles—selective catheterization findings. *Journal of Steroid Biochemistry*, **20**, 901.

Morimoto, I., Edmiston, A., Hawks, D. & Horton, R. (1981) Studies on the origin of androstanediol and androstanediol glucuronide in young and elderly men. *Journal of Clinical Endocrinology and Metabolism*, **52**, 772.

Mowszowicz, I., Riahi, M., Wright, F., Bouchard, P., Kuttenn, F. & Mauvais-Jarvis, P. (1981) Androgen receptor in human skin cytosol. *Journal of Clinical Endocrinology and Metabolism*, **52**, 338.

Mowszowicz, I., Melanitou, E., Kirchhoffer, M-O. & Mauvais-Jarvis, P. (1983) Dihydrotestosterone stimulates 5α-reductase activity in pubic skin fibroblasts. *Journal of Clinical Endocrinology and Metabolism*, **56**, 320.

Murad, S., Hodgins, M.B., Simpson, N.B., Oliver, R.F. & Jahoda, C. (1985) Androgen receptors and metabolism in cultured dermal papilla cells from human hair follicles (Abstract). *British Journal of Dermatology*, **113**, 768.

Reiter, E.O., Fuldauer, V.G. & Root, A.W. (1977) Secretion of the adrenal androgen dehydroepiandrosterone sulphate, during normal infancy, childhood, and adolescence, in sick infants, and children with endocrinological abnormalities. *Journal of Pediatrics*, **90**, 766.

Rich, B.H., Rosenfield, R.L., Lucky, A.W., Helke, J.C. & Otto, P. (1981) Adrenarche: changing adrenal response to adrenocorticotrophin. *Journal of Clinical Endocrinology and Metabolism*, **52**, 1129.

Rittmaster, R.S. (1988) Differential suppression of testosterone and estradiol in hirsute women with the superactive gonadotrophin-releasing hormone agonist leuprolide. *Journal of Clinical Endocrinology and Metabolism*, **67**, 651.

Rosenfeld, R.S., Rosenburg, B.J., Fukushima, D.K. & Hellman, L. (1975) 24-Hour secretory pattern of dehydroisoandrosterone and dehydroisoandrosterone sulphate. *Journal of Clinical Endocrinology and Metabolism*, **40**, 850.

Rosenfield, R.L. (1971) Plasma 17-ketosteroids and 17β-hydroxysteroids in girls with premature development of sexual hair. *Journal of Pediatrics*, **79**, 260.

Sansone-Bazzono, G., Reisner, R.M. & Bazzano, G. (1972) Conversion of testosterone-1,2- ³H to androstenedione-³H in the isolated hair follicle of man. *Journal of Clinical Endocrinology and Metabolism*, **34**, 521.

Sawaya, M.E., Mendez, A.J., Lewis, C.A. & Hsia, S.L. (1988) Two forms of androgen receptor protein in human hair follicles and sebaceous glands: variation in transitional and bald scalp (Abstract). *Journal of Investigative Dermatology*, **90**, 606.

Scanlon, M.J., Whorwood, C.B., Franks, S., Reed, M.J. & James, V.H.T. (1988) Serum androstanediol glucuronide concentrations in normal and hirsute women and patients with thyroid dysfunction. *Clinical Endocrinology*, **29**, 529.

Schweikert, H.U. & Wilson, J.D. (1974a) Regulation of human hair growth by steroid hormones. I. Testosterone metabolism in isolated hairs. *Journal of Clinical Endocrinology and Metabolism*, **38**, 811.

Schweikert, H.U. & Wilson, J.D. (1974b) Regulation of human hair growth by steroid hormones. II. Androstenedione metabolism in isolated hairs. *Journal of Clinical Endocrinology and Metabolism*, **39**, 1012.

Schweikert, H.U., Milewich, L. & Wilson, J.D. (1975) Aromatisation of androstenedione by isolated human hairs. *Journal of Clinical Endocrinology and Metabolism*, **40**, 413.

Sklar, C.A., Kaplan, S.L. & Grumbach, M.M. (1980) Evidence for dissociation between adrenarche and gonadarche: studies in patients with idiopathic precocious puberty, gonadal dysgenesis, isolated gonadotrophin deficiency, and constitutionally delayed growth and adolescence. *Journal of Clinical Endocrinology and Metabolism*, **51**, 548.

Takayasu, S. & Adachi, K. (1972) The conversion of testosterone to 17β-hydroxy-5α-androstan-3-one (dihydrotestosterone) by human hair follicles. *Journal of Clinical Endocrinology and Metabolism*, **34**, 1098.

Vermeulen, A. & Verdonck, L. (1976) Plasma androgen levels during the menstrual cycle. *American Journal of Obstetrics and Gynecology*, **125**, 491.

Vermorken, A.J.M., Goos, C.M.A.A., Henderson, P. Th. & Bloemendal, H. (1979) Hydroxylation of dehydroepiandrosterone in human scalp hair follicles. *British Journal of Dermatology*, **100**, 693.

Wilson, E.M. & French, F.S. (1976) Binding properties of androgen receptors: evidence for identical receptors in rat testis, epididymis, and prostate. *Journal of Biological Chemistry*, **211**, 5620.

Wilson, S.C., Oakey, R.E. & Scott, J.S. (1988) Evidence for secondary 5α-reductase deficiency in genital and supra-pubic skin of subjects with androgen insensitivity syndrome. *Acta Endocrinologica*, **117**, 353.

Androgen pathophysiology in hirsuties (References p. 98)

Hirsuties is a response of the hair follicles to androgenic stimulation and increased hair growth is therefore often seen in endocrine disorders characterized by hyperandrogenism. These disorders may be due to abnormalities of either the ovaries or adrenal glands. It is likely that the majority of hirsute women have underlying polycystic ovary syndrome (PCO). A small proportion of hirsute women have no detectable hormonal abnormality and are usually classified as 'idiopathic' hirsuties. This subgroup is gradually becoming smaller as diagnostic techniques become more refined, and is probably due to more subtle forms of ovarian or adrenal hypersecretion, alterations in serum androgen-binding proteins or in the cutaneous metabolism of androgens (see Table 4.2).

Table 4.2 Causes of hirsuties

Ovarian causes:	polycystic ovary syndrome, ovarian tumours
Adrenal causes:	congenital adrenal hyperplasia, Cushing's disease, prolactinoma
Gonadal dysgenesis	
Androgen therapy	
Idiopathic hirsuties	
?? Stress	

Although many hirsute women are obese the role of adipose tissue is undefined but it is clinically recognized, though undocumented, that weight loss by obese hirsute women with menstrual irregularities results in regulation of menses and a reduction in body hair growth.

Ovarian overproduction

Polycystic ovary syndrome (PCO). The perception of PCO has changed dramatically since it was first described by Stein & Leventhal (1935). They defined a syndrome consisting of obesity, amenorrhoea, hirsutism and infertility associated with bilaterally enlarged polycystic ovaries. This disorder has been a controversial diagnosis as it is defined by the appearance of organs that are difficult to visualize. This has led to the use of multiple diagnostic formulations based on clinical and biochemical abnormalities. A more fundamental issue relating to the nosology of the disorder has been raised by modern imaging techniques which have revealed the presence of polycystic ovaries in apparently normal women (Polson *et al.* 1988a).

Ideas concerning the pathogenesis of PCO have been as controversial as the diagnosis and different authorities embrace the belief that it is primarily due to either an ovarian abnormality (Jacobs 1987), inappropriate gonadotrophin secretion (Pehrson *et al.* 1986), a disorder of the adrenal glands (Yen 1980) or to increased peripheral aromatase activity resulting in hyperoestronaemia (McKenna 1988).

The relationship between PCO and the source of the increased serum androgen production is still quite unclear. Loughlin *et al.* (1986) have consistently found that the hyperandrogenism in PCO is adrenal in origin and they consider this to be the cause of PCO. Polson *et al.* (1988b) have found no evidence for increased adrenal androgen production as assessed by 11β- hydroxyandrostenedione, which they claim is predominantly an adrenal androgen. This debate is not even clarified by selective catheterization of the adrenal and ovarian veins (see p. 98).

The pattern of clinical features of patients with PCO will depend to an extent on the diagnostic definition of the disorder and upon the presenting symptom, be it dermatological, endocrine or gynaecological. Using ultrasound visualization of polycystic ovaries as the diagnostic criterion (Fig. 4.7), Conway *et al.* (1990) found the following clinical features in a series of 556 patients: hirsuties (61%), acne

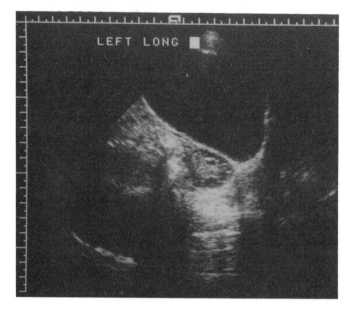

Fig. 4.7 High resolution ultrasound scan of the ovary demonstrating multiple peripherally located cysts (courtesy of T. Rae, St Mary's Hospital, London).

(24%), alopecia (8%), acanthosis nigricans (2%) (see p. 102), obesity (35%), menorrhagia (1%), oligomenorrhoea (45%), amenorrhoea (26%), and infertility (>29%). However, those patients who present to a dermatologist will almost invariably have acne and/or hirsuties.

Laboratory investigations in PCO usually reveal an elevated level of luteinizing hormone, often with an increased luteinizing:follicle-stimulating hormone ratio, and testosterone, androstenedione and oestradiol levels are often raised (Coney 1984). The demonstration by ultrasound examination of multiple peripheral ovarian cysts around a dense central core will depend on the expertise of the operator. Adams *et al.* (1986) report that they can detect these features in as many as 92% of hirsute women with normal menstrual cycles but this is not a universal experience.

Ovarian tumours. Hirsuties is a nearly universal feature in virilizing ovarian tumours; however, ovarian tumours are a rare cause of hirsuties, and functioning tumours which cause virilization represent approximately 1% of ovarian tumours (Woodruff & Parmley 1983). Amenorrhoea or oligomenorrhoea develop in all premenopausal patients and alopecia, cliteromegaly, deepening of the voice and a male habitus develop in about half of the patients (Sandberg & Jackson 1963; Moltz *et al.* 1984b). The features of virilization usually develop rapidly; however it is important to note that many cases present after years of hirsutism and menstrual disturbances (German *et al.* 1961). The majority of patients with virilizing ovarian tumours have raised plasma testosterone levels (Woodruff & Parmley 1983; Moltz *et al.* 1984b).

Hirsuties in pregnancy. Hirsuties has only rarely been reported to develop during pregnancy; it may be due to the development of PCO or a virilizing tumour. PCO has been reported to present with virilization during the first or third trimester and may regress post partum (Shortle *et al.* 1987; Magendantz *et al.* 1972; Fayez *et al.* 1974). Androgens freely cross the placenta and virilization of a female foetus may occur (Fayez *et al.* 1974). The range of tumours occurring during pregnancy has been reviewed by Novak *et al.* (1970). The features of virilization may regress after the surgical removal of the tumour (Novak *et al.* 1970).

Stoddard (1945) described two cases of apparent hirsutism during pregnancy. In both cases, the hair growth developed within the first 8 weeks of pregnancy and grew throughout pregnancy over the entire body, particularly affecting the forehead, cheeks and under the ears. The hair fell spontaneously at 8 weeks post partum in one case and in the other case was considerably reduced at this time. The published clinical photographs, however, demonstrate fine, silky hair and this, together with the history, suggests that the diagnosis may be an undescribed form of acquired hypertrichosis lanuginosa.

Trotter (1935) measured the rates of hair growth in pubic, perineal and lumbar hairs in 7 normal women during and after pregnancy and could detect no differences.

Adrenal overproduction

Congenital adrenal hyperplasia. Cholesterol is metabolized in the adrenal cortex via a complex pathway into aldosterone, cortisol, androgens and oestrogens. A defect in a pathway results in a reduction of the product of the pathway involved with a redistribution of the precursors to other pathways, which results in overproduction of the other hormones. Complete absence of a particular enzyme may be incompatible with life and severe reduction in enzyme activity is usually apparent at birth or early childhood due to dehydration with a salt-losing state and/or virilization.

Partial reduction in enzyme activity may present after childhood and during the past decade a small proportion of women presenting with post-pubertal hirsuties have been demonstrated to have subtle forms of 'late-onset' congenital adrenal hyperplasia (CAH). The diagnosis cannot be made clinically and dynamic endocrine investigations are required to differentiate between PCO and idiopathic hirsuties (Chrousos *et al.* 1982). Women with late-onset CAH may have normal menstrual cycles (Medina *et al.* 1986); however, approximately 80% will have polycystic ovaries (Hague *et al.* 1986).

21-Hydroxylase deficiency is the commonest defect associated with late-onset CAH. As many as 3–6% of women presenting with hirsuties may be affected with this form (Chetkowski *et al.* 1984; Kutten *et al.* 1985). This form is an allelic variant of the classic childhood salt-wasting type; the classic form is associated with HLA-Bw47 and the late-onset form with HLA-B14 (Gordon *et al.* 1985). Of women with this abnormality 75% will present with hirsutism with or without menstrual irregularities (Dewailly *et al.* 1986).

3β- and *11β- Hydroxylase* deficiencies are less common forms of CAH and are consequently less frequently found in hirsute women (Pang *et al.* 1985; Cathelineau. *et al.* 1980)

Acquired adrenocortical disease. Adrenal carcinomata usually present with abdominal swelling or pain; however, 10% of both adenomata and carcinomata may present with isolated virilization (Bennett *et al.* 1971; King & Lack 1979). The combination of virilization and Cushing's syndrome strongly suggests the presence of a carcinoma. The testosterone level is usually markedly raised in the latter.

Patients with Cushing's syndrome are said to have both hypertrichosis, a generalized diffuse growth of fine hair due to hypercortisolaemia, and androgen-induced coarse hair in the usual male pattern (Griffing & Melby 1983).

Gonadal dysgenesis

Moltz *et al.* (1981) described six patients with 46,XY gonadal dysgenesis. All had unambiguously female genitalia but male skeletal characteristics; wide span, broad shoulders and chest. Two were hirsute, two had temporal recession and three had deep voices. Rosen *et al.* (1988) reported a further 30 patients with gonadal dysgenesis of whom three (with Y chromosome material) presented with slowly progressive hirsuties and secondary amenorrhoea.

Hyperprolactinaemia

The exact relationship between prolactin and hirsuties is not clear. The incidence of hirsuties in the amenorrhoea–galactorrhoea syndrome has been reported to be 22–60% (Robyn & Tukumbane 1983). This may be due to a direct effect of prolactin on adrenal androgen production (Pepe & Albrecht 1985) or to PCO with which it is frequently associated (Lavric 1969). Prolactin has also been reported to attenuate cutaneous 5α-reductase activity both *in vivo* and *in vitro* (Serafini & Lobo 1986).

Idiopathic hirsuties

Idiopathic hirsuties is the diagnostic category given to those hirsute women in whom no underlying endocrine disorder can be detected. The frequency with which this diagnosis is made will therefore depend upon the curiosity of the physician and, in the case of PCO, the breadth of the diagnostic criteria.

There are a number of subtle dynamic alterations in the androgen metabolism of hirsute women compared with non-hirsute women. Firstly, daily testosterone production is increased by 3.5–5-fold (Bardin & Lipsett 1967). Secondly, the majority of androgen is secreted as testosterone (hirsute 75% vs. normal <40%) rather than as androstenedione (Bardin & Lipsett 1967; Kirshner & Bardin 1972; Kirschner *et al.* 1976). Thirdly, increased androgens in hirsute women are associated with lower levels of SHBG which binds less testosterone and increases its free level (Hauner *et al.* 1988). More free testosterone is, therefore, available for peripheral metabolism and clearance; these two factors disguise the increased rates of testosterone production (Rosenfield & Moll 1983). Free testosterone is a more sensitive measure of testosterone status (Cumming & Wall 1985) and is approximately threefold greater in hirsute than non-hirsute women (Rosenfield & Moll 1983).

Normal values for total testosterone are found in 25–60% of hirsute women and in 80% of those with regular menstrual cycles (Abraham *et al.* 1975; Mathur *et al.* 1981; Wild *et al.* 1983). This may be due to the effect of SHBG or to the wide fluctuations in plasma testosterone seen in hirsute women. Consequently, multiple measurements are often required to detect the increased levels (Rosenfield 1979). Some women will, however, not demonstrate elevations of testosterone despite exhaustive investigation. Paradoxically, in these women, the growth of hair by their skin is the only, and most sensitive, androgen bioassay.

The source of increased androgen production by hirsute women is often unclear. In order to clarify the source, investigators have selectively catheterized the ovarian and adrenal veins and measured the effluent androgen concentrations;

Table 4.3 Source of androgens (%) in hirsute women as determined by ovarian and adrenal vein catheterization

	Sample size	Ovarian	Adrenal	Combined	Other
Unselected patients					
Oake *et al.* (1974)	5	–	60	20	20
Northrop *et al.* (1975)	19	38	5	58	–
Kirschner *et al.* (1976)	44	95	5	–	–
Farber *et al.* (1978)	13	31	23	46	–
Moltz *et al.* (1984)	60	27	12	41	20
PCO patients					
Stahl *et al.* (1973)	20	–	40	45	15
Wajchenberg *et al.* (1986)	12	100	–	–	–

the results may be seen in Table 4.3. The findings are not uniform, but there is a suggestion that in the majority of women with established hirsuties, the source of androgen production is both adrenal and ovarian. Other investigators have attempted to delineate the site by dexamethasone suppression of the adrenals, but Kirshner *et al.* (1976) have demonstrated that ovarian androgen production is also suppressed which may invalidate all of the suppression studies.

References

Abraham, G.E., Chakmakjian, Z.H., Buster, J.E. & Marshall, J.R. (1975) Ovarian and adrenal contributions to peripheral androgens in hirsute women. *Obstetrics and Gynecology*, **46**, 169.

Adams, J., Polson, D.W. & Franks, S. (1986) Prevalence of polycystic ovaries in women with anovulation and idiopathic hirsutism. *British Medical Journal*, **293**, 355.

Bardin, C.W. & Lipsett, M.B. (1967) Testosterone and androstenedione blood production rates in normal women and in women with idiopathic hirsuties or polycystic ovaries. *Journal of Clinical Investigations*, **46**, 891.

Bennett, A.H., Harrison, J.H. & Thorn, G.W. (1971) Neoplasms of the adrenal gland. *Journal of Urology*, **106**, 607.

Cathelineau, G., Brerault, J.-L., Fiet, J., Julien, R., Dreux, C. & Canivet, J. (1980) Adrenocortical 11-beta-hydroxylation defect in adult women with postmenarchial onset of symptoms. *Journal of Clinical Endocrinology and Metabolism*, **51**, 287.

Chetkowski, R.J., DeFazio, J., Shamonki, I., Judd, H.L. & Chang, R.J. (1984) The incidence of late-onset congenital adrenal hyperplasia due to 21-hydroxylase deficiency among hirsute women. *Journal of Clinical Endocrinology and Metabolism*, **58**, 595.

Chrousos, G.P., Loriaux, D.L., Mann, D.L. & Cutler, G.B. (1982) Late-onset 21-hydroxylase deficiency mimicking idiopathic hirsutism or polycystic ovarian disease. *Annals of Internal Medicine*, **96**, 143.

Coney, P. (1984) Polycystic ovarian disease: current concepts of pathophysiology and therapy. *Fertility and Sterility*, **42**, 667.

Conway, G.S., Honour, J.W. & Jacobs, H.S. (1989) Heterogeneity of the polycystic ovary syndrome: clinical, endocrine and ultrasound features in 556 patients. *Clinical Endocrinology*, **30**, 459.

Cumming, D.C. & Wall, S.R. (1985) Non sex-hormone binding globulin-bound testosterone as a marker for hyperandrogenism. *Journal of Clinical Endocrinology and Metabolism*, **61**, 873.

Dewailly, D., Vantyghem-Haudiquet, M.-C., Sainsard, C., Buvat, J., Cappoen, J.P., Ardaens, K.,

Racadot, A., Lefebre, J. & Fossati, P. (1986) Clinical and biological phenotypes in late-onset 21-hydroxylase deficiency. *Journal of Clinical Endocrinology and Metabolism*, **63**, 418.

Farber, M., Millan, V.G., Turksoy, R.N., & Mitchell, G.W. Jr. (1978) Diagnostic evaluation of hirsutism in women by selective bilateral adrenal and ovarian venous catheterisation. *Fertility and Sterility*, **30**, 283.

Fayez, J.A., Bunch, T.R. & Miller, G.L. (1974) Virilization in pregnancy associated with polycystic ovary disease. *Obstetrics and Gynecology*, **44**, 511.

German, E., Horowitz, H., Wiele, R.V. & Torack, R.M. (1961) Leydig-cell tumor of the ovary: case report and review. *Journal of Clinical Endocrinology and Metabolism*, **21**, 91.

Gordon, M.T., Conway, D.I., Anderson, D.C. & Harris, R. (1985) Genetics and biochemical variability of variants of 21-hydroxylase deficiency. *Journal of Medical Genetics*, **22**, 354.

Griffing, G.T. & Melby, J.C. (1983) Cushing's syndrome. In *Hirsutism and Virilism*, p. 63, eds. V.B. Mahesh & R.B. Greenblatt. John Wright PSG, Boston.

Hague, W.M., Adams, J., Rodda, C., Brook, C.G.D., Dewhurst, C.J. & Jacobs, H.S. (1986) Prevalence of ultrasonically detected polycystic ovaries in females with congenital adrenal hyperplasia. *Journal of Endocrinology*, **111** (supplement), 46.

Hauner, H., Ditschuneit, S.B., Pal, S.B., Moncayo, R. & Pfeiffer, E.F. (1988) Fat distribution, endocrine and metabolic profile in obese women with and without hirsutism. *Metabolism*, **37**, 281.

Jacobs, H.S. (1987) Polycystic ovaries and polycystic ovary syndrome. *Gynecologic Endocrinology*, **1**, 113.

King, D.R. & Lack, E.E. (1979) Adrenal cortical carcinoma: a clinical and pathologic study of 49 cases. *Cancer*, **44**, 239.

Kirschner, M.A. & Bardin, C.W. (1972) Androgen production and metabolism in normal and virilised women. *Metabolism*, **21**, 667.

Kirschner, M.A., Zucker, I.R. & Jespersen, D. (1976) Idiopathic hirsutism: an ovarian abnormality. *New England Journal of Medicine*, **294**, 637.

Kutten, F., Couillin, P., Girard, F., Billaud, L., Vicens, M., Boucekkine, C., Thalabard, J.-C., Maudelonde, T., Spritzer, P., Mowszowicz, I., Boue, A. & Mauvais-Jarvis, P. (1985) Late-onset adrenal hyperplasia in hirsutism. *New England Journal of Medicine*, **313**, 224.

Lavric, M.V. (1969) Galactorrhea and amenorrhea with polycystic ovaries. *American Journal of Obstetrics and Gynecology*, **104**, 814.

Loughlin, T., Cunningham, S., Moore, A., Culliton, M., Smythe, P.P.A. & McKenna, T.J. (1986) Adrenal abnormalities in polycystic ovary syndrome. *Journal of Clinical Endocrinology and Metabolism*, **62**, 142.

Magendantz, H.G., Jones, D.E.J. & Schomberg, D.W. (1972) Virilisation during pregnancy associated with polycystic ovary disease. *Obstetrics and Gynecology*, **40**, 156.

Mathur, R.S., Holtz, G., Baker, E.R., Moody, L.O., Landgrebe, S.C., Rust, P.F. & Williamson, H.O. (1981) Plasma androgens, 17β-estradiol, and sex hormone binding globulin in patients with hirsutism and/or cliteromegaly. *Fertility and Sterility*, **36**, 188.

McKenna, T.J. (1988) Current concepts: pathogenesis and treatment of polycystic ovary syndrome. *New England Journal of Medicine*, **318**, 558.

Medina, M., Herrera, J., Flores, M., Martin, O., Bermudez, J.A. & Zarate, A. (1986) Normal ovarian function in a mild form of late-onset 3-beta-hydroxysteroid dehydrogenase deficiency. *Fertility and Sterility*, **46**, 1021.

Moltz, L., Schwartz., U., Pickartz, H., Hammerstein, J. & Wolf, U. (1981) XY gonadal dysgenesis: aberrant testicular differentiation in the presence of H–Y antigen. *Obstetrics and Gynecology*, **58**, 17.

Moltz, L., Schwartz, U., Sorensen, R., Pickartz, H. & Hammerstein, J. (1984a) Ovarian and adrenal vein steroids in patients with non-neoplastic hyperandrogenism: selective catheterisation findings. *Fertility and Sterility*, **42**, 69.

Moltz, L., Pickartz, H., Sorensen, R., Schwartz, U. & Hammerstein, J. (1984b) Ovarian and adrenal vein steroids in seven patients with androgen-secreting ovarian neoplasms: selective catheterization findings. *Fertility and Sterility*, **42**, 585.

Northrop, G., Archie, J.T., Patel, S.K. & Wilbanks, G.D. (1975) Adrenal and ovarian vein androgen levels and laparoscopic findings in hirsute women. *American Journal of Obstetrics and Gynecology,* **122**, 192.

Novak, D.J., Lauchlan, S.C., McCawley, J.C. & Faiman, C. (1970) Virilization during pregnancy: case report and review of literature. *American Journal of Medicine,* **49**, 281.

Oake, R.J., Davies, S.J., McLachlan, M.S.F. & Thomas, J.P. (1974) Plasma testosterone in adrenal and ovarian vein blood of hirsute women. *Quarterly Journal of Medicine,* **43**, 603.

Pang, S., Lerner, A.J., Stoner, E., Levine, L.S., Oberfield, S.E., Engel, I. & New, M.I. (1985) Late-onset adrenal steroid 3-beta-hydroxysteroid dehydrogenase deficiency. 1. A cause of hirsutism in pubertal and postpubertal women. *Journal of Clinical Endocrinology and Metabolism,* **60**, 428.

Pehrson, J.J., Vaitukaitis, J. & Longcope, C. (1986) Bromocriptine, sex steroid metabolism, and menstrual patterns in the polycystic ovary syndrome. *Annals of Internal Medicine,* **105**, 129.

Pepe, G.J. & Albrecht, E.D. (1985) Prolactin stimulates adrenal androgen secretion in infant baboons. *Endocrinology,* **117**, 1968.

Polson, D.W., Adams, J., Wadsworth, J. & Franks, S. (1988a) Polycystic ovaries—a common finding in normal women. *Lancet,* **i**, 870.

Polson, D.W., Reed, M.J., Franks, S., Scanlon, M.J. & James, V.H.T. (1988b) Serum 11-beta-hydroxy-androstenedione as an indicator of the source of excess androgen production in women with polycystic ovaries. *Journal of Clinical Endocrinology and Metabolism,* **66**, 946.

Robyn, C. & Tukumbane, M. (1983) Hyperprolactinemia and hirsuties. In *Hirsutism and Virilism,* p. 189, eds. V.B. Mahesh & R.B. Greenblatt. John Wright PSB, Boston.

Rosen, G.F., Kaplan, B. & Lobo, R.A. (1988) Menstrual function and hirsutism in patients with gonadal dysgenesis. *Obstetrics and Gynecology,* **71**, 677.

Rosenfield, R.L. (1979) Plasma free androgen patterns in hirsute women and their diagnostic implications. *American Journal of Medicine,* **66**, 417.

Rosenfield, R.L. & Moll, G.W. Jr. (1983) The role of proteins in the distribution of plasma androgens and estradiol. In *Androgenisation in Women,* p. 25, eds. G.M. Molinatti, L. Martini & V.H.T. James. Raven Press, New York.

Sandberg, E.C. & Jackson, J.R. (1963) A clinical analysis of ovarian virilising tumors. *American Journal of Surgery,* **105**, 784.

Serafini, P. & Lobo, R.A. (1986) Prolactin modulates peripheral androgen metabolism. *Fertility and Sterility,* **45**, 41.

Shortle, B.E., Warren, M.P. & Tsin, D. (1987) Recurrent androgenicity in pregnancy: a case report and literature review. *Obstetrics and Gynecology,* **70**, 462.

Stahl, N.L., Teeslink, C.R. & Greenblatt, R.B. (1973) Ovarian, adrenal, and peripheral testosterone levels in the polycystic ovary syndrome. *American Journal of Obstetrics and Gynecology,* **117**, 194.

Stein, I.F. & Leventhal, M.C. (1935) Amenorrhoea associated with bilateral polycystic ovaries. *American Journal of Obstetrics and Gynecology,* **29**, 181.

Stoddard, F.J. (1945) Hirsutism in pregnancy. *American Journal of Obstetrics and Gynecology,* **49**, 417.

Trotter, M. (1935) The activity of hair follicles with reference to pregnancy. *Surgery, Gynecology and Obstetrics,* **60**, 1092.

Wajchenberg, B.L., Achando, S.S., Okada, H., Czeresnia, C.E., Peixoto, S., Lima, S.S. & Goldman, J. (1986) Determination of the source(s) of androgen overproduction in hirsutism associated with polycystic ovary syndrome by simultaneous adrenal and ovarian venous catheterization. Comparison with the dexamethasone suppression test. *Journal of Clinical Endocrinology and Metabolism,* **63**, 1204.

Wild, R.A., Umstsot, E.A., Andersen, R.N., Ranney, G.B. & Givens, J.R. (1983) Androgen parameters and their correlation with body weight in 138 women thought to have hyperandrogenism. *American Journal of Obstetrics and Gynecology,* **146**, 602.

Woodruff, J.D. & Parmley, T.H. (1983) Virilizing ovarian tumors. In *Hirsutism and Virilism: Pathogenesis and Management,* p. 129, eds. V.B. Mahesh & R.B. Greenblatt. Wright PSG, London.

Yen, S.S.C. (1980) The polycystic ovary syndrome. *Clinical Endocrinology,* **12**, 177.

The skin and hyperandrogenism: 'Cutaneous Virilism' (References p. 102)

Alterations in the cutaneous sensitivity to androgens is the reason cited for the existence of hirsuties in the presence of normal serum androgens and the lack of hirsuties in women with raised androgens. However, there has been no systematic study of hyperandrogenized non-hirsute women to determine whether or not they have other cutaneous features of androgen excess. The skin is a complex structure containing many different tissues and it is now recognized that all the structures within the skin are modified by androgens. The eccrine and sebaceous glands are more active, and the skin is thicker and contains more collagen in men than in women (Shuster 1982). Inflammation of the apocrine glands in hidradenitis suppurativa is associated with hyperandrogenism (Mortimer *et al.* 1986) as is occlusion of the follicular duct both in vellus (Knutson 1974) and terminal hairs (Barth *et al.* 1988a). It is possible therefore that the skin of non-hirsute hyperandrogenized women does respond to androgens, but not by the development of terminal hairs.

The ability of the skin to metabolize androgen would suggest a biological role. Kirschner *et al.* (1983) have proposed that the skin is an integral part of the androgen clearance mechanism which operates when the clearance ability of the liver is exceeded. In non-hirsute women, the skin does not play a role; however, in both hirsute women and men up to 50% of androgen clearance is performed by an extra-splanchnic site which they suggest is the skin. They further propose that 5α-reductase activity is stimulated by the increase in testosterone to perform the increased clearance and that it metabolizes testosterone 'at the expense of hair follicle stimulation'.

Shuster (1972) has proposed a primary role for the skin. He suggested that in some individuals, the genetically determined level of cutaneous enzymes is sufficiently active to produce a negative feedback on the ovaries and adrenals and so enhance androgen production; he offered no evidence to support this hypothesis. However, studies by Toscano *et al.* (1983) have provided data for a primary increase in cutaneous androgen metabolism. They noted that the only androgen abnormality in women who have a very short history of hirsuties (less than 1 year) is an increase in the cutaneous androgen products (dihydrotestosterone (DHT) and 3α-androstanediol).

Cutaneous metabolism of androgens in hirsute women
The metabolic activity of skin in hirsuties is increased both in direct incubation assays of skin and by measurements *in vivo*, for example 3α-androstanediol glucuronide. Whole skin homogenates from genital (Serafini & Lobo 1985) and pubic skin (Kuttenn *et al.* 1977) of hirsute women have been demonstrated to express increased conversion of testosterone to DHT. However, isolated hair follicles from hirsute women do not appear to have different enzyme activities from controls (Miyazaki *et al.* 1978; Glickman & Rosenfield 1984). As the

pilosebaceous unit contains considerable androgen metabolizing ability, the increased conversion of testosterone by whole skin homogenates may merely reflect the increased mass of pilosebaceous tissue in hirsute women. Furthermore, the reduction in conversion of testosterone by skin after therapy with anti-androgens (Mowszowicz *et al.* 1984; Serafini *et al.* 1985) may similarly reflect the reduction in size of the pilosebaceous unit.

3α-Androstanediol glucuronide has been proposed to be a specific marker of cutaneous androgen metabolism; early studies suggested that it was raised only in hirsute women with polycystic ovaries but not in controls or non-hirsute women with polycystic ovaries (Lobo *et al.* 1983). There has been little con-firmatory work and a recent study has cast doubt on its infallibility (Scanlon *et al.* 1988).

Metabolic and physical abnormalities of hirsute women
Hirsute women have a number of systemic abnormalities which suggest that hirsuties is not only a cosmetic disability but may have a more serious prognosis. Hirsute women have body shapes that tend towards the male shape (Ferriman *et al.* 1957; Evans *et al.* 1988) and with this, they have altered lipid profiles that would suggest an increased risk of cardiovascular disease (Hauner *et al.* 1988).

Hyperandrogenism, acanthosis nigricans and insulin resistance (HAIR–AN)
A relationship between diabetes and hyperandrogenism in women or 'Diabetes of Bearded Women' has been recognised for many years (Achard & Thiers 1921). However, it has now been established that the disordered carbohydrate metabolism is due to insulin resistance (IR) (Flier *et al.* 1979). Furthermore, acanthosis nigricans (AN) acts as a cutaneous marker for the IR. The combination of AN and IR occurs in 5% of women with hyperandrogenism (HA) (Flier *et al.* 1985) and in 7% of women presenting with hirsuties (Barth *et al.* 1988b). Women with HAIR–AN have marked features of virilism, namely muscular physique, acne, alopecia and hidradenitis suppurativa (Barth *et al.* 1988b; Dunaif *et al.* 1985).

Insulin may have an important role in the pathogenesis of hyperandrogenism. Studies *in vitro* have demonstrated that insulin exerts a stimulatory effect on ovarian androgen production (Hernandez *et al.* 1988) and that it inhibits the synthesis of sex hormone-binding globulin by the liver (Plymate *et al.* 1988). Its mode of action may be through the receptors for insulin-like growth factors which are present both on the ovaries and in the skin. Stimulation of the latter may result in AN. It is, however, unknown whether the hyperinsulinaemia and insulin resistance are primary or secondary.

References
Achard, C. & Thiers, S. (1921) Insuffisance glycolytique associée au virilisme pilaire (diabète des femmes à barbe). *Bulletin de l'Academie Nationale de Médecine*, **cxxxvi**, 58.
Barth, J.H. Wojnarowska, F. & Dawber, R.P.R. (1988a) Is keratosis pilaris another androgen-dependent dermatosis? *Clinical and Experimental Dermatology*, **13**, 240.

Barth J.H., Ng, L.L., Wojnarowska, F. & Dawber, R.P.R (1988b) Acanthosis nigricans, insulin resistance and cutaneous virilism. *British Journal of Dermatology*, **118**, 613.

Dunaif, A., Hoffman, A.R., Scully, R.E. Flier, J.S., Longcope, C., Levy, L.J. & Crowley, W.F. Jr. (1985) Clinical, biochemical, and ovarian morphologic features in women with acanthosis nigricans and masculinisation. *Obstetrics and Gynecology*, **66**, 545.

Evans, D.J., Barth, J.H. & Burke, C.W. (1988) Body fat topography in women with androgen excess. *International Journal of Obesity*, **12**, 157.

Ferriman, D., Thomas, P.K. & Purdie, A.W. (1957) Constitutional virilism. *British Medical Journal*, **ii**, 1410.

Flier, J.S., Kahn, C.R. & Roth, J. (1979) Receptors, antireceptor antibodies and mechanisms of insulin resistance. *New England Journal of Medicine*, **300**, 413.

Flier, J.S., Eastman, R.C., Minaker, K.L., Matteson, D. & Rowe, J.W. (1985) Acanthosis nigricans in obese women with hyperandrogenism: characterization of an insulin-resistant state distinct from the type A and B syndromes. *Diabetes*, **34**, 101.

Glickman, S.P. & Rosenfield, R.L. (1984) Androgen metabolism by isolated hairs from women with idiopathic hirsutism is usually normal. *Journal of Investigative Dermatology*, **82**, 62.

Hauner, H., Ditschuneit, S.B., Pal, S.B., Moncayo, R. & Pfeiffer, E.F. (1988) Fat distribution, endocrine and metabolic profile in obese women with and without hirsuties. *Metabolism*, **37**, 281.

Hernandez, E.R., Resnick, C., Holtzclaw, W.D., Payne, D.W. & Adashi, E.Y. (1988) Insulin as a regulator of androgen biosynthesis by cultered rat ovarian cells: cellular mechanism(s) underlying physiological and pharmacological hormonal actions. *Endocrinology*, **122**, 2034.

Kirschner, M.A., Samoljlik, E. & Silber, D. (1983) A comparison of androgen production and clearance in hirsute and obese women. *Journal of Steroid Biochemistry*, **19**, 607.

Knutson, D.D. (1974) Ultrastructural observations in acne vulgaris: the normal sebaceous follicle and acne lesions. *Journal of Investigative Dermatology*, **62**, 288.

Kuttenn, F., Mowszowicz, I., Schaison, G. & Mauvais-Jarvis, P. (1977) Androgen production and skin metabolism in hirsutism. *Journal of Endocrinology*, **75**, 83.

Lobo, R.A., Goebelsmann, U. & Horton, R. (1983) Evidence for the importance of peripheral tissue events in the development of hirsutism in the polycystic ovary syndrome. *Journal of Clinical Endocrinology and Metabolism*, **57**, 393.

Miyazaki, M., Takayasu, S., Karakawa, T., Aono, T., Kurachi, K. & Matsumoto, K. (1978) Activity of testosterone 5-alpha-reductase in the hair follicles of women with polycystic ovaries. *Journal of Endocrinology*, **78**, 445.

Mortimer, P.S., Dawber, R.P.R., Gales, M.A. & Moore, R.A. (1986) Mediation of hidradenitis suppurativa by androgens. *British Medical Journal*, **292**, 245.

Mowszowicz, I., Wright, F., Vincens, M., Rigaud, C., Nahoul, K., Mavier, P., Guillemant, S., Kuttenn, F. & Mauvais-Jarvis, P. (1984) Androgen metabolism in hirsute patients treated with cyproterone acetate. *Journal of Steroid Biochemistry*, **20**, 757.

Plymate, S.R., Matej, L.A., Jones, R.E. & Friedl, K.E. (1988) Inhibition of sex hormone-binding globulin production in the human hepatoma (Hep G2) cell line by insulin and prolactin. *Journal of Clinical Endocrinology and Metabolism*, **67**, 460.

Scanlon, M.J., Whorwood, C.B., Franks, S., Reed, M.J. & James, V.H.T. (1988) Serum androstanediol glucuronide in normal hirsute women and patients with thyroid dysfunction. *Clinical Endocrinology*, **29**, 529.

Serafini, P. & Lobo, R.A. (1985) Increased 5-alpha-reductase activity in idiopathic hirsutism. *Fertility and Sterility*, **43**, 74.

Serafini, P.C., Catalino, J. & Lobo, R.A. (1988) The effect of spironolactone on genital skin 5-alpha-reductase activity. *Journal of Steroid Biochemistry*, **23**, 191.

Shuster, S. (1972) Primary cutaneous virilism or idiopathic hirsuties? *British Medical Journal*, **ii**, 285.

Shuster, S. (1982) The sebaceous glands and primary cutaneous virilism. In *Androgens and Anti-Androgen Therapy*, p. 1, ed. S.L. Jeffcoate. John Wiley, Chichester.

Toscano, V., Adamo, M.V., Caiola, S., Foli, S., Petrangeli, E., Casilli, D. & Sciarra, F. (1983) Is hirsutism an evolving syndrome? *Journal of Endocrinology*, **97**, 379.

Diagnostic approach to the hirsute woman

Most hirsute women have probably been aware of excess hair since puberty; some will give a shorter history but it will still be in the order of years. Some women are so good at cosmetic procedures that they do not appear hirsute at all. It is important to obtain facts from the history regarding patterns of hirsuties and alopecia or other features of cutaneous virilism and evidence for PCO, for example, irregular menses or infertility. A family history of childhood dehydration or precocious puberty in a brother might be a feature of congenital adrenal hyperplasia. A drug history may point to an ingested source of androgens, for example glucocorticoid or anabolic steroids. The progestogenic components of many contraceptive preparations are relatively androgenic and this is often cited as a cause of hirsuties but this has not been a relevant factor in our experience.

The cutaneous examination will include the pattern and severity of hair growth and the associated presence of acne, androgenic alopecia, obesity and acanthosis nigricans. Features suggestive of systemic virilization will include a deepening of the voice, increased muscle bulk and loss of the smooth skin contours, hypertension, striae distensae and cliteromegaly. This last feature, cliteromegaly, is probably the most important physical sign pointing towards systemic virilization. The implication of systemic virilization, especially where there is a short history (for example less than 1 year), is that there is a tumourous cause which is quite different from 'cutaneous virilism'.

The extent to which it is necessary for hirsute women to be investigated is debatable. The following recommendations for investigation have been proposed (Crosignani & Rubin 1990):

1 Long-standing mild hirsutism with regular menstrual cycles and no features of systemic virilism. These patients require no further investigation.

2 Moderate hirsuties with or without menstrual cycle disturbances. Most of these patients probably have polycystic ovary disease. This may be confirmed by ultrasound examination and a plasma testosterone may be valuable. These patients only require further investigation if their hair growth fails to respond to adequate anti-androgen therapy.

3 Severe hirsuties and virilization with a short history or very severe hirsuties with a long history. These signs should be suspected to be due to an androgen-secreting tumour and the patient should be thoroughly investigated.

The main reason for the depth of investigation of hirsute women is the inability to differentiate between IH, PCO and CAH on clinical grounds and it is out of this quagmire that the standard of over-investigation has arisen. The therapeutic tools available at present are too clumsy to warrant such diagnostic definition.

Reference

Crosignani, P.G. & Rubin, B. (1989) Strategies for the treatment of hirsutism. *Hormone Research*, **4**, 651.

Therapy for hirsuties (References p. 110)

Most women will be satisfied with the assurance that they are not 'turning into men' and may not require any medical help or may only need advice about local destructive measures; however, many women will already have tried these methods.

Cosmetic measures for the removal of excessive hair
The easiest measure is to bleach the hair with hydrogen peroxide. This produces a yellow hue due to the native colour of keratin and may be as unacceptable as the original colour. Hair plucking is widely performed but the act of plucking not only removes the hair shaft but also stimulates the root into the anagen phase and there is only a brief delay whilst the shaft grows through the epidermis. Shaving avoids this problem by removing all the hairs but is followed by growth only of the hairs which were previously in anagen. This effect may be important if facial hair has a long telogen phase.

Waxing is performed by the application of a sheet of soft wax onto the skin and, as soon as it has hardened with the hair shafts embedded, it is abruptly peeled off the skin removing all the shafts. This is a painful method and is often complicated by folliculitis. Certain natural sugars, long used in parts of the Middle East, are becoming popular in place of waxes as they appear to depilate as effectively but with less trauma.

Electrolysis is the only permanent method for removal of hair (Peereboom-Wynia 1975; Richards *et al.* 1986). A fine electrical wire is introduced down the hair shaft to the papilla which is destroyed by an electrical current. Techniques with either direct or alternating currents, or both, have been employed (Wagner *et al.* 1985). Complications, unusual in skilled hands, include local and systemic infection (Daneshmend 1984) and local scarring.

Systemic anti-androgen therapy
Since hirsuties is a condition mediated by androgens, attempts have been made to ameliorate the growth of hair with drugs with anti-androgenic properties. The complete spectrum of therapeutic agents evaluated in the treatment of hirsuties has been reviewed in this section. It is, however, our practice to use cyproterone acetate and spironolactone as first line therapy for those women whose hirsuties is so severe as to warrant systemic therapy.

It is important that hirsute women are carefully selected prior to initiating therapy for the following reasons. Firstly, the effect on hair growth takes several months to become apparent and only partial improvements may be expected. Secondly, anti-androgens feminize male foetuses and it is essential that the women do not become pregnant. Thirdly, these drugs only have a suppressive, and not curative, effect which wears off a few months after cessation of therapy and therapy may need to be taken indefinitely if a favourable improvement occurs. Finally, the long-term safety of these drugs is unknown and tumours in laboratory animals have been reported with several of the following agents.

Cyproterone acetate. Cyproterone acetate (CPA) is both an anti-androgen and an inhibitor of gonadotrophin secretion. It reduces androgen production, increases the metabolic clearance of testosterone (Mowszowicz *et al.* 1984) and binds to the androgen receptor (Eil & Edelson 1984); in addition, long-term therapy is associated with a reduction in the activity of cutaneous 5α-reductase (Mowszowicz *et al.* 1984). Cyproterone acetate is a potent progestogen but does not reliably inhibit ovulation. It is usually administered with cyclical oestrogens in order to maintain regular menstruation and to prevent conception in view of the risk of feminizing a male foetus.

Several dose regimens have been advocated. Low dose therapy (Dianette® Schering AG) is an oral contraceptive containing 35 µg ethinyl oestradiol and 2 mg CPA taken daily for 21 days in every 28. However, all of the dose-ranging and efficacy studies were performed using the preparation which contained 50 µg ethinyl oestradiol; this may be relevant as only the higher dose of oestrogen increases sex hormone-binding globulin (Pogmore & Jequier 1979). High dose therapy consists of Dianette® taken for 21 days with CPA 50–100 mg taken only for the first 10 days (the reverse sequential regimen of Hammerstein *et al.* (1975)). This regimen was designed to allow for CPA stores to be cleared from adipose tissue by the end of the cycle. Other regimens have been designed using intra-muscular oestrogens and/or CPA (Hammerstein 1980).

Current dosage recommendations for CPA usually advise that 50 or 100 mg CPA should be administered for 10 days/cycle (Hammerstein *et al.* 1975). However, there have now been three dose-ranging studies which suggest that there is no dose effect. A large multicentre study performed in Canada reported that after 12 months therapy the mean reduction in hirsuties score with Diane® was 25%, whereas with Diane® plus 100 mg CPA the reduction was marginally greater at 31% (Belisle & Love 1986). An open Italian study of Diane® in four dose schedules could show no difference (Molinatti *et al.* 1983). Finally, our studies comparing Dianette® with and without CPA similarly found no difference, either in the reduction of the overall hirsuties grades or in the reduction in hair shaft diameters (Barth *et al.* 1990).

The direct effect of CPA (100 mg in reverse sequential regimen) on thigh hair growth was first quantitatively investigated by Ebling *et al.* (1977) in a single hirsute woman. After 6 months therapy linear growth was reduced by 12% and diameter reduced by 24%; although they only examined one woman, their results are similar to larger studies. Peereboom-Wynia (1980) noted a 10% reduction in thigh hair shaft diameter and a hair density reduction of 24% after over 3 months. These changes in density may reflect a reduction in the length of the hair cycle (Peereboom-Wynia & Beek 1977).

Holdaway (Holdaway *et al.* 1985a,b) has measured linear hair growth on the sideburn area of the face in two studies comprising 68 women who took CPA (100 mg) and found a reduction of 12–19% after 3 months. The site at which facial growth measurements are taken may be important as Jones *et al.* (1981) measured linear hair growth on the chin and could only detect a reduction in 2 out of 10 patients taking CPA (50 mg). Similarly Peereboom-Wynia and Boekhorst (1980) could demonstrate no change in shaft diameter with 100 mg CPA but there was a fall in hair density of 50%. The effect of a higher dose of CPA (150 mg continuously) has been investigated by Jones *et al.* (1987) who reported a reduction in linear growth rates of 40% after 12 months on hair measured either on the face or abdomen.

Side effects of CPA include weight gain, fatigue, loss of libido, mastodynia, nausea, headaches and depression. All these side effects are more frequent with a higher dose. Contra-indications to its use are the same as for the contraceptive pill and include cigarette smoking, age, obesity and hypertension (Hammerstein *et al.* 1983).

Spironolactone. Spironolactone has several anti-androgenic pharmacological pro-perties. It reduces the bioavailability of testosterone by interfering with its production (Menard *et al.* 1974) and increases its metabolic clearance (Rose *et al.* 1977). It binds to the androgen receptor (Eil & Edelson 1984) and, like cyproterone acetate, long-term therapy is associated with a reduction in cutaneous 5α-reductase activity (Serafini *et al.* 1985). It was an act of serendipity that demonstrated its therapeutic advantage in hirsuties. A 19-year-old hirsute woman with polycystic ovary syndrome was treated with spironolactone (200 mg daily) for concurrent hypertension and she noted after 3 months that she needed to shave less frequently (Ober & Hennessy 1978). This report was soon followed by a study demonstrating that spironolactone reduced testosterone production and subjectively reduced hair growth in six hirsute women (Boiselle & Tremblay 1979). These authors commented on a delay of about 3–4 months before the effect on hair growth became apparent. There have subsequently been several clinical studies.

Different dose schedules of spironolactone have been studied, varying between 50–200 mg taken either daily or cyclically (daily for 3 weeks in every 4). A daily dose of 200 mg produces a reduction in subjective hair growth grades of approximately 40% after 6 months' therapy with little further effect (Shapiro & Evron 1980; Cumming *et al.* 1982; Burke & Cunliffe 1985; Evans & Burke 1986; Barth *et al.* 1989). At doses below 200 mg per day, there have been conflicting reports of efficacy. Studies using daily doses of 150 and 100 mg have demonstrated less than 20% improvement in subjective score (Dorrington-Ward *et al.* 1985; Chapman *et al.* 1986) but such results may lie within the range of observer error. A study of 50 mg daily was enthusiastically reported to offer an improvement in 71% of patients (Nielsen 1982).

Objective measurements of hair growth give a less clear picture of the efficacy of spironolactone. Cumming *et al.* (1982), using 200 mg daily, noted a 40% reduction in hair shaft diameter of facial hair after 6 months' therapy. Our own studies (Barth *et al.* 1989) with 200 mg daily have revealed a reduction of 25–35% in daily growth rates and a 20% reduction in hair shaft diameter on the face, abdomen and thighs after 12 months' therapy. Lobo *et al.* (1985) compared 100 mg with 200 mg; they noted a reduction in hair shaft diameter of facial and abdominal hairs but no significant difference between doses. Spandri *et al.* (1984) used 100 mg daily and noted a reduction of 20% after 4 and 12 months in the weight of thigh hair shavings. These findings contrast with those of Dorrington-Ward *et al.* (1985) who used 150 mg daily; they measured both the linear growth rate and shaft diameter of thigh hair but noted no overall change after 11 months' therapy.

The main side effects of spironolactone are breast soreness and menstrual irregularities but there is considerable variation in their reported incidence. Menstrual irregularities result in 8–56% of patients stopping therapy (Evans & Burke 1986; Helfer *et al.* 1988). This effect can probably be ameliorated by the concomitant use of an oral contraceptive containing either cyproterone acetate or desogestrel as the gestagen. Breast tenderness has been reported to occur in 0–39% of patients (Helfer *et al.* 1988; Hughes & Cunliffe 1988).

Comparison of cyproterone acetate with spironolactone. There have been no formal clinical trials between the two treatments but comparative reports claim that both agents are equally effective (Suraci *et al.* 1983; Thomas *et al.* 1985). Lunde and Djoseland (1987) suggested that spironolactone (50 mg daily) is more effective than Diane® and Rubens & Vermeulen (1987) reported that 50 mg cyproterone acetate given in the reverse sequential regimen is similar to spironolactone (100 mg daily). It is not known whether the two agents have an additive effect.

Corticosteroids. Corticosteroids are first-line therapy for congenital adrenal hyperplasia and were the first endocrine therapy to be employed in the treatment of hirsuties with the rationale of suppressing the production of adrenal androgens. Corticosteroids are effective in reducing plasma androgen levels but there are contradictory reports regarding their therapeutic effect on hair growth. Subjective assessment with dexamethasone (0.25–1.0 mg daily) suggested a reduction of 30–70% in hair growth (Ettinger *et al.* 1973; Abraham *et al.* 1981; Cunningham *et al.* 1983). However, these clinical impressions of improvement have not been supported by direct measurements of hair growth (Casey *et al.* 1966). Oral prednisolone therapy gives no clinical improvement (Rittmaster & Givner 1988).

Medroxyprogesterone acetate. Medroxyprogesterone acetate (MPA) is a synthetic progestogen which was introduced as an anovulatory agent due to its ability to block gonadotrophin secretion. It reduces androgen levels by reducing the production of testosterone and increasing its metabolic clearance (Gordon *et al.* 1972). There have been subjective reports suggesting a reduction of hair growth in 50–95% of patients (Ettinger *et al.* 1973; Correa de Oliveira *et al.* 1975).

Schmidt *et al.* (1985) compared topical (0.2% ointment) with systemic therapy either by intra-muscular injection of MPA (150 mg every 6 weeks) or sub-cutaneous injection (100 mg every 6 weeks). They state that the majority of patients gained a beneficial response. Direct measurements of facial hair shaft diameter were made for four patients in each group; the average hair shaft diameter was reduced by 38% over the subcutaneous injection site after 9 weeks and a similar reduction was produced after intra-muscular administration after 19 weeks, but only by 23% after topical administration after 21 weeks. No response was seen in 20% and in 10 out of 13 patients given topical therapy there was no change in hair diameter.

Medroxyprogesterone acetate given alone may result in menorrhagia (Correa de Oliveira *et al.* 1975) but this may be prevented by cyclical administration with ethinyl oestradiol (Ettinger *et al.* 1973).

Desogestrel. Desogestrel is the progestogen used in the Marvelon® contraceptive pill (Organon Ltd) which contains 30 µg ethinyl oestradiol and 150 mg desogestrel. There have been three studies of its efficacy in hirsuties (Dewis *et al.* 1985; Cullberg *et al.* 1985; Ruutiainen 1986). All have reported subjective and/or objective reductions in hair growth of 20–25% after 6–9 months' therapy with a high degree of patient satisfaction.

Ketoconazole. Ketoconazole is a potent inhibitor of adrenal and ovarian steroid synthesis (Sonino 1987). There have only been isolated reports of its use in hirsuties but these have demonstrated a marked reduction in hair growth after 6 months (Carvalho *et al.* 1985; Pepper *et al.* 1987; Martikainen *et al.* 1988). This treatment cannot be recommended in view of the risks of hepatic toxicity during long-term therapy.

Flutamide. Flutamide acts as a pure anti-androgen and works by binding to androgen receptors. However, it has no anti-gonadotrophic effect and the result of binding to central androgen receptors is that it prevents the negative feedback effect of testosterone and consequently androgen levels rise (Balzono *et al.* 1987). There has been a single study in hirsuties in which flutamide (250 mg b.d.) was administered with an oral contraceptive for 7 months; 12 out of 13 patients demonstrated a subjective improvement in hair growth and acne (Cusan *et al.* 1988).

Gonadotrophin-releasing hormone agonists. Gonadotrophin-releasing hormone (Gn-RH) agonists inhibit LH production and this results in profound suppression of ovarian function and therefore androgen production. These agents are presently under investigation, but preliminary studies suggest that they effectively reduce hair growth and acne in women with PCO after a minimum of 6 months' therapy (Andreyko *et al.* 1986; Couzinet *et al.* 1986; Rittmaster 1988).

Cimetidine. Cimetidine is a weak anti-androgen mediated by androgen receptor binding (Eil & Edelson 1984). There have been two reports of its use in the treatment of hirsuties. The first study of four patients with idiopathic hirsuties demonstrated a marked reduction in hair growth using hair weight (Vigersky *et al.* 1980) whereas a placebo controlled study demonstrated no such effect (Grandesso *et al.* 1984).

Bromocriptine. The irregularity of LH secretion in PCO may be due to abnormalities in hypothalamic dopamine. Bromocriptine is a dopamine agonist and long-term therapy with bromocriptine regulates menstrual cycle length, but 12 months' therapy produces no measurable effect on linear hair growth in women with polycystic ovaries (Murdoch *et al.* 1987).

References

Abraham, G.E., Maroulis, G.B., Boyers, S.P., Buster, J.E., Magyar, D.M. & Elsner, C.W. (1981) Dexamethasone suppression test in the management of hyperandrogenised patients. *Obstetrics and Gynecology,* **57**, 158.

Andreyko, J.L., Monroe, S.E. & Jaffe, R.B. (1986) Treatment of hirsutism with a gonadotrophin-releasing hormone agonist (Nafarelin). *Journal of Clinical Endocrinology and Metabolism,* **63**, 854.

Balzano, S., Migliari, R., Sica, V., Scarpa, R.M., Pintus, C., Loviselli, A., Usai, E. & Balestrieri, A. (1987) The effect of androgen blockade on pulsatile gonadotrophin release and LH response to naloxone. *Clinical Endocrinology,* **27**, 491.

Barth, J.H., Cherry, C.A., Wojnarowska, F. & Dawber, R.P.R. (1989) Spironolactone is an effective and well tolerated systemic anti-androgen therapy for hirsute women. *Journal of Clinical Endocrinology and Metabolism,* **68**, 966.

Barth, J.H., Cherry, C.A., Wojnarowska, F. & Dawber, R.P.R. (1990) Cyproterone acetate for severe hirsutism: results of a double-blind dose-ranging study. (Submitted for publication.)

Belisle, S. & Love, E.J. (1986) Clinical efficacy and safety of cyproterone acetate in severe hirsutism: results of a multicentred Canadian study. *Fertility and Sterility,* **46**, 1015.

Boiselle, A. & Tremblay, R.R. (1979) New therapeutic approach to the hirsute patient. *Fertility and Sterility,* **32**, 276.

Burke, B.M. & Cunliffe, W.J. (1985) Oral spironolactone therapy for female patients with acne, hirsutism or androgenic alopecia. *British Journal of Dermatology,* **112**, 124.

Carvalho, D., Pignatelli, D. & Resende, C. (1985) Ketoconazole for hirsutism. *Lancet,* **ii**, 560.

Casey, J.H., Burger, H.G., Kent, J.R., Kellie, A.E., Moxham, A., Nabarro, J. & Nabarro, J.D.N. (1966) Treatment of hirsutism by adrenal and ovarian suppression. *Journal of Clinical Endocrinology and Metabolism,* **26**, 1307.

Chapman, M.G., Dowsett, M., Hague, W., Jeffcoate, S.L. & Dewhurst, C.J. (1986) Spironolactone in the treatment of hirsutism. *Acta Obstetricia et Gynecologica Scandinavica,* **65**, 349.

Correa de Oliveira, R.E., Novaes, L.P., Lima, M.B., Rodrigues, J., Franco, S., Khenaifes, A.I. & Francalanci, C.P. (1975) A new treatment for hirsutism. *Annals of Internal Medicine,* **83** 817.

Couzinet, B., Le Strat, N., Brailly, S. & Schaison, G. (1986) Comparative effects of cyproterone acetate or a long-acting gonadotrophin-releasing hormone agonist in polycystic ovarian disease. *Journal of Clinical Endocrinology and Metabolism,* **63**, 1031.

Cullberg, G., Hamberger, L., Mattsson, L.-A., Mobacken, H. & Samisoe, G. (1985) Effects of a low-dose desogestrel-ethinylestradiol combination on hirsutism, androgens and sex hormone binding globulin in women with a polycystic ovary syndrome. *Acta Obstetricia et Gynecologica Scandinavica,* **64**, 195.

Cumming, D.C., Young, J.C., Rebar, R.W. & Yen, S.S.C. (1982) Treatment of hirsutism with spironolactone. *Journal of the American Medical Association,* **247**, 1295.

Cunningham, S.K., Loughlin, T., Culliton, M. & McKenna, T.J. (1983) Plasma sex hormone-binding globulin and androgen levels in the management of hirsute patients. *Acta Endocrinologica*, **104**, 365.

Cusan, L., Dupont, A., Tremblay, R., & Labrie, F. (1988) Treatment of hirsutism with the pure antiandrogen flutamide. *Proceedings of the International Society of Gynecology and Endocrinology*, (Crans-Montana: Switzerland) March 6–12 (in press).

Daneshmend, T.K. (1984) Need for antibiotic prophylaxis during hair electrolysis? *British Medical Journal*, **289**, 1693.

Dewis, P., Petsos, P., Newman, M. & Anderson, D.C. (1985) The treatment of hirsutism with a combination of desogestrel and ethinyl oestradiol. *Clinical Endocrinology*, **22**, 29.

Dorrington-Ward, P., McCartney, A.C.E., Holland, S., Scully J., Carter, G., Alaghband-Zadeh, J. & Wise, P. (1985) The effect of spironolactone on hirsutism and female androgen metabolism. *Clinical Endocrinology*, **23**, 161.

Ebling, F.J., Thomas, A.K., Cooke, I.D., Randall, V.A., Skinner, J. & Cawood, M. (1977) Effect of cyproterone acetate on hair growth, sebaceous secretion and endocrine parameters in a hirsute subject. *British Journal of Dermatology*, **97**, 371.

Eil, C. & Edelson, S.K. (1984) The use of human skin fibroblasts to obtain potency estimates of drug binding to androgen receptors. *Journal of Clinical Endocrinology and Metabolism*, **59**, 51.

Ettinger, B., Goldfield, E.B., Burrill, K.C., Von Werder, K. & Forsham, P.H. (1973) Plasma testosterone stimulation–suppression dynamics in hirsute women. *American Journal of Medicine*, **54**, 195.

Evans, D.J. & Burke, C.W. (1986) Spironolactone in the treatment of idiopathic hirsutism and the polycystic ovary syndrome. *Journal of the Royal Society of Medicine*, **79**, 451.

Gordon, G.G., Southern, A.L., Calanog, A., Olivio, J. & Rafii, F. (1972) The effect of medroxyproges terone acetate on androgen metabolism in the polycystic ovary syndrome. *Journal of Clinical Endocrinology and Metabolism*, **35**, 444.

Grandesso, R., Spandri, P., Gangemi, M., Nardelli, G.B., Ambrosio, G.B., Conte, G., de Salvia, D. & Meneghetti, G. (1984) Hormonal changes and hair growth during treatment of hirsutism with cimetidine. *Clinical and Experimental Obstetrics and Gynecology*, **11**, 105.

Hammerstein, J. (1980) Possibilities and limits of endocrine therapy. In *Androgenisation in Women*, p. 221, eds. J. Hammerstein, U. Lachnit-Fixen, F. Neumann & G. Plewig. Excerpta Medica, Amsterdam.

Hammerstein, J., Moltz, L. & Schartz, U. (1983) Antiandrogens in the treatment of acne and hirsutism. *Journal of Steroid Biochemistry*, **19**, 591.

Hammerstein, J., Meckies, J., Leo-Rossberg, I., Moltz, L. & Zielske, F. (1975) The use of cyproterone acetate (CPA) in the treatment of acne, hirsutism and virilism. *Journal of Steroid Biochemistry*, **6**, 827.

Helfer, E.L., Miller, J.L. & Rose, L.I. (1988) Side effects of spironolactone therapy in the hirsute woman. *Journal of Clinical Endocrinology and Metabolism*, **64**, 208.

Holdaway, I.M, Fraser, A., Sheehan, A., Croxson, M.S., France, J.T. & Ibbertson, H.K. (1985a) Objective assessment of treatment response in hirsutism. *Hormone Research*, **22**, 253.

Holdaway, I.M., Croxson, M.S., Ibbertson, H.K., Sheehan, A., Knox, B. & France, J.T. (1985b) Cyproterone acetate as initial treatment and maintenance therapy for hirsutism. *Acta Endocrinologica*, **109**, 522.

Hughes, B.R. & Cunliffe, W.J. (1988) Tolerance of spironolactone. *British Journal of Dermatology*, **118**, 687.

Jones, K.R., Katz, M., Keyzer, C. & Gordon, W. (1981) Effect of cyproterone acetate on rate of hair growth in hirsute females. *British Journal of Dermatology*, **105**, 685.

Jones, D.B., Ibraham, I. & Edwards, C.R.W. (1987) Hair growth and androgen responses in hirsute women treated with continuous cyproterone acetate and cyclical ethinyl oestradiol. *Acta Endocrinologica*, **116**, 497.

Lobo, R.A., Shoupe, D., Serafini, P., Brinton, D. & Horton, R. (1985) The effects of two doses of spironolactone on serum androgens and anagen hair in hirsute women. *Fertility and Sterility*, **453**, 200.

Lunde, O. & Djoseland, O. (1987) A comparative study of Aldactone and Diane in the treatment of hirsutism. *Journal of Steroid Biochemistry*, **28**, 161.

Martikainen, H., Heikkinen, J., Ruokonen, A. & Kauppila, A. (1988) Hormonal and clinical effects of ketoconazole in hirsute women. *Journal of Clinical Endocrinology and Metablism*, **66**, 987.

Menard, H., Stripp, B. & Gillette, J.R. (1974) Spironolactone and testicular cytochrome P-450: decreased testosterone formation in several species and changes in hepatic drug metabolism. *Endocrinology*, **94**, 1628.

Molinatti, G.M., Messina, M., Manieri, C., Massuchetti, C. & Biffignandi, P. (1983) Current approaches to the treatment of virilizing syndromes. In *Androgenization in Women*, p. 79, eds. G.M. Molinatti, L. Martini & V.H.T. James. Raven Press, New York.

Mowszowicz, I., Wright, F., Vincens, M., Rigaud, C., Nahoul, K., Mavier, P., Guillemant, S., Kuttenn, F. & Mauvais-Jarvis, P. (1984) Androgen metabolism in hirsute patients treated with cyproterone acetate. *Journal of Steroid Biochemistry*, **20**, 757.

Murdoch, A.P., McClean, K.G., Watson, M.J., Dunlop, W. & Kendall Taylor, P. (1987) Treatment of hirsutism in polycystic ovary syndrome with bromocriptine. *British Journal of Obstetrics and Gynaecology*, **94**, 358.

Nielsen, P.G. (1982) Treatment of idiopathic hirsutism with spironolactone. *Dermatologica*, **165**, 194.

Ober, K.P. & Hennessy, J.F. (1987) Spironolactone therapy for hirsutism in a hyperandrogenic woman. *Annals of Internal Medicine*, **98**, 643.

Peereboom-Wynia, J.D.R. (1975) The effect of electrical epilation on the beard hair of women with idiopathic hirsutism. *Archives of Dermatological Research*, **254**, 15.

Peereboom-Wynia, J.D.R. & Beek, C.H. (1977) The influence of cyproterone-acetate orally on the hair root status in women with idiopathic hirsutism. *Archives of Dermatological Research*, **260**, 137.

Peereboom-Wynia, J.D.R. & Boekhorst, J.C. (1980) Effect of cyproterone acetate orally on hair density and diameter and endocrine factors in women with idiopathic hirsutism. *Dermatologica*, **160**, 7.

Pepper, G.M., Poretsky, L., Gabrilove, J.L. & Ariton. M.M. (1987) Ketoconazole reverses hyperandrogenism in a patient with insulin resistance and acanthosis nigricans. *Journal of Clinical Endocrinology and Metabolism*, **65**, 1047.

Pogmore, J.R. & Jequier, A.M. (1979) Effect of varying amounts of ethinyl oestradiol in the combined oral contraceptive on plasma sex hormone binding globulin capacity in normal women. *British Journal of Obstetrics and Gynecology*, **86**, 563.

Richards, R., McKenzie, M.A. & Meharg, G.E. (1986) Electroepilation in hirsutism. *Journal of the American Academy of Dermatology*, **15**, 693.

Rittmaster, R.S. (1988) Differential suppression of testosterone and estradiol in hirsute women with the superactive gonadotrophin-releasing hormone agonist leuprolide. *Journal of Clinical Endocrinology and Metabolism* **67**, 651.

Rittmaster, R.S. & Givner, M.L. (1988) Effect of daily and alternate day low dose prednisolone on serum cortisol and adrenal androgens in hirsute women. *Journal of Clinical Endocrinology and Metabolism*, **67**, 400.

Rose, L.I., Underwood, R.H., Newmark, S.R., Kisch, E.S. & Williams, G.H. (1977) Pathophysiology of spironolactone-induced gynecomastia. *Annals of Internal Medicine*, **87**, 398.

Rubens, R. & Vermeulen, A. (1987) Clinical assessment of two antiandrogen treatments, cyproterone acetate combined with ethinyl estradiol and spironolactone in hirsutism. In *New Developments in Biosciences 3*, p. 133, ed. A.E. Schindler. W. de Gruyter, Berlin.

Ruutiainen, K. (1986) The effect of an oral contraceptive containing ethinylestradiol and desogestrel on hair growth and hormonal parameters of hirsute women. *International Journal of Gynaecology and Obstetrics*, **24**, 361.

Schmidt, J.B., Huber, J. & Spona, J. (1985) Medroxyprogesterone acetate therapy in hirsutism. *British Journal of Dermatology*, **113**, 161.

Serafini, P., Catalino, J. & Lobo, R.A. (1985) The effect of spironolactone on genital skin 5α-reductase activity. *Journal of Steroid Biochemistry*, **23**, 191.

Shapiro, G. & Evron, S. (1980) A novel use of spironolactone: treatment of hirsutism. *Journal of Clinical Endocrinology and Metabolism*, **51**, 429.

Sonino, N. (1987) The use of ketoconazole as an inhibitor of steroid production. *New England Journal of Medicine*, **317**, 812.

Spandri, P., Gangemi, M., Nardelli, G.B., Meneghetti, G., Grandesso, R., de Salvia, D., Ambrosio, G.B. & Predebon, O. (1984) Testosterone, 17KS, $17\beta E_2$ FSH–LH variations and hirsutism modifications during spironolactone therapy. *Clinical and Experimental Obstetrics and Gynecology*, **11**, 49.

Suraci, C., Costa, C. & de Pedrini, P. (1983) Ciproterone acetato e spironolattone a confronto nella terapia dell'irsutismo femminile. *Clinica Terapeutica*, **104**, 463.

Thomas, A.K., Slobodniuk, R., Taft, J., Cooper, M., Montalto, J. & Jerums, G. (1985) The treatment of hirsutism: experience with cyproterone acetate and spironolactone. *Australian Journal of Dermatology*, **26**, 19.

Vigersky, R.A., Mehlman, I., Glass, A.R. & Smith, C.E. (1980) Treatment of hirsute women with cimetidine. *New England Journal of Medicine*, **303**, 1042.

Wagner, R.F. Jr., Tomich, J.M. & Grande D.J. (1985) Electrolysis and thermolysis for permanent hair removal. *Journal of the American Academy of Dermatology*, **12**, 441.

Common baldness

History and nomenclature (References p. 114)

Common baldness is a genetically determined physiological event in the lives of most men and women. There is perhaps no normal phenomenon that has been so widely regarded as abnormal by physician and layman alike. An ancient Egyptian papyrus from 4000 years ago records the anxieties of males at the time (Giacometti 1967) and it is reasonable to assume that men and women have sought help and cure for as long as society has existed.

Our understanding of the process started with the studies of Hamilton (1942), although there have been many dozens of theories over the past two centuries. Erasmus Wilson described 'calvities' which he thought was due to a tightly bound scalp; however, he also mentioned heredity as one of many 'remote causes'. Hebra & Kaposi (1874) sought to establish a link between pityriasis capitis, seborrhoea and baldness. The discovery of *Pityrosporum* organisms in dandruff and seborrhoea allowed Elliott & Merrill (1895) to propose that premature alopecia was secondary to seborrhoeic dermatitis due to *Pityrosporum* in 316 of 320 patients. King (1868) suggested that 'continuous wearing of caps or close fitting unventilated hats was important' and this was supported by Jackson & McMurty (1913) who also felt that 'cerebral congestion' might explain the occurrence of baldness in sedentary workers. Further improbable theories included Ellinger's (1879) finding that lack of care of the hair was the active cause and Parker's (1907) opinion that a 'toxin' developed in expired air and therefore premature alopecia could be avoided by taking deep breaths.

Hamilton (1942) established beyond doubt that common baldness is a normal process induced in the genetically predisposed hair follicle following exposure to androgen at or around the time of puberty. Montagna and other workers (Montagna & Uno 1968) have confirmed Hamilton's work in man and other primates.

The contemporary nomenclature for common baldness is confusing. In some countries 'seborrhoeic alopecia' is favoured. This term is unfortunate in that it has misleading aetiological connotations. 'Male pattern alopecia' is perhaps the most widely used term, but it is descriptively misleading when applied to common baldness in women. 'Pattern baldness' and 'androgenetic baldness' are unobjectionable but have not found favour. 'Common baldness' has the advantage of emphasizing that, except in a minority of affected women, the loss of hair is a normal phenomenon.

References

Ellinger, L. (1879) Zur Aetiologie und Prophylaze der Alopecia praematura. *Virchows Archiv für pathologische Anatomie und Physiologie*, **77**, 549.

Elliott, G.T. & Merrill, W.H. (1895) A further study of alopecia praematura or praesenilic and its most frequent cause—eczema seborrhoicum, and a preliminary bacteriological report on eczema seborrhoicum. *New York Medical Journal*, **62**, 525.

Giacometti, L. (1967) Facts, legends and myths about the scalp throughout history. *Archives of Dermatology*, **95**, 629.

Hamilton, J. (1942) Male hormone stimulation is prerequisite and an incitant in common baldness. *American Journal of Anatomy*, **71**, 451.

Hebra, F. & Kaposi, M. (1874) *On Disease of the Skin*, vol. III, p. 203, trans. by W. Tay. New Sydenham Society, London.

Jackson, G.T. & McMurty, C.W. (1913) *Treatise on Diseases of the Hair*. Henry Kimpton, London.

King, A.F.A. (1868) On the causes of alopecia and its greater frequency in males than females. *American Journal of Medical Science*, **55**, 416.

Montagna, W. & Uno, H. (1968) The phylogeny of baldness. In *Biopathology of Pattern Alopecia*, p. 9, eds. A. Baccareda-Boy, G. Moretti & J.R. Fray. Karger, Basel.

Parker, D.L. (1907) Common baldness: its cause and treatment. *American Journal of Dermatology and Genito-urinary Diseases*, **11**, 261.

Phylogeny of common baldness (Reference p. 115)

Man is not the only primate species in which baldness is a natural phenomenon associated with sexual maturity (Montagna & Uno 1968). The orang-utan (*Pongo pygmaeus*) and the chimpanzee (*Pan troglodytes*) both show some degree of baldness when they reach maturity. In the juveniles long hair extends from the level of the eyebrows to merge imperceptibly with the scalp, whereas in the adult the forehead and the frontal region of the scalp bear only fine vellus hair. Other species showing this phenomenon include the uakari (*Cacajao* sp.) and the stump-tailed macaque (*Macaca arctoides*). The latter species has been studied extensively by Montagna, Uno and their colleagues at the Oregon Primate Center who established the essential similarity of the balding process between the macaque and man. These studies have demonstrated clearly that common baldness is a physiological process in genetically predisposed individuals whether simian or human. Terminal follicles are progressively transformed into 'vellus' follicles, which differ from true vellus follicles in that they may still have the remnants of fibres of the arrector pili muscles attached to them.

Reference

Montagna, W. & Uno, H. (1968) The phylogeny of baldness. In *Biopathology of Pattern Alopecia*, p. 9, eds. A. Baccareda-Boy, G. Moretti & J.R. Fray. Karger, Basel.

Prevalence and genetics (References p. 118)

The prevalence of common baldness in any population has not been accurately recorded but it probably approaches 100% in the Caucasoid races. In other words, the replacement of some terminal follicles by vellus type follicles from puberty onwards is a universal phenomenon. A number of investigations have been carried out to record the extent of balding, but few studies have made any real attempt at quantification.

Hair patterns

Hamilton (1951) produced the first useful grading scale after examining 312 white males and 214 white females aged 20–89. This classification was modified by Norwood (1975) who added grades IIIa, III vertex, IVa and Va to the Hamilton scale (Fig. 4.8). The Norwood scoring system has been used extensively in clinical trials of regrowth particularly with regard to topical minoxidil.

Hamilton described the natural progression of the normal prepubertal scalp pattern (Type I) in both sexes to Type II in 96% of men and 79% of women after

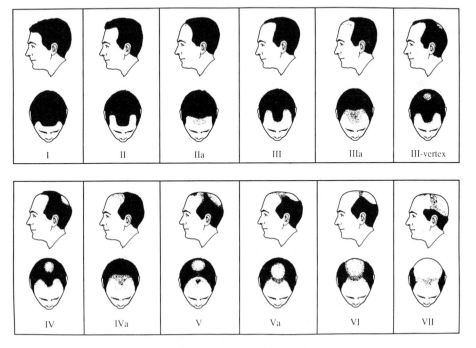

Fig. 4.8 Patterns of hair loss in males. (After Norwood 1975.)

puberty. He also observed patterns Type V to VIII in 58% of men aged over 50 years with the extent of baldness tending to increase to the age of 70. About 25% of women developed Type IV scalps by the age of 50, after which there was no further increase in balding. Indeed, after 50 some women who had developed Type II at puberty revert to Type I. Types V to VIII were not found in any women.

Although, as these figures show, the male pattern of baldness occurs in females with some frequency, androgenetic alopecia in women more often assumes a diffuse form (Ludwig 1977) (Fig. 4.9).

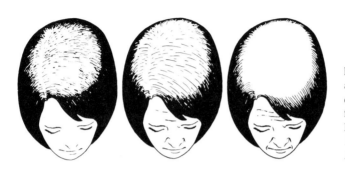

Fig. 4.9 Patterns of androgenetic alopecia commonly occurring in the female (courtesy of Professor Ludwig and the Editor of the *British Journal of Dermatology*).

Venning & Dawber (1988) have shown a change of patterning in 100% of 564 women over 20 years old. In this study these workers carefully wetted the vaultal hair and observed from above. They analysed their patients by decade and found that 87% of premenopausal women showed vaultal thinning of the Ludwig pattern I–III and 13% had Hamilton type II–IV. Post-menopausal women showed an increased tendency to the male patterning with 63% of Ludwig I–III and 37% of Hamilton II–V including some women with deep M-shaped bitemporal frontoparietal recession.

Other observations, much less accurately recorded, tended to group together Hamilton's types II, III and IV, and are therefore of interest only in confirming the great frequency of common baldness in other populations of Caucasoids. For example, Buschke & Grenepert (1926) in Germany found bitemporal recession in 62.5% of men aged 20–40. Beek (1946) in Holland found baldness in 27% of women aged 35–40 and 64% in those aged 40–70. Figures from Italy (Binazzi & Wierolis 1962) also serve to emphasize the frequency of baldness in women of Caucasoid descent.

Setty (1970) reported that a full head of hair—Hamilton Type I—was four times more frequent in Negroes than in Caucasoids. Hamilton found that Type I scalp was retained after puberty by most Chinese in whom baldness is uncommon, mild and of late-onset. Japanese males develop common baldness approximately one decade later than Caucasians and in each decade of life have 1.4 times lower incidence (Takashima *et al.* 1981).

Venning & Dawber's work (1988) suggests that separating hair patterns into the eight Hamilton and three Ludwig types is only of use in defining a population for the purpose of clinical trial evaluation. The grades are imprecise measures of a continuum of hair patterns that are seen in adults of both sexes. The single consistent finding is a change from the prepubertal pattern in all adults. The magnitude and rate of that change is influenced by genetic predisposition and by sex hormone levels in both sexes (*vide infra*).

Inheritance

The very high frequency of common baldness has complicated the many attempts to establish its mode of inheritance. Moreover, it is by no means clear that common baldness is genetically homogeneous; some authorities differentiate between early onset (before the age of 30 in men) and the same pattern 20 years later. Osborn (1916) thought that baldness was determined by a single pair of sex-influenced factors and Snyder & Yingling (1935) considered that both gene frequency studies and family histories supported this hypothesis. Harris (1946) insisted that early baldness must be distinguished from late baldness, and that the former was transmitted by a single autosomal dominant gene. He assumed that the heterozygous female was normally not affected, but was uncertain about the homozygous female.

In a small study of first-degree relatives of 56 women with ordinary baldness Smith & Wells (1964) showed that 54% of males and 23% of females over the age of 30 were similarly affected. These authors considered that baldness could apparently develop in the heterozygous female and they postulated that was either dominant inheritance with increased penetrance in the male or multifactorial inheritance. The concept of multifactorial inheritance was supported by Salamon (1968), although the question remains unanswered. It is still unclear whether early and late-onset baldness are inherited separately. It is nevertheless certain that both are inherited and that both depend upon androgenic stimulation of susceptible follicles. In a search for a biochemical marker of baldness, Hodgins *et al.* (1985) plucked scalp hair follicles from young adults not yet expressing baldness but with a strong family history of baldness and found two populations, one with high 17β-hydroxysteroid dehydrogenase activity and one with low enzyme activity. Low enzyme activity seemed to be related to retention of hair and a family history of hair retention. Extension of this type of work is essential to arrive at a precise definition of the mode of inheritance.

The association of baldness with an increased susceptibility or resistance to certain diseases has been claimed, but the evidence is unsatisfactory. Bruchner *et al.* (1964) reported a fourfold decrease in the incidence of carcinoma of the bronchus but an increased incidence of coronary artery disease in bald men. Cooke (1979) could not confirm the association of baldness with coronary artery disease.

There is no association between baldness and dense hair patterns on the trunk and limbs (Burton *et al.* 1979); nor is there an association between hair loss and increased fertility (Damon *et al.* 1965).

References

Beek, C.H. (1946) Calvities frontalis bei Frauen. *Dermatologica*, **93**, 213.

Binazzi, M. & Wierolis, T. (1962) Les Alopécies féminines Hypooestrogéniques. *Annales de Dermatologie et de Syphiligraphie*, **89**, 382.

Bruchner, H.A., Brown, M. & Tretsea, R.J. (1964) Baldness and emphysema. *Journal of the Louisiana State Medical Society*, **116**, 34.

Burton, J.L., Ben Halim, M.M. & Meyrick, G. (1979) Male pattern alopecia and masculinity. *British Journal of Dermatology*, **100**, 507.

Buschke, A. & Grenepert, M. (1926) Zur Kenntnis des Sexualcharakters der Kopfhaarkleiden. *Klinische Wochenschrift*, **5**, 18.

Cooke, M.T. (1979) Male pattern alopecia and coronary artery disease in men. *British Journal of Dermatology*, **101**, 455.

Damon, A., Burr, W.A. & Gerson, D.E. (1965) Baldness, fertility and number and sex ratio of children. *Human Biology*, **37**, 366.

Hamilton, J.B. (1951) Patterned long hair in man: types and incidence. *Annals of the New York Academy of Science*, **53**, 708.

Harris, H. (1946) The inheritance of premature baldness in man. *Annals of Eugenics*, **13**, 172.

Hodgins, M.B., Murad, S. & Simpson, N.B. (1985) A search for variation in hair follicle androgen metabolism which might be linked to male pattern baldness (Abstract). *British Journal of Dermatology*, **113**, 794.

Ludwig, E. (1977) Classification of the types of androgenic alopecia (common baldness) arising in the female sex. *British Journal of Dermatology*, **97**, 249.

Norwood, O' T.T. (1975) Male pattern baldness: Classification and incidence. *Southern Medical Journal*, **68**, 1359.

Osborn, D. (1916) Inheritance of baldness. *Journal of Heredity*, **7**, 347.

Salamon, T. (1968) Genetic factors in male pattern alopecia. In *Biopathology of Pattern Alopecia*, p. 39, eds. A. Baccaradda-Boy, G. Moratti & J.R. Fray. Karger, Basel.

Setty, L.R. (1970) Hair patterns of the scalp of white and Negro males. *American Journal of Physical Anthropology*, **33**, 49.

Smith, M.A. & Wells, R.S. (1964) Male type alopecia, alopecia areata and normal hair in women. *Archives of Dermatology*, **89**, 95.

Snyder, L.H. & Yingling, H.C. (1935) The application of the gene frequency method of analysis to sex-influenced factors with special reference to baldness. *Human Biology*, **7**, 608.

Takashima, T., Iju, M. & Sudo, M. (1981) Alopecia androgenetica—its incidence in Japanese and associated conditions. In *Hair Research*, p. 287, eds. C.E. Orfanos, W. Montagna & G. Stüttgen. Springer-Verlag, Berlin.

Venning, V.A. & Dawber, R. (1988) Patterned androgenic alopecia. *Journal of the American Academy of Dermatology*, **18**, 1073.

Experimental models (References p. 119)

Common baldness is found in other primates and these animals have been studied extensively by Montagna, Uno and colleagues at the Oregon Primate Center (Uno *et al.* 1969). Much of the work has been conducted on the stump-tailed macaque (*Macaca arctoides*) but this is a protected species. Limited results from the andro-chronogenetic mouse look promising (Matias *et al.* 1989).

Plucked human anagen scalp hairs have been used extensively for analysis of androgenic activity and other enzyme systems *in vitro* but it has proved difficult to localize androgen receptors and/or enzyme systems in the hair follicle. The plucked anagen hair leaves behind some precortical matrix and all of the dermal papilla. Accumulated evidence of the controlling influence of the dermal papilla in the induction and maintenance of hair growth (Oliver 1966, 1970; Jahoda *et al.* 1984) has led to the use of cultured dermal papilla cells *in vitro* as a model for androgen metabolism and other enzyme activity. Much of this work has only been reported in abstract form and is therefore not available for complete criticism. Human cultured dermal papilla cells are capable of androgen interconversion and possess androgen receptors (Murad *et al.* 1985, 1986; Messenger *et al.* 1988; Itami *et al.* 1990).

References

Itami, S., Kurata, S. & Takayasu, S. (1990) 5 α-Reductase activity in cultured human dermal papilla cells from beard compared with reticular dermal fibroblasts. *Journal of Investigative Dermatology*, **94**, 150.

Jahoda, C.A.B., Horne, K.A. & Oliver, R.F. (1984) Induction of hair growth by implantation of cultured dermal papilla cells. *Nature*, **311**, 560.

Matias, J.R., Malloy, V. & Orentreich, N. (1989) Animal models of androgen-dependent disorders of the pilosebaceous apparatus. 1. The androchronogenetic alopecia (AGA) mouse as a model for male pattern baldness. *Archives of Dermatological Research*, **281**, 247.

Messenger, A.G., Thornton, M.J., Elliott, K. & Randall, V.A. (1988) Androgen responses in cultured human hair papilla cells (Abstract). *Journal of Investigative Dermatology*, **91**, 382.

Murad, S., Hodgins, M.B., Simpson, N.B., Oliver, R.F. & Jahoda, C. (1985) Androgen receptors and metabolism in cultured dermal papilla cells from human hair follicles (Abstract). *British Journal of Dermatology*, **113**, 768.

Murad, S., Hodgins, M.B., Oliver, R.F. & Jahoda, C.A. (1986) Comparative studies of androgen receptors and metabolism in dermal papilla cells cultured from human and rat hair follicles (Abstract). *Journal of Investigative Dermatology*, **87**, 158.

Oliver, R.F. (1966) Whisker growth after removal of the dermal papilla and length of the follicle in the hooded rat. *Journal of Embryology and Experimental Morphology*, **15**, 331.

Oliver, R.F. (1970) The induction of hair follicle formation in the adult hooded rat by vibrissa dermal papillae. *Journal of Embryology and Experimental Morphology*, **23**, 219.

Uno, H., Adachi, K. & Montagna, W. (1969) Morphological and biochemical studies of hair follicle in common baldness of stump-tailed macaque (*Macaca speciosa*). In *Advances in Biology of the Skin*, vol. 9, *Hair Growth*, p. 221, eds. W. Montagna & R.L. Dobson. Pergamon Press, Oxford.

Pathology (References p. 120)

The earliest histological change is focal perivascular basophilic degeneration in the lower third of the connective tissue sheath of otherwise normal anagen follicles. This is followed by a perifollicular lymphohistiocytic infiltrate at the level of the sebaceous duct. The basophilic sclerotic remains of the connective tissue sheath can be seen early in the process as 'streamers' (Kligman 1988). The destruction of the connective tissue sheath may account for the irreversibility of hair loss. In about a third of biopsies multinucleate giant cells are seen surrounding fragments of hair (Domnitz & Silvers 1979). The errector pili muscle decreases in size more slowly than the follicle (Maguire & Kligman 1962; Lattenand & Johnson 1975). In the scalp which appears totally bald most of the follicles are short and small with some quiescent terminal follicles.

As the balding scalp loses its protective covering of hair so solar degenerative changes may be seen (Singh & McKenzie 1961; Allegra 1968). There is no correlation between the thickness of the scalp and the development of baldness (Garn *et al.* 1954). The reduction of blood supply has been confirmed by modern methods (Klemp *et al.* 1989), but whether it follows (Cormia & Ernyey 1961) or precedes baldness is unknown. When the follicles become small or disappear, their unsupported nerve networks coil and twist and come to resemble encapsulated end-organs (Giacometti & Montagna 1968).

The development of baldness is associated with shortening of the anagen phase of the hair cycle and consequently with an increase in the proportion of telogen hairs, which may be detected in trichograms of the frontovertical region before baldness is evident (Braun-Falco & Christophers 1968; Vogelsberg *et al.* 1980). This is no doubt the explanation of the recorded differences in the force required to extract hairs from various regions of the adult male scalp (Light 1951).

The reduction in the size of the affected follicles, which is the essential histological feature of ordinary baldness, necessarily results in a reduction in the diameter of the hairs they produce. This reduction is said to be greater in women than in men (Silvestri 1967; Jackson *et al.* 1972). Balding patients showed a wide spread of hair shaft diameters with peaks at 0.04 and 0.06 mm, while non-bald subjects showed a symmetrical distribution with a single peak at 0.08 mm. The studies of the shaft in common baldness showed no abnormality on electron microscopy (Puccinelli *et al.* 1968) and preliminary studies have shown no abnormality in its chemical composition (Salamon 1971).

References

Allegra, F. (1968) Histology and histochemical aspects of the hair follicles in pattern alopecia. In *Biopathology of Pattern Alopecia*, p. 155, eds. A. Baccaradda-Boy, G. Moratti & J.R. Fray. Karger, Basel.

Braun-Falco, O. & Christophers, E. (1968) Hair root patterns in male pattern alopecia. In *Biopathology of Pattern Alopecia*, p. 141, eds. A. Baccaradda-Boy, G. Moratti & J.R. Fray. Karger, Basel.

Cormia, F.E. & Ernyey, A. (1961) Circulatory changes in alopecia. Preliminary report with a summary of the cutaneous circulation of the normal scalp. *Archives of Dermatology*, **84**, 772.

Domnitz, J.M. & Silvers, D.N. (1979) Giant cells in male pattern alopecia—a histological marker and pathogenic clue. *Journal of Cutaneous Pathology*, **6**, 108.

Garn, S.M. Selby, S. & Young, R. (1954) Scalp thickness and the fat-loss theory of balding. *AMA Archives of Dermatology and Syphilology*, **79**, 601.

Giacometti, L. & Montagna, W. (1968) The nerve fibres in male pattern alopecia. In *Biopathology of Pattern Alopecia*, p. 208, eds. A. Baccaradda-Boy, G. Moratti & J.R. Fray. Karger, Basel

Jackson, D., Church, R.E. & Ebling, F.J. (1972) Hair diameter in female baldness. *British Journal of Dermatology*, **87**, 361.

Klemp, P., Peters, K. & Hansted, B. (1989) Subcutaneous blood flow in early male patten baldness. *Journal of Investigative Dermatology*, **92**, 725.

Kligman, A.M. (1988) The comparative histopathology of male-pattern baldness and senescent baldness. *Clinics in Dermatology*, **6**, 108.

Lattenand, A. & Johnson, W.C. (1975) Male pattern alopecia. A histopathologic and histochemical study. *Journal of Cutaneous Pathology*, **2**, 58.

Light, A.F. (1951) Patterned loss of hair in man; pathogenesis and prognosis. *Annals of the New York Academy of Science*, **53**, 729.

Maguire, H.C. & Kligman, A.M. (1962) The histopathology of common male baldness. *Proceedings of the XII International Congress of Dermatology*, Washington, p. 1438.

Puccinelli, V.A., Caputo, R. & Casinelli, T. (1968) Electron microscopic studies of the hair shaft in normal and alopecic subjects. In *Biopathology of Pattern Alopecia*, p. 129, eds. A. Baccaradda-Boy, G. Moratti & J.R. Fray. Karger, Basel.

Salamon, T. (1971) Comparative chemical investigations on hair of various areas of the capillitium in subjects with 'normal' hair and with alopecia seborrhoeica. *Folia Medica Facultatis Medicinae Universitatis Saravenesis*, **5**, 241.

Silvestri, U. (1967) Studio fisico del capello in causistica de alopecia su base seborrhoica. *Archivio Italiano di Dermatologia, Venereologia e Sessuologia*, **34**, 405.

Singh, M. & McKenzie, J. (1961) The histology and histochemistry of the diseases of hairy and non hairy parts of the human skin with special reference to baldness. *Journal of Anatomy*, **95**, 569.

Vogelsberg, H., Klarner, W. & Rupec, M. (1980) Einige Beobachtungen zur Frage der androgenetischen Alopezie der Frau. *Zeitschrift für Hautkrankheiten*, **55**, 125.

Pathogenesis (References p. 124)

Any unifying hypothesis for common baldness has to explain all of the following: the occurrence in man and simian species, strong autosomal inheritance, the involvement of both sexes, geographical patterning of hair loss on the scalp, and the co-existence of greasy skin, acne and hirsutism in some women.

Hamilton (1942) showed that baldness did not develop in 10 eunuchoids, 10 men castrated at puberty and 34 men castrated during adolescence. Following administration of testosterone baldness developed in those who were genetically predisposed; when testosterone was discontinued the baldness did not progress although it did not reverse. In further studies Hamilton (1958) showed that the time interval between puberty and castration was crucial to the development of the beard in males. Castration before puberty prevented the development of a beard, while between 16 and 20 years of age it partially prevented the full development of a beard and after age 20 it had no effect on beard development. Testosterone administration at any stage following castration allowed full growth of beard. Hamilton (1942) showed that the development of baldness after castration followed a similar pattern of events to the beard, albeit in the reverse direction. Males suffering from syndromes of androgen insensitivity such as families with 5α-reductase deficiency and Rifenstein's syndrome lack beard hair and fail to develop temporal recession after puberty (Petersen *et al.* 1977). Very high doses of testosterone caused some virilization with beard growth (Price *et al.* 1984) but there is no record of change in scalp hair pattern. It appears that the magnitude of the response of hair to androgens may be set permanently by modification of gene expression following puberty (Shuster 1982).

The discovery of the importance of exposure to androgen in the pathogenesis of baldness led to claims for increased sexuality and androgens in balding males. Scientific support for this fanciful hypothesis is lacking. Phillipou & Kirk (1981) failed to find a correlation with testosterone levels but noticed a weak correlation between baldness and urinary dehydroepiandrosterone and Pitts (1987) found elevated serum dehydroepiandrosterone sulphate but normal testosterone levels in

18 balding males compared with non-balding controls. The improvement in technology and the ability to measure free and bound androgens has shown that normal male levels of androgen are sufficient to make manifest the degree of baldness determined genetically for the individual. The situation in women is different and it has become apparent that the degree of baldness may be related to circulating androgen levels (Apostalakis *et al.* 1965; Binazzi & Calandra 1968; Ludwig 1968; Kuhn 1972; Miller *et al.* 1982; De Villez & Dunn 1986; Moltz 1988). In addition, up to 48% of women presenting to an endocrine clinic with diffuse vaultal alopecia had evidence of polycystic ovarian disease (Futterweit *et al.* 1988).

All adult women show a change from the prepubertal hair pattern (Venning & Dawber 1988). The maximum change in hair pattern occurs after the menopause when oestrogen levels decline and a more 'androgenic' environment exists. Androgens, in the normal female range, induce baldness only in premenopausal women with a strong genetic predisposition. In women with a less strong genetic predisposition baldness develops only when androgen production is increased or drugs with androgen-like activity are taken—such as some progestogens in the oral contraceptive. In these women the severity of baldness is probably related to the extent of increased androgenicity but this remains unproven. In a third group of women even grossly abnormal levels of androgen cause no clinically significant baldness, although all such patients are necessarily hirsute.

The evidence for the association between androgens and ordinary baldness is strong and theories identifying the mechanism of this association are discussed below.

Sebaceous glands
The association of seborrhoea and common baldness led to the erroneous theories of the 19th century. The 'seborrhoea' probably has more to do with the refatting kinetics of fine hair than with any change in sebaceous gland activity except in a few women. During the course of baldness the total number of sebaceous glands decreases significantly (Rampini *et al.* 1968).

Sebaceous glands are under androgenic control and in men seem to be under maximal stimulation from normal circulating androgen levels. In women, however, increased sebum production occurs following a small increase in circulating androgens. It is not surprising, therefore, that many young women with higher grades of baldness, who have demonstrable abnormalities in circulating androgens, also have greasier skins. Maibach *et al.* (1968) found no differences in the casual level or hourly production of sebum on the bald or hairy scalp of balding men and the scalp of fully haired subjects. Skin surface lipids are unchanged qualitatively in the balding areas of males (Bloom *et al.* 1955). A theory that auto-oxidation of hair lipids within the follicle gave rise to depilatory substances (Kuchinska 1973 (reviewed by Thiele 1975)) met with little support because it failed to explain the selective nature of pattern hair loss.

The metabolism of hair follicles

The weight of evidence strongly supports the opinion that the essential inherited factor responsible for ordinary baldness concerns the manner in which certain follicles in the frontovertical region of the scalp react to androgens. The ability of the pilosebaceous unit to metabolize a wide range of androgens has been established beyond doubt (Fazekas & Sandor 1973; Bingham & Shaw 1973; Hay & Hodgins 1973, 1974, 1978; Schweikert & Wilson 1974 a,b; Itami & Takayasu 1982). The interconversion of androgens within the pilosebaceous unit has been discussed on pp. 88–91. The same androgens are responsible for the seborrhoea of acne, the conversion of vellus to terminal hair in the beard, pubic area and axillae and, paradoxically, the opposite effect on hair in the balding process in both sexes. Sebaceous gland androgen metabolism has been studied extensively, but even within the pilosebaceous unit we cannot with certainty extrapolate results from the sebaceous gland to the hair follicle or vice versa. The presence of androgen receptors has been established in sebocytes of the hamster flank organ (Adachi 1974; Lucky *et al.* 1985) but it has been much more difficult to localize androgen receptors or androgen metabolising enzyme systems in the hair follicle. Part of the problem has been methodological; plucked anagen hair follicles fracture and leave behind some of the germinative matrix and precortex and all of the dermal papilla. The presence of androgen receptors on dermal papillary cells in culture (Messenger *et al.* 1988) and the ability of dermal papilla cells to metabolize a range of androgens (Murad *et al.* 1985, 1986) suggest that this area will hold much promise for further investigation.

Schweikert and Wilson (1974 a,b) studied the metabolism of testosterone and androstenedione in individual plucked hair roots of balding and hairy scalp areas and found a higher concentration of 5α-reduced metabolites and 17-oxosteroid metabolites in balding males but were unable to determine whether these changes were primary or secondary to the balding process. Similarly, difference in sebaceous gland 3β-hydroxysteroid dehydrogenase Δ^{4-5} isomerase activity between bald and non-bald scalp (Sawaya *et al.* 1988) may be due to geographical influences in the balding areas or related to slight elevations of plasma dehydroepiandrosterone and dehydroepiandrosterone sulphate in some balding males (Pitts 1987).

If individual variation in androgen metabolism was linked causally to hair loss or retention it should be apparent in women and in young men before the onset of baldness. Hodgins *et al.* (1985) have reported two populations of high and low activity variants of the enzyme 17β-hydroxysteroid dehydrogenase in plucked hair roots. Enzyme activity appeared to be linked to the presence or absence of a strong family history of baldness. This work is a promising approach but needs to be confirmed.

The differential effect of castration at varying intervals after puberty (*vide supra*) and the fact that anti-androgens fail to reverse the process (*vide infra*) suggests that a change occurs in genetically prone follicles following exposure to androgens at puberty. From this time a 'genetic clock' is set running which eventually leads the follicle to undergo cycles of decreasing length producing finer and finer hair until full vellus change occurs. The genetic 'switch' would appear to be an irreversible process; however the tendency for some follicles to appear to regrow during treatment with minoxidil has cast some doubt on the true irreversibility of common baldness. This work is described in the next section.

There is no evidence that the non-sexual hormones are in any way involved in causing ordinary baldness (Stüttgen & Goerz 1968), but the changes resulting from such states as hypothyroidism may occur in chance association with ordinary baldness.

References

Adachi, K. (1974) Receptor proteins for androgen in hamster sebaceous glands. *Journal of Investigative Dermatology*, **62**, 217.

Apostolakis, M., Ludwig, E. & Voigt, K.-D. (1965) Testosteron-Oestrogen, und Gonadotropenausscheidung bei diffuser unerblicher Alopecia. *Klinische Wochenschrift*, **43**, 9.

Binazzi, M. & Calandra, P. (1968) Testosterone elimination in female patients with acne, chronic alopecia and hirsutism. *Italian General Review of Dermatology*, **8**, 241.

Bingham, K.D. & Shaw, D.A. (1973) The metabolism of testosterone by human male scalp skin. *Journal of Endocrinology*, **57**, 111.

Bloom, R.E., Wood, S. & Nicolaides, N. (1955) Hair fat composition in early male pattern alopecia. *Journal of Investigative Dermatology*, **24**, 97.

De Villez, R.L. & Dunn, J. (1986) Female androgenic alopecia. The 3α,17β-androstanediol glucuronide/sex hormone binding globulin ratio as a possible marker for female pattern baldness. *Archives of Dermatology*, **122**, 1011.

Fazekas, A.G. & Sandor, T. (1973) The metabolism of dehydroepiandrosterone by human scalp hair follicles. *Journal of Clinical Endocrinology*, **36**, 582.

Futterweit, W., Dunif, A., Yeh, H.-C. & Kingsley, P. (1988). The prevalence of hyperandrogenism in 109 consecutive female patients with diffuse alopecia. *Journal of the American Academy of Dermatology*, **19**, 831.

Hamilton, J.B. (1942) Male hormone stimulation is prerequisite and an incitement in common baldness. *American Journal of Anatomy*, **71**, 451.

Hamilton, J.B. (1948) The role of testosterone secretions as indicated by the effect of castration in man and by studies of pathological conditions and the short life-span associated with maleness. *Recent Progress in Hormone Research*, **3**, 257.

Hamilton, J.B. (1958) Age, sex and genetic factors in the regulation of hair growth in man: a comparison of Caucasian and Japanese populations. In *The Biology of Hair Growth*, p. 399, eds. W. Montagna & R.A. Ellis. Academic Press, New York.

Hamilton, J.B. (1960) Effect of castration in adolescent and young adult males upon further changes in the proportions of bare and hairy scalp. *Journal of Clinical Endocrinology*, **20**, 1309.

Hay, J.B. & Hodgins, M.B. (1973) Metabolism of androgens *in vitro* by human facial and axillary skin. *Journal of Endocrinology*, **59**, 475.

Hay, J.B. & Hodgins, M.B. (1974) Metabolism of androgens by human skin in acne. *British Journal of Dermatology*, **91**, 123.

Hay, J.B. & Hodgins, M.B. (1978) Distribution of androgen metabolising enzymes in isolated tissues of human forehead and axillary skin. *Journal of Endocrinology*, **79**, 29.

Hodgins, M.B., Murad, S. & Simpson, N.B. (1985) A search for variation in hair follicle androgen metabolism which might be linked to male pattern baldness (Abstract). *British Journal of Dermatology*, **113**, 794.

Itami, S. & Takayasu, S. (1982) Activity of 3β-hydroxysteroid dehydrogenase Δ^{4-5} isomerase in human skin. *Archives of Dermatological Research*, **274**, 289.

Kuchinska, R. (1973) Chemische Aspekte des Haarausfalls und ihre kosmetologischen Bedeutung. *Kosmetologie*, **5**, 177.

Kuhn, B.H. (1972) Male pattern alopecias and/or androgenetic hirsutism in females. Part III: definition and etiology. *Journal of the American Medical Women's Association*, **27**, 357.

Ludwig, E. (1968) The role of sexual hormones in pattern alopecia. In *Biopathology of Pattern Alopecias*, p. 50, eds. A. Baccaradda-Boy, G. Moratti & J.R. Fray. Karger, Basel.

Lucky, A.W., Eisenfeld, A.L. & Visintin, I. (1985) Autoradiographic localisation of tritiated dihydrotestosterone in the flank organ of the albino hamster. *Journal of Investigative Dermatology*, **84**, 122.

Maibach, H.I., Feldman, R., Payne, B. & Hutshell, T. (1968) Scalp and forehead sebum production in male pattern alopecia. In *Biopathology of Pattern Alopecias*, p. 171, eds. A. Baccaradda-Boy, G. Moratti & J.R. Fray. Karger, Basel.

Messenger, A.G., Thornton, M.J., Elliott, K. & Randall, V.A. (1988) Androgen responses in cultured human hair papilla cells (Abstract). *Journal of Investigative Dermatology*, **91**, 382.

Miller, J.A., Darley, C.R., Karkavitsas, K., Kirby, J.D. & Munro, D.D. (1982) Low sex-hormone binding globulin levels in young women with diffuse hair loss. *British Journal of Dermatology*, **106**, 331.

Moltz, L. (1988) Hormonale Diagnostik der sogenannten androgenetischen Alopezie der Frau. *Geburtshilfe-Frauenheilkunde*, **48**, 203.

Murad, S., Hodgins, M.B., Oliver, R.F. & Jahoda, C.A. (1986) Comparative studies of androgen receptors and metabolism in dermal papilla cells cultured from human and rat hair follicles (Abstract). *Journal of Investigative Dermatology*, **87**, 158.

Murad, S., Hodgins, M.B., Simpson, N.B., Oliver, R.F. & Jahoda, C. (1985) Androgen receptors and metabolism in cultured dermal papilla cells from human hair follicles (Abstract). *British Journal of Dermatology*, **113**, 768.

Peterson, R.E., Imperato-McGinley, J., Gautier, T. & Sturla, E. (1977) Male pseudohermaphroditism due to steroid 5α-reductase deficiency. *American Journal of Medicine*, **62**, 170.

Phillipou, G. & Kirk, J. (1981) Significance of steroid measurements in male pattern alopecia. *Clinical and Experimental Dermatology*, **6**, 53.

Pitts, R.L. (1987) Serum elevation of dehydroepiandrosterone sulfate associated with male pattern baldness in young men. *Journal of the American Academy of Dermatology*, **16**, 571.

Price, P., Wass, J.A.H., Griffin, J.E., Leshin, M., Savage, M.O., Large, D.M., Bullock, D.E., Anderson, D.C., Wilson, J.D. & Besser, G.M. (1984) High dose androgen therapy in male pseudohermaphroditism due to 5α-reductase deficiency and disorders of the androgen receptor. *Journal of Clinical Investigation*, **74**, 1496.

Rampini, E., Bertamino, R. & Moretti, G. (1968) Size and shape of sebaceous glands in male pattern alopecia. In *Biopathology of Pattern Alopecia*, p. 155, eds. A. Baccaradda-Boy, G. Moratti & J. R. Fray. Karger, Basel.

Sawaya, M.E., Honig, L.S., Garland, L.D. & Hsia, S.L. (1988) Δ^5-3β-hydroxysteroid dehydrogenase activity in sebaceous glands of scalp in male-pattern baldness. *Journal of Investigative Dermatology*, **91**, 101.

Schweikert, H.U. & Wilson, J.D. (1974b) Regulation of human hair growth by steroid hormones. II. Testosterone metabolism in isolated hairs. *Journal of Clinical Endocrinology and Metabolism*, **38**, 811.

Schwiekert, H.U. & Wilson, J.D. (1974b) Regulation of human hair growth by steroid hormones. II. Androstenedione metabolism in isolated hairs. *Journal of Clinical Endocrinology and Metabolism*, **39**, 1012.

Shuster, S. (1982) The sebaceous glands and primary cutaneous virilism. In *Androgens and Antiandrogen Therapy*, p. 1, ed. S.L. Jeffcoate. John Wiley & Sons, Chichester.

Stüttgen, G. & Goerz, G. (1968) Non sexual hormones and male pattern alopecia. In *Biopathology of Pattern Alopecias*, p. 61, eds. A. Baccaradda-Boy, G. Moratti & J.R. Fray. Karger, Basel.

Thiele, F.A.I. (1975) Chemical aspects of hair loss and its cosmetological significance. *British Journal of Dermatology*, **92**, 355.
Venning, V.A. & Dawber, R. (1988) Patterned androgenic alopecia. *Journal of the American Academy of Dermatology*, **18**, 1073.

Clinical features (References p. 128)

Until further genetic studies have clarified the situation ordinary baldness of early and of late-onset must be regarded as variants of a single clinical syndrome. The very high incidence of some degree of common baldness, and the great frequency of many disorders of hair growth, in particular the temporary and reversible disturbance of the hair cycle, inevitably results in the frequent fortuitous association of one or more disorders with common baldness.

The essential clinical feature of common baldness in both sexes is the replacement of terminal hairs by progressively finer hairs, which are eventually short and virtually unpigmented. This process may begin at any age after puberty and may become clinically apparent by the age of 17 in the normal male and by 25–30 in the endocrinologically normal female. The reduction in the size of the follicles is accompanied by shortening of anagen and by increased shedding of telogen hairs. This shedding often attracts the patient's attention and induces him or her to seek advice.

Males
The replacement of terminal by smaller hairs occurs characteristically in a distinctive pattern, which spares the posterior and lateral scalp margins, even in the most advanced cases, and even in old age. The sequence of patterns in the male has been described by Hamilton (see Fig. 4.8). Bitemporal recession is followed by balding of the vertex. Eventually more uniform frontal recession joins the bald areas and the entire frontovertical region bears only inconspicuous secondary vellus hair, which may also finally be lost. Variations in the pattern are governed at least in part by genetic factors, as can be confirmed in any large collection of family portraits. The rate of progression too is probably determined by heredity; however, in the absence of evidence it would be wrong to exclude the possible influence of other factors.

Females
The use of the term 'male pattern alopecia' must be held partly responsible for the frequent failure to appreciate that in its earlier stages common baldness in women need not conform to the 'male pattern'. As in the male, increased shedding of telogen hairs accompanies the reduction of shaft diameter, but the follicles first affected are more widely distributed over the frontovertical region. As a result many secondary vellus hairs are interspersed with hairs still normal and others only slightly reduced in diameter. Partial baldness is sometimes first apparent on the vertex, but the most frequent presentation of common baldness in women is as a diffuse alopecia (Maguire & Kligman 1963; Vadasz & Debreczeni 1967). Ludwig

(1977) has classified the succession of patterns which occur in women to produce the distinctive clinical features of 'female pattern alopecia' (Figs 4.9, 4.11 & 4.12). However, Venning & Dawber (1988) have shown that all women display a change of scalp hair pattern after puberty. The rate of change of patterning is very slow but accelerates during and after the menopause. These workers also showed that hair patterns of the classical male type shown by Hamilton (Fig. 4.8) occur with increasing frequency after the menopause with some women showing extensive Hamilton patterns V–VII. The occurrence of Ludwig pattern II–III or Hamilton pattern IV or greater in a premenopausal woman is unlikely to occur in the absence of abnormal circulating androgens (Miller *et al.* 1982; De Villez & Dunn 1986; Moltz *et al.* 1988; Futterweit *et al.* 1988). Androgens also stimulate sebaceous gland activity. The frequent complaint of greasy scalp and seborrhoea (Fig. 4.12) made by women with thinning hair may be due to the refatting kinetics of fine hair as no true increase in sebum production has been demonstrated. A full medical history and examination are essential, and in many cases endocrinological investigation is desirable in all women with common baldness of rapid onset, even if it be an isolated abnormality, and in women with common baldness of gradual onset but accompanied by menstrual disturbance, hirsutism or recrudescence of acne. Hair loss of Hamilton Type IV may occur in women without hirsutism but more extensive baldness (Type V–VII) is always accompanied by hirsutism (Fig. 4.10).

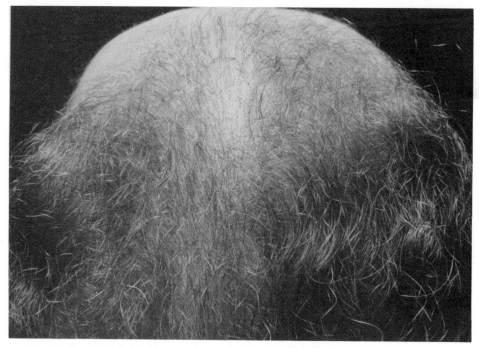

Fig. 4.10 Male pattern baldness in a woman with an ovarian tumour.

References

De Villez, R.L. & Dunn, J. (1986) Female androgenic alopecia. The 3α,17β-androstanediol glucu-ronide/sex hormone binding globulin ratio as a possible marker for female pattern baldness. *Archives of Dermatology*, **122**, 1011.

Futterweit, W., Dunif, A., Yeh, H.-C. & Kingsley, P. (1988) The prevalence of hyperandrogenism in 109 consecutive female patients with diffuse alopecia. *Journal of the American Academy of Dermatology*, **19**, 831.

Ludwig, E. (1977) Classification of the types of androgenic alopecia (common baldness) occurring in the female sex. *British Journal of Dermatology*, **97**, 247.

Maguire, H.C. & Kligman, A.M. (1963) Common baldness in women. *Geriatrics*, **18**, 329.

Miller, J.A., Darley, C.R., Karkavitsas, K., Kirby, J.D. & Munro, D.D. (1982) Low sex-hormone binding globulin levels in young women with diffuse hair loss. *British Journal of Dermatology*, **106**, 331.

Moltz, L. (1988) Hormonale Diagnostik der sogenannten androgenetischen Alopezie der Frau. *Geburtshilfe-Frauenheilkunde*, **48**, 203.

Vadasz, E. & Debreczeni, M. (1967) Untersuchungen zur Ätiologie der androgenetischen Alopecie der Frau. *Hautarzt*, **18**, 454.

Venning, V.A. & Dawber, R. (1988) Patterned androgenic alopecia. *Journal of the American Academy of Dermatology*, **18**, 1073.

Diagnosis

Males

In the male over 25 years of age, the characteristic pattern of the baldness usually makes diagnosis a simple matter, provided that the possible co-existence of hair loss of a different type is constantly borne in mind. Such a possibility may be suggested by a history of recent rapid deterioration. It is frequently necessary to see the patient on several occasions over a period of some weeks before a definite conclusion can be reached, and investigations to exclude the known causes of diffuse hair loss may be required.

In the younger male, the diagnosis may be difficult. He often complains principally not of baldness, but of increased shedding, particularly when he washes his hair. In such patients it is not always easy to determine whether shedding is really excessive or whether introspection born of depression has made him abnormally apprehensive of physiological shedding. Sometimes he may complain of baldness which is not evident to the observer. Such patients should not be dismissed with casual reassurance, but should be re-examined at intervals, after a detailed medical and social history has been taken. A strong family history may support a diagnosis of common baldness, but the absence of such a history does not exclude the diagnosis. The presence or absence of seborrhoea is not of diagnostic significance, for this is a genetic variable, and seborrhoea is evidence merely of normal sexual maturation in a susceptible subject.

Very rare cases may include hyperprolactinaemic states in which a small but distinctive group of young adult males present a history of increased shedding of head hair and also some loss of body and pubic hair. The patient is usually depressed and may also complain of loss of libido and partial impotence. Sometimes the distribution of subcutaneous fat approaches the female pattern.

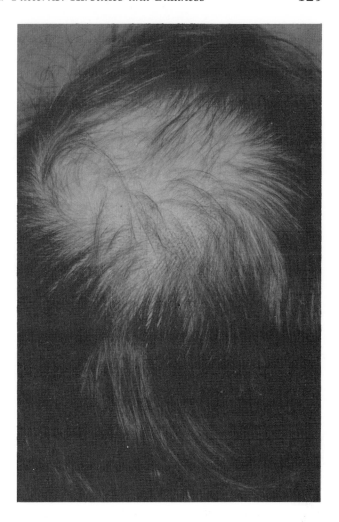

Fig. 4.11 Androgenetic
alopecia of well over 20
years' duration in a woman
aged 60.

Females

In women, the diagnosis of common baldness may be difficult. The most frequent
presentation is a diffuse frontovertical thinning and the patient may complain
that her hair has become finer and greasier. In all cases it should be regarded as
one of three cutaneous manifestations of androgenic stimulation and the presence
of acne and/or hirsutism should be noted. In the presence of such changes
endocrinological assessment may be desirable. In their absence, particularly if
there is a strong family history of baldness, the diagnosis may present no problems.
As in men the association of common baldness with other forms of hair loss is
frequently encountered, and many cases require careful evaluation over a period
of weeks. An accurate diagnosis is of importance in prognosis, and at times a
biopsy may be useful.

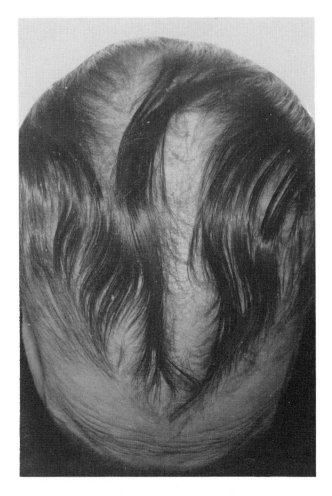

Fig. 4.12 Androgenetic alopecia in a woman accompanied by gross seborrhoea.

Therapy (References p. 133)

There is effective treatment which prevents further transformation of terminal into vellus hair for many women in whom the severity of their baldness is the result of abnormal androgen metabolism. In many countries there is a topical preparation which prevents further progression and may even appear to reverse common baldness in males. The available procedures, surgical and medical are discussed below.

Surgery

All surgical procedures are attempts to spread parietal and occipital hairs thinly over the rest of the scalp. Hair transplantation involves the removal of plugs of bald scalp by punch biopsy followed by insertion of hair-bearing punches (Orentreich 1959). Correct orientation of each punch is essential. Hair will only grow in the transplanted area, which on a very bald scalp may lead to a 'dolls head' or toothbrush appearance. Rotation flaps from the parietal to the frontal area may give a better appearance to the frontal hair line (Juri 1975; Elliot 1977; Dardour 1985). Reduction of the bald area by removal of an ellipse from the vault or repeated such operations may cover the top of the head by stretching the remaining parietal scalp (Bell 1982). However, the over-enthusiastic operator may produce necrosis of the remaining scalp from excessive tension on the sutures. Tissue expansion techniques for breast reconstruction have been used successfully to restore post-traumatic alopecia and more recently for common baldness in men (Manders *et al.* 1987; Masser 1988). The technique involves implantation of inflatable bags under the skin of the scalp. These bags are inflated progressively over 6 weeks with resultant stretching of the overlying scalp. It is then possible to excise the bald central area and to oppose the expanded tissue and suture to close the deficit. While patients and surgeons alike are pleased with the result of this technique the expansion phase distorts the subject's appearance to such an extent that he may wish to remain indoors for as long as 2–3 months.

Wigs
In women the baldness is usually too diffuse for transplantation surgery to be possible. If the hair loss is extensive, only a wig will conceal it. In addition, there are various procedures by which small wigs are interwoven with the pre-existing terminal hair in men and the cosmetic result is sometimes satisfactory. However, subjects should be warned that their hair will continue to grow and tend to 'lift off' the interwoven wig necessitating frequent readjustment which is expensive. The patient who seeks advice from his doctor before embarking on some such procedure should be assessed in the same way as a patient considering surgery and the issue must be addressed as to whether baldness is really the problem. The subject should be advised to obtain a written statement of the probable cost of the initial procedure and subsequent regular maintenance. Tension on the patient's surviving terminal hair has occasionally led to patchy scarring alopecia (Perlstein 1969).

Anti-androgens
The side effects of anti-androgens preclude their use in men. There is little scientific evidence for regrowth of hair in women with cyproterone acetate but the drug in doses of 50–100 mg per day with ethinyl oestradiol may prevent further progression (Ekoe *et al.* 1980; Mortimer *et al.* 1984). Burke & Cunliffe (1985) reported a subjective improvement with oral spironolactone and Aram (1987) claimed success with high dose cimetidine which also has anti-androgenic activity. Topical anti-androgens are ineffective in the human but Rittmaster *et al.* (1987) reported that a topical 5α-reductase inhibitor prevented the onset of baldness in four stump-tailed macaques.

Non-hormonal therapy
Groveman *et al.* (1985) were the first to demonstrate a definite placebo response after centuries of unsuccessful patent remedies for baldness. Claims for regrowth of

hair in common baldness as part of a general hypertrichosis have been made for oral minoxidil (Zappacosta 1980), benoxaprofen (Fenton *et al.* 1982), cyclosporin A (Harper *et al.* 1984) and PUVA (Singh & Lal 1967). With the exceptions of minoxidil and tretinoin, topical use of these drugs has produced sporadic and disappointing results.

Minoxidil is a piperidinopyrimidine derivative and a potent vasodilator which is effective orally for severe hypertension. When applied topically as a solution in an alcohol and water base containing 10% propylene glycol, minoxidil has shown conversion of vellus to terminal hair in up to 30% of individuals (Vanderveen *et al.* 1984; De Villez 1985; Olsen *et al.* 1985, 1987; Shupak *et al.* 1987; Reitschel & Duncan 1987; Savin 1987; Civatte *et al.* 1987). Terminal hair appeared to regrow at the margins but complete covering of the bald areas was seen in less than 10% of responders. De Villez (1985) suggested that bald men who responded best to minoxidil were those in whom the balding process was at an early stage with a maximum diameter of the bald area less than 10 cm and in whom the pretreatment hair density was in excess of 20 hairs/cm^2. There was an increasing dose response up to 2% minoxidil using the recommended 1 ml twice daily regimen (Olsen *et al.* 1987; Shupak *et al.* 1987).

The mode of action of minoxidil is unknown but a shortening of the vellus hair cycle with histological thickening of growing hairs with maintenance of anagen has been seen in the scalps of stump-tailed macaques (*Macaca arctoides*) (Uno *et al.* 1985, 1987). Minoxidil does not have anti-androgenic properties (Nuck *et al.* 1987) and there is no effect on sebaceous gland activity (Simpson & Stewart 1987). Wester *et al.* (1984) found an increase in the cutaneous blood flow of the scalp in a small study but failed to demonstrate a dose–response and did not include a positive control. However, Bunker and Dowd (1988) found no change in cutaneous blood flow in a well-designed experiment using a similar technique and a positive control. Minoxidil sulphate may be an active metabolite following oral administration (Johnson *et al.* 1982); skin demonstrates sulphatase and sulpho-transferase activity, but this aspect has yet to be explored scientifically.

Topical minoxidil appears to be a safe therapy with side effects only of local irritation and a low incidence of contact dermatitis (Tosti *et al.* 1985). Withdrawal of therapy leads to regression of enlarged follicles in the stump-tailed macaque (Uno *et al.* 1987) and clinical regression in man occurs after 3 months to the state of baldness that would have existed if no treatment had been applied (Olsen & Weiner 1987; Shrank 1989). Patients should be warned that in order to maintain any beneficial effect applications must continue twice daily for ever (Olsen *et al.* 1990). The effectiveness of topical minoxidil in women with common baldness is unproven but could be expected to match results seen in males. Combination therapies may prove to be beneficial in the future; Bazzano *et al.* (1986) found in a 1-year study that topical tretinoin and 0.5% minoxidil was as efficient as 2% minoxidil alone. Vermoken (1983) failed to show synergism with the anti-androgen cyproterone acetate and minoxidil and Pestana *et al.* (1987) found no additional effect of ultraviolet light and topical minoxidil in advanced male-pattern baldness.

Summary

The availability of a topical treatment which appears to some extent to reverse the problem of common baldness in males has encouraged many young men to seek medical help. These men should be counselled carefully and made aware of the need for continuous use to maintain any effect. It is preferable that treatment advice be given by qualified medical practitioners who are fully aware of the pitfalls of treatment so that these vulnerable individuals may be kept away from commercial centres where profit is the only motivation. Each patient needs careful medical assessment to ensure that the diagnosis is beyond doubt. He or she should then be given a detailed explanation of the nature and significance of common baldness. Most men, if they are mildly affected, will accept the situation philosophically. Many, however, when baldness first becomes manifest at a stressful stage of their career, may attempt to lay the blame for any lack of success, socially or at work, on their baldness, even when this is of minimal extent. Such patients should be encouraged to discuss their problem in full. In the course of doing so they often become aware that they have not seen their baldness in its proper perspective, but may be enabled to do so. However, in some patients this lack of insight is only one of the many manifestations of a depressive illness which may require treatment.

References

Aram, H. (1987) Treatment of female androgenetic alopecia with cimetidine. *International Journal of Dermatology*, **26**, 128.

Bazzano, G.S., Terezakis, N. & Gaylon, W. (1986) Topical tretinoin for hair growth promotion. *Journal of the American Academy of Dermatology*, **15**, 880.

Bell, M.L. (1982) Role of scalp reduction in the treatment of male pattern baldness. *Plastic and Reconstructive Surgery*, **69**, 272.

Bunker, C.B. & Dowd, P.M. (1988) Alterations in scalp blood flow after the epicutaneous application of 3% minoxidil and 0.1% hexylnicotinate in alopecia (Correspondence). *British Journal of Dermatology*, **117**, 668.

Burke, B. & Cunliffe, W.J. (1985) Oral spironolactone therapy for female patients with acne, hirsutism or androgenic alopecia (Correspondence). *British Journal of Dermatology*, **112**, 124.

Civatte, J., Laux, B., Simpson, N.B. & Vickers, C.F.H. (1987) 2% topical minoxidil solution in male-pattern baldness: preliminary European results, *Dermatologica*, **175** (suppl. 2), 42.

Dardour, J.C. (1985) Treatment of male pattern baldness with a one stage flap. *Aesthetic Plastic Surgery*, **9**, 109.

De Villez, R.L. (1985) Topical minoxidil therapy in hereditary androgenetic alopecia. *Archives of Dermatology*, **121**, 197.

Ekoe, J.K., Burckhardt, P. & Ruedi, B. (1980) Treatment of hirsutism, acne and alopecia with cyproterone acetate. *Dermatologica*, **160**, 398.

Elliot, R.A. (1977) Lateral scalp flaps for instant results in male pattern baldness. *Plastic and Reconstructive Surgery*, **60**, 699.

Fenton, D.A., English, J.S. & Wilkinson, J.D. (1982) Reversal of male pattern baldness, hypertrichosis and accelerated hair and nail growth in patients receiving benoxaprofen. *British Medical Journal*, **284**, 1228.

Groveman, H.D., Ganiats, T. & Klauber, M.R. (1985) Lack of efficacy of polysorbate 60 in the treatment of male pattern baldness. *Archives of Internal Medicine*, **145**, 1454.

Harper, J.I., Kendra, J.R., Desai, S., Staughton, R.C.D., Barrett, A.J. & Hobbs, J.R. (1984) Dermatological aspects of the use of cyclosporin A for prophylaxis of graft versus host disease. *British Journal of Dermatology*, 110, 469.

Johnson, G.A., Barsuhn, K.J. & McCall, J.M. (1982) Sulfation of minoxidil by liver sulfotransferase. *Biochemical Pharmacology*, 31, 2949.

Juri, J. (1975) Use of parieto-occipital flaps in the surgical treatment of baldness. *Plastic and Reconstructive Surgery*, 55, 456.

Manders, E.K., Au, V.K. & Wong, R.K. (1987) Scalp expansion for male pattern baldness. *Clinics of Plastic Surgery*, 14, 469.

Masser, M.R. (1988) A twin tissue expander used in the elimination of alopecia. *Plastic and Reconstructive Surgery*, 81, 444.

Mortimer, C.H., Rushton, H. & James, K.C. (1984) Effective medical treatment for common baldness in women. *Clinical and Experimental Dermatology*, 9, 342.

Nuck, B.A., Fogelson, S.L. & Lucky, A.W. (1987) Topical minoxidil does not act as an anti-androgen in the flank organ of the golden Syrian hamster. *Archives of Dermatology*, 123, 59.

Olsen, E.A., Weiner, M.S., Delong, E.R. & Pinnell, S.R. (1985) Topical minoxidil in early male pattern baldness. *Journal of the American Academy of Dermatology*, 13, 185.

Olsen, E.A., Delong, E.R. & Weiner, M.S. (1987) Long-term follow-up of men with male pattern baldness treated with topical minoxidil. *Journal of the American Academy of Dermatology*, 16, 688.

Olsen, E.A. & Weiner, M.S. (1987) Topical minoxidil in male pattern baldness; effects of discontinuation of treatment. *Journal of the American Academy of Dermatology*, 17, 97.

Olsen, E.A., Weiner, M.S., Amara, I.A. & Delong, E.R. (1990) Five year follow-up of men with androgenetic alopecia treated with topical minoxidil. *Journal of the American Academy of Dermatology*, 22, 643.

Orentreich, N. (1959) Autografts in alopecias and other selected dermatological conditions. *Annals of the New York Academy of Sciences*, 83, 463.

Perlstein, H.H. (1969) Traction alopecia due to hair weaving. *Cutis*, 5, 440.

Pestana, A., Olsen, E.A., Delong, E.R. & Murray, J.C. (1987) Effect of ultraviolet light on topical minoxidil-induced hair growth in advanced male pattern baldness. *Journal of the American Academy of Dermatology*, 16, 971.

Reitschel, R.L. & Duncan, S.H. (1987) Safety and efficacy of topical minoxidil in the management of androgenetic alopecia. *Journal of the American Academy of Dermatology*, 16, 677.

Rittmaster, R.S., Uno, H., Povar, M.L., Mellin, T.N. & Loriaux, D.L. (1987) The effects of N, N-Diethyl-4-methyl-3-oxo-4-aza-5α-androstane-17β-carboxamide, a 5α-reductase inhibitor and antiandrogen on the development of baldness in the stumptail macaque. *Journal of Clinical Endocrinology and Metabolism*, 65, 188.

Savin, R.C. (1987) Use of topical minoxidil in the treatment of male pattern baldness. *Journal of the American Academy of Dermatology*, 16, 696.

Shupak, J.L., Kassimir, J.J., Thirumoorthy, T., Reed, M.L. & Jondreau, L. (1987) Dose–response study of topical minoxidil in male pattern alopecia. *Journal of the American Academy of Dermatology*, 16, 673.

Shrank, A. (1989) Treating young men with hair loss. *British Medical Journal*, 298, 847.

Simpson, N.B. & Stewart, E.J.C. (1987) Scalp sebum excretion is unaffected by topical minoxidil. *Abstracts of the XVII World Congress of Dermatology, Berlin, 24–29 May 1987.*

Singh, G. & Lal, S. (1967) Hypertrichosis and hyperpigmentation with systemic psoralen treatment. *British Journal of Dermatology*, 79, 501.

Tosti, A., Bardazzi, F., De Padova, M.P., Caponeri, G.M., Melino, M. & Veronesi, S. (1985) Contact dermatitis to minoxidil. *Contact Dermatitis*, 13, 275.

Uno, H., Kappas, A. & Brigham, P. (1987) Action of topical minoxidil in the bald stump-tailed macaque. *Journal of the American Academy of Dermatology*, 16, 657.

Uno, H., Kappas, A. & Schlagel, C. (1985) Cyclic dynamics of hair follicles and the effect of minoxidil on the bald scalps of stump tailed macaques. *American Journal of Dermatopathology*, 7, 283.

Vanderveen, E.C., Ellis, C.N., Kang, S., Case, P., Headington, J.T., Voorhees, J.J. & Swanson, N.A. (1984) Topical minoxidil for hair regrowth. *Journal of the American Academy of Dermatology*, 11, 416.

Vermoken, A.J.M. (1983) Reversal of androgenetic alopecia by minoxidil: lack of effect of simultaneously administered doses of cyproterone acetate. *Acta Dermato-Venereologica,* **63**, 268.

Wester, R.C., Maibach, H.I., Guy, R.H. & Novak, E. (1984) Minoxidil stimulates cutaneous blood flow in human balding scalps: Pharmacodynamics measured by laser doppler velocimetry and photopulse plethysmography. *Journal of Investigative Dermatology,* **82**, 515.

Zappacosta, A.R. (1980) Reversal of baldness in a patient receiving minoxidil for hypertension. *New England Journal of Medicine,* **303**, 1480.

Chapter 5
Diffuse Alopecia: Endocrine, Metabolic and Chemical Influences on the Follicular Cycle

History and nomenclature
(References p. 143)

Diffuse shedding of hair has been called 'symptomatic alopecia', or defluvium capillorum. Some authors, for example Sabouraud (1932), restricted the latter term to sudden diffuse loss of hair following shortly after a severe emotional shock, while others applied it to all forms of alopecia.

Kligman (1961), in a lucid and influential article, studied the pathodynamics of one common pattern of response of hair follicles to a variety of insults and named it telogen effluvium. Kligman cannot be held responsible for the frequent misuse of this term by some authors. During the 1950s many authors described 'chronic diffuse alopecia' in women (e.g. Sulzberger *et al.* 1960). This syndrome was differentiated from acute diffuse reversible alopecia, attributable in most cases to a readily identifiable cause. The majority of such patients have common (androgenetic) baldness, undiagnosed because of the misleading use of the term male pattern alopecia (see Chapter 4).

In this chapter we are concerned with the clinical syndrome of diffuse alopecia in either sex. Many of the conditions which can give rise to the various forms of the syndrome are discussed in greater detail in other chapters.

Pathogenesis
(References p. 143)

The daily shedding of telogen hairs diffusely distributed over the scalp is a physiological process. Follicles which have shed their hairs normally re-enter anagen, the trichogram remains unchanged and no alopecia results. If, however, a significant number of hair follicles prematurely enter catagen and thence telogen, the excessive shedding of hair inevitably takes place some 2–3 months later. The hair is temporarily sparse but regrows normally if the insult is not repeated. This is the mechanism of 'telogen effluvium', which may be induced by childbirth, high fever, haemorrhage, sudden starvation, accidental or surgical trauma, severe emotional stress, and by certain drugs.

The sudden diffuse shedding of telogen hairs is one of the responses of the hair follicles to the unknown insult or insults of alopecia areata (see Chapter 10).

Follicles which shed their hairs at the end of a normal telogen may temporarily fail to re-enter anagen. Diffuse thinning of the scalp hair then develops slowly in the absence of any increase in the rate of hair shedding. This form of diffuse alopecia is seen in iron deficiency (Quinones & Garcia Munoz 1963; Aquilera Maruri 1966). Malnutrition, whether primary or secondary, is accompanied by diffuse shedding of telogen hairs, usually in association with changes in shaft diameter and pigmentation. The mechanism of hair loss in hypothyroidism and hypopituitarism may well be similar, but has not been adequately studied. The metabolic disturbances that accompany severe impairment of liver function may be associated with increased shedding of telogen hairs (Zaun *et al.* 1969).

The gross metabolic disturbance following resection of a large part of the liver for a massive hepatoma was associated with severe alopecia. In one such case (Starzl *et al.* 1975) hair loss developed within a few days post-operatively. The liver gradually regenerated, and the hair regrew in 9 months.

Hair loss in patients with malignant disease has been relatively little investigated by modern methods; it is diffuse, with increased shedding of telogen hair. It was formerly attributed to a hypothetical 'cancer toxin', but it may well be the result of iron deficiency or hypoproteinaemia. Alopecia has occurred as an early sign of Hodgkin's disease (Klein *et al.* 1973) (see also Chapter 16).

The problem of so-called idiopathic chronic diffuse alopecia in women has already been mentioned. Most such women have ordinary baldness, periods of progression of which are always preceded and accompanied by increased shedding of telogen hairs (see Chapter 4). Common baldness is common in many races and frequently occurs in association with hair loss of other origins. Multifactorial alopecia is often encountered (Steigleder & Mahrle 1973) and a double or even a treble diagnosis may be appropriate.

Diffuse alopecia caused by drugs or other chemicals will be considered in some detail on pp. 153–161 and will be discussed here only as a problem in differential diagnosis.

The role of psychological factors in diffuse alopecia is controversial and very difficult to assess. There is circumstantial evidence that acute stress may precipitate acute reversible hair loss (Sabouraud 1932; Kligman 1961). Androgenetic common baldness in women may be associated with depression (Eckert 1975); the patient may blame the alopecia for the depression, but there are some patients in whom depression antedates or exactly coincides with the onset of alopecia. Depression may lead a patient to become aware of, and concerned about, hair shedding of physiological degree.

The association of alopecia with organic lesions of the central nervous system has been the subject of many case reports but no consistent picture emerges. Head injuries, particularly in children, have been followed by diffuse alopecia, often associated with reversible hirsutism, which may be asymmetrical (Tarnow 1971). Total alopecia has been seen in association with postencephalitic damage to the brain stem, and with a glioma of the hypothalamus (Hoff & Riehl 1937–8). Recurrent annual hair loss in a patient with syringo-encephalia and syringobulbia remains mysterious (Mikula & Steidl 1961). Our almost complete ignorance of the effects of the central nervous system on hair growth is further emphasized by the report of frequent episodes of generalized piloerection in a patient with a deep parietal glioblastoma (Brody *et al.* 1960).

Incidence
(References p. 143)

The incidence of diffuse alopecia is high in both sexes, but most episodes of increased shedding are transitory and cause little or no concern. Shedding, whether acute or chronic, which leads to a significant degree of baldness is also common and although large numbers of such patients are referred to dermatologists these represent only a small proportion of those affected, many of whom do not even consult their own doctor. Hospital statistics are therefore biased, but no others are available.

Alexander (1965) studied 98 women with diffuse alopecia, excluding cases in which the hair loss was of 'male pattern'. She found that the alopecia had followed fever in 10, childbirth in 10, and was a manifestation of alopecia areata in nine. Drugs were incriminated in five cases. External trauma from self-inflicted cosmetic procedures was involved in no fewer than 36 cases, and in six the physical or chemical trauma had been inflicted by hairdressers. In five the alopecia was associated with anaemia and in one case it was caused by syphilis. Sixteen patients remained unclassified. Bergfeld (1978) confirmed the importance of trauma. Patchy baldness with broken hairs and eventually some scarring may be produced by the excessively frequent application of hair dyes over a long period (Brown & Brayles 1980).

Eckert and her colleagues (1967) excluded cases of alopecia areata from their series of 150 women with diffuse alopecia. They found only seven patients with alopecia of the male pattern. Cosmetic trauma was the cause of the hair loss in 11, seven had seborrhoeic dermatitis and two had icthyosis involving the scalp. In 14 the alopecia had followed parturition, in four it was post-febrile. Two patients had systemic lupus erythematosus and eight were iron deficient. In six cases amphetamines were incriminated. Endocrine disorders were present in 21 cases; hypothyroidism in 16, hyperthyroidism in two, and hypopituitarism in three. Three patients developed alopecia after oophorectomy, but, as the authors pointed out, there was no evidence that the menopause was a factor in diffuse alopecia. In 68 patients no associated factors, local or systemic, could be found.

These authors failed to find a cause in 16 to over 45% of patients. Most of these women probably had common baldness (see Chapter 4). In over 350 cases of diffuse alopecia in women at Cambridge more than 60% had the diffuse type of common baldness. In 5% no cause whatever could be established, but many of these cases may well have had common baldness.

The scarcity of publications on diffuse alopecia in men is due to the fact that the large proportion who have common baldness are readily recognized as such, although diagnosis may be delayed in young men who present with diffuse shedding and have as yet no patterned baldness. After common baldness the most frequent causes of diffuse alopecia in young males are alopecia areata, fevers and drugs, and in older males drugs and malignant disease.

Aetiology
(References p. 143)

Post-febrile alopecia (Fig. 5.1)
It is said that the fever must exceed 39°C (Sabouraud 1932). In the days before antibiotics typhoid and tuberculosis were the classical causes. Recurrent bouts of fever have a more marked effect than a single bout, for each damages follicles at the same susceptible stage of their cycle. Fever of any origin has a similar effect; diffuse alopecia may follow febrile episodes in ulcerative colitis (Schwenzner & Walther 1961) and after influenza, malaria, glandular fever, pneumonia and brucellosis. Erysipelas of the scalp may lead to early shedding of hair from the affected region with more delayed loss from the remainder of the scalp (Sabouraud 1932). Post-febrile alopecia begins 8–10 weeks after the first damaging bout of fever; it may be severe but is never total. Full recovery is the rule, but is not invariable particularly when the fever has been prolonged or recurrent (Alexander 1965).

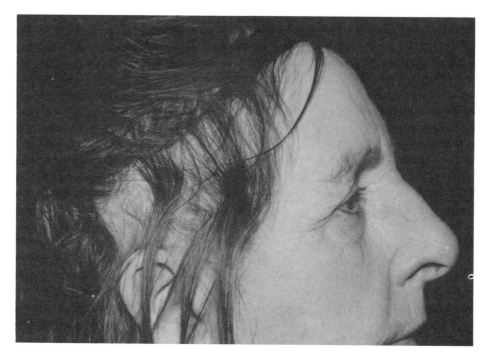

Fig. 5.1 Diffuse post-febrile alopecia.

Postpartum alopecia

Some postpartum increase in hair loss is probably universal, but hair loss sufficient to cause anxiety to the patient is not uncommon, and occasionally quite severe alopecia may occur. The increased loss of hair becomes obvious 1 month after childbirth in some women but only after 2–3 months in the majority, and may occasionally be delayed until after 4 months (Schiff & Kern 1963; Skelton 1966). For unknown reasons the loss is usually most marked in the frontal and temporal regions, but may be generalized; it is never total. Full spontaneous recovery takes 3–12 months.

Drug-induced alopecia

In the presence of diffuse alopecia a careful history of all recent medication is essential and the possibility of industrial or accidental exposure to chemicals must be considered. Microscopy of shed and growing hairs (see Chapter 19) may reveal the type of injury to the follicles and thus help to incriminate a particular type of chemical.

Stress-induced alopecia

Severe hair loss beginning 2 weeks after severe stress, as reported by Sabouraud (1932) and other authors, requires further study; some at least of such cases may be alopecia areata.

Desai and Roaf (1984) reported telogen effluvium in a patient after prolonged surgery with regrowth after 4 months. This would appear to differ from the patchy alopecia after long operations which has been presumed to be due to localized pressure (Abel & Lewis 1960).

Alopecia and food deprivation
Alopecia and the other hair changes associated with primary or secondary malnutrition are not easily overlooked. Acute voluntary starvation in young women is common and may be missed as a cause of hair loss. Obese adolescents sometimes inflict upon themselves a diet of salads and fruit, even when they do not have anorexia nervosa. Rooth and Carlström (1970) noted hair loss and weakness in 20 obese patients on a 200-calorie diet or total fast, but these changes were prevented by the addition of a small amount of protein.

Hypoproteinaemia
Hypoprotinaemia of metabolic as well as of dietary origin may lead to the premature onset of telogen in some follicles. This possibly accounts for the temporary diffuse loss of hair which may follow blood loss, including voluntary blood donation.

Iron deficiency
Iron deficiency, even in the absence of anaemia, may be a factor in diffuse alopecia, but it is a common condition and its fortuitous association with common baldness is therefore to be expected. However, if iron deficiency is discovered its cause should be established and it should be treated.

Alopecia in malignant disease, in renal failure and in hepatic insufficiency
The diffuse hair loss has no distinctive feature.

Diffuse alopecia areata (see also Chapter 10)
Rapid onset of diffuse alopecia may be the first sign of alopecia areata, particularly in young patients (Fig. 5.2). Diagnostic changes may be lacking, for alopecia areata may cause widespread precipitation into telogen. The diagnosis can then only be suspected, and perhaps confirmed by the subsequent course.

Syphilis
Diffuse hair loss may occur in secondary syphilis, in which the classical 'moth-eaten' appearance is not always present.

Traumatic alopecia (see Chapter 9)
In this book we do not apply the term diffuse alopecia to the patchy or widespread damage to hair shafts by physical or chemical agents but many authors (Alexander 1965; Eckert *et al.* 1967) include it among the diagnostic

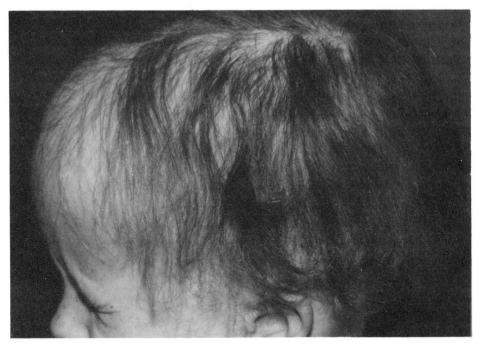

Fig. 5.2 Diffuse alopecia in a child. The cause was not established. The diffuse form of alopecia areata is probable, but a toxic origin could not be excluded. Spontaneous recovery took place.

possibilities. Certainly it must be excluded by a careful history, supported by microscopy of the damaged hairs and it must be remembered that misguided 'treatment' of diffuse alopecia of any origin may add variations to the clinical picture.

The compulsive plucking of hair in psychologically disturbed women may denude the scalp almost completely, leaving only a carpet of 1-cm stumps.

Diagnosis

The diagnosis of diffuse alopecia is time consuming and often cannot be accomplished in a single consultation. A detailed general medical history is essential. First, common baldness must be excluded. Microscopy of growing and of shed hair should always be carried out. It may reveal evidence of physical and chemical damage to hair shafts; it may show dystrophic anagen hairs, the fractured hairs of cytotoxic injury, or the unsuspected presence of a congenital defect of shaft formation which has rendered the hair unduly susceptible to trauma.

Treatment

Treatment is the treatment of the cause, when this can be established.

References

Abel, R.R. & Lewis, G.M. (1960) Post operative (pressure) alopecia. *AMA Archives of Dermatology*, **81**, 34.

Alexander, S. (1965) Diffuse alopecia in women. *Transactions of the St John's Hospital Dermatological Society*, **51**, 99.

Aquilera Maruri, C. (1966) Alopecia diffusa feminina e hiposideremia. *Actas Dermo-Sifiliograficas*, **57**, 169.

Bergfeld, W. (1978) Diffuse hair loss in women. *Cutis*, **22**, 190.

Brody, I.A., Odom, G.L. & Kunkle, E.C. (1960) Pilomotor seizures. *Neurology*, **10**, 993.

Brown, A.C. & Brayles, J.A. (1980) Accumulative scarring of the scalp due to hair dyes. In *Hair, Trace Elements and Human Illness*, p. 348, eds. A.C. Brown & R.G. Crounse. Praeger, New York.

Desai, S.P. & Roaf, E.R. (1984) Telogen effluvium after anesthesia and surgery. *Anesthesia and Analgesia*, **63**, 83.

Eckert, J. (1975) Diffuse hair loss and psychiatric disturbance. *Acta Dermato-Venereologica*, **55**, 147.

Eckert, J., Church, R.E., Ebling, F.L. & Munra, D.S. (1967) Hair loss in women. *British Journal of Dermatology*, **79**, 543.

Hoff, H. & Riehl, G. (1937-8) Zur Frage der durch Erkrankung des Zentralnervensystems bedingter Alopecie. *Archiv für Dermatologie und Syphilologie*, **176**, 191.

Klein, A.W., Rudolph, R.I. & Leyden, J.J. (1973) Telogen effluvium as a sign of Hodgkin's disease. *Archives of Dermatology*, **108**, 702.

Kligman, A.M. (1961) Pathologic dynamics of reversible hair loss in human. I. Telogen effluvium. *AMA Archives of Dermatology*, **83**, 175.

Mikula, F. & Steidl, L. (1961) Ein Beitrag zur Ätiopathogenase der periodischer Alopezie. *Dermatologische Wochenschrift*, **143**, 543.

Quinones, P.A. & Garcia Munoz, C.M. (1963) El metabolismo del hierro en las alopecias—Alopecias difusas femininas y 'ferropenia latente'. *Actas Dermo-Sifiliograficas*, **54**, 425.

Rooth, G. & Carlström, S. (1970) Therapeutic fasting. *Acta Medica Scandinavica*, **187**, 455.

Sabouraud, R. (1932) *Diagnostic et Traitement des Affections du Cuir Chevelu*, p. 342. Masson, Paris.

Schiff, B.L. & Kern, A.B. (1963) Study of postpartum alopecia. *AMA Archives of Dermatology*, **87**, 609.

Schwenzner, G. & Walther, H. (1961) Alopecia diffusa bei Colitis ulcerosa und nach allgemeiner zytostatischer Therapie mittles Endoxan. *Zeitschrift für Haut und Geschlectskrankheiten*, **31**, 211.

Skelton, J.B. (1966) Postpartum alopecia. *American Journal of Obstetrics and Gynecology*, **94**, 125.

Starzl, T.E. Putnam, C.W., Groth, C.G., Corman, J.L. & Taubman, J. (1975) Alopecia, ascites and incomplete regeneration after 85–95% liver resection. *American Journal of Surgery*, **129**, 587.

Steigleder, G.K. & Mahrle, G. (1973) Haarausfall als polyätiologisches Symptom. *Fortschritte der praktischen Dermatologie und Venereologie*, **7**, 237.

Sulzberger, M.B., Witten, V.H. & Kopf, A.W. (1960) Diffuse alopecia in women. *AMA Archives of Dermatology*, **81**, 556.

Tarnow, G. (1971) Haarkleidstörungen nach schweren Hirntraumen. *Journal of Neuro-Visceral Relations*, suppl. x, 549.

Zaun, H., Müting, D. & Steinmann, I. (1969) Wachstumsstörungen der Kopfhaare als Folge von Hepatopathien. *Archiv für klinische und experimentelle Dermatologie*, **235**, 386.

The hair in pregnancy
(References p. 144)

When the extent and complexity of the endocrine changes of pregnancy are considered (Hytten & Leitch 1971) their relatively small effects on hair growth seem surprising. However, there is considerable individual variation in these effects and further quantitative investigations are needed.

Many women maintain that their hair is particularly attractive and healthy during pregnancy. Trichograms show no increase in density, but during the second half of pregnancy, the percentage of anagen hairs increases from the normal 85% to about 95% (Lynfield 1960; Pecoraro *et al.* 1969); in order words, the normal shedding of telogen hairs is reduced. At this time the percentage of hairs of large shaft diameter is higher than in non-pregnant women of the same age (Pecoraro *et al.* 1969).

The rate of hair growth is slightly reduced during pregnancy (Pecoraro *et al.* 1969; Bosse 1971. A few women complain that the hair is sparse, especially in the parietal regions. Some follicles which enter a normal telogen phase may fail to re-enter anagen (Bosse 1971), and this, rather than increased shedding, accounts for the clinically evident thinning.

After parturition the follicles, in which anagen has been prolonged, rapidly enter catagen and thus telogen. Increased shedding is evident after a few weeks (1–4 months) (Schiff & Kern 1963; Skelton 1966) and may continue for several months, since shedding that will restore the pre-pregnancy equilibrium is supplemented by further shedding precipitated by the psychophysical trauma of labour, with blood loss, low plasma protein and sometimes also anticoagulants, as contributory factors (Bosse 1971). Full recovery is usual in 4–9 months providing the patient is not debilitated by breast feeding and poor dietary intake. No treatment is available or necessary.

All the changes so far described tend to be less severe in subsequent pregnancies (Pecoraro *et al.* 1969).

The rate of growth of body hair is not normally affected (Trotter 1935). However, hirsutism may develop, usually during the last trimester. In such cases irreversible frontovertical baldness accompanies it in women genetically predisposed to common baldness.

References

Bosse, K. (1971) Haarwachstum und Schwangerschaft. *Schriften der Alfred-Marchionini-Stiftung*, **2**, 59.

Hytten, F.E. & Leitch, I. (1971) *The Physiology of Human Pregnancy*, 2nd edn. Blackwell Scientific Publications, Oxford.

Lynfield, Y.L. (1960) Effect of pregnancy on the human hair cycle. *Journal of Investigative Dermatology*, **35**, 323.

Pecoraro, V., Barman, J.M. & Astore, I. (1969). The normal trichogram of pregnant women. In *Advances in Biology of Skin*, vol. IX, *Hair Growth*, p. 203, eds. W. Montagna & R.L. Dobson. Pergamon Press, Oxford.

Schiff, B.L. & Kern, A.B. (1963) Study of postpartum alopecia. *AMA Archives of Dermatology*, **87**, 609.

Skelton, J.B. (1966) Postpartum alopecia. *American Journal of Obstetrics and Gynecology*, **94**, 125.

Trotter, M. (1935) The activity of hair follicles with reference to pregnancy. *Surgery, Gynecology and Obstetrics*, **60**, 1092.

Oral contraceptives and the hair

Most contraceptive pills consist of a mixture of an oestrogen and a progestogen. Many progestogens possess androgenic activity; therefore, any pill will have a net oestrogenic or androgenic potential. The formulation of oral contraceptives has changed in the last 10 years in an attempt to reduce thromboembolic side effects by providing lower doses of oestrogens. Published observations on the effects of 'the pill' on hair growth have unfortunately been uncontrolled, and have also failed to take into account the nature or the dose of the hormones. Reports such as those of Cormia (1967) and Greenwald (1970) are difficult to evaluate. Both authors noted diffuse alopecia in five women while they were taking, or after they had stopped taking, a contraceptive pill. Other causes of hair loss were not excluded.

Zaun and Gerber (1969) studied 50 women who were taking a contraceptive pill of the combined type. Many patients showed no significant change in the proportion of anagen to telogen scalp follicles. A temporary increase in the proportion of telogen follicles was shown by 25, but the ratio returned to normal by the sixth month. Eleven patients whose telogen percentage was high showed a steady return to normal. Dystrophic changes in hair roots were occasionally seen. In a similar investigation of 51 women taking a sequential contraceptive pill, essentially the same changes were observed but there were no dystrophic hairs (Zaun & Ruffing 1970). In neither group of patients were there clinically evident changes while the pill was being taken. The lack of clinically evident hair loss was confirmed by Griffiths (1973).

Triphasic oestrogen pills are popular because of suppression of the mid-cycle surge of luteinizing hormone, but the net balance of these pills may be androgenic during one or more of the three phases of prescription. 'Pills' with net androgenic activity may induce or worsen acne, hirsutism (Zaun 1972) and common baldness in genetically predisposed women. Women prone to these problems should be prescribed contraceptive pills containing desorgestrol, gestodene or cyproterone acetate as the progestogen.

The observation (Cormia 1967; Greenwald 1970) that many women show increased shedding of hair from 2 weeks to 3–4 months after they stop taking an oral contraceptive has also been confirmed (Dawber & Connor 1971; Griffiths 1973). This hair loss simulates that which is commonly seen after parturition; it seldom results in more than a mild degree of diffuse alopecia, but it varies greatly in degree. Recovery occurs spontaneously.

References

Cormia, F.E. (1967) Alopecia from oral contraceptives. *Journal of the American Medical Association,* **201,** 635.

Dawber, R.P.R. & Connor, B.L. (1971) Pregnancy, hair loss and the pill. *British Medical Journal,* **iv,** 234.

Greenwald, A.E. (1970) Anovulatorias-y-alopecie. *Dermatologia ibero latina-americana*, **12**, 29.

Griffiths, W.A.D. (1973) Diffuse hair loss and oral contraceptives. *British Journal of Dermatology*, **88**, 31.

Zaun, H. (1972) *Ovulationshemmer in der Dermatologia*. Thieme, Stuttgart.

Zaun, H. & Gerber, T. (1969) Die Wirkung monophasis der Ovulationshemmer auf das Wachsstem der Kopfhaare. *Archiv für klinische und experimentelle Dermatologie*, **234**, 353.

Zaun, H. & Ruffing, H. (1970) Untersuchungen über der Einfluss antikonzeptioner Zuriphasen–Hormonpräparate auf das Wachsstem der Kopfhaare. *Archiv für klinische und experimentelle Dermatologie*, **238**, 197.

Thyroid influences on hair growth
(References p. 147)

Epidermal thickness is reduced in patients with hypothyroidism, and the rates of epidermal cell division and anabolic activity in the epidermis are increased in thyrotoxicosis (Holt *et al.* 1976). The changes observed in both hypothyroid and hyperthyroid states are reversible when the euthyroid state is restored. Epidermal receptors for thyroid hormone appear to be specific for tri-iodothyronine (Holt & Marks 1977).

Hypothyroidism

In severe hypothyroidism of long duration the skin appendages are almost completely absent. When the changes are less severe the number of appendages in the atrophic epidermis is reduced and horny plugs are seen in orifices of sweat ducts and follicles (Saito *et al.* 1976).

There is no consistent correlation between the degree and duration of hypothyroidism and the severity of alopecia, probably because the thyroid, apart from its direct effect on the hair cycle, has other metabolic activities which can directly or indirectly affect hair growth (Saito *et al.* 1976). Whilst a mildly scaly skin and diffuse sparsity of scalp and body hair are commonly seen in cretins (Butterworth 1954) and in myxoedema, diffuse alopecia may be the only cutaneous sign of hypothyroidism (Church 1965). The cases of hypothyroid alopecia most likely to come to the notice of the dermatologist are of this type (Chapman & Main 1967).

The alopecia in hypothyroidism is diffuse and of very gradual onset. Microscopy of plucked hairs shows a marked increase in the proportion in telogen. The telogen ratio drops rapidly when thyroxine is administered and resting follicles re-enter anagen (Freinkel & Freinkel 1972). The routine history taken from the patient with diffuse hair loss without obvious cause should include questions concerning gain in weight, cold tolerance, energy and initiative. Even in the absence of such symptoms of hypothyroidism the thyroid radio-iodine uptake and the blood thyroxine level should be estimated.

Longstanding hypothyroidism may be accompanied, in the genetically predisposed, by common baldness, hirsutism and acne. The mechanism is presumed to be due to an increase in plasma free androgens. Sex hormone-binding globulin levels are decreased in hypothyroidism (Cavaliere *et al.* 1988; Sarne *et al.* 1988).

Hypothyroid alopecia responds promptly to replacement therapy with thyroxine, unless it is of very long duration and some follicles have atrophied. However, alopecia in a patient who is biochemically hypothyroid is not necessarily wholly or even partly the result of impaired thyroid function. Patients with common baldness have been treated for long periods with thyroxine on the basis of borderline biochemical findings, or even of a so-called 'clinical diagnosis' of hypothyroidism based on gain in weight and perhaps an elevated serum cholesterol level, neither of which is an acceptable diagnostic criterion.

Frankel and Frankel (1964) reported myxoedema of the scalp presenting as diffuse thickening with the consistency 'of a rubber pillow'. The scalp hair was normal. The diagnosis was confirmed histologically and biochemically. An unusual and unexplained temporary diffuse alopecia occurred in a child aged 10 months with myxoedema, 17 days after starting treatment with thyroxine (Achten *et al.* 1960).

Thyrotoxicosis

Severe thyrotoxicosis is said to cause diffuse alopecia of the scalp. The evidence for this and the claim that decreased axillary hair is a feature of about 50% of cases of thyrotoxicosis (Williams 1947) is at best circumstantial.

References

Achten, G., Ledoux-Corbusier, M., Van der Meiren, L. & Wolter, R. (1960) Défluvium chez un enfant myxoedémateux traité. *Archiv Belges de Dermatologie et de Syphiligraphie*, **16**, 209.

Butterworth, T. (1954) Dermatological aspects of cretinism. *Archives of Dermatology and Syphilology*, **70**, 565.

Cavaliere, H., Abalin, N. & Madeiros-Neto, G. (1988) Serum levels of total testosterone and sex hormone binding globulin in hypothyroid patients and normal subjects treated with incremental doses of L-T_4 or L-T_3. *Journal of Andrology*, **9**, 215.

Chapman, R.S. & Main, R.A. (1967) Diffuse thinning of the hair in iodine-induced hypothyroidism. *British Journal of Dermatology*, **79**, 103.

Church, R.E. (1965) Hypothyroid hair loss. *British Journal of Dermatology*, **77**, 661.

Frankel, E.B. & Frankel, A.R. (1964) Localised myxoedema of the scalp and hypothyroidism. *Archives of Dermatology*, **90**, 460.

Freinkel, R.K. & Freinkel, N. (1972) Hair growth and alopecia in hypothyroidism. *Archives of Dermatology*, **106**, 349.

Holt, P.J.A., Lazarus, J. & Marks, R. (1976) The epidermis in thyroid disease. *British Journal of Dermatology*, **95**, 513.

Holt, P.J.A. & Marks, R. (1977) The epidermal responses to changes in thyroid status. *Journal of Investigative Dermatology*, **68**, 299.

Saito, R., Hori, Y. & Kuribayashi, T. (1976) Alopecia in hypothyroidism. In *Biology and Diseases of the Hair*, p. 279, eds. T. Kobori & W. Montagna. University Park Press, Baltimore.

Sarne, D.H., Refetoff, S., Rosenfield, R.L. & Farriaux, J.P. (1988) Sex hormone binding-globulin in the diagnosis of peripheral tissue resistance to thyroid hormone: the value of changes after short term triiodothyronine administration. *Journal of Clinical Endocrinology and Metabolism,* **66,** 740.

Williams, R.H. (1947) Thyroid and adrenal interrelations with special reference to hypotrichosis axillaris in thyrotoxicosis. *Journal of Clinical Endocrinology and Metabolism,* **7,** 52.

Nutritional influences on hair growth
(References p. 150)

Malnutrition has an important effect on hair growth. The most widespread is protein–calorie malnutrition, which is common in many developing countries, but is not unknown in countries with a high standard of living. The more specific dietary deficiencies, affecting hair growth, are the predictable products of 'sophisticated' techniques of artificial feeding and should no longer be seen to be due to supplementation of proprietary products.

Protein–calorie malnutrition (PCM)
PCM is classified in four degrees of severity:

1 nutritional growth retardation

⎫
⎬   deficiency of good quality protein.
⎭

2 kwashiorkor

3 marasmic kwashiorkor

⎫
⎬   protein and calorie deficiency
⎭

4 nutritional marasmus

In PCM the hair becomes dry and lifeless in appearance. Partial loss of pigment from black hair gives patches which are reddish or pale in colour (Hennington *et al.* 1958). The hair roots show a prompt response to protein deficiency. The proportion of roots in telogen increases. Anagen follicles show dystrophic changes with reduction in the diameter of the hair bulb and in the contour of the shaft (Bradfield 1968; Bradfield *et al.* 1969). Both internal and external root sheaths are markedly reduced (Crounse *et al.* 1970). There is a gross reduction in the rate of hair growth (Sims 1968). Other clinical aspects of kwashiorkor are discussed by Gillman & Gillman (1951) and by Lowry and Meilman (1975).

Secondary protein deficiency has occurred after severe diarrhoea some years after a gastrectomy (Silverblatt & Brown 1960) and in ulcerative colitis (Melnikoff 1957). In both patients black hair became reddish and sparse.

Marasmus is severe chronic malnutrition, in which the child adapts to the stress by failing to grow (Bradfield 1974). Follicles in telogen conserve nitrogen. The hair is also fine and dry but almost no anagen follicles remain, and if the marasmic state continues, the hair becomes very sparse as the telogen hairs are shed.

In kwashiorkor a relatively acute shortage of protein interrupts a period of more normal growth. Linear growth of hair may continue, but the calibre of the hair shaft is reduced, and some anagen follicles become dystrophic. Intermediate stages are also seen (Bradfield & Bailey 1968; Bradfield *et al.* 1969). Johnson *et al.* (1976) assessed the value of changes in hair root morphology in nutrition surveys. Significant differences in shaft diameter and in anagen/telogen ratio were found only between well-nourished and severely malnourished children. The different stages of PCM could not be reliably differentiated in a field survey by the examination of hair morphology. Nevertheless such changes constitute an important physical sign in the individual child.

Essential fatty acid deficiency
Deficiency of essential fatty acids is liable to arise in patients who receive prolonged parenteral alimentation without supplementation. Cutaneous changes by this deficiency have been reported in infants (Caldwell *et al.* 1972) and adults (Riella *et al.* 1975; Skolnik *et al.* 1977). After 2–4 months of deficient alimentation the patient develops redness and scaling in the scalp and eyebrows. Most hair is shed, and what remains is dry, unruly and lighter in colour.

The suspected diagnosis can be confirmed by demonstrating a high serum level of the fatty acid eicosatrianoic acid, and a low concentration of arachidonic acid. The cutaneous changes are reversed by the topical application of safflower oil which contains 60–70% lineolic acid (Skolnik *et al.* 1977).

Zinc deficiency
Zinc deficiency occurs as a result of an inborn defect of zinc absorption, or from dietary deficiency of this element, or as the results of long-continued parenteral alimentation.

Acrodermatitis enteropathica
This uncommon hereditary disorder of zinc metabolism is determined by an autosomal recessive gene (Moynahan 1974). The onset. of symptoms often coincides with weaning. There are erythema and scaling plaques, partially covered with bullae and vesicles. These skin changes characteristically occur on the extremities and around the mouth and anus. The hair may be sparse, dry and brittle or may be shed completely. The child is listless and apathetic and growth is retarded. The symptoms respond rapidly to zinc sulphate (50 mg three times daily).

Environmental zinc deficiency
In the absence of an adequate intake of zinc, such as occurs in some areas of Egypt and Iran as a result of a diet of unleavened wholemeal wheat bread, which is high in phosphate, growth and sexual maturation are retarded in some prepubertal males (Ronaghy *et al.* 1974). Hair growth in such individuals has not been investigated, but there are no gross clinical changes.

Zinc deficiency after parenteral alimentation.

Acute zinc deficiency is characterized by a dermatitis resembling that of acrodermatitis enteropathica, and associated with diarrhoea, apathy and alopecia (Kay
& Tasman-Jones 1975). Chronic zinc deficiency in patients receiving only
parenteral feeding (Wexler & Pace 1977) gave rise to skin changes after about 2
months. Redness and scaling developed in the nasolabial folds and at the corners
of the mouth. Red scaly patches appeared on the knees, with bullae on the hands
and feet, followed by perianal erosions and sparseness of the hair of the scalp and
eyebrows. In another patient similar but less severe changes occurred after 16
months of hyperalimentation. Many other cases have been reported (Weismann
et al. 1976). The symptoms which should suggest the possibility of zinc deficiency
are peri-occipital redness and scaling, bullae and hair loss. The subject has been
fully reviewed by Weismann (1980), Prasad (1985) and Evans (1986).

References

Bradfield, R.B. (1968) Changes in hair root morphology and hair diameter associated with protein–
    calorie malnutrition. In *Protein Deficiencies and Calorie Deficiencies*, p. 213, eds. R.A. McCance &
    E.M. Widdowson. Churchill, London.
Bradfield, R.B. (1974) Hair tissue as a medium for the differential diagnosis of protein calorie
    malnutrition: a commentary. *Journal of Pediatrics*, **84**, 294.
Bradfield, R.B. & Bailey, M.A. (1968) Hair root response to protein undernutrition. In *Advances in
    Biology of Skin*, vol. IX, *Hair Growth*, p. 109, eds. W. Montagna & R.C. Dobson. Pergamon Press,
    Oxford.
Bradfield, R.B. Cordano, A. & Graham, G.G. (1969) Hair-root adaptation to marasmus in Andean
    Indian children. *Lancet*, **ii**, 1395.
Caldwell, M.D., Jonsson, H.T. & Otherson, H.B. (1972) Essential fatty acid deficiency in an infant
    receiving prolonged parenteral alimentation. *Journal of Pediatrics*, **8**, 894.
Crounse, R.G., Bollet, A.J. & Owens, S. (1970) Tissue assay of human protein malnutrition using
    scalp hair roots. *Transactions of the Association of American Physicians*, **83**, 185.
Evans, G.W. (1986) Zinc and its deficiency diseases. *Clinical Physiology and Biochemistry*, **4**, 94.
Gillman, J. & Gillman, T. (1951) *Perspectives in Human Malnutrition*. Grune & Stratton, New York.
Hennington, V.M., Caroe, E., Derbes, V. & Kennedy, B. (1958) Kwashiorkor. *Archives of Dermatology*,
    78, 157.
Johnson, A.A., Latham, M.C. & Ron, D.A. (1976) An evaluation of the use of changes in hair root
    morphology in the assessment of protein–calorie malnutrition. *American Journal of Clinical
    Metabolism*, **29**, 502.
Kay, R.G. & Tasman-Jones, C. (1975) Acute zinc deficiency in man during intravenous alimenta-
    tion. *Australian and New Zealand Journal of Surgery*, **292**, 879.
Lowry, G. & Meilman, I. (1975) Kwashiorkor, aspectes clinicos e dermatologicos. *Medicina cutanea*,
    ILE, **3**, 181.
Melnikoff, G.M. (1957) Temporary reddening of the hair in ulcerative colitis. *American Journal of
    Digestive Diseases (and Nutrition)*, **2**, 738.
Moynahan, E.J. (1974) Acrodermatitis enteropathica. A lethal inherited human zinc deficiency
    disorder. *Lancet*, **ii**, 399.
Prasad, A.S. (1985) Clinical, endocrinological and biochemical effects of zinc deficiency. *Clinics in
    Endocrinology and Metabolism*, **14**, 567.
Riella, M.C., Broviac, J.W., Wells, M. & Scribner, B.H. (1975) Essential fatty acid deficiency in
    human adults during total parenteral nutrition. *Annals of Internal Medicine*, **83**, 786.

Ronaghy, H.A., Reinhold, J.G., Malhoudji, M., Ghavasni, P., Spivey Fox, N.R. & Halsted, J.A. (1974) Zinc supplementation of malnourished schoolboys in Iran: increased growth and other effects. *The American Journal of Clinical Nutrition*, **27**, 112.

Silverblatt, C.W. & Brown, H.E. (1960) 'Kwashiorkor-like' syndrome associated with burning feet syndrome in an adult male. *American Journal of Medicine*, **28**, 847.

Sims, R.T. (1968) The measurement of hair growth as an index of protein synthesis in malnutrition. *British Journal of Nutrition*, **22**, 229.

Skolnik, P., Eaglstein, W.H. & Zibouh, V.A. (1977) Human essential fatty-acid deficiency. *Archives of Dermatology*, **113**, 939.

Weismann, K. (1980) Zinc metabolism and the skin. In *Recent Advances in Dermatology*, p. 109, eds. A. Rook & J.A. Savin. Churchill Livingstone, Edinburgh.

Weismann, K., Hjorth, N. & Fischer, A. (1976) Zinc depletion syndrome with acrodermatitis during long-term intravenous feeding. *Clinical and Experimental Dermatology*, **1**, 237.

Wexler, D. & Pace, W. (1977) Acquired zinc deficiency disease of the skin. *British Journal of Dermatology*, **96**, 669.

Malabsorption

There are numerous causes of malabsorption states (Dyer & Dawson 1968) and there are wide quantitative and qualitative variations in the nature and degree of absorption failure. It follows that the clinical manifestations of malabsorption may be equally diverse.

Classical symptoms, not all present in every patient, are frequent loose, pale and bulky stools. Weight loss is usual. If the malabsorption begins in childhood there will be short stature and hypogonadism. Cutaneous changes are common (Wells 1962) but are rarely progressive. Most frequent are ichthyosis and follicular keratosis. The scalp is scaly and the hair somewhat sparse. The tongue may be sore, red and smooth. Less frequently there may be eczema, which can be extensive but without distinctive features (Friedman & Hare 1965). Uncommonly the eczema occurs in large, scaly plaques, which are followed by conspicuous pigmentation. If these plaques are in the scalp there may be extensive temporary shedding of the hair in the affected areas (Lachapelle & Rook 1967), and this circumscribed severe loss is superimposed on the existing diffuse alopecia.

Detailed studies by modern methods of the hair changes in malabsorption states have not been reported. When sparse hair and growth retardation are associated with the symptoms mentioned above each case should be thoroughly investigated for malabsorption. The response to appropriate treatment, for example, a gluten-free diet in gluten enteropathy, is impressive.

References

Dyer, N.H. & Dawson, A.M. (1968) Malabsorption. *British Medical Journal*, ii, 161.

Friedman, M. & Hare, P.J. (1965) Gluten-sensitive enteropathy and eczema. *Lancet*, i, 521.

Lachapelle, J.-M. & Rook, A.J. (1967) Les manifestations cutanées des états de malabsorption. *Archives Belges de Dermatologie et de Syphiligraphie*, **23**, 267.

Wells, G.C. (1962) Skin disorders in relation to malabsorption. *British Medical Journal*, ii, 937.

Pancreatic disease of the tropics

A form of pancreatic disease affecting predominantly young adult males occurs widely in East Africa (Klaus 1980). Its cause is unknown. The principal manifestations of pancreatic disease of the tropics are steatorrhoea, upper abdominal pain, the symptoms of diabetes mellitus and malnutrition. Malabsorption may result in weakness, oedema and ascites.

In Uganda about one third of patients with this disease develop small irregular areas of fine scaling which gradually become generalized and are associated with pigment dilution. The hair becomes soft, fine and reddish-brown in colour. Diffuse alopecia develops on the vertex and pubic and axillary hair become sparse.

Reference

Klaus, S.N. (1980) Acquired pigment dilution of the hair and skin. *International Journal of Dermatology*, **19**, 508.

Chronic renal failure and maintenance haemodialysis

Chronic renal failure is frequently associated with cutaneous changes (Scoggins & Harlan 1967; Lubach 1980). Pigmentation is increased and the skin generally is ichthyotic and pruritic. Maintenance haemodialysis does not reverse these changes and often gives rise to additional abnormalities, particularly of the hair and nails. The scalp hair becomes dry, brittle and rather sparse and there is thinning of body hair, including pubic and axillary hair. The nails are brittle and may be deformed. The mechanisms underlying the effect on hair is unknown.

References

Lubach, D. (1980) Dermatologische Veränderungen bei Patienten mit Langzeithämodialyse. *Hautarzt*, **31**, 82.
Scoggins, R.B. & Harlan, W.R. Jr. (1967) Cutaneous manifestations of hyperlipidemia and uraemia. *Postgraduate Medicine*, **41**, 357.

Cronkhite–Canada syndrome
(References p. 153)

History and nomenclature
This rare but well-defined syndrome is conveniently linked eponymously to Cronkhite & Canada (1955) as its pathogenesis is still uncertain.

Pathology
Diffuse gastrointestinal polyposis is a frequent finding, but it has been suggested (Johnson *et al.* 1972) that the essential abnormality is a diffuse, potentially reversible, gastroenterocolitis with the formation of inflammatory pseudopolyps.

Malabsorption and exudative enteropathy are constant features and hypoproteinaemia may be extreme (Shibuya 1972; Mielke 1973). Reported cases have occurred in several different races, aged between 30 and 75 at the onset of symptoms. Complete remission of both gastrointestinal and cutaneous features has been described (Russell *et al.* 1983; Peart *et al.* 1984).

Clinical features

The principal symptoms are severe diarrhoea, weakness, oedema, and loss of weight. Cutaneous symptoms may precede but commonly follow the onset of diarrhoea. Loss of head hair is usually diffuse and may be severe. In one case (Johnston *et al.* 1962) it was described as 'extensive alopecia areata' and in some cases it becomes total. Body hair becomes sparse. The pathodynamics of the hair loss have not been adequately studied.

Most finger and toe nails show a distinctive though not pathognomonic dystrophy. The humped appearance suggests the formation of ventral nail in the absence of normal nail formation by the matrix (Cunliffe & Anderson 1967). Pigmentation may affect the palmar aspect of the fingers and may be widespread (Herzberg & Kaplan 1990), but does not involve the mucous membranes.

References

Cronkhite, L.W. & Canada, W.J. (1955) Generalized gastrointestinal polyposis: an unusual syndrome of polyposis, pigmentation, alopecia and onychatrophia. *New England Journal of Medicine,* **252,** 1011.

Cunliffe, W.J. & Anderson, J. (1967) Case of Cronkhite–Canada syndrome and associated jejunal diverticulosis. *British Medical Journal,* iv, 601.

Herzberg, A.J. & Kaplan, D.L. (1990) Cronkhite–Canada syndrome. Light and electron microscopy of the cutaneous pigmentary abnormalities. *International Journal of Dermatology,* **29,** 121.

Johnson, G.K., Soergel, K.H., Hensby, G.T., Dodds, W.J. & Hogan, W.J. (1972) Cronkhite–Canada syndrome: gastrointestinal pathophysiology and morphology. *Gastroenterology,* **63,** 140.

Johnston, M.N., Vosburgh, J.W., Wiens, A.T. & Walsh, G.C. (1962) Gastrointestinal polyposis associated with alopecia, pigmentation and atrophy of the fingernails and toenails. *Annals of Internal Medicine,* **56,** 935.

Mielke, F.W. (1973) Diffuse polyposis ventriculi, polyposis intestinali—Cronkhite–Canada syndrome. *Zeitschrift für Gastroenterologie,* **11,** 529.

Peart, A.G. Jr., Sivak, M.V. Jr., Rankin, G.B., Kish, L.S. & Steck, W.D. (1984) Spontaneous improvement of Cronkhite–Canada syndrome in a postpartum female. *Digestive Diseases and Sciences,* **29,** 470.

Russell, D.M., Bhathal, P.S. & St-John, D.J. (1983) Complete remission in Cronkhite–Canada syndrome. *Gastroenterology,* **85,** 180.

Shibuya, C. (1972) An autopsy case of Cronkhite–Canada's syndrome—generalised gastrointestinal polyposis, pigmentation, alopecia and onychatrophia. *Acta pathologica japonica,* **22,** 171.

Alopecia and pigmentary changes induced by chemicals
(References p. 161)

Many chemicals which are capable of inducing alopecia are frequently used in therapeutics. Man is only rarely and accidentally exposed to some chemicals but others are occupational hazards. Together they account for a small but increasing proportion of cases of diffuse alopecia. The role of environmental chemical contamination in causing alopecia and other disturbances of hair growth is probably underestimated. Exposure to boric acid, for example (see below), is seldom considered amongst diagnostic possibilities. There are a number of reports of alopecia with polyneuritis and optic atrophy (Euzière *et al.* 1951; Symonds 1953) and in which a toxic cause was suspected but never proved. Exposure to a chemical should always be considered as a possible cause of unexplained hair loss.

The mode of action of many chemicals on the hair cycle is known and the clinical features and course of the alopecia can be correlated with the nature of the changes produced in the growing follicles. Flesch (1963) reviewed the subject at length and differentiated drugs which inhibit mitosis, those that disturb keratinization and those which precipitate premature catagen. These distinctions are important clinically, but a single drug may interfere with hair growth in different ways according to the degree of damage it inflicts. The clinical effect of a given dose is influenced by the ratio of anagen to telogen (A/T) follicles in the scalp when it is administered; the greater the proportion of anagen follicles, the greater the hair loss. The A/T ratio is generally higher in the young but the proportion of telogen hairs is increased in many diseases, including most neoplastic diseases.

For many drugs the non-specific nature of increased shedding of telogen hairs can be related to the administration of the drug only circumstantially. All dermatologists see patients in whom diffuse alopecia clearly related to an acute febrile illness has been wrongly attributed to the drugs prescribed to treat it. On the other hand it is probable that drugs are often overlooked as a cause of increased shedding of hair.

Although a provisional classification of the mechanisms of drug action on hair follicles is possible, there are so many drugs, the mode of action of which is unknown, that it is more practical to classify the drugs into groups according to their pharmacological activity.

Cytostatic agents
Inhibition of mitosis in the hair papilla leads either to narrowing of the hair shaft, which fractures readily at this point, or to complete failure of hair formation. In either case so-called 'anagen alopecia' results and dystrophic hairs are shed within days of the first administration of an adequate dose of the drug. The same drug may produce broken shafts and anagen shedding in some follicles and premature catagen, followed by telogen shedding in others (Zaun 1964). A study of the trichograms of 40 patients receiving cytostatic drugs (Orfanos & Gerstein 1976) showed that qualitative changes such as broken shafts, disordered keratin structure and melanin distribution were regularly found; the proportion of such hairs and of telogen hairs varied with the drug and with the dose. In a further

study of 49 patients who developed hair loss after receiving cytostatic drugs, Gerstein & Orfanos (1976) showed that most developed hair loss 10 days to 6 weeks after starting treatment. Of these patients 31 were carefully followed; six developed total baldness of the scalp and 29 developed some generalized hair loss which became universal in four. The rate of hair growth was reduced and the male patients needed to shave less frequently.

Cyclophosphamide (also known as Endoxan) has been very thoroughly investigated (Braun-Falco 1961). With this drug and with methotrexate and actinozine D (Crounse & Van Scott 1960) 4–6 days after an adequate dose there was diminution of the diameter of the bulb or of the keratogenic zone leading to constriction and fracture of the hair. Continued therapy with two or more cytostatic drugs has a greater effect than a larger dose of only one. The occasional delay of the onset of alopecia to 3 months after the start of cytostatic therapy has been reported (Falkson & Schulz 1960, 1964). The so-called 'universal' alopecia of cytostatic therapy is due to telogen shedding.

Colchicine produces changes similar to cyclophosphamide (Malkinson & Lynfield 1959; Harms 1980). With high dosage there is anagen alopecia and matrix atrophy. With low dosage there is increased telogen shedding. High dosage of desacetyl methyl colchicine led to loss of 90% of scalp hair in 2 weeks (Mikkelson *et al.* 1956). The sensitivity of cells to injury by colchicine depends on the mitosis rate.

Cytostatic drugs taken to induce abortion have produced anagen alopecia, with diagnostic broken, tapered hair shafts (Maibach & Maguire 1964), which could be of medico-legal importance. Cantharidine administered with criminal intent, or taken accidentally, causes an anagen alopecia, with fracture of dystrophic anagen hairs (Pinetti & Biggio 1967).

Hair loss from cyclophosphamide is less under continuous low dosage than with intermittent high dosage regimes (Stoll 1974). Scalp cooling has been helpful in minimizing alopecia. The application of ice packs to the scalp for 30 minutes before injection produced considerable benefit with doxorubicin alone, or in combination with cyclophosphamide, and some patients did not require wigs (Luce *et al.* 1973; Dean *et al.* 1979). A slightly different technique using a cooling gel pack for 15 minutes before, and at least 30 minutes after, doxorubicin treatment, was effective in preventing hair loss or reducing it to a cosmetically acceptable level (Anderson *et al.* 1981). Symonds *et al.* (1986) reported success with a vortex refrigeration tube giving cold air cooling to the scalp. The effect of cooling is related to the metabolic effects of hypothermia rather than due to reduced blood flow (Bulow *et al.* 1985).

The combination of azathioprine and prednisone, prescribed for renal transplant patients, the collagen diseases and in bullous disorders, leads to thinning and breaking of scalp hair, beginning after 1–3 weeks. When the hair is allowed to regrow it may be darker, greyer or more curly than before immunosuppression (Koranda 1974).

Cassady and Jaffe (1974) recorded that hair which had regrown after irradiation, was protected from the epilatory effect of subsequent radiotherapy.

Many plant species contain cytostatic chemicals. The accidental ingestion of the tubers of *Gloriosa superba*, a member of the lily family which contains colchicine, was followed by a severe acute alopecia (Gooneratne 1966). Cytostatic agents capable of provoking acute anagen alopecia occur in a number of leguminous plants which may be accidentally eaten by man. Various spines of *Lecythis* contain selenocystothionine (Kerdel Vegas 1964). *Leucaena glauca* contains mimosine, which has caused alopecia in women (Crounse *et al.* 1962). Abrin, present in the seeds of *Abrus precatorius*, has a similar effect (Vignolo-Lutasi 1962). As the coloured seeds of this plant are worn as necklaces the possibility of accidental exposure, especially in children, may arise in countries in which the plant itself does not occur.

Anticoagulants

Heparin, the heparinoids and the coumarins all cause diffuse alopecia in about 50% of patients. Hair loss usually begins after about 8 weeks (3–20 weeks) and lasts for about 6 months (Fischer *et al.* 1953). The incidence of alopecia tends to be highest when large doses have been given over a short period (Tudhope *et al.* 1958) but shows some variation in different series (Hirschback *et al.* 1954). A polyhexuronic ester, a synthetic heparinoid, produced alopecia in 70%, beginning after 3–4 weeks; up to 75% of hair was lost from the vertex, but less from the sides and back of the scalp (Field *et al.* 1961). The precise mode of action of anticoagulants on the hair follicle is uncertain. From studies in man and in the rat (Miki 1960 a,b) an anti-mitotic effect on anagen follicles has been suggested.

Coumarin, in the form of warfarin, is used as a rat poison. Children have developed alopecia after eating poisoned food put down as bait (Cornbleet & Hoit 1957).

Thallium

Thallium salts have been widely used to kill rodents and cockroaches, and contaminated food stores have caused outbreaks of poisoning in dogs and cats and in man. Thallium salts have been used for homicide (Truhaut 1958) and political assassination (McCormack & McKinney 1983), and were prescribed in medicine, first to control sweats in tuberculosis, and later to produce epilation in the treatment of ringworm. An early report of hair loss (Combemale 1898, cit. Heyroth 1947) was the consequence of the prescription of thallium to a tuberculous patient. There is an extensive early literature on such disasters (Buschke & Peiser 1931).

Investigations in the rat (Thyresson 1951) showed that thallium was taken up by anagen follicles and disturbed keratinization. Tactile hairs in rats (Thyresson 1952) showed vacuolization of matrix cells after about 3 days; later the hair shafts showed nodular enlargements through which some shafts broke. The addition of 1–2% cystine to the diet of rats (Gross *et al.* 1948) delayed the development of alopecia in chronic thallium poisoning and reduced the mortality in acute poisoning.

In accidental poisoning in dogs and cats (Skelley & Gabriel 1964) hair loss began after 12–14 days; in some cases erythema and necrosis of the skin occurred, especially around the muzzle and in the large flexures.

Thallium salts are no longer prescribed in medicine, and are not contained pesticides available in Britain but in many parts of the world outbreaks of poisoning have occurred from contamination of food, for example in Brussels (Achten 1962), South Africa (Heyl & Barlow 1989), Texas (Chamberlain *et al.* 1958; Reed *et al.* 1963), New York (Frank & Hirsch 1952) and California (Munch *et al.* 1933). Contamination of cocaine has produced poisoning in some addicts (Insley *et al.* 1986). With growing awareness of the dangers of these tasteless poisons, large-scale outbreaks are likely to be less frequent, but pesticides containing the salts are still available in many countries.

Schwartzman and Kirschbaum (1962) recorded the early induction of telogen. A study of the dynamics of thallium alopecia (Arnold *et al.* 1964) confirmed that the initial alopecia wa due to intra-follicular breaking of growing hairs, but a week after the onset of alopecia 80% of follicles were in catagen. The tapered end of the broken hair shows a distinctive dark zone (Ludwig 1961; Eberhartinger 1962). These areas are due to gaseous material within the medulla (Metter & Vock 1984; Kijewski 1984).

The symptoms of thallium poisoning are very variable. The features have been reviewed by Saddique and Peterson (1983). Nausea and vomiting may occur early, and weakness, ataxia and tremor somewhat later, but alopecia, fatigue and pains in the legs are the most frequent manifestations (Munch *et al.* 1933; Chamberlain *et al.* 1958). In the more acute forms the initial gastrointestinal symptoms are rapidly followed by delirium, convulsions and coma (Report 1957). In patients exposed to smaller doses there may be fatigue, weight loss and aching limbs, but alopecia may be the only symptom (Hubler 1959, 1966). The hair loss which is diffuse and may become total develops in the second and third weeks; it is a most important diagnostic feature, whether it occurs alone or with more vague and non-specific symptoms (Gettler & Weiss 1943). Treatment consists of Prussian blue, forced diuresis and charcoal haemoperfusion (Heath *et al.* 1983).

In one Texas outbreak (Reed *et al.* 1963) 13% of 72 cases were fatal. Death results from damage to the central nervous system and to the kidneys, and some survivors have permanent neurological defects (Steinberg 1961; Reed *et al.* 1963). Most victims of less severe poisoning make a complete recovery. Generalized hyperaminoacidosis of renal type has been reported in some cases (Fischl 1966).

Unexplained diffuse alopecia, if the commoner causes can be excluded, should lead to a suspicion of thallium poisoning even if no source of thallium can be traced. The suspicion is verified if the alopecia is accompanied by neurological symptoms or signs (Webster *et al.* 1958). Thallium is excreted in the urine and faeces over a period of many weeks; any thallium present is abnormal.

Thyreostatic drugs

These drugs may cause hair loss by inducing hypothyroidism, but there are reports also of diffuse hair loss in patients who were still hyperthyroid (Wilburne 1951). Levy (1950) reported pronounced hair loss in a woman whose basal metabolic rate was reduced from +55 to 0 by propylthiouracil. Seven patients with thyrotoxicosis treated with thiouracil developed a myxoedematoid syndrome of which diffuse alopecia was one component (Lundbaek 1946). Carbimazole produced hair loss in five patients, 4–40 weeks after starting treatment (Papadopoulos & Harden 1966). The mechanism was not studied.

Allopurinol

Auerbach & Orentreich (1968) reported dramatic hair fall with many dystrophic telogen hairs associated with allopurinol therapy.

Borax

Borates may be ingested accidentally as a result of the excessive use of proprietary mouth washes containing boric acid (Stein *et al.* 1973), or from occupational exposure to sodium borate (Tan 1970). The alopecia is diffuse and of gradual onset. Serum boric acid levels are elevated.

Hypolipidaemic agents

Triparanol and other drugs given to reduce hypercholesterolaemia also reduce cholesterol biosynthesis in epidermis (Flesch 1963). The skin gradually becomes dry and ichthyotic. The hair becomes sparse, dry and paler in colour (Achor *et al.* 1961; Winkelmann *et al.* 1963). Cataracts may develop (Kirby *et al.* 1962). Clofibrate has been reported to cause hair loss but the mechanism is unknown (De Gennes *et al.* 1965).

Hypervitaminosis A

The ingestion of excessive doses of vitamin A is usually the consequence of misguided medical prescribing or of cranky self-medication, but acute vitamin A poisoning has occurred in polar explorers eating the livers of seals, huskies and polar bears (Cleland & Southcott 1969). In acute poisoning a febrile illness with headache, drowsiness, vertigo, vomiting and diarrhoea is followed by generalized exfoliation and loss of hair.

Chronic hypervitaminosis A in adults was first described by Sulzberger and Lazar (1951) in a women who for 18 months had taken 600,000 i.u. of vitamin A daily. She had a dry, rough, scaly skin, with sparse, coarse, brittle scalp hair, and absent eyebrows, eyelashes, pubic and axillary hair and vellus body hair. These changes were reversed when she stopped taking vitamin A. Other cases Raaschou-Nielsen 1961; Stimson 1961; Solen-Bechera & Soscia 1963) have shown similar changes. Fatigue, weight loss, bone and joint pains, and headache, have been the other principal manifestations.

When hair loss occurs with retinoid therapy it is generally diffuse (Mahrle *et al.* 1979) and affects up to 70% of patients on acitretin (Gupta *et al.* 1989). Specific hair dystrophies have been claimed for isotretinoin (Shalita *et al.* 1983) and etretinate (Graham *et al.* 1985). These changes consist of kinking to produce a false curly appearance. The changes seem to be due to a dynamic effect on hair moulding and keratinization at the level of the inner root sheath (Graham *et al.* 1985). Heilgemeir *et al.* (1982) reported that the trichogram was unchanged by isotretinoin. Isotretinoin caused curly hair after 1 year in a single case (Bunker *et al.* 1990); Barth-Jones *et al.* (1990) noted alopecia in 22 patients on etretinate.

Chloroprene
Condensation products of monomeric chloroprene have caused diffuse reversible alopecia in workers manufacturing synthetic rubber (Polemann 1954; Lijhancova 1967). Hair loss occurred also in workers engaged in the polymerization of chlorobutadin to elastomers of the neoprene class (Ritter & Carter 1948).

Levodopa
Levodopa has been held responsible for severe diffuse alopecia developing 6 weeks to 3 months after starting a daily dose of 2.5–3 g (Marshall & Williams 1971).

Beta-blockers
Propranolol (Martin *et al.* 1973) and metoprolol (Graeber & Lapkin 1981) may cause diffuse alopecia after 3 months. The mechanism is thought to be a telogen effluvium with slow regrowth on cessation of therapy. Shelley & Shelley (1985) reported alopecia accompanied by scalp dermatitis due to nadolol with rapid regrowth and settling of dermatitis following drug withdrawal.

Butyrophenone
Cutaneous changes were produced in those patients receiving high doses (Simpson *et al.* 1964). The skin became dry and ichthyotic, and the hair, which was shed diffusely, also became lighter in colour.

Potassium thiocyanate
This drug, formerly prescribed in the treatment of hypertension, can cause diffuse alopecia, beginning after about 3 months' treatment (Hollander *et al.* 1949).

Antimalarial drugs
Mepacrine (quinacrin) causes a severe lichenoid eruption in some individuals with an irreversible cicatricial alopecia (Bauer 1981).

Chloroquine has caused bleaching of normally blonde or reddish hair (Marten 1957; Saunders *et al.* 1959). The bleaching was first apparent in the eyebrows or at the temples.

Proguanil may cause non-scarring patchy hair loss (Hanson & Kuylen 1989).

Mercury (including acrodynia)

Occupational exposure to mercury is now strictly regulated in most countries, and mercury poisoning occurs either accidentally or from cosmetics. Some bleaching creams contain mercury and there may be sufficient percutaneous absorption to cause diffuse loss of hair and systemic symptoms such as weight loss and restlessness. In one such case the nails were hyperpigmented (Wüstner & Orfanos 1975).

Medicaments containing mercury were prescribed frequently for infants as teething powders, as antibacterial applications and for a variety of infections. The symptoms of mercury poisoning in infancy were known as 'pink disease' but the syndrome was named acrodynia by Chardon in 1830. Affected children, usually between 6 months and 2 years of age, first suffered from unexplained febrile symptoms, restlessness and hypotonia. The hands, feet and nose became swollen, pink and exfoliated. Sweating was profuse. Some diffuse shedding of hair occurred and alopecia was occasionally severe with loss of nails (Warkany 1966).

The diagnosis is confirmed by estimating the levels of mercury in the urine.

Anticonvulsants

Hydantoin derivatives cause hypertrichosis (Livingston *et al.* 1955) but sporadic reports of diffuse alopecia have occurred. Holowach and Sanden (1960) described alopecia due to troxidone and reversal following cessation of therapy. Shuper *et al.* (1985) recorded similar findings for carbamazapine. Transient hair loss occurs in 0.5–4% of patients on sodium valproate and is most commonly seen when hydantoin derivatives are also taken (Jeavons & Clarke 1974). Hair loss occurs after 1–4 months of valproate and regrowth occurs with continued treatment in the majority but the mechanism is unknown (Koch-Weser & Browne 1980).

Bromocriptine

Bromocriptine, used in hyperprolactinaemia and in acromegaly, caused increased hair loss from the beginning of treatment in all of 14 women but in none of 10 men. The hair loss did not become severe even after 3 years of treatment (Blum & Leiba 1980).

Lithium salts

Dawber & Mortimer (1982) reported alopecia due to lithium salts.

Mephenesin

Mephenesin has caused depigmentation of dark hair (Spillane 1963).

Para-aminosalicylate

This has caused a lichenoid eruption leaving cicatricial alopecia (Piñol Aguadé *et al.* 1968; Kutty *et al.* 1982).

Thiamphenicol
Thiamphenicol caused diffuse alopecia in 10 of 155 patients; in two the baldness became complete. After 8 weeks, at the end of treatment, the hair had regrown in six but the alopecia persisted in two; one patient had died, and one had been lost to observation (Manchlin *et al.* 1974).

Anti-rheumatic drugs
Sporadic claims of hair loss have been reported for gold (Gordon *et al.* 1975), ibuprofen (Mayer 1979), diclofenac and indomethacin (Martindale 1982) but this group of diseases is also associated uncommonly with alopecia. Earlier reports of alopecia due to penicillamine may have been due to contamination of D-penicillamine by L-penicillamine which has an anti-cysteine effect (Walshe 1968).

Miscellaneous
There remain a number of drugs for which occasional reports of alopecia have been filed. These reports are unsubstantiated and drawn from correspondence columns. The mechanisms of action are unknown but they are worthy of further study. Such drugs include;
1 Amiodarone (Samanta *et al.* 1983).
2 Cimetidine (Ahmad 1979; Khalsa *et al.* 1983; Vircburger *et al.* 1981; Tullio & Roberts 1985).
3 Danazol (Duff & Meyer 1981).
4 Gentamicin (Yoshioka & Matsuda 1970).
5 Itraconazole (Heilesen 1986).
6 Metyrapone (Harris 1986).
7 Pyridostigmine bromide (Field 1980).
8 Sulphasalazine (Breen & Donnelly 1986), and
9 Terfenadine (Jones & Morley 1985).

Diagnosis of alopecia caused by chemicals

Before loss of hair is attributed to a chemical, the physician must establish that the type of alopecia (for example, anagen, telogen, dystrophic) is appropriate to the chemical in question and the time intervals between exposure to the chemical and onset of hair loss are compatible.

If the suspected chemical has not previously been incriminated as causing alopecia, recovery of the hair loss on discontinuing the exposure and further recurrence on re-exposure may be required before the evidence can be considered convincing.

References
Achor, R.W.P., Winkelmann, R.K. & Perry, H.O. (1961) Cutaneous side effects from use of triparanol (Mer-29): preliminary data on ichthyosis and loss of hair. *Proceedings of Staff Meetings of the Mayo Clinic*, **36**, 217.

Achten, G. (1962) L'Intoxication thallique. *Archives Belges de Dermatologie et Syphiligraphie*, **18**, 300.

Ahmad, S. (1979) Cimetidine and alopecia (letter). *Annals of Internal Medicine*, **91**, 930.

Anderson, J.E., Hunt, J.M. & Smith, I.E. (1981) Prevention of doxorubicin-induced alopecia by scalp cooling in patients with advanced breast cancer. *British Medical Journal*, **282**, 423.

Arnold, W., Herzberg, J.J., Ludwig, E. & Sturde, H. (1964) Die Dynamik des Haarausfalls bei Thallium-Vergiftung. *Archiv für klinische und experimentelle Dermatologie*, **218**, 396.

Auerbach, R. & Orentreich, N. (1968) Alopecia and ichthyosis secondary to allopurinol. *American Archives of Dermatology*, **98**, 104.

Bauer, F. (1981) Quinacrine hydrochloride drug eruption (tropical lichenoid dermatitis). *Journal of the American Academy of Dermatology*, **4**, 239.

Barth-Jones, J., Shuttleworth, D. & Hutchinson, P.E. (1990) A study of etretinate alopecia. *British Journal of Dermatology*, **122**, 751.

Blum, I. & Leiba, S. (1980) Increased hair loss as the side effect of bromocriptine treatment. *New England Journal of Medicine*, **303**, 1418.

Braun-Falco, O. (1961) Klinik und Pathomechanismus der Endoxan-Alopecie als Beitrag zur Wesen cytostatischer Alopecie. *Archiv für klinische und experimentelle Dermatologie*, **212**, 194.

Breen, E.G. & Donnelly, S. (1986) Alopecia associated with sulphasalazine (unreviewed report). *British Medical Journal*, **292**, 802.

Brown, W.O. & Seed, L. (1945) Effect of colchicine on human tissues. *American Journal of Clinical Pathology*, **65**, 189.

Bulow, J., Friberg, L., Gaardsting, O. & Hansen, M. (1985) Frontal subcutaneous blood flow, and epi- and subcutaneous temperatures during scalp cooling in normal man. *Scandinavian Journal of Clinical and Laboratory Investigation*, **45**, 505.

Bunker, C.B., Maurice, P.D.L. & Dowd, P.M. (1990) Isotretinoin and curly hair. *Clinical and Experimental Dermatology*, **15**, 143.

Buschke, A. & Peiser, B. (1931) Die biologische Wirkung und die praktische Bedeutung des Thalliums. *Ergebnisse der allgemeiner Pathologie*, **25**, 1.

Cassady, J.R. & Jaffe, N. (1974) Protection from chemotherapeutic epilation by pure irradiation. *Radiology*, **112**, 197.

Chamberlain, P.H., Stavinoha, W.B., Davis, H., Kniker, W.T. & Panos, T.C. (1958) Thallium poisoning. *Pediatrics*, **22**, 1170.

Chardon, Fils (1830) De l'acrodynie. *Revue Médicale Française*, **3**, 51.

Cleland, J. & Southcott, R.V. (1969) Hypervitaminosis A in the Australasian Antarctic Expedition of 1911–1914. *Medical Journal of Australia*, **i**, 1337.

Cornbleet, T. & Hoit, L. (1957) Alopecia from coumarin. *Archives of Dermatology*, **75**, 440.

Crounse, R.G. & Van Scott, E.J. (1960) Changes in scalp hair roots as a measure of toxicity from cancer therapeutic drugs. *Journal of Investigative Dermatology*, **35**, 83.

Crounse, R.G., Maxwell, J.D. & Blank, H. (1962) Inhibition of growth of hair by mimosine. *Nature*, **194**, 694.

Dawber, R.P.R. & Mortimer, P. (1982) Hair loss during lithium treatment. *British Journal of Dermatology*, **107**, 124.

Dean, J.C., Salmon, S.E. & Griffith, K.S. (1979) Prevention of doxorubicine-induced hair-loss with scalp hypothermia. *New England Journal of Medicine*, **301**, 1427.

DeGennes, J.C., Maunand, B., Salmon, S., Laudate, Ph. & Truffert, J. (1965) Résultats de traitement par l'atromide en CPIB avec on sans androstérone dans les hyperlipidémies (110 essais thérapeutiques sur deux ans). *Bulletins et Mémoires de la Société Médicale des Hôpitaux de Paris*, **11**, 759.

Duff, P. & Meyer, A.R. (1981) Generalised alopecia: an unusual complication of danazol therapy. *American Journal of Obstetrics and Gynecology*, **141**, 349.

Eberhartinger, C. (1962) Die diagnostische Bedeutung bon Haarveränderungen bei Thallium-vergiftung. *Wiener medizinische Wochenschrift*, **112**, 329.

Euzière, J., Pages, P. & Coulier, C. (1951) Polynévrites récidivantes avec alopécie et atrophie optique *Revue neurologique*, **84**, 343.

Falkson, G. & Schultz, E.J. (1960) Endoxan alopecia. *British Journal of Dermatology*, **72**, 296.

Falkson, G. & Schultz, E.J. (1964) Skin changes caused by cancer chemotherapy. *British Journal of Dermatology*, **76**, 309.

Field, L.M. (1980) Toxic alopecia caused by pyridostigmine bromide (letter). *Archives of Dermatology*, **116**, 1103.

Field, J.B., Attyah, A.M., Ramsay, G.D. & Levitt, H. (1961) The chemical intoxication caused by a heparinoid. *American Journal of Medical Science*, **241**, 637.

Fischer, R., Bircher, J. & Reith, T. (1953) Der Haarausfall nach antikoagulierender Therapie. *Schweizeriche Medizinische Wochenschrift* **82**, 509.

Fischl, J. (1966) Aminoacidosis in thallium poisoning. *American Journal of the Medical Sciences*, **251**, 40.

Flesch, P. (1963) Inhibition of keratinizing structures by systemic drugs. *Pharmacological Reviews*, **15**, 653.

Frank, S.B. & Hirsch, D.R. (1952) Thallium intoxication. Report of two cases. *Journal of the American Medical Association*, **150**, 586.

Gerstein, E. & Orfanos, C.G. (1976) Haarausfall nach Zytostatica. *Artzliche Kosmetologie*, **6**, 54.

Gettler, A.O. & Weiss, L. (1943) Thallium poisoning. III. Clinical toxicology of thallium. *American Journal of Clinical Pathology*, **13**, 422.

Gooneratne, B.W.N. (1966) Massive generalised alopecia after poisoning by *Gloriosa superba*. *British Medical Journal* i, 1023.

Gordon, M.H., Tiger, L.H. & Ehrlich, G.E. (1975) Gold reactions are not more common in Sjögren's syndrome. *Annals of Internal Medicine*, **82**, 47.

Graeber, C.W. & Lapkin, R.A. (1981) Metoprolol and alopecia. *Cutis*, **28**, 633.

Graham, R.M., James, M.P., Ferguson, D.J. & Guerrier, C.W. (1985) Acquired kinking of the hair associated with etretinate therapy. *Clinical and Experimental Dermatology*, **10**, 426.

Gross, P., Runne, E. & Wilson, J.W. (1948) Studies on the effect of thallium poisoning on the rat. The influence of cystine and methionine on alopecia and survival periods. *Journal of Investigative Dermatology*, **10**, 119.

Gupta, A.K., Goldfarb, M.T., Ellis, C.N. & Voorhees, J.J. (1989) Side-effect profile of acitretin therapy in psoriasis. *Journal of the American Academy of Dermatology*, **20**, 1088.

Hanson, S.N. & Kuylen, K. (1989) Hair loss and scaling with proguanil. *Lancet*, **225**, corresp.

Harms, M. (1980) Haarausfall unter Haarverändermazen. *Hautarzt*, **31**, 161.

Harris, P.L. (1986) Alopecia associated with long-term metyrapone use. *Clinical Pharmacy*, **5**, 66.

Heath, A., Ahlmen, J., Branegard, B., Lindstedt, S., Wickstrom, I. & Anderson, O. (1983) Thallium poisoning—toxin elimination and therapy in three cases. *Journal of Toxicology and Clinical Toxicology*, **20**, 451.

Heilgemeir, G.P., Braun-Falco, O., Plewig, O. & Sund, M. (1982). Einfluss der 13-cis-Retinsäure auf das Haarwachstum. *Hautarzt*, **33**, 533.

Heilesen, A.M. (1986) Hair loss during itraconazole treatment. *British Medical Journal*, **293**, 825.

Heyl, T. & Barlow, R.J. (1989) Thallium poisoning: a dermatological perspective. *British Journal of Dermatology*, **121**, 787.

Heyroth, F.F. (1947) Thallium. *Reports of the US Public Health Service*, Suppl. 197.

Hirschback, J.S., Madison, F.W. & Pischiotta, A.V. (1954) Alopecia and other toxic effects of heparin and synthetic heparoids. *American Journal of Medical Science*, **227**, 278.

Hollander, L., Evans, G.F. & Krugh, F.J. (1949) Multiple cutaneous effects of potassium sulfocyanate. *AMA Archives of Dermatology and Syphilology*, **59**, 112.

Holowach, J. & Sanden, H.V. (1960) Alopecia as a side effect of treatment of epilepsy with trimethadione. *New England Journal of Medicine*, **263**, 1187.

Hubler, W.R. (1959) Partial alopecia due to thallium. *AMA Archives of Dermatology*, **80**, 137.

Hubler, W.R. (1966) Hair loss as a symptom of chronic thallotoxicosis. *Southern Medical Journal*, **59**, 436.

Insley, B.M., Grufferman, S. & Ayliffe, H.E. (1986) Thallium poisoning in cocaine abusers. *American Journal of Emergency Medicine*, **4**, 545.

Jeavons, P.M. & Clarke, J.E. (1974) Sodium valproate in the treatment of epilepsy. *British Medical Journal*, 2, 584.

Jones, S.K. & Morley, W.N. (1985) Terfenadine causes hair loss (unreviewed report). *British Medical Journal*, 291, 940.

Kerdel Vegas, F. (1964) Generalised hair loss due to the ingestion of 'Coco de Mono' (*Lecythis ollaria*). *Journal of Investigative Dermatology*, 42, 91.

Khalsa, J.H., Graham, C.F. & Jones, J.K. (1983) Cimetidene-associated alopecia (letter). *International Journal of Dermatology*, 22, 202.

Kijewski, H. (1984) Zur Natur der Schwarzungszonen in Haaren nach Thalliumaufnahme. *Archiv für Kriminologie*, 173, 36.

Kirby, T.J., Achor, R.W.P., Perry, H.O. & Winkelmann, R.K. (1962) Cataract formation after triparanol therapy. *Archives of Ophthalmology*, 68, 486.

Koch-Weser, J. & Browne, T.R. (1980) Drug therapy: valproic acid. *New England Journal of Medicine*, 302, 661.

Koranda, F.C. (1974) Hair changes in immunosuppressed patients. *First Human Hair Symposium*, p. 91, ed. A.C. Brown. Medcom Press, New York.

Kutty, P.K., Raman, K.R., Hawken, K. & Barrowman, J.A. (1982) Hair loss and 5-aminosalicylic acid enemas (letter). *Annals of Internal Medicine*, 97, 785.

Levy, L.K. (1950) Loss of hair following use of propylthiouracil. *Journal of the American Medical Association*, 147, 860.

Lijhancova, G. (1967) Berufsbedingte Haarausfall durch Chloroprene. *Berufsdermatosen*, 15, 280.

Livingston, S., Peterson, D. & Boks, L.L. (1955) Hypertrichosis occurring in association with dilantin therapy. *Journal of Pediatrics*, 47, 351.

Luce, J.K., Raffetto, T.J., Crisp, I.M. & Grief, G.C. (1973) Prevention of alopecia by scalp-cooling in patients receiving adriamycin. *Cancer Chemotherapy Reports*, 57, 108.

Ludwig, E. (1961) Pathognomonische Haarbefunde bei Thallium-Vergiftung und dem Deutung. *Hautarzt*, 12, 456.

Lundbaek, K. (1946) Toxic, allergic and myxoedematoid symptoms in the treatment of thyrotoxicosis with antithyroid substances. *Acta medica Scandinavica*, 124, 266.

Mahrle, G., Orfanos, C.E., Ippen, H. & Hofbauer, M. (1979) Haarwachstum, Leberwerte und Lichtempfindlichkeit unter oraler Retinoid-Therapie bei Psoriasis. *Deutsche Medizinische Wochenschrift*, 104, 473.

Maibach, H.I. & Maguire, H.C. (1964) Acute hair-loss from drug-induced abortion. *New England Journal of Medicine*, 270, 1112.

Malkinson, F.D. & Lynfield, Y.L. (1959) Colchicine alopecia. *Journal of Investigative Dermatology*, 33, 371.

Manchlin, S., Novotny, Z., Koller, F. & Ruefli, P. (1974) Cytostatic side effects of thiamphenicol: alopecia and reversible cytopenia. *Schweizerische medizinische Wochenschrift*, 104, 384.

Marshall, A. & Williams, M.J. (1971) Alopecia and levodopa. *British Medical Journal*, ii, 47.

Marten, R.H. (1957) Hair bleaching during chloroquine treatment. *Transactions of the St John's Hospital Dermatological Society*, 39, 45.

Martin, C.M., Southwick, E.G. & Maibach, H.I. (1973) Propranolol-induced alopecia. *American Heart Journal*, 86, 236.

Martindale, (1982) *The Extra Pharmacopoeia*, ed. J.E.F. Reynolds. The Pharmaceutical Press, London.

Mayer, H.C. (1979) Alopecia associated with ibuprofen. *Journal of the American Medical Association*, 242, 142.

McCormack, J. & McKinney, W. (1983) Thallium poisoning in group assassination attempt. *Postgraduate Medicine*, 74, 239.

Metter, D. & Vock, R. (1984) Untersuchungen über die Haarstruktur bei Thalliumvergiftung. *Zeitschrift für Rechtsmedizin*, 91, 201.

Miki, Y. (1960a) Alopecia from heparin. *Medical Journal of Osaka University*, 11, 315.

Miki, Y. (1960b) The effect of heparin on hair growth of rats. *Medical Journal of Osaka University*, 11, 325.

Mikkelson, W.M., Salin, R.W. & Duff, I.F. (1956) Alopecia totalis after desacetylmethylcolchicine therapy of acute gout. *New England Journal of Medicine*, **255**, 766.

Munch, J.G., Ginsberg, H.M. & Nixon, C.E. (1933) The 1932 thallotoxicosis outbreak in California. *Journal of the American Medical Association*, **100**, 1315.

Orfanos, C.G. & Gerstein, E. (1976) Haarausfall nach Zytostatica. *Ärztliche Kosmetologie*, **6**, 96.

Papadopoulos, S. & Harden, R.N. (1966) Hair loss in patients treated with carbimazole. *British Medical Journal*, **ii**, 1502.

Pinetti, P. & Biggio, P. (1967) Contributo alla conoscenza delle alopecie tossiche con particolare riguardo alle alopecie conseguenti ad avvelenamento da cantaridina. *Rassegna Medica Sarda*, **70**, 433.

Piñol Aguadé, J., Castellas Mas, A., Lecha, M., Mascaro, J.M., Gimarz-Camerase, J.M., Harch, P. de, Gras, J., Tuset, N. & Castalls Rodallas, A. (1968) Gran dermatitis liquenoide con alopecia irreversible z beta alanuria en pacientes tratados con tuberculostaticos. *Medicina cutanea*, **3**, 275.

Polemann, G. (1954) Depilationswirkung ungesättigter Verbindenger als Beitrag zur Alopezieproblem. *Dermatologica*, **108**, 98.

Raaschou-Nielsen, W. (1961) Chronic intoxication with vitamin A in adults. *Dermatologica*, **123**, 293.

Reed, D., Crawley, J., Faro, S.N., Pieper, S.J. & Kurland, L.T. (1963) Thallotoxicosis. *Journal of the American Medical Association*, **183**, 516.

Report to the Council on Drugs of the American Medical Association (1957) Thallotoxicosis—a recurring problem. *Journal of the American Medical Association*, **165**, 1566.

Ritter, W.L. & Carter, A.S. (1948) Hair loss in neoprene manufacturers. *Journal of Industrial Hygiene (and Toxicology)*, **30**, 192.

Saddique, A. & Peterson, C.D. (1983) Thallium poisoning: a review. *Veterinary and Human Toxicology*, **25**, 16.

Samanta, A., Jones, G.R. & Burden, A.C. (1983) Adverse reactions during treatment with amiodarone hydrochloride (letter). *British Medical Journal*, **287**, 503.

Saunders, T.S., Fitzpatrick, T.B., Seiji, M. Brunet, P. & Rosenbaum, E.E. (1959) Decrease in human hair color and feather pigment of fowl following chloroquine diphosphate. *Journal of Investigative Dermatology*, **33**, 87.

Schwartsman, R.M. & Kirschbaum, J.O. (1962) The cutaneous histopathology of thallium poisoning. *Journal of Investigative Dermatology*, **39**, 169.

Shalita, A.R., Cunningham, W.J., Leyden, J.J., Pochi, P.E. & Strauss, J.S. (1983) Isotretinoin treatment of acne and related disorders: an update. *Journal of the American Academy of Dermatology*, **9**, 629.

Shelley, E.D. & Shelley, W.B. (1985) Alopecia and drug eruption of the scalp associated with a new beta-blocker, nadolol. *Cutis*, **35**, 148.

Shuper, A., Stahl, B. & Wietz, R. (1985) Carbamazapine induced hair loss. *Drug Intelligence and Clinical Pharmacy*, **19**, 924.

Simpson, G.M., Blair, J.H. & Cranswick, C.H. (1964) Cutaneous effects of a new butyrophenone drug. *Clinical Pharmacological Therapy*, **5**, 310.

Skelley, J.F. & Gabriel, K.L. (1964) Thallium intoxication in the dog. *Annals of the New York Academy of Science*, **111**, 612.

Solen-Bechera, J. & Soscia, J.L. (1963) Chronic hypervitaminosis A. *Archives of Internal Medicine*, **112**, 462.

Spillane, J.D. (1963) Brunette to blonde. Depigmentation of human hair during oral treatment with mephenesin. *British Medical Journal*, **i**, 997.

Stein, K.M., Odom, R.B., Justice, G.R. & Martin, G.C. (1973) Toxic alopecia from ingestion of boric acid. *Archives of Dermatology*, **108**, 95.

Steinberg, H.J. (1961) Accidental thallium poisoning in adults. *Southern Medical Journal*, **54**, 6.

Stimson, W.H. (1961) Vitamin A intoxication in adults. *New England Journal of Medicine*, **265**, 369.

Stoll, B.A. (1974) Evaluation of cyclophosphamide dosage schedules in breast cancer. *British Journal of Cancer*, **24**, 475.

Sulzberger, M.B. & Lazar, M.P. (1951) Hypervitaminosis A. Report of a case in an adult. *Journal of the American Medical Association*, **140**, 788.

Symonds, W.J.C. (1953) Alopecia, optic atrophy and peripheral neuritis of probably toxic origin. *Lancet*, **ii**, 1338.

Symonds, R.P., McCormick, C.V. & Maxted, K.J. (1986) Adriamycin alopecia prevented by cold air scalp cooling. *American Journal of Clinical Oncology*, **9**, 454.

Tan, T.G. (1970) Occupational toxic alopecia due to borax. *Acta Dermato-Venereologica*, **50**, 55.

Thyresson, N. (1951) Experimental induction of thallium poisoning in the rat. *Acta Dermato-Venereologica*, **31**, 3 and 133.

Thyresson, N. (1952) Effect of thallium on the growth of tactile hairs in the white rat. *Acta Dermato-Venereologica*, Suppl. 29, 370.

Truhaut, R. (1958) L'Intoxication par le thallium. *Annales de Médecine légale*, **38**, 189.

Tudhope, G.R., Cohn, H. & Meikle, R.W. (1958) Alopecia following treatment with dextran sulphate and other anticoagulant drugs. *British Medical Journal*, **i**, 1034.

Tullio, C.J. & Roberts, M.A. (1985) Cimetidine induced alopecia (letter). *Clinical Pharmacy*, **4**, 145.

Vignolo-Lutasi, K. (1962) Über die experimentelle Alopecie durch Abain. *Archiv für Dermatologie und Syphilologie*, **111**, 549.

Vircburger, M.I., Prelevic, G.M., Brkic, S., Andrejevic, M.M. & Peric, L.A. (1981) Transitory alopecia and hypergonadotrophic hypogonadism during cimetidine treatment (letter). *Lancet*, **i**, 1160.

Walshe, J.M. (1968) Toxic reactions to penicillamine in patients with Wilson's disease. *Postgraduate Medical Journal*, **44**, Suppl. 11, 6.

Warkany, J. (1966) Acrodynia—postmortem of a disease. *American Journal of Diseases of Children*, **112**, 146.

Webster, J.R., Huff, S. & Gecht, M.C. (1958) Thallotoxicosis. *AMA Archives of Dermatology*, **78**, 278.

Wilburne, M. (1951) Hair loss and pigmentation due to thiouracil derivatives. *Journal of the American Medical Association*, **147**, 379.

Winkelmann, R.K., Perry, H.O., Achor, R.W.P. & Kirby, T.J. (1963) Cutaneous syndromes produced as side effects of triparanol therapy. *Archives of Dermatology*, **87**, 372.

Wüstner, H. & Orfanos, C.E. (1975) Nagelsverfärbung und Haarausfall: Leitsymptome einer Quecksilbervergiftung durch kosmetiche Bleichmittel. *Deutsche medizinische Wochenschrift*, **100**, 1694.

Yoshioka, H. & Matsuda, J. (1970) Loss of hair related to gentamicin treatment. *Journal of the American Medical Association*, **211**, 123.

Zaun, H. (1964) Tierexperimentelle Untersuchungen zur Pathophysiologie der 'gemischten' Alopecie. *Archiv für klinische und experimentelle Dermatologie*, **221**, 75.

Chapter 6
Hereditary and Congenital Alopecia and Hypotrichosis

History and nomenclature
(References p. 171)

Case reports of individuals who have been almost or totally hairless throughout life can be found in the early literature but these reports and some more recent ones are of limited value because they include no histological information and an inadequate account of associated defects; there is at the most a note to the effect that the nails and teeth were or were not normal.

There have been numerous attempts to classify the conditions characterized by congenital alopecia or hypotrichosis. Bonnet (1892) proposed a classification which was widely used for the next 40 years and which was said to be based on embryological principles.

1 Congenital absence of hair, with associated defects of teeth and nails.
2 Congenital absence of hair with normal teeth and nails.
3 Congenital absence of hair with partial or complete recovery at puberty.

Ideally one would like a complete, logical classification of hair abnormalities and any associated changes based on dysmorphology (Kingston 1989) with clearcut malformations, disruptions, deformations, etc., together with the specific follicular, scalp and hair shaft faults worked out to biochemical level. In practice one is confronted by often unique, sporadic and ill-studied entities with little detailed mechanistic investigation for many moral and ethical reasons.

Cockayne (1933) in attempting a more critical analysis of the literature, was aware that this oversimplification was no longer helpful. Each of Bonnet's groups can be shown to contain a number of genetically distinct entities as well as many

167

cases which cannot yet be categorized. Although there are now many conditions which are so well defined that they can be diagnosed on clinical features alone, there are many more which are still of questionable status, and will remain so until adequate histological studies of the scalp and electron microscopic studies of shafts of any hairs that may be present have been combined with analysis of the chemical and physical properties of such hairs, and the detailed examination of the patient for structural and metabolic defects involving other organs.

As a working classification which allows the known syndromes to be identified, and provides a provisional status for those not yet characterized, the following modification of Muller's (1973) proposals has been found useful.

1 Congenital alopecia or hypotrichosis without associated defects.

2 Congenital alopecia or hypotrichosis as a major feature of well-defined hereditary syndromes.

3 Congenital alopecia or hypotrichosis as a major feature of uncharacterized syndromes.

4 Congenital alopecia or hypotrichosis as a major or inconstant feature of hereditary syndromes.

Bertilino and Freedberg (1988) have used these subsections to produce charts outlining most of the syndromes described up to 1987.

Any classification of congenital and hereditary alopecias must be tentative. However, the work of Baden & Kubilus (1980) suggests that it may eventually be possible to differentiate congenital alopecias which are due to an abnormality in the formation of the follicle from those due to an abnormality in some component of hair differentiation; for example defects of keratinocyte migration and keratins produced.

The ectodermal dysplasias
(References p. 171)

The term 'ectodermal dysplasia' was originally applied to anhidrotic ectodermal dysplasia in which hair, teeth, nails and sweat glands are defective. As more and more syndromes have been described (Burton & Rook 1986) their nomenclature has become confused and complex and 'ectodermal dysplasia' has been applied loosely and inconsistently to a wide variety of states such as aplasia cutis congenita, local dermal hypoplasia etc. In general, ectodermal dysplasias should be congenital and affect at least two tissues of ectodermal origin, according to Paller (1989).

Freire-Maia (1977) has drawn attention to these difficulties of classification and nomenclature and has suggested a provisional classification based on the ectodermal derivatives which show a primary defect; conditions in which the ectodermal changes are secondary, as in xeroderma pigmentosum, are thus excluded from the ectodermal dysplasias. According to Freire-Maia's classification (1) is a hair dysplasia, (2) a dental dysplasia, (3) a nail dysplasia, (4) a sweat gland defect, and (5) a defect of other ectodermal structures (Freire-Maia & Pinheiro 1985). Anhidrotic ectodermal dysplasia thus falls into subgroup 1, 2, 3, 4, hidrotic ectodermal dysplasia into subgroup 1, 2, 3, and any syndrome in which hair dysplasia is the only defect, into subgroup 1 (Solomon & Keuer 1980).

Hereditary alopecia without associated defects
(References p. 171)

Recessive forms

There are several apparently distinctive genotypes. Most commonly reported is a total and permanent absence of hair (Fig. 6.1), probably determined by an autosomal recessive gene. Two brothers (Calvo Melendro 1955) whose parents were consanguineous, came of a family in which 261 individuals could be traced through over a century; 3.04% were affected. Lundbäck (1944) reported nine cases

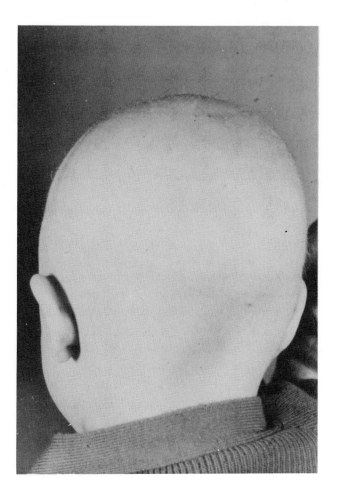

Fig. 6.1 Congenital alopecia without associated defects.

in two families. The hair was normal at birth, but was soon shed and never replaced. Hair follicles were absent, but sebaceous glands were normal in number, but small. In the family reported by Birke (1954) two of three children of consanguineous parents were bald from birth; a third child was born with some head hair, which was soon lost. A biopsy showed short follicles containing horny plugs; there were no milia or papules. Two of four German siblings showed essentially the same clinical and histological changes (Kauftheil 1926) as did the patients reported by Kraus (1903). A similar condition, with universal absence of hair, was reported in three of four Yugoslav siblings (Bunton & Fettich 1974) and in three of five Punjabi siblings (Sein 1936). Other authors who have reported one or more cases of what appears to be the same condition include Bettman (1902), Stein (1925), Klövekorn (1928), Henckel (1935), Janssen and Kox (1947), Friederich (1930), Tillman (1952), Linn (1964), Shy and Treister (1968) and Cantu *et al.* (1980). The siblings reported by Porter (1973) probably had the same syndrome; histological and histochemical investigations suggested that the essential defect was dyskeratosis of the hair shaft.

Dominant forms

Several pedigrees have been published showing autosomal dominant inheritance of hypotrichosis as an apparently isolated defect. There are differences in the clinical features and more than one genotype is involved.

Peterson (1915) described a family in which nine individuals were affected in three generations. From about the age of 5 the previously normal scalp hair was replaced by short, sparse hair of a lighter colour.

Jeanselme & Rimé (1924) observed a family in which 14 individuals in four generations were affected. Towards the end of the first year normal hair was shed and was partially replaced by sparse and brittle hair in all hairy regions including the brows and lashes.

A pedigree covering eight generations of a Spanish family was well documented by Toribio & Quiñones (1974). The hair was normal until the age of 5–12 years when retardation of hair growth was first noted and diffuse thinning began. By the age of 25 only a few hairs remained on the scalp, but hair elsewhere was not affected. Histologically the number of follicles is found not to be decreased but they fail progressively to re-enter anagen. The hair shafts appear normal with the light microscope and in the electron microscope show focal cuticular defects which are not distinctive and may be the result of normal weathering.

A similar condition in four generations of a family was reported by Bentley-Phillips and Grace (1979). The hair was apparently normal until the age of 7–13 when there was progressive shedding of scalp hair, and eyebrows and lashes were lost. Eventually only a few wispy hairs remained in the atrophic scalp. Teeth, nails and eyes were normal. In the scanning electron microscope the hairs show weathering with partial or complete absence of cuticular scales.

A few other pedigrees also suggest apparent dominant transmission of congenital alopecia (Pajtas 1950; Tillman 1952).

Congenital triangular alopecia may be a localized form of these total scalp problems (Tosti 1987).

Madarosis

The congenital absence or underdevelopment of the eyelashes occurs sporadically, but autosomal dominant inheritance has been reported (Bergsma 1979). The eyebrows and scalp hair may also be absent, but nails and sweat glands are normal.

References

Baden, H.P. & Kubilus, J. (1980) Analysis of hair from alopecia congenita. *Journal of the American Academy of Dermatology*, **3**, 623.

Bentley-Phillips, B. & Grace, H.J. (1979) Hereditary hypotrichosis. *British Journal of Dermatology*, **101**, 331.

Bergsma, D. (1979) Madarosis. In *Birth Defects Compendium*, 2nd edn., p. 676, ed. D. Bergsma. Macmillan, London.

Bertilino, A.P. & Freedberg, I.M. (1988) Disorders of epidermal appendages and related disorders. In *Dermatology in General Medicine*, 3rd edn., p. 636, eds. T.B. Fitzpatrick, A.Z. Eisen, K. Wolff *et al.* McGraw-Hill, New York.

Bettman, S. (1902) Über angeborenen Haarmangel. *Archiv für Dermatologie und Syphilologie*, **60**, 348.

Birke, G. (1954) Über Atrichia congenita und ihren Erbgang. *Archiv für Dermatologie und Syphilologie*, **197**, 322.

Bonnet, R. (1892) Ueber Hypotrichosis congenita universalis. *Anatomische Hefte*, **I**, 233.

Bunton, S. & Fettich, J. (1974) Atrichia congenita universalis. *Acta Dermato-Venereologica Jugoslav*, **I**, 97.

Burton, J.L. & Rook, A.J. (1986) Genetics in dermatology. In *Textbook of Dermatology*, p. 130, eds. A. Rook, J. Ebling, D.S. Wilkinson, R. Champion & J.L. Burton. Blackwell Scientific Publications, Oxford.

Calvo Melendro, J. (1955) Atriquia congenita total y permanente. *Medicina Clinica*, **24**, 253.

Cantu, J.M., Sanchez-Corona, J., Gonzalez-Mendoza, A., Martinez, R.M. & Garcia-Crez, D. (1980) Autosomal recessive inheritance of atrichia congenita. *Clinical Genetics*, **17**, 209.

Cockayne, A.E. (1933) *Inherited Abnormalities of the Skin and its Appendages*, p. 229. Oxford University Press, Oxford.

Freire-Maia, N. (1977) Ectodermal dysplasia revisited. *Acta Genetico Medico e Gemellologia*, **26**, 12.

Freire-Maia, N. & Pinheiro, M. (1985) *Ectodermal Dysplasias*. Alan R. Liss, New York.

Friederich, H.C. (1930) Zur Kenntnis der kongenitale Hypotrichosis. *Dermatologische Wochenschrift*, **121**, 408.

Henckel, K.O. (1935) Hypotrichosis congenita bei einegen Drillingen. *Klinische Wochenschrift*, **14**, 428.

Janssen, T.A.E. & Kox, W. (1947) Alopecia universalis congenita and hypoplasia renum in a newborn. *Acta Paediatrica (Stockholm)*, **34**, 289.

Jeanselme, A. & Rimé, G. (1924) Un cas d'alopécie congénitale familiale. *Bulletin de la Société française de Dermatologie et de Syphiligraphie*, **31**, 79.

Kauftheil, L. (1926) Über einen Fall von Atrichia congenita. *Dermatologische Zeitschrift*, **48**, 267.

Kingston, H.M. (1989) Dysmorphology and teratogenesis. *British Medical Journal*, **298**, 1235.

Klövekorn, B. (1928) Totale kongenitale alopecie. *Archiv für Dermatologie und Syphilologie*, **155**, 328.

Kraus, A. (1903) Beiträge zur Kenntnis der Alopecia congenita familiaris. *Archiv für Dermatologie und Syphilologie*, **66**, 369.

Linn, H.W. (1964) Congenital atrichia, *Australian Journal of Dermatology*, **7**, 223.

Lundbäck, H. (1944) Total congenital hereditary alopecia. *Acta Dermato-Venereologica*, **25**, 189.

Muller, S.A. (1973) Alopecia: syndromes of genetic significance. *Journal of Investigative Dermatology.* **60**, 475.

Pajtas, J. (1950) Totale familiäre hereditäre Hypotrichosis in 4 Generationen. *Dermatologica*, **101**, 90.

Paller, A.S. (1989) Hereditary diseases of the skin, hair, nails and skin structure. In *Textbook of Paediatric Dermatology*, p. 85, eds. R.R. Maldonado, L.C. Parish & J.M. Beare. Grune & Stratton, Philadelphia.

Peterson, H. (1915) Kongenitale familiäre hereditäre Alopezie auf der Basis irres Hypothyroidismus. *Dermatologische Zeitschrift*, **22**, 202.

Porter, P.S. (1973) Genetic disorders of hair growth. *Journal of Investigative Dermatology*, **60**, 493.

Sein, M. (1936) Congenital and familial absence of hair from the whole surface of the body. *Lancet*, **ii**, 564.

Shy, W.S. & Treister, M. (1968) Isolated Congenital Hypotrichosis. i. Recessive Hairlessness in Man. ii. Mendelian Inheritance in Man. 2nd edn., ed. V.A. McKusick. Johns Hopkins Press, Baltimore.

Solomon, L.M. & Keuer, E.J. (1980) The ectodermal dysplasias. *Archives of Dermatology*, **116**, 1295.

Stein, R.O. (1925) Alopecia totalis congenita. *Zeitschrift für Haut und Geschlechtskrankheiten*, **18**, 520.

Tillman, W.G. (1952) Alopecia congenita: report of two families. *British Medical Journal*, **ii**, 428.

Toribio, J. & Quiñones, P.A. (1974) Hereditary hypotrichosis siplex of the scalp. *British Journal of Dermatology*, **91**, 687.

Tosti, A. (1987) Congenital triangular alopecia. *Journal of the American Academy of Dermatology*, **16**, 991.

The hair in ectodermal dysplasias
(References p. 180)

The term ectodermal dysplasia is used here as defined by Solomon & Keuer (1980). Freire-Maia & Pinheiro (1985) have recorded very many types and sub-types.

The following criteria must be met: (i) the disease is congenital; (ii) it is diffuse and involves the epidermis and at least one of the appendages; (iii) it is not progressive. The hair defect is in almost all ectodermal dysplasias a reduction in the number and size of the follicles, producing hypotrichosis or alopecia, but in some, for example the CHAND syndrome, the hair is curly but otherwise normal.

The ectodermal dysplasias, thus defined, are here classified provisionally in accordance with Freire-Maia's suggestion:
Subgroup 1, 2, 3, 4 *Hair, teeth, nails and sweating defects*
    Anhidrotic ectodermal dysplasia
    Rapp–Hodgkin hypohidrotic ectodermal dysplasia
    Ectrodactyly, ectodermal dysplasia and cleft lip or palate
    Popliteal web syndrome
    XTE syndrome
Subgroup 1, 2, 3 *Hair, teeth and nail defects*
    Clouston's hidrotic ectodermal dysplasia
    Trichodento-osseous syndrome
    Ellis–van Creveld syndrome
    AEC syndrome
    Basan syndrome
    Tooth–nail syndrome

Subgroup 1, 3, 4 *Hair, nails and sweating defects*
   Freire-Maia syndrome
Subgroup 1, 2 *Hair and teeth defects*
   Orofaciodigital syndrome I
   Sensenbrenner syndrome
   Trichodental syndrome
Subgroup 1, 3 *Hair and nail defects*
   CHAND syndrome
   Onychotrichodysplasia with neutropenia
Subgroup 1 *Hair defects*
   Trichorhinophalangeal syndromes I and II
   Dubowitz syndrome
   Moynahan syndrome
These groupings and the sub-types within them can never hope to be complete as new 'unique' associations seem to be described frequently.

Anhidrotic ectodermal dysplasia (Christ–Siemens–Touraine syndrome; hereditary ectodermal polydysplasia)
The inheritance of this uncommon syndrome is usually determined by an X-linked recessive gene (Kerr *et al.* 1966). Girls who present with the disorder appear to inherit it in an autosomal recessive pattern or occasionally may represent heterozygotes with maximum expression of diseases features. Sweat gland and other skin appendages are absent or few in number. The full syndrome occurs only in males. Scalp hair is short, fine and very sparse and often light in colour, but may increase in quantity after puberty (Reed *et al.* 1970). In the scanning electron microscope (Porter & Aoyagi 1974) the hairs may show unusual overlapping and furrowing of cuticular scales, occasional irregular bulging of the shaft, and some longitudinal ridging, though many have normal or fine hair. Eyebrows and eyelashes may also be sparse or absent but may be relatively little affected. Body hair may be sparse or absent. The prominent square forehead, saddle nose, the thick lower lip and the pointed chin produce a distinctive facies. The skin around the eyes is finely wrinkled and may be pigmented. The teeth may be absent or few in number; characteristically the canines and incisors are conical. The absent or reduced sweating leads to heat intolerance, and unexplained pyrexia may be the presenting symptom in infancy (Norval *et al.* 1988). Carrier females may be clinically normal but may show in some degree one or more of the features of the syndrome, e.g. conical teeth, hypotrichosis or heat intolerance. Otherwise apparently normal carriers may show dermatoglyphic abnormalities, the presence of which may be of value in diagnosis (Verbov 1970). Just as eccrine gland function may be defective so may other 'ectodermal' glands; affected children may develop many nasal, sinus, pharyngeal and laryngeal problems and infections (Myer 1987).

Anhidrotic ectodermal dysplasia may sometimes depend on an autosomal recessive gene, in which case the full syndrome may be found in the female. It is not yet certain whether, as is probable, cases so inherited differ in some respects from those determined by a sex-linked recessive gene (Passarge *et al.* 1966; Crump & Danks 1971).

Children with hypohidrotic ectodermal dysplasia have an increased frequency of atopic dermatitis and other atopic disorders. The high incidence of mental retardation in some species may be the results of episodes of hyperpyrexia.

Rapp–Hodgkin hypohidrotic ectodermal dysplasia
In this syndrome originally described in three members of one family, the inheritance is determined by an autosomal dominant gene; hypohidrosis may be severe enough to lead to heat intolerance. The hair is sparse and the nails are narrow and dystrophic; pili torti may be associated (Cirillo *et al.* 1982). Short stature, a cleft lip and palate and hypospadia are other features (Schroeder & Sybert 1987). The hair is light in colour and may be of the texture of steel wool.

EEC syndrome
The association of Ectrodactyly (lobster-claw deformity), Ectodermal dysplasia, and Cleft lip and palate in a syndrome of autosomal dominant inheritance is now well documented (Brill *et al.* 1972). However, the expressivity of the gene is very variable and there are numerous reports of cases or pedigrees of complex syndromes which are probably genetically distinct but which show some of the main features of the EEC syndrome. All cases in which ectrodactyly or syndactyly and/or cleft lip or palate are associated with ectodermal defects are worthy of full investigation so that the genetic pattern of these syndromes may be elucidated.

Cases reported as the EEC syndrome show sparse hair, malformed teeth with early caries, ectrodactyly, cleft lip and/or palate, lacrimal duct stenosis and renal anomalies, but not all defects are present in all affected individuals within a single family (Brill *et al.* 1972; Preuss & Fraser 1973).

Other cases are reported in which hypotrichosis as one manifestation of ectodermal dysplasia is associated with cleft lip or palate and a variety of other defects, and the presence of such an association should suggest the need for a search of the rapidly growing genetic literature in which such syndromes are gradually being characterized.

Popliteal web syndrome

History and nomenclature. This rare syndrome was first reported by Trilet in 1869, but has been widely recognized only in the last three decades (Roselli & Gulienetti 1961). It has been referred to as the popliteal pterygium syndrome or the popliteal web syndrome.

Aetiology. Most pedigrees show autosomal dominant inheritance determined by a gene of variable expressivity (Hecht & Jarvinen 1967), but Bartsocas and Papas (1972) suggest that a form with more severe manifestations including mental retardation may be determined by an autosomal recessive gene.

Clinical features. The principal features of the syndrome are a cleft palate, with or without a cleft lip, lip-pits, popliteal and other webs, hypodontia, enamel defects and toe nail dysplasia. Genital and perineal defects vary greatly in degree. There may be a large clitoris, a bifid scrotum or aplasia of the labia majora. Syndactyly has been present in some cases. An inconsistent feature is absence of eyebrows and eyelashes, with brittle, short, sparse, light-coloured head hair.

Xeroderma, talipes and enamel defect: XTE syndrome
This autosomal dominant syndrome is characterized by dry skin, readily forming blisters in the spring season, talipes and defective enamel. The sweat glands are small and few in number. The scalp hair is coarse and sparse, the eyelashes are absent and the nails are dystrophic.

Clouston's hidrotic ectodermal dysplasia
This hereditary syndrome, which is not excessively rare, is determined by an autosomal dominant gene (Clouston 1929, 1939; Williams & Fraser 1967). A structural gene for a matrix polypeptide is probably implicated (Gold & Scriver 1971). It is alternatively known as Fischer–Jacobsen–Clouston syndrome and is most commonly seen in French-Canadian families. Keratinization is disturbed, resulting in abnormal hair and nails and reduced surface desquamation, most evident on palms and soles. The alopecia is such a striking feature of this syndrome that many pedigrees have been published under the diagnosis of congenital alopecia (e.g. Bazant-Gavalowski 1921; Stevanovic 1959).

Detailed studies of the hair (Gold & Scriver 1972) which is abnormal in 75% of cases has shown reduced elasticity and tensile strength. Birefringence also was reduced; the shaft had a loose structure and the normal parallel longitudinal striation was distorted. However, on X-ray diffraction the α helical structure of the keratin fibres was intact. Biochemically, serine, proline and cystine residues were decreased and tyrosine and phenylalanine residues were increased. A reduced disulphide content was not compensated by a thiol increase. It was postulated that there was depletion of matrix proline and disruption of, or failure of, some disulphide bonds in the remaining keratin. In the scanning electron microscope (Wilsch *et al.* 1977) numerous structural abnormalities are seen in variation in diameter, splitting of the cuticle, fracture without node formation, and an abnormal cuticular pattern (Pierard *et al.* 1979).

Head hair is very sparse, fine, pale and brittle; it may be totally absent. Eyebrows are sparse or absent and eyelashes are few and small. Pubic and axillary hair, and vellus, are sparse or absent. Although the hair changes are inconstant and variable they are present at least in some degree in the majority of cases (Clouston 1929;

Lopez *et al.* 1970; Dethlep & Tronnier 1972). In only 20% of individuals with nail changes is the hair apparently normal (Wilkinson 1974). Sweating is normal. There is often some keratoderma of palms and soles, which may be red, scaly and fissured (Escobar 1983).

General physical development and sexual maturation are normal, but some degree of mental retardation is frequent. The teeth are usually normal. The nails are consistently dystrophic from birth, being thickened, ridged and discoloured or, less frequently, thin and brittle.

The diagnosis is made on the association of alopecia with nail dystrophy, with or without palmoplantar keratoderma, but with normal sweating and no distinctive dental defect. The biochemical and biophysical defects of the hair appear to be diagnostic.

Trichodento-osseous syndrome (TDO syndrome)

All children who subsequently show the distinctive features of this syndrome are born with a full head of tightly curled hair, which tends to become straighter during childhood. Microscopically the structure of the shaft is seen to be normal. The eyelashes also are curly.

The teeth are small and widely spaced, pitted on account of defective enamel, and soon eroded and discoloured. Early caries is inevitable. Dolichocephaly combined with frontal bossing and a square jaw give a distinctive facies. Bone density is slightly to moderately increased. Physical development is normal.

The syndrome is determined by an autosomal dominant gene (Quattromani *et al.* 1983).

Ellis–van Creveld syndrome (chondroectodermal dysplasia)

The principal features of this autosomal recessive syndrome are chondrodysplasia of the long bonds giving rise to acromegalic dwarfism, congenital heart disease in about 50% and ectodermal dysplasia. The latter includes oligodontia and attachment of the upper lip to the anterior gingival margin, small hypoplastic nails and sparse hair, but the hair defect may be mild in degree.

AEC syndrome (Hay–Wells syndrome)

This autosomal dominant syndrome has been identified in seven patients in four families (Hay & Wells 1976). Ankyloblepharon is associated with Ectodermal defects, and Cleft lip and palate (Spiegel & Cotton 1985).

The hair is wiry and sparse, or absent. On electron microscopy the hair shafts show changes similar to those found in the Marie Unna syndrome i.e. longitudinal fluting and focal defects of the cuticle. Skin sections show decreased numbers of hair follicles and sebaceous glands. The nails are absent or dystrophic. The teeth are pointed and widely spaced and are soon eroded or lost, and sweating is diminished. The broad nasal bridge and sunken maxilla produce a facies which is striking rather than pathognomonic.

Inconstantly associated defects include lacrimal duct stenosis, supernumerary nipples, syndactyly and deformities of the auricle.

Basan syndrome

Aetiology. This rarely reported hereditary ectodermal defect is determined by an autosomal dominant gene.

Clinical features. Body hair, eyebrows and eyelashes are sparse throughout life. Scalp hair may at first be normal in quantity, but coarse, and is shed during the second decade. The skin generally is very dry, with sweating reduced to a degree sufficient to give rise to moderate intolerance of heat.

The mucous membranes are dry, and severe dental caries develop early.

Tooth and nail syndrome (Ellis–Dawber syndrome)
In this autosomal dominant syndrome hypodontia, with peg-shaped milk teeth and agenesis of permanent teeth, is accompanied by hypoplastic nails. The hair is sparse with some twisting but not pili torti.

In one family (Ellis & Dawber 1980) there was 50% reduction of palmar sweat pore patency, but the number of sweat pores was normal. Sweating was normal on the trunk and limbs.

Orofaciodigital syndrome I

Aetiology. The inheritance of this syndrome is determined by an X-linked dominant gene, linked in the male.

Clinical features. Oral and skeletal defects dominate the syndrome. The tongue is lobed, the lower lateral incisor teeth fail to develop and the palate is cleft.

In 90% of cases there is brachydactyly, syndactyly or clinodactyly. There are numerous milia on the skin at birth and the hair is frequently fine, sparse, dry and dull. Milia and decreased numbers of sebaceous glands are present (Solomon *et al.* 1970).

Abnormalities of the skin and hair are not features of Orofaciodigital syndrome II; this is inherited as an autosomal recessive disorder.

Sensenbrenner syndrome (Sensenbrenner et al. 1975)
This rarely reported syndrome is probably determined by an autosomal recessive gene. The affected children are small and dolichocephalic. The facies is unusual with frontal bosses, hypertelorism, epicanthic folds, antimongoloid palpebral fissures, full rounded cheeks and eversion of the lower lip. The hair is short and very fine. The teeth are small, grey and widely spaced.

Coffin–Siris syndrome
An autosomal dominant condition with sparse scalp hair, eyebrows and eyelashes but hypertrichosis on limbs, forehead and back. Other major signs include abnormal phalanges and nails, dermatoglyphic changes and delayed dentition with microdontia.

Trichodental syndrome
In a large pedigree the inheritance of this syndrome was determined by an autosomal dominant gene. The scalp hair is fine, dry and lustreless and grows slowly. In the electron microscope the cuticular scale pattern is abnormal. The outer halves of the eyebrows are missing. There is hypodontia.

Curly hair, ankyloblepharon nail dysplasia (CHAND) syndrome
This autosomal dominant syndrome is characterized by curly hair, dysplastic nails and ankyloblepharon.

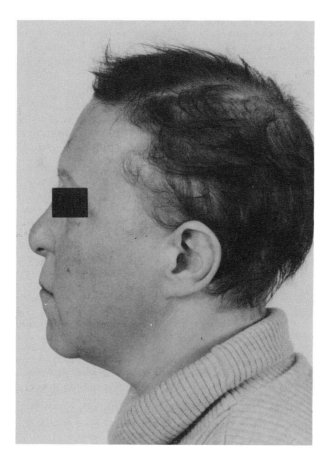

Fig. 6.2 Trichorhinophal-angeal syndrome Type I showing distinctive facies (Professor Hunter, Edinburgh).

Onychotrichodysplasia with neutropenia
In this syndrome, apparently determined by an autosomal recessive gene, sparse hair and dystrophic nails are associated with mild mental retardation and with chronic neutropenia.

Trichorhinophalangeal syndrome, Type I
The inheritance of this syndrome is usually determined by an autosomal dominant gene of variable expressivity, but there may also be a recessive form (Pashyon *et al.* 1974). The principal features are: (i) a distinctive facies provided by a pear-shaped nose and a high philtrum, with a receding chin (Fig. 6.2); (ii) brachyphalangeal dysostosis, which results in fusiform swelling of the proximal interphalangeal joints (Fig. 6.3); and (iii) fine, brittle, sparse hair (Fig. 6.4). The sparse hair is often the symptom for which the patients seek medical advice. The medial halves of the eyebrows are denser than the lateral halves.

Trichorhinophalangeal syndrome, Type II
All reported cases of this syndrome have been sporadic. The nose is bulbous, the philtrum is elongated and prominent, the upper lip is thin and the ears are large and protruding. The scalp hair is sparse. There is some degree of microcephaly and mild to moderate mental retardation.

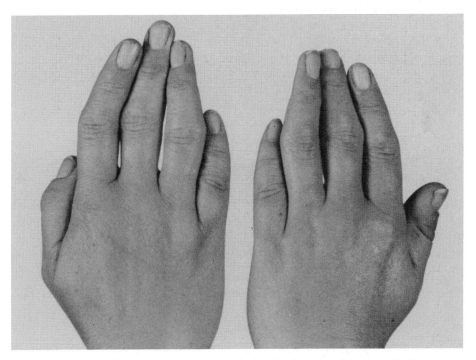

Fig. 6.3 Trichorhinophalangeal syndrome Type I—brachyphalangeal dysostosis (Professor Hunter, Edinburgh).

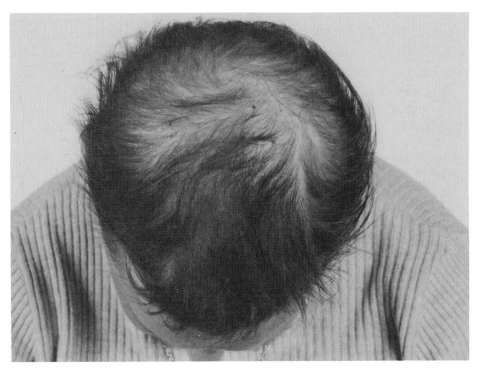

Fig. 6.4 Trichorhinophalangeal syndrome Type I — fine brittle sparse hair (Professor Hunter, Edinburgh.)

Multiple cartilaginous exostoses develop from childhood.

Parizel *et al.* (1987) described a 'hybrid' type of trichorhinophalangeal syndrome with clinical and radiological evidence of Type I but an abnormal karyotype consistent with Type II.

Moynahan syndrome

This very rare syndrome is characterized by absence of hair at birth, and the development of very sparse fine hair later.

Epilepsy and severe mental retardation are present.

References

Bartsocas, C.S. & Papas, C.V. (1972) Popliteal pterygium syndrome. *Journal of Medical Genetics*. **9**, 222.

Basan, M. (1965) Ektodermale dysplasie. Fehlendes Papillanmuster. Nagelveränderungen und Vierfingerfurche. *Archiv für klinische und experimentelle Dermatologie*, **222**, 546.

Baughman, F.A. (1971) CHANDS: the Curly Hair–Ankyloblepharon–Nail Dysplasia Syndrome. *Birth Defects Original Article Series*, **7**, 100.

Bazant-Gavalowski, K. (1921) Hypotrichosis universalis congenita. *Archiv für Dermatologie und Syphilologie*, **137**, 174.

Brill, C.R., Hsu, L.Y.F. & Hirschhorn, K. (1972) The syndrome of ectrodactyly, ectodermal dysplasia and cleft lip and palate: report of a family demonstrating a dominant inheritance pattern. *Clinical Genetics*, **3**, 295.

Cirillo, S.M., Davi, G.F., Bianco, R. *et al.* (1982) Distinctive hair changes (Pili torti) in R.–H. ectodermal dysplasia. *Clinical Genetics,* **21,** 297.

Clouston, H.R. (1929) A hereditary ectodermal dystrophy. *Canadian Medical Association Journal,* **21,** 18.

Clouston, H.R. (1939) The major forms of hereditary ectodermal dysplasia. *Canadian Medical Association Journal,* **40,** 1.

Crump, I.A. & Danks, D.M. (1971) Hypohidrotic ectodermal dysplasia. *Journal of Pediatrics,* **78,** 466.

Dethlep, B. & Tronnier, H. (1972) Beitrag zum Krankheitsbild der hydrotischen (Minor-) Form des Ectodermalen Dysplasia. *Hautarzt,* **23,** 541.

Ellis, J. & Dawber, R.P.R. (1980) Ectodermal dysplasia syndrome: a family study. *Clinical and Experimental Dermatology,* **5,** 295.

Escobar, V.H. (1983) Clouston syndrome: an ultrastructural study. *Clinical Genetics,* **24,** 140.

Freire-Maia, N. & Pinheiro, M. (1985) *Ectodermal Dysplasias.* Alan R. Liss, New York.

Giansanti, J.S., Long, S.M. & Rankin, J.L. (1974) The 'tooth and nail' type of autosomal dominant ectodermal dysplasia. *Oral Surgery,* **37,** 576.

Giedion, A., Burdea, M., Fruchter, Z., Meloni, T. & Trox, V. (1973) Autosomal-dominant transmission of the tricho-rhino-phalangeal syndrome. *Helvetica paediatrica Acta,* **28,** 249.

Gold, R.J.M & Scriver, C.R. (1971) The characterization of hereditary abnormalities of keratin. *Birth Defects, Original Article Series,* **7,** 91.

Gold, R.J.M. & Scriver, C.R. (1972) Properties of hair keratin in an autosomal dominant form of ectodermal dysplasia. *American Journal of Human Genetics,* **24,** 549.

Gorlin, R.J. & Psaume, J. (1962) Orodigitofacial dysostosis: a new syndrome: a study of 22 cases. *Journal of Pediatrics,* **61,** 520.

Gorlin, R.J., Pindborg, J.J. & Colen, M.M. (1976) Chondroectodermal dysplasia. In *Syndromes of the Head and Neck,* 2nd edn., p. 80, eds. R.J. Gorlin, J.J. Pindborg and M.M. Cohen. McGraw-Hill, New York.

Hall, J.G. (1979) Tricho-rhino-phalangeal syndrome type II. In *Birth Defects Compendium,* 2nd edn., p. 1043, ed. D. Bergsma. Macmillan, London.

Hay, R.J. & Wells, R.S. (1976) The syndrome of ankyloblepharon, ectodermal defects and cleft lip and palate: an autosomal dominant condition. *British Journal of Dermatology,* **94,** 277.

Hecht, F. & Jarvinen, J.M. (1967) Hereditable dysmorphic syndrome with normal intelligence. *Journal of Pediatrics,* **70,** 927.

Hernandez, A., Olivares, F. & Carter, J.N. (1979) Autosomal recessive onychotrichodysplasia chronic neutropenia and mental retardation: delineation of the syndrome. *Clinical Genetics,* **15,** 147.

Kerr, C.B., Wells, R.S. & Cooper, K.E. (1966) Gene effect in carriers of anhidrotic ectodermal dysplasia. *Journal of Medical Genetics,* **3,** 169.

Lichtenstein, J., Warson, R., Jorgenson, R., Dorst, R.P. & McKusick, V.A. (1972) The Tricho–Dento-Osseous (TDO) syndrome. *American Journal of Human Genetics,* **24,** 569.

Lopez, D.A., Reed, W.B., Berke, M. & Morales, R.A. (1970) Displasio ectodermico congenita de tepo hidrotico. *Medicina cutanea,* **4,** 335.

Lucaya, J., Garcia-Conesa, J.A., Bosch-Banyera, J.M. *et al.* (1981) Coffin–Siris syndrome: a report of four cases and review of the literature. *Pediatric Radiology,* **11,** 35.

Melnick, N., Shields, E.D. & El-Kafrawy, A.H. (1977) Trichodentoosseous syndrome: a scanning electron microscopic analysis. *Clinical Genetics,* **12,** 17.

Moynahan, E.J. (1970) XTE syndrome (Xeroderma, Talipes and Enamel defect): a new heredofamilial syndrome. Two cases. Homozygous inheritance of a dominant gene. *Proceedings of the Royal Society of Medicine,* **63,** 447.

Moynahan, E.J. (1979) Moynahan Syndrome. In *Birth Defects Compendium,* 2nd edn., p. 723, ed. D. Bergsma. Macmillan, London.

Myer, C.M. (1987) Role of the otolaryngologist in the care of ectodermal dysplasia. *Pediatric Dermatology,* **4,** 34.

Norval, E.J.G., Van Wyk, C.W., Basson N.J. & Coldrey, J. (1988) Hypohidrotic ectodermal dysplasia: a genealogic, stereo microscope and scanning electron microscope study. *Pediatric Dermatology,* **5** (3), 159.

Parizel, D.M., Dumon, T., Vasson, P. *et al.* (1987) The trichorhinophalangeal syndrome revisited. *European Journal of Radiology*, **7**(2), 154.

Pashyon, H.M., Solomon, L. & Chan. G. (1974) The tricho-rhino-phalangeal syndrome. *American Journal of Diseases of Children*, **127**, 257.

Passarge, E., Nuzum, C.T. & Schubert, W.K. (1966) Anhidrotic ectodermal dysplasia as autosomal recessive trait in an inbred kindred. *Humangenetik*, **3**, 181.

Pierard, G.E., Van Neste, D. & Letot, B. (1979) Hidrotic ectodermal dysplasia. *Dermatologica*, **158**, 168.

Porter, P.S. & Aoyagi, T. (1974) Classification of genetic abnormalities of hair growth. *First Human Hair Symposium*, p. 205, ed. A. Brown. New York.

Preuss, M. & Fraser, F.C. (1973) The lobster claw defect with ectodermal defects, cleft lip and palate, tear duct anomaly and renal anomalies. *Clinical Genetics*. **4**, 369.

Quattromani, F., Shapiro, S.D., Young, R.S. *et al.* (1983) Clinical heterogeneity in the **TDO** syndrome. *Human Genetics*, **64**, 116.

Rapp, R.S. & Hodgkin, W.E. (1968) Anhidrotic ectodermal dysplasia: autosomal dominant inheritance with palate and lip anomalies. *Journal of Medical Genetics*, **5**, 219.

Reed. W.B., Lopez, D.A. & Landing, B. (1970) Clinical spectrum of anhidrotic ectodermal dysplasia. *Archives of Dermatology*, **102**, 134.

Robinson, G.C., Miller, J. & Worth, H.M. (1966) Hereditary manual hypoplasia: its association with characteristic hair structure. *Pediatrics*, **37**, 498.

Roselli, D. & Gulienetti, R. (1961) Ectodermal dysplasia. *British Journal of Plastic Surgery*, **14**, 190.

Salinas, C.F. & Spector, M. (1980) Trichodental syndrome. In *Hair, Trace Elements and Human Illness*, p. 290, eds. A.C. Brown & R.G. Crounse. Praeger, New York.

Schroeder, H.W. & Sybert, V.P. (1987) Rapp–Hodgkin ectodermal dysplasia. *Journal of Pediatrics*, **110**, 72.

Sensenbrenner, J.A., Dorst, J.P. & Owens, R.P. (1975) New syndrome of skeletal, dental and hair anomalies. *Birth Defects*, **11**, 372.

Solomon, L.M. & Keuer, E.J. (1980) The ectodermal dysplasias. *Archives of Dermatology*, **116**, 1295.

Solomon, L.M., Fretzin, D. & Pruzansky, S. (1970) Pilosebaceous dysplasia in the oro-facio-digital syndrome. *Archives of Dermatology*, **102**, 508.

Spiegel, J. & Cotton, A. (1985) AEC syndrome: ankyloblepharon, ectodermal defect and cleft lip and palate. *Journal of the American Academy of Dermatology*, **12**, 810.

Stevanovic, D.V. (1959) Alopecia congenita. *Acta Genetica*, **9**, 127.

Summitt, R.L. & Hiatt, R.L. (1971) Hypohidrotic ectodermal dysplasia with multiple associated anomalies. *Birth Defects*, **7**, 121.

Verbov, J. (1970) Hypohidrotic (or anhidrotic) ectodermal dysplasia. An appraisal of diagnostic methods. *British Journal of Dermatology*, **83**, 341.

Wamarachue, N., Hall, B.D. & Smith, D.W. (1972) Ectodermal dysplasia with multiple defects (Rapp–Hodgkin type). *Journal of Pediatrics*, **81**, 1217.

Wilkinson, R.D. (1974) Hidrotic ectodermal dysplasia of Clouston: clinical and histopathological features. *First Human Hair Symposium*, p. 61, ed. A. Brown. Medcon, New York.

Williams, M. & Fraser, F.C. (1967) Hidrotic ectodermal dysplasia—Clouston's family revisited. *Canadian Medical Association Journal*, **96**, 36.

Wilsch, L., Haneke, E. & Schaidt, G. (1977) Structural hair abnormalities in hidrotic ectodermal dysplasia. *Archives of Dermatological Research*, **259**, 101.

Hereditary hypotrichosis: Marie Unna type
(References p. 185)

History and nomenclature

Marie Unna of Hamburg published in 1925 an account of a family in which 27 individuals in seven generations were affected by a previously unreported type of hypotrichosis. Ludwig (1953) found three more cases among the descendants of a member of this same family and Borelli (1954) found two more in another branch of the family. The syndrome is distinctive and most subsequent authors have associated it eponymously with Marie Unna.

Cases have now been reported from Hungary (Kemeny & Csontos 1967), Yugoslavia (Stevanovic 1970), Britain (Peachey & Wells 1971) and the United States (Solomon *et al.* 1971).

Ullmo's (1944) patients were a brother and sister with similar hair changes, but as they also had keratosis pilaris and mental retardation they may not have had the same syndrome.

Aetiology

The inheritance of this form of hypotrichosis is determined by an autosomal dominant gene (Rijzewijk 1988). This mode of inheritance has been noted in all pedigrees in which the diagnosis is beyond question. There may be minor differences between families (Peachey & Wells 1971) but the main features of the syndrome are remarkably consistent.

Pathology

The histological changes in the balding scalp are not pathognomonic. The number of follicles is markedly reduced; granulomatous reactions may be seen around partially destroyed follicles. Solomon *et al.* (1971) found proliferation of the internal root sheath and horn cyst formation in the lower third of some follicles, but Stevanovic (1970) noted proliferation of the external root sheath in the region of the keratogenous zone, with a tendency for it to bulge into the internal root sheath.

With the light microscope the hairs are coarse and flattened, and are twisted at irregular intervals. The shaft diameter may be up to 100 µm as compared with 65–75 µm in normal relations (Ludwig 1953).

In the scanning electron microscope the hair shafts are ridged and the scale pattern is lost, particularly in the valleys between the ridges (Peachey & Wells 1971) (Fig. 6.5). On routine electron microscopy (Solomon *et al.* 1971) there are intra-cellular fractures of cuticular cells and an increase in interfibrillar matrix. On chemical analysis a small decrease in cysteine–cystine and an increase in methionine are found.

Clinical features

The hair may be normal at birth and be shed during infancy, but more frequently is sparse or absent at birth, and remains fine and sparse for the first years of life. During the third year coarse twisted hair grows on the scalp, but with the approach of puberty is progressively lost from the vertex and scalp margins (Fig. 6.6). The ultimate extent of the scarring alopecia shows some variation, and it tends to be more severe in males. It is often patchy (Fig. 6.7). Rijzewijk (1988) noted that if

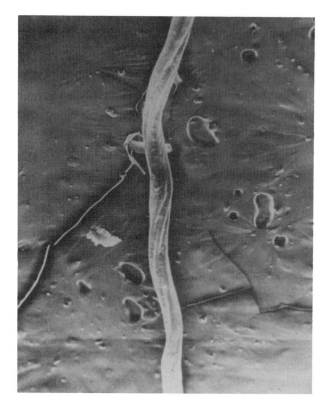

Fig. 6.5 Hair from Marie Unna syndrome: scanning electron micrograph.

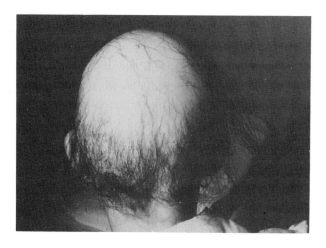

Fig. 6.6 Extensive alopecia in the Marie Unna syndrome.

individual hairs are pulled gently they develop kinks similar to those produced by stretching an iron wire.

Eyebrows and eyelashes and body hair are typically absent or scanty from birth, and after puberty axillary and pubic and beard hair are also sparse.

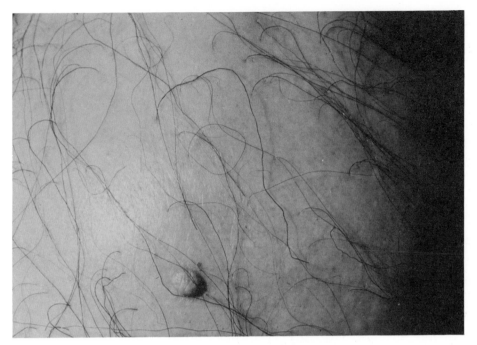

Fig. 6.7 Sparse hair of horse-hair texture in Marie Unna syndrome.

Affected individuals are usually otherwise normal; facial milia were present at birth in all of eight cases in one family (Solomon *et al.* 1971).

Differential diagnosis
Despite the reported variations in the age of onset and degree of severity of the alopecia, the growth of coarse twisted hair in early childhood and its subsequent destruction with scarring on the vertex and the scalp margins cannot be confused with any other syndrome. The histopathological changes are not diagnostic. The defects in the structure of the hair shaft support the clinical diagnosis.

Treatment
There is no effective treatment, but avoidance of trauma may bring some cosmetic benefit as the abnormal hairs may be brittle and are also easily extracted. When folliculitis is troublesome, long-term antibiotic treatment may be useful (Peachey & Wells 1971).

References
Borelli, S. (1954) Hypotrichosis congenita hereditaria Marie-Unna. *Hautarzt*, **5**, 18.
Kemeny, P. & Csontos, E. (1967) Hypotrichosis congenita hereditaria (Unna syndrome). *Kinderärtzliche Praxis*, **35**, 29.
Ludwig, E. (1953) Hypotrichosis congenita hereditaria. Typ. M. Unna. *AMA Archives of Dermatology and Syphilology*, **196**, 261.

Peachey, R.D.G. & Wells, R.S. (1971) Hereditary hypotrichosis (Marie-Unna type). *Transactions of the St John's Hospital Dermatological Society*, **57**, 157.

Rijzewijk, J. (1988) Congenital hereditary hypotrichosis of the Marie-Unna type. *British Journal of Dermatology*, **119**, 129.

Solomon, L.M., Esterly, M.B. & Medenica, M. (1971) Hereditary trichodysplasia: Marie Unna's hypotrichosis. *Journal of Investigative Dermatology*, **57**, 387.

Stevanovic, D.V. (1970) Hereditary hypotrichosis congenita: Marie Unna type. *British Journal of Dermatology*, **83**, 331.

Ullmo, A. (1944) Un nouveau type d'agénésie et de dystrophie pilaire familiale et héréditaire. *Dermatologica*, **90**, 75.

Unna, M. (1925) Über Hypotrichosis congenita hereditaria. *Dermatologische Wochenschrift*, **81**, 1167.

Hallermann–Streiff syndrome
(References p. 187)

History and nomenclature
It was the curious pattern of sutural alopecia which first attracted attention to this syndrome (Aubry 1893). It was subsequently described by others under various designations which emphasized the ocular defects (Lamy *et al.* 1965). Two of at least four such reports were published by Hallermann (1948) and Streiff (1950) who differentiated the syndrome from mandibulofacial dysostosis. François (1958) reviewed the literature thoroughly and gave a good description of the syndrome, which is now known as mandibulo-oculo-facial dyscephaly or, eponymously, as the Hallermann–Streiff syndrome, the Hallermann–Streiff–François syndrome, or the François syndrome.

Aetiology
This complex of ectodermal and mesodermal defects has not been proved to be hereditary, and most cases have been sporadic. However, it has been reported in a father and son (Guyard *et al.* 1962), and may be determined by a dominant gene, most cases being new mutations.

Pathology
The atrophic skin shows loosely woven collagen and frequent abnormal elastic fibres (François & Pierard 1971). The hair shafts show, in the scanning electron microscope, circumferential grooving of the cuticle, which in places is deficient (Golomb & Porter 1975).

Clinical features
Dyscephaly, a beaked nose and a hypoplastic mandible give the patient a bird-like profile. Physical and mental development is retarded. Microphthalmia and congenital cataracts are the concomitant of many ocular defects (François 1958). Dental defects also are frequent and numerous (Hutchinson 1971); teeth may be absent, hypoplastic or irregularly implanted.

The scalp hair may be normal at birth but soon becomes diffusely sparse and brittle, with frontal baldness, baldness of lateral and posterior scalp margins or, most characteristically, following the lines of the cranial sutures. Eyebrows and eyelashes are scanty or absent and pubic and axillary hair also may be sparse (Golomb & Porter 1975). The case described by Gratton *et al.* (1989) showed well-defined areas of alopecia in the frontal and parietal scalp which did not obviously follow suture lines; eyebrows and eyelashes were normal. The scalp within the areas of alopecia appeared wrinkled and atrophic although some fine vellus hairs were still present.

The skin of the face is atrophic, particularly in the central area, where telangiectasia may be marked. The subcutaneous veins may be conspicuously visible.

Diagnosis
Association of hair loss with distinctive facies should establish the diagnosis. In progeria alopecia is diffuse and the cutaneous atrophy is generalized.

Treatment
Little can be offered but regular ophthalmic and dental supervision and the provision of a wig.

References
Aubry, M. (1893) Variété singulaire d'alopécie congénitale: Alopécie suturale. *Annales de Dermatologie et de Syphiligraphie*, **4**, 399.
François, J. (1958) A new syndrome: dyscephalia with bird face and dental anomalies, nanism, hypotrichosis, cutaneous atrophy, micro-ophthalmia and congenital cataract. *Archives of Ophthalmology*, **60**, 842.
François, J. & Pierard, J. (1971) François dyscephalic syndrome and skin manifestations. *American Journal of Ophthalmology*, **71**, 1241.
Golomb, R.S. & Porter, P.S. (1975) A distinct hair shaft abnormality in the Hallermann–Streiff syndrome. *Cutis*, **16**, 122.
Gratton, C.E.H., Liddle, B.J. & Willshaw, H.E. (1989) Atrophic alopecia in the Hallermann–Streiff syndrome. *Clinical and experimental Dermatology*, **14**, 250.
Guyard, M., Perdriel, G. & Cerutti, F. (1962) Sur deux cas de syndrome dyscéphalique à tête d'oiseau. *Bulletin de la Société ophtalmique de France*, **62**, 433.
Hallermann, W. (1948) Vogelgesicht und Cataracta congenita. *Klinische Monatschrifte für Augenheilkunde*, **113**, 315.
Hutchinson, D. (1971) Oral manifestations of oculomandibulodyscephaly with hypotrichosis. *Oral Surgery*, **31**, 234.
Lamy, M., Jammet, M.-L., Marateaux, P. & Ajjan, N. (1965) Le Dyscephalu. *Archives françaises de Pédiatrie*, **22**, 929.
Streiff, E.B. (1950) Dysmorphie mandibulo-faciale (tête d'oiseau) et altérations oculaires. *Ophthalmologie*, **120**, 79.

Atrichia with papular lesions
(References p. 188)

History and nomenclature
Under this descriptive term Damsté & Prakken (1954) of Amsterdam described in their patients a distinctive association of atrichia with numerous follicular

keratinous cysts. A few years later Loewenthal & Prakken (1961) reported another very similar case. The few cases since published have been observed in Germany, in Spain or in Latin American countries. The mode of inheritance is uncertain but two Mexican patients were sisters (Castillo *et al.* 1974). Two affected brothers were the children of an incestuous relationship (Fonseca Moreton *et al.* 1972). Three German patients were brothers (Czarnecki & Stiegl 1980). Autosomal recessive inheritance is therefore probable.

Although all cases show lack of hair in association with keratinous cysts, there is considerable variation between them and it cannot yet be established whether one or more genotypes are concerned.

Pathology
The papules are keratin-filled follicular cysts. The scalp shows normal sebaceous glands and horn plugs in the follicular orifices (Castillo *et al.* 1974).

Clinical features
The first of the three cases of Damsté & Prakken (1954) was a women aged 26. She had been born with normal hair which was soon shed and never replaced. She had sparse eyebrows, normal lashes and no body hair. She began to develop horny papules on her face at 18 and they gradually spread to other parts of the body. In the two other patients described by these authors the hair loss was similar but the papules began to appear at the age of 5 or 6. In some cases the papules have developed as early as the second year (Castillo *et al.* 1974). The papules are pin-head sized, smooth and white (Loewenthal & Prakken 1961).

The patient reported by Ledo *et al.* (1973) was a boy who showed essentially the same features as did the two Spanish brothers (Fonseca Moreton *et al.* 1972), who also had severe acne.

The three patients reported by Czarnecki & Stiegl (1980) were hairless from birth, and developed follicular cysts from the age of 7; they also showed retarded ossification and abnormal dental implantation.

Physical and mental development have been normal except in two sisters (Castillo *et al.* 1974) who were mentally retarded.

A case reported under this diagnosis from the Argentine (Krinaa 1955) gives insufficient detail for classification. The patient was bald from birth and had also atrophoderma vermiculata of the cheeks. His grandmother and maternal aunt were similarly affected.

A Japanese patient also had extensive polyposis throughout the gastrointestinal tract (Ishii *et al.* 1979).

References
del Castillo, V., Ruiz-Maldonado, R. & Carvale, A. (1974) Atrichia with papular lesions and mental retardation in two sisters. *International Journal of Dermatology*, **13**, 261.
Czarnecki, N. & Stiegl, S. (1980) Atrichia congenita mit Hornzysten—Variante einer partiellen ektodermalen Dysplasia. *Zeitschrift für Hautkrankheiten*, **55**, 210.

Damsté, J. & Prakken, J.R. (1954) Atrichia with papular lesions: a variant of congenital ectodermal dysplasia. *Dermatologica*, **108**, 14.

Fonseca Moreton, A., Aguilar, R., Franil, P., Balsa, T., Oubiña, N. & Prado, C. (1972) Atriquia familiae con pápulas. *Medicins cutanea*, **6**, 407.

Ishii, Y., Kremhara, T. & Nagata, T. (1979) Atrichia with papular lesions associated with gastrointestinal polyposis. *Journal of Dermatology* (Tokyo), **6**, 111.

Krinaa, J. (1955) Atriquia congenita familiae con lesiones papulosas y atrofodermia vermiculata de las surjillas. *Archivos Argentinos de Dermatologia*, **5**, 196.

Ledo, A., Jaqueti, G. & Gallago, J.R. (1973) Atriquia con lesiones papulosas. *Medicina cutanea*, **7**, 339.

Loewenthal, J.A. & Prakken, J.R. (1961) Atrichia with papular lesions. *Dermatologica*, **122**, 85.

Hair in the premature ageing syndromes
(References p. 191)

Sparse scalp and body hair is a feature of progeria. Scalp hair is sparse and fine in metageria, and premature greying followed by loss of hair are usual in Werner's syndrome—pangeria.

A prematurely aged appearance is usual in poikiloderma congenitale and in some forms of bird-headed dwarfism and in Cockayne's syndrome.

Progeria (De Busk 1972)
The inheritance of progeria (Hutchinson–Gilford syndrome) is possibly determined by an autosomal recessive gene but affected subjects do not reproduce and proof is lacking. During the first year the child appears to be more or less normal, though there may be scleroderma-like changes on the abdomen, flanks or thighs and mid-facial cyanosis. During the second year somatic growth becomes retarded and subcutaneous fat is progressively lost. Alopecia becomes total, apart from a few downy blonde or white hairs, and eyebrows and lashes are sometimes shed. The child comes to resemble a little old man and early death from premature arteriosclerosis is inevitable. Insulin resistance is common but diabetes is rare (Rosenbloom *et al.* 1983); other abnormalities described include variable serum lipid abnormalities, increased metabolic rate, abnormal collagen and decreased fibroblast lifespan in culture.

The syndrome is rare, only approximately 80 cases having been described (Paller 1989)

Metageria
This recently described autosomal recessive syndrome (Gilkes *et al.* 1974) is characterized by normal physical and mental development, lack of subcutaneous fat, and a thin face with a prominent broad nose. During the second decade mottled pigmentation and telangiectases develop. The scalp hair is fine and sparse.

Werner's syndrome (pangeria)
The inheritance of this uncommon but widely distributed syndrome is determined by an autosomal recessive gene. It has been described also as pangeria of the adult

and as pangeria (Gilkes *et al.* 1974), terms which underline its status as one of the spectrum of syndromes characterized by features of premature ageing.

Growth ceases at about the age of 12 years, and the stature remains small.

Greying of the hair at the temples usually begins between the ages of 12 and 14, but onset as early as 8 has been recorded (Maeder 1949). The greying gradually becomes more extensive and may be complete by 20, and is soon associated with progressive alopecia, bitemporal at first, but gradually more diffuse, and the increasing sparsity of the hair is accentuated by a reduction in the diameter of the hair shaft. The ultimate extent of the alopecia is very variable. The body hair also is sparse, and hypogonadism is usual, but not constant.

Other skin changes are usually first noticed between 18 and 30. The lower legs and feet, the forearms and hands are most severely affected, the face and neck less so. The shiny, tense, adherent skin shows mottled pigmentation and telangiectasia. Subcutaneous fat is lost on the face and limbs, and the bird-like facies and spindly limbs contrast with an often obese trunk. Ulcers of the legs are frequent. Cataract develops in some cases between 20 and 35. Diabetes occurs in over 20%, and abnormal glucose tolerance in many more. Early generalized arteriosclerosis shortens life, as does the high incidence of malignant disease (Schumacher *et al.* 1969); Usui *et al.* (1984) described soft tissue sarcomas in three siblings with Werner's syndrome.

Poikiloderma congenitale (Rothmund–Thomson syndrome)
This hereditary syndrome is determined by an autosomal recessive gene. In early infancy erythema of the face and ears and of the extensor aspects of the limbs is

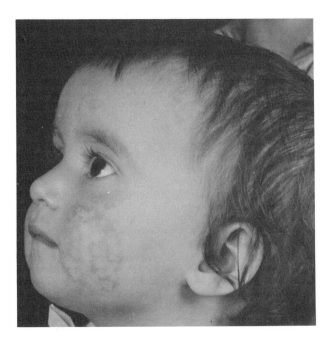

Fig. 6.8 Poikiloderma congenitale — sparse fine hair (Dr Harvey Baker, London Hospital).

followed by mottled pigmentation, depigmentation, atrophy and telangiectasia.

Associated defects may include hypogonadism and cataracts. Scalp, axillary and pubic hair may be sparse or almost absent (Fig. 6.8) and eyebrows and eyelashes are often scanty (Rook *et al.* 1959; Gorlin *et al.* 1976).

Bird-headed dwarfism (Fitch *et al.* 1970)

A beaked nose, micrognathia and low-set ears give these children a distinctive bird-like facies. Dwarfism and microcephaly are characteristic. The hair becomes grey prematurely and hair loss in the male pattern is well advanced by 18.

Cockayne's syndrome (Lasser 1972)

Growth retardation becomes evident during the second year. The limbs are long, with large hands and feet. Photosensitivity results in the early development of solar degenerative changes which increase the aged appearance. Mental as well as physical retardation is usual. The scalp hair is sparse and fine.

References

De Busk, F.L. (1972) The Hutchinson–Gilford progeria syndrome. *Pediatrics*, **80**, 697.

Fitch, N., Pinsky, L. & Lachance, R.C. (1970) A form of bird headed dwarfism with premature senility, *American Journal of Diseases of Children*, **120**, 210.

Gilkes, J.J.H., Sharvill, D.E. & Wells, R.S. (1974) The premature ageing syndrome. *British Journal of Dermatology*, **91**, 243.

Gorlin, R.J., Pindborg, J.J. & Cohen, M.M. (1976) *Syndromes of the Head and Neck*, 2nd edn, p. 652. McGraw-Hill, New York.

Lasser, A.E. (1972) Cockayne's syndrome. *Cutis*, **10**, 143.

Maeder, G. (1949) Le Syndrome de Rothmund et le Syndrome de Werner. *Annales d'Oculistique*, **182**, 809.

Paller, A.S. (1989) Ectodermal dysplasias. In *Textbook of Paediatric Dermatology*, p. 95, eds. R. Ruize-Maldonado, L.C. Parish & J.M. Beare. Grune & Stratton, Philadelphia.

Rook, A., Davis, R.A. & Stevanovic, D. (1959) Poikiloderma congenitale. Rothmund–Thomson Syndrome. *Acta Dermato-Venereologica*, **39**, 392.

Rosenbloom, A.L., Kappy, M.S. & De Busk, F.L. (1983) Progeria: insulin resistance and hyperglycaemia. *Journal of Pediatrics*, **80**, 697.

Schumacher, K., Rodermund, O.E. & Doerfman, R. (1969) Das Werner-Syndrom. *Archiv für klinische Medizin*, **216**, 116.

Usui, M., Ishii, I. & Yamawaki, S. (1984) The occurrence of soft tissue sarcoma in 3 siblings with Werner's syndrome. *Cancer*, **54**, 2580.

Hair defects and skeletal abnormalities
(References p. 194)

Hypotrichosis is a feature of several syndromes in which skeletal abnormalities occur:

1 cartilage–hair hypoplasia
2 chondrodysplasia punctata
3 focal dermal hypoplasia
4 hypomelia–hypotrichosis–facial haemangioma syndrome

Cartilage–hair hypoplasia (metaphyseal dysplasia, McKusick type)
This syndrome is determined by an autosomal recessive gene. It is unexpectedly frequent in Finland (Virolainen *et al.* 1978). A metaphyseal dysostosis from cartilage hypoplasia results in a high degree of dwarfism (McKusick *et al.* 1965). Many affected children showed increased susceptibility to certain infections, and an impaired cell-mediated respone (Lux *et al.* 1970; Virolainen *et al.* 1978). Pierce and Polmar (1982) described marked lymphocyte dysfunction in this syndrome, suggesting that there is a cell cycle specific defeat in T-cell growth. Abnormal elastic tissue was noted in the skin of one patient who also had anergy to common skin test antigens, decreased phytohaemagglutinin responsiveness and increased numbers of natural killer cells (Brennan & Pearson 1988).

The hair is short, sparse, fine and silky, and lighter in colour than in unaffected siblings. There is considerable variation in hair shaft calibre, but if many hairs are measured the hairs of patients are significantly finer and show less variation than those of control subjects (Dapuzzo & Jon 1972). In some affected individuals there may be almost complete baldness.

The appearance of the hair in the electron microscope is normal, apart from decreased diameter and increased spaces between overlapping cuticular cells (Brown 1971; Blackston & Brown 1980). The tensile strength of the hair is disproportionately reduced (Coupe & Lowry 1970). Stress–strain curves are markedly abnormal. The filamentous and matrix proteins of the hair have no gross structural defects, and it has been suggested that decreased reactivity of some disulphide bonds may be responsible for the hair's abnormal properties (Kelling *et al.* 1973).

Chondrodysplasia punctata
Punctate calcification of the long bones, carpal and tarsal bones, the processes of the vertebrae and the ischiopubic bones is present as a radiological change in infancy. During childhood there is asymmetrical shortening of the long bones, with epiphyseal defects in regions which formerly showed punctate calcification.

These skeletal abnormalities form part of two, possibly three, syndromes in which changes of skin and scalp occur in a significant proportion of cases (Sprenger *et al.* 1971).

Chondrodysplasia punctata—Conradi–Hänemann type. Many cases are sporadic but autosomal dominant inheritance is usual (Bergstrom *et al.* 1972). X-linked dominant inheritance also is reported (Happle 1980).

At birth and in early infancy in about 25% of cases extensive erythema and scaling are frequently present, and are succeeded by ichthyosis. A saddle nose and a high arched palate are also found and congenital cataracts are present in 20%. Characteristic stippling of the epiphyses is seen on radiological examination, but tends to disappear after the age of 6 months (Bodian 1966; Tasker *et al.* 1970).

Relatively few reports have been published of children over the age of 5 with this disease, but a high proportion of such patients have shown follicular atrophoderma of the distal extremities, and coarse head hair with patchy cicatricial alopecia (Comings *et al.* 1968; Edidin *et al.* 1977). The hair is lustreless and irregularly twisted. Eyebrows and lashes are sparse and irregular.

Chondrodysplasia punctata—rhizomelic type (Sprenger *et al.* 1971). The inheritance of this disorder is determined by an autosomal recessive gene. The skin changes occur with approximately the same frequency as in the above syndrome, but there are also lymphoedema of the face and microcephaly. Cataracts are present in 80%.

Most affected children die in infancy; those that survive to childhood are severely retarded.

Focal dermal hypoplasia
This is a rare syndrome probably transmitted by an autosomal dominant gene, with lethality in the male (Ruiz-Maldonado *et al.* 1974) for almost all cases have been female. There is widespread dysplasia of mesodermal and ectodermal structures.

The destructive skin lesions are of three types: there are irregular linear streaks of telangiectasia, atrophy and pigmentation; groups, often linear, of soft fatty nodules; and papillomas of the lips and sometimes of the vulva and anus. Skeletal malformations and ocular defects complete the main characteristics of the syndrome (Hall & Terezhalmy 1983; Lawlor & Charles-Holmes 1989).

The scalp hair is usually sparse and brittle and may be lacking completely from small areas of aplasia cutis, which may be present also in the pubic region (Goltz *et al.* 1970). In some cases there may be more extensive cicatricial alopecia (Gomez Orbaneja & de Castro Torres 1967). Two girls (Howell 1965) had generally sparse hair, with linear or oval areas of cicatricial alopecia.

The incidence of hypotrichosis in the syndrome is difficult to estimate reliably. The analysis of 41 case reports (Ishibashi & Kurihara 1972) gave an incidence of 24%, but if only those reports in which the state of the hair is specifically mentioned are included, the incidence is over 80%.

Hypomelia–hypotrichosis–facial haemangioma syndrome
Four cases of this distinctive syndrome, probably inherited as an autosomal recessive trait, were described by Herrmann *et al.* (1969) in two pairs of siblings. The limb defects suggested the designation 'pseudothalidomide syndrome'. The report of a further sporadic case (Hall & Greenberg 1972; Ruiz Gomez *et al.* 1982) emphasized the constancy of its principal features. These are limb reduction defects, a mid-facial capillary naevus, and sparse silver-blonde hair.

The nasal bridge is high, the alae and septum are hypoplastic and the nares are retroverted. These defects in combination with micrognathia give a distinctive facies.

No reports on the electron microscopic appearance or chemical composition of the hair have been published.

References

Bergstrom, K., Gustavson, K.-H. & Jorulf, H. (1972) Chondrodystrophia calcificans congenita (Conradi's disease) in a mother and her child. *Clinical Genetics*, **3**, 158.

Blackston, R.D. & Brown, A.C. (1980) Cartilage–hair hypoplasia. In *Hair, Trace Elements and Human Illness*, p. 257, eds. A.C. Brown & R.G. Crounse. Praeger, New York.

Bodian, E.L. (1966) Skin manifestations of Conradi's disease. *Archives of Dermatology*, **94**, 743.

Brennan, T.E. & Pearson, R.W. (1988) Abnormal elastic tissue in cartilage–hair hypoplasia. *Archives of Dermatology*, **124**, 1411.

Brown, A.C. (1971) Congenital hair defect. *Birth Defects, Original Article Series* VII, 52.

Comings, D.E., Papazian, C. & Schoeme, H.R. (1968) Conradi's disease. *Journal of Pediatrics*, **72**, 63.

Coupe, R.L. & Lowry, R.B. (1970) Abnormality of the hair in cartilage–hair hypoplasia. *Dermatologica*, **141**, 329.

Dapuzzo, V. & Jon, E. (1972) Metaphysale Dysostose und Hypoplasie der Haar: Knorpel-Haar Hypoplasie. *Helvetica Pediatrica Acta*, **27**, 241.

Edidin, D.V., Esterly, N.P., Banzais, A.K. & Fretzin, D.F. (1977) Chondrodystrophia punctata. *Archives of Dermatology*, **113**, 1931.

Goltz, R.W., Henderson, R.R., Hitch, J.M. & Ott, J.E. (1970) Focal dermal hypoplasia syndrome. *Archives of Dermatology*, **101**, 1.

Gomez Orbaneja, J. & de Castro Torres, A. (1967) Un nuevo caso de hipoplasia dérmica focal. *Actas Dermo-Sifiliograficas*, **58**, 93.

Hall, B.D. & Greenberg, M.H. (1972) Hypomelia, hypotrichosis–facial hemangioma syndrome. *American Journal of Diseases of Children*, **123**, 602.

Hall, E.H. & Terezhalmy, G.T. (1983) Focal dermal hypoplasia syndrome. Case report and review of the literature. *Journal of the American Academy of Dermatology*, **93**, 443.

Happle, R. (1980) X-gekoppelt dominante Chondrodystrophia punctata. *Monatschrift für Kinderheilkunde*, **128**, 203.

Herrmann, J., Feingold, M. & Tuffli, G.A. (1969) A familial dysmorphogenetic syndrome of limb deformation, characteristic facial appearance, and associated anomalies: the pseudothalidomide or SC syndrome. *Birth Defects, Original Article Series*, **5**, 81.

Howell, J.B. (1965) Nevus angiolipomatas vs. focal dermal hypoplasia. *Archives of Dermatology*, **92**, 328.

Ishibashi, A. & Kurihara, Y. (1972) Goltz's syndrome: focal dermal dysplasia syndrome. *Dermatologica*, **144**, 156.

Kelling, C., Goldsmith, L.A. & Baden, H.P. (1973) Biophysical and biochemical studies of the hair in cartilage–hair hypoplasia. *Clinical Genetics*, **4**, 500.

Lawlor, F. & Charles-Holmes, S. (1989) Focal dermal hypoplasia syndrome in the neonate. *Journal of the Royal Society of Medicine*, **82**, 165.

Lux, S.E., Johnston, R.B., August, C.S., Say, B., Penchaszadeh, V.B., Rosen, F.S. & McKusick, V.A. (1970) Chronic neutropenia and abnormal cellular immunity in cartilage–hair hypoplasia. *New England Journal of Medicine*, **282**, 231.

McKusick, V.A., Eldridge, R., Hostatler, J.A., Ruangwrt, U. & Egeland, J.A. (1965) Dwarfism in the Amish. *Bulletin of the Johns Hopkins Hospital*, **116**, 285.

Pierce, G.F. & Polmar S.H. (1982) Lymphocyte dysfunction in cartilage–hair hypoplasia. II. Evidence for a cell cycle specific defect in T-cell growth. *Clinical and Experimental Immunology*, **50**, 621.

Ruiz-Maldonado, R., Carnevale, A., Tamayo, L. & Milonas de Montiel, E. (1974) Focal dermal hypoplasia. *Clinical Genetics*, **6**, 36.

Ruiz Gomez, M., Perez Brena, E., Lopez Sanchez, C. *et al.* (1982) H–H–FH syndrome. *Anales Espanoles de Pediatria*, **17**, 229.

Sprenger, J.W., Opitz, J.M. & Bidder, U. (1971) Heterogeneity of chondrodysplasia punctata. *Humangenetik*, **11**, 190.

Tasker, W.C., Mastri, A.R. & Gold, A.P. (1970) Chondrodystrophia calcificans congenita (Dysplasia epiphysalis punctata). *American Journal of Diseases of Children*, **119**, 122.

Virolainen, M., Savilahti, E., Kaitela, I. & Perhecutana, J. (1978) Cellular and humoral immunity in cartilage–hair hypoplasia. *Pediatric Research*, **12**, 961.

Hypotrichosis in other hereditary syndromes
(References p. 197)

Hypotrichosis is reported in some patients with dyskeratosis congenita and has also been associated with hypomelanosis of Ito, and, exceptionally, with xeroderma pigmentosum.

Dyskeratosis congenita
Pachyonychia congenita
Xeroderma pigmentosum
Bazex's syndrome
Hypomelanosis of Ito
Dubowitz syndrome
Johanson–Blizzard syndrome
Dystrophia myotonica
Hypotrichosis, nail, retinal angioma syndrome

Dyskeratosis congenita (Zinsser–Engman–Cole syndrome;
Cole–Rauschkolb–Toomey syndrome)

The inheritance of this syndrome is determined by an autosomal dominant or X-linked gene. Most reported cases have been males, but the full syndrome and partial forms have occurred also in females.

The affected child is usually apparently normal for its first 5 years. During the next 10 years the essential features make their appearance; nail dystrophy and destruction following episodes of infection; leukoplakia leading eventually to carcinoma; reticulate pigmentation most marked on neck and thighs (Bazex & Dupré 1957). Haematological abnormalities are frequent. Llistosella *et al.* (1984) detected macular cutaneous amyloid deposits in dyskeratosis congenita.

The hair is often normal, but may be fine and dry and sparse (Bazex & Dupré 1957). Premature canities has been reported (Connan & Trague 1981; Sorrow & Hitch 1963). Two patients had cicatricial alopecia (Milgrom *et al.* 1964; Nazarro *et al.* 1971).

Pachonychia congenita

The inheritance of this rare syndrome is determined by an autosomal dominant gene of variable expressivity. Present in all cases, and in some degree even at birth, is the pachyonychia, which is strictly a thickening of the nail bed which imparts a pronounced transverse curve to the overlying nail (Baran & Dawber 1984).

Other features are palmoplantar keratoderma, at pressure points, and hyperhidrosis. Leukoplakia, sometimes leading to malignancy, develops on the oral, nasopharyngeal or anal mucous membranes from the second decade onwards.

Hypotrichosis, which may be severe, is present in over 10% of cases (Moldenhauer & Ernst 1968), and may be associated with 'kinky' hair (Soderquist & Reed 1968) or other defects of the hair shafts. Hypotrichosis may be generalized (Vogt *et al.* 1971) or confined to the scalp.

Xeroderma pigmentosum
This term is applied to a group of hereditary disorders all characterized in varying degree by increased susceptibility to light damage, with the early onset of pigmentary changes, atrophy, keratoses and malignant tumours on light-exposed skin (Reed *et al.* 1969). The hair is usually clinically normal, but no biochemical or biophysical studies have been reported. One patient with xeroderma pigmentosum had no hair (Diem & Fritsch 1973), but the association of these defects may have been fortuitous.

Bazex's syndrome (Bazex *et al.* 1964; Somasundaran *et al.* 1988)
The mode of inheritance of this complex syndrome is uncertain. The characteristic features are follicular atrophoderma, localized anhidrosis or generalized hypo-hidrosis, multiple basal-cell carcinomas, and hypotrichosis. In one family in which eight individuals in three generations were known to be affected (Viksnins & Berlin 1977) the hair was normal, but in other reported cases the sparsity of hair has been a striking feature (Cabrera *et al.* 1980; Plosila *et al.* 1981). The hair shafts are defective and may show pili torti (Meynadier *et al.* 1979).

The follicular atrophoderma is present on the dorsa of hands and feet and on the elbows. There may be multiple facial milia at birth. Basal-cell carcinomas of the face develop from adolescence or early adult life.

Hypomelanosis of Ito
This rare syndrome was first reported from Japan, where it is perhaps less un-common than elsewhere, under the name of 'incontinentia pigmenti achromians'. It is characterized by the development of infancy, or later in childhood, of depigmentation which is like a negative image of the pigmentation of 'inconti-nentia pigmenti'. Most cases occur in females and some have ocular and dental defects.

In one reported case (Hamada *et al.* 1967) the scalp hair was said to be sparse.

Dubowitz syndrome (Dubowitz 1965)

Aetiology. The inheritance of this rarely reported syndrome is determined by an autosomal recessive gene.

Clinical features. Low birthweight and retardation of postnatal growth and some degree of mental retardation are associated with a distinctive facies. The hair is sparse and fine. There is a high sloping forehead and flat supra-orbital ridges and a broad nasal bridge. The palpebral fissures are short and the mouth is small. Eczema may develop.

Johanson–Blizzard syndrome

Sparse, fine, hypopigmented hair is associated with aplasia cutis of the scalp and with multiple defects.

Dystrophia myotonica (Steinert's disease) (Slatt 1961)

This rare disorder is inherited as an autosomal dominant trait. It becomes clinically apparent during the third decade with myotonia and muscle wasting. Premature greying of the hair accompanies frontoparietal baldness and reduction in body hair. The subcutaneous fat is diminished. The skin becomes dry as sebum secretion is reduced. There is testicular atrophy.

The average age of onset is 27 years, but the disease can be recognized in infancy (Bell & Smith 1972).

Retinal angiomas, hair and nail syndrome

Tolmie *et al.* (1988) described two sisters with bilateral Coats reaction of the retina, intra-cranial calcification, sparse hair and dysplastic nails; one subject also had retinal angiomas.

References

Baran, R. & Dawber, R.P.R. (1984) *Diseases of the Nail and Their Management*, 1st edn., p. 303. Blackwell Scientific Publications, Oxford.

Bazex, A. & Dupré, A. (1957) Dyskeratose congénital. *Annales de Dermatologie et de Syphiligraphie*, **84**, 497.

Bazex, A., Dupré, A. & Christol, B. (1964) Génodermatose complexe de type indeterminé associant une hypotrichose, un état atrophodermique généralisé et des dégénérescences cutanées multiples (épithéliomas basocellulaires). *Bulletin de la Société française de Dermatologie et de Syphiligraphie*, **71**, 206.

Bell, D.B. & Smith, D.W. (1972) Myotonic dystrophy in the neonate. *Journal of Pediatrics*, **81**, 83.

Cabrera, H.N., Ferreyra, M. & Costa, J.A. (1980) Sindrome de Bazex–Dupré–Christol. *Revista Argentina de Dermatología*, **61**, 97.

Connan, J.M. & Trague, R.H. (1981) Dyskeratosis congenita. Report of a large kindred. *British Journal of Dermatology*, **105**, 321.

Diem, E. & Fritsch, P. (1973) Xeroderma pigmentosum, universelle. Haarlösigkeit und assoziente neuro-oculäre Symptomatik. *Hautarzt*, **24**, 204.

Dubowitz, V. (1965) Familial low birthweight, dwarfism with an unusual facies and a skin eruption. *Journal of Medical Genetics*, **2**, 12.

Hamada, T., Saito, T., Sugai, T. & Morita, Y. (1967) Incontinentia pigmenti achromians (Ito). *Archives of Dermatology*, **96**, 673.

Jelinek, J.E., Bart, R.S. & Schiff, G.M. (1973) Hypomelanosis of Ito. *Archives of Dermatology*, **107**, 596.

Llistosella, E., Moreno, A. & Moragas, J.M. (1984) Dyskeratosis congenita with macular cutaneous amyloid deposits. *Archives of Dermatology*, **120**, 1381.

Meynadier, J., Guilhou, J.-J., Barnéon, G., Malbos, S. & Guillot, B. (1979) Atrophodermie folliculaire hypotrichose, grains de milium multiples associés à des dystrophies ostéocartilagineuses minimes *Annales de Dermatologie et de Syphiligraphie*, **106**, 497.

Milgrom, H., Stoll, H.L. & Crissey, J.T. (1964) Dyskeratosis congenita. *Archives of Dermatology*, **89**, 345

Moldenhauer, E. & Ernst, K. (1968) Das Jadassohn–Lewandowsky Syndrom. *Hautarzt,* **19,** 441.

Nazzaro, P., Argenturi, R., Bassetti, F., Leonetti, F. & Fuzio, M. (1971) La discheratosi congenita di Zinsser–Cole–Engman. *Bollettino dell'Istituto Dermatologico S. Gallicano,* **7,** 3.

Plosila, M., Kiistala, R. & Niemi, K.-M. (1981) The Bazex syndrome; follicular atrophoderma, with multiple basal cell carcinomas, hypotrichosis and hypohidrosis. *Clinical and Experimental Dermatology,* **6,** 31.

Reed, W.B., Landing, B., Sugarman, G., Cleaver, J.E. & Melnyk, J. (1969) Xeroderma pigmentosum. *Journal of the American Medical Association,* **207,** 2073.

Slatt, B. (1961) Myotonia dystrophia: a review of 17 cases. *Canadian Medical Association Journal,* **85,** 250.

Soderquist, N.A. & Reed, W.B. (1968) Pachyonychia congenita with epidermal cysts and other congenital dyskeratoses. *Archives of Dermatology,* **97,** 31.

Solomon, L.M. & Keuer, E.J. (1980) Johanson–Blizzard syndrome. *Archives of Dermatology,* **116,** 1295.

Somasundaram, V., Premalatha, S., Raghuveera Rao, N. *et al.* (1988) Basex syndrome with unusual clinical manifestations. *International Journal of Dermatology,* **27,** 508.

Sorrow, J.M. & Hitch, J.M. (1963) Dyskeratosis congenita. *Archives of Dermatology,* **88,** 340.

Tchou, P.-K. & Kohn, T. (1982) Dyskeratosis congenita: an autosomal dominant disorder. *Journal of the American Academy of Dermatology,* **6,** 1034.

Tolmie, J.L., Browne, B.H., McGettrick, P.M. & Stephenson, J.B.P. (1988) A familial syndrome with Coats reaction retinal angiomas, hair and nail defects and intracranial calcification. *Eye,* **2,** 297.

Viksnins, P. & Berlin, A. (1977) Follicular atrophoderma and basal cell carcinomas. *Archives of Dermatology,* **113,** 948.

Vogt, H.-J., Calap, J. & Müller-Jensen, K. (1971) Jadassohn–Lewandowsky–Syndrom mit Miterophthalmos. *Hautarzt,* **22,** 294.

Hypotrichosis in chromosomal abnormalities
(References p. 199)

Down's syndrome

In Down's syndrome (mongolism) which occurs once in about 700 births, and the incidence of which increases with the age of the mother, some 95% of cases are due to trisomy 21, and the remainder to other chromosomal abnormalities.

The most frequent cutaneous changes are vascular (Desmons *et al.* 1974): fixed erythema of the cheeks and livedo reticularis of the limbs. Keratosis pilaris and other keratotic lesions are common. The skin is soft and velvety in infancy, but during childhood becomes progressively drier and more scaly.

Skin infections occur frequently and infection and trauma partly account for the chronic cheilitis seen in well over 50%, and increasing in incidence with age (Butterworth *et al.* 1960).

The hair may be normal, but is often fine and may become sparse and dry. The most comprehensive study of the hair in Down's syndrome was reported by Vivot (1968) in his thesis. His figures show that sparsity of pubic and axillary hair is less often found than some authors have suggested, but the horizontal pattern of pubic hair is usual in both sexes. He confirms the high incidence of alopecia areata in Down's syndrome. This is unexplained; the incidence of eczema, asthma and hay fever is lower in these children than in their unaffected siblings (Coghlan & Evans 1964).

Klinefelter's syndrome

The karyotype of this syndrome is 47XXY: it occurs once in about 400 male births.

There are no clinical manifestations before puberty, which tends to be delayed. The testes remain small, but the external genitalia usually develop normally, although they may be small in some patients. Fertility is low. In one series of 50 cases (Becker *et al.* 1966) diminished facial and body hair was a horizontal pubic escutcheon. Gynaecomastia frequently occurs. The urinary gonadotrophin excretion is above normal.

The sparsity of facial hair sometimes brings these patients to a dermatologist, since the wearing of full beards has again become fashionable amongst the young in some countries.

The diagnosis can be confirmed by establishing the karyotype.

References

Becker, K.L., Hoffman, D.L., Albert, A., Underdahl, L.O. & Mason, H.L. (1966) Klinefelter's syndrome. *Archives of Internal Medicine*, **118**, 314.

Butterworth, T., Leoni, E.P., Burmon, H., Wood, M.G. & Shear, L.P. (1960) Cheilitis of mongolism. *Journal of Investigative Dermatology*, **35**, 247.

Coghlan, M.K. & Evans, P.R. (1964) Infantile eczema, asthma and hay fever in Mongolism. *Guy's Hospital Reports*, **113**, 223.

Desmons, F., Bar, J. & Brandt, A. (1974) Les signes cutanés du mongolisme (Trisomie 21). *Bulletin de la Société française de Dermatologie et de Syphiligraphie*, **80**, 232.

Vivot, N.A. (1968) *Alteraciones cutaneas en el Sindrome de Down (Mongolismo)*. Direccion Nacional de Sanidad Escolar. Buenos Aires.

Chapter 7
Defects of the Hair Shaft

Introduction
(References p. 201)

Structural defects of the hair shaft may be sufficient in degree to cause significant cosmetic disability, or they may render the hair abnormally susceptible to injury by minor degrees of trauma. They may also be the result of hereditary or acquired metabolic disorders, to the diagnosis of which they afford valuable clues.

Price (1979) classifies anomalies of the shaft into those which are associated with increased fragility, and those which are not. This distinction is useful because only the former present clinically as patchy or diffuse alopecia. Price's classification will be followed throughout the present chapter. Whiting (1987) has published a detailed and authoritative outline of all the major structural defects. Birnhaum and Baden (1987) have also carefully reviewed the rarer structural abnormalities.

References

Birnhaum, P.S. & Baden, H.P. (1987) Heritable disorders of hair. *Dermatology Clinics*, 5(1), 137.

Price, V.H. (1979) Strukuranomalien de Haarschaftes. In *Haar und Haarkrankheiten*, p. 387, ed. C.E. Orfanos. Fischer, Stuttgart.

Whiting, D.A. (1987) Structural abnormalities of the hair shaft. *Journal of the American Academy of Dermatology*, 16, 1.

Structural defects of the shaft with increased fragility

Monilethrix (References p. 206)

History and nomenclature

Walter Smith of Dublin first published in 1879 a description of 'A Rare Nodose Condition of the Hair', for which Radcliffe Crocker subsequently suggested the term monilethrix, which has been generally accepted. Luce in France independently described the same defect in his Paris thesis entitled 'Un cas curieux d'alopécie innominée'. Alternative names to monilethrix such as Spindelhaare and Alopecia pilorum intermittens have failed to find favour. Many other cases were reported during the next 2 years and the condition was firmly established as an entity at the International Medical Congress in London in 1881. Nevertheless some early reports, and even some more recent ones, confuse monilethrix with other shaft defects. The condition is so distinctive and easily diagnosed by routine light microscopy that sporadic examples are now rarely the subject of a paper—it is probably more common than literature suggests.

Aetiology

The hereditary nature of monilethrix was recognized soon after the condition was first identified. Autosomal dominant transmission has been demonstrated in numerous large pedigrees (Alexander & Grant 1958; Bartosova & Jorda 1973; Beare 1956; Norgaard 1957; Rodemund 1969; Salamon & Schneyder 1962; Solomon & Green 1963; Tomkinson 1932).

The alleged occurrence of normal carriers of the dominant gene has not been proven, for a parent with only 5% of abnormal follicles is easily passed as normal (Deraemaeker 1957). The gene appears to have high penetrance but variable expressivity.

Cockayne (1933) reviewed the evidence that monilethrix may be determined also by an autosomal recessive gene. Several pedigrees suggested this possibility and some more recently published pedigrees do likewise (Hanhart 1955). If the existence of a second genotype is established, it is likely that phenotypic differences can be shown to be present.

Pathology
The hair shaft is beaded and brittle as the result of a developmental defect. Elliptical nodes. 0.7–1.0 mm apart are separated by narrower internodes at which the medulla is lacking. The width of the nodes and the distance between them show some variation within a single family but interfamily variation is probably not significant (Korn-Heydt *et al.* 1967). In the scanning electron microscope (Fig. 7.1)

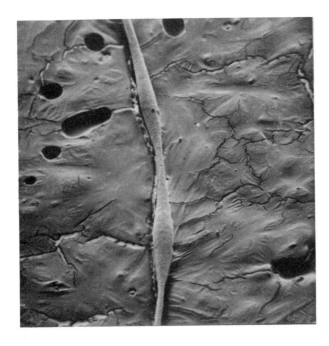

Fig. 7.1 Monilethrix — scanning electron micrograph.

the nodes and some of the internodes show a normal imbricated scale pattern, but most internodes show longitudinal ridging (Dawber & Comaish 1970). This ridging is acquired and progressive as internodes move away from the scalp (Dawber 1980). X-ray diffraction studies (Malt 1965) show α-keratin less well accentuated than in normal hair.

Histologically the follicle shows wide and narrow zones corresponding to the nodes and internodes, but the general structure of the follicle is otherwise traditionally said to be normal (Borda & Abulafia 1952; Salamon & Schneyder 1962). However, the follicles are abnormally distributed and there is no whorl formation. Gummer and Dawber (1981) in a detailed electron microscopic study, noted that changes were visible in the zone of keratinization; the cell membranes of the deeper hair shaft cuticular cells are thrown into folds, particularly at the narrower internodes where breakage occurs. The adjacent inner root sheath was also abnormal.

Attempts have been made to investigate the mechanism of node formation and to relate it to the diurnal rate of hair growth. Behrend (1885) suggested that the nodes were formed at night and the internodes by day. Martin-Scott (1950) was unable to confirm this. Klingmüller (1954) claimed to have found a 48-hour cycle in two patients. Baker (1962) studied four cases in one family in which inheritance was of autosomal dominant type; he found that a complete nodal complex was formed in 24 hours. Comaish (1969) studied two patients autoradiographically and found no daily rhythm and no simple time-cycle; the rate of growth of beaded hair was greater than that of normal hair in the same subject. A recent study (Lubach & Traintos 1979) also showed no regular rhythm of node formation.

Intermittent administration of an anti-mitotic agent can give rise to zones of constriction alternating with zones of normal diameter (Van Scott *et al.* 1957). Mimosine causes similar changes in sheep (Reis *et al.* 1975).

Studies in the electron-microscope (Dawber 1977) have shown that increased susceptibility of the hair shaft to the effects of trauma—premature weathering—is an important factor in the failure of the hair to attain a normal length.

Clinical features

Monilethrix shows considerable variation in age of onset, severity and course. There is not yet sufficient information to establish whether these variations are in part consistently correlated with different genotypes. There is, however, much variation even within the more commonly reported autosomal dominant form, but some of it is merely apparent: vigorous hair brushing may reveal a defect, the presence of which would otherwise have been overlooked.

The hair may be obviously abnormal at birth but is most commonly normal, and is progressively replaced by abnormal hair during the first months of life (Beare 1956): in other cases the normal hair is succeeded by horny follicular papules from the summit of which emerge brittle beaded hairs (Fig. 7.2). The follicular keratosis and the abnormal hairs are most frequent on the nape and occiput but may involve the entire scalp. However, the keratosis is not directly related to the beading and either change may precede the other and the keratosis is sometimes absent. In

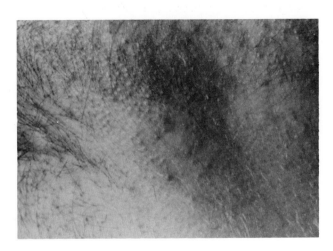

Fig. 7.2 Monilethrix. Follicular keratosis of the nape.

a typical case the short stubble of broken hairs and rough horny plugs gives a distinctive appearance. However, the apparent onset of monilethrix may occur in early childhood or even as late as 17 (Gilchrist 1898). Severe alopecia may develop (Fig. 7.3) or only a few affected hairs may be present, which may be overlooked unless they are carefully sought.

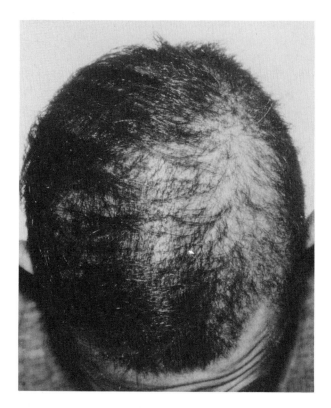

Fig. 7.3 Monilethrix. Moderately severe alopecia.

In some cases the eyebrows and eyelashes, pubic and axillary hair and general body hair may be affected, or one or more of these sites may show few of many abnormal hairs, when the scalp is normal.

In cases of early onset the degree of baldness tends to increase during childhood, but only to a limited extent if trauma is avoided. In many patients the condition persists with little change throughout life (Alexander & Grant 1958), though there may be some temporary improvement in pregnancy (Solomon & Green 1963) (Fig. 7.4). Spontaneous improvement or complete recovery have occurred (Heydt 1964; Solomon & Green 1963). Temporary improvement has followed an epilating dose of X-rays (Ingram 1934) and has been reported during pregnancy (Summerly & Donaldson 1962). Griseofulvin also has temporarily restored normal hair growth (Keipert 1973).

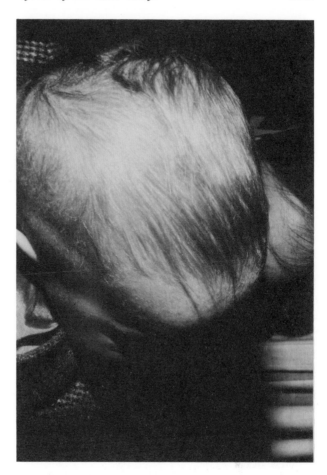

Fig. 7.4 Monilethrix.
Growth of some normal hair
during pregnancy.

Associated defects

Only one of 134 patients with monilethrix had oligophrenia and schizophrenia: genetic linkage is improbable (Korn-Heydt 1967). However, other investigators (Salamon & Schneyder 1962) thought the association with oligophrenia and with nail and tooth defects was significant. Two affected girls also had a delayed and incomplete second dentition (Strandberg 1922). It is possible that such associations may be a feature of the recessive phenotype, since oligophrenia and poor physical development were noted also in two siblings with monilethrix (Sfaello & Hariga 1967). In another family in which the authors (Bartosova & Jorda 1973) suggested that inheritance was of the autosomal recessive type, two of five affected individuals were oligophrenic, and one epileptic. An association with juvenile cataract has been reported on a number of occasions (Thiel 1959).

Reports on abnormalities in amino acid metabolism are conflicting. Argininosuccinicacidura was reported in a number of cases (Grosfeld *et al.* 1964; Barthowick *et al.* 1967; Sobolawska & Wilmanska 1968; Rondon Lugo *et al.* 1977), but a technical error was subsequently detected (Efron & Hoefnagel 1966). No abnormality in the urinary amino-acid pattern was found in a family presenting the autosomal dominant type investigated by Summerly & Donaldson (1962) or in an isolated case in a sickly child (Mäder & Rose 1969). An apparent excess of aspartic acid and of arginine in the urine of an affected mother and daughter (Marques Llagaria *et al.* 1973) remains unexplained.

Diagnosis

The differential diagnosis from other developmental shaft defects must be based on careful microscopical study of affected hairs.

Treatment

None is available but Tamayo (1983) has suggested that oral retinoids can induce some hair regrowth—this may however relate to effects on follicles obstructed by keratosis pilaris. Reduction of hairdressing trauma may be followed by some improvement in the less severely affected cases.

References

Alexander, J. O'D. & Grant, P.W. (1958) Monilethrix. *Scottish Medical Journal*, **3**, 351.

Baker, H. (1962) An investigation of monilethrix. *British Journal of Dermatology*, **74**, 24.

Barthowick, K., Pawkaczyk, B., Sochacka, K. & Spalona, M. (1967) Monilethrix. *Przeglad Dermatologiczny*, **54**, 689.

Bartosova, L. & Jorda, V. (1973) Monilethrix. *Ceskoslovenská Dermatologie*, **48**, 232.

Beare, J.M. (1956) Monilethrix. *Ulster Medical Journal*, **25**, 98.

Behrend, G. (1885) Ueber Knotenbildung am Haarschaft. *Berliner klinische Wochenschrift*, **22**, 270.

Borda, J.M. & Abulafia, J. (1952) Monilethrix. *Archivos Argentinos de Dermatologia*, **2**, 337.

Cockayne, E.A. (1933) *Inherited Abnormalities of the Skin and its Appendages*, p. 144. Oxford University Press, Oxford.

Comaish, S. (1969) Autoradiographic studies of hair growth and rhythm in monilethrix. *British Journal of Dermatology*, **81**, 443.

Dawber, R.P.R. (1977) Weathering of hair in monilethrix and pili torti. *Clinical and Experimental Dermatology*, **2**, 271.

Dawber, R.P.R. (1980) Weathering of hair in some genetic hair shaft abnormalities. In *Hair: Trace Elements and Human Illness*, eds. A. Brown & R.G. Crosin. Praeger, New York.

Dawber, R.P.R. & Comaish, S. (1970) Scanning electronmicroscopy of normal and abnormal hair shafts. *Archives of Dermatology*, **101**, 316.

Deraemaeker, R. (1957) Monilethrix: Report of a family with special reference to some problems concerning inheritance. *American Journal of Human Genetics*, **9**, 195.

Efron, M.L. & Hoefnagel, D. (1966) Argininosuccinic acid in monilethrix. *Lancet*, **i**, 321.

Gilchrist, T.C. (1898) A case of monilethrix with an unusual distribution. *Journal of Cutaneous Diseases*, **16**, 157.

Grosfeld, J.C.M., Mighorst, J.A. & Moolhuysen, T.M.G.F. (1964) Argininosuccinic aciduria in monilethrix. *Lancet*, **ii**, 789.

Gummer, C.L., Dawber, R.P.R. & Swift, J.A. (1981) Monilethrix: an electron microscopic and electron histochemical study. *British Journal of Dermatology*, **105**, 529.

Hanhart, E. (1955) Erstmaliger Hinweis auf das Vorkommen iners Monohybrid-rezessivere Erbgangs bei Monilethrix (Moniletrichosis). *Archiv Julius-Klaus Stiftung für Vererbungsforschung*, **30**, 1.

Heydt, G.E. (1964) Intrafamiliäre Expressivitätshaarkanger des Monilethrix-Gens. *Archiv für klinische und experimentelle Dermatologie*, **219**, 415.

Ingram, J.T. (1934) Monilethrix. *British Journal of Dermatology*, **46**, 272.

Keipert, J.A. (1973) The effect of griseofulvin on hair growth in monilethrix. *Medical Journal of Australia*, **ii**, 1236.

Klingmüller, G. (1954) Monilethrix mit 48 Stunden-Rhythmus. *Hautarzt*, **5**, 23.

Korn-Heydt, G.E. (1967) Uber einem Fall von Monilethrix mit Schwadsinen und Schizophrenia. *Archiv für klinische und experimentelle Dermatologie*, **228**, 445.

Korn-Heydt, G.E., Dinger, R. & Ihen, P. (1967) Statistische Untersuchungen zur intra und inter familiären Variabilität des Monilethrix-Gens. *Archiv für klinische und experimentelle Dermatologie*, **229**, 256.

Lubach, D. & Triantos, N. (1979) Untersuchungen über die Monilethrix. *Hautarzt*, **30**, 253.

Mäder, A.K. & Rose, H-J. (1969) Monilethrix und Argininbersteinsaüre-Ausscheidung. *Dermatologische Monatschrift*, **155**, 409.

Malt, R.A. (1965) Keratin in monilethrix. *Journal of Investigative Dermatology*, **44**, 364.

Marques Llagaria, E., Calap Calatynd, J. & Torres Peris, V. (1973) Monilethrix: Estudio aproposito de dos casos familiares. *Actas Dermo-Sifiligrafícas*, **64**, 203.

Martin-Scott, I. (1950) Monilethrix. *British Journal of Dermatology*, **62**, 35.

Norgaard, O. (1957) Monilethrix i fem generationer. *Nordisk Medicin*, **58**, 1082.

Reis, P.J., Downes, A.M. & Chapman, R.E. (1976) The influence of chemical defleecing agents in the properties of wool. In *Proceedings, 5th International Wool Research Conference, Aachen, 1975*, vol. 4, p. 24, ed. K. Ziegler. Deutsches Wollforschungsinstitut Technische Hochschule, Aachen.

Rodemund, O.E. (1969) Zur Monilethrix. *Zeitschrift für Haut und Geschlectkrankheiten*, **44**, 291.

Rondon Lugo, A.J., Piquero, J., Moullo, J. & Hernandez, P. (1977) Caso de Monilethrix con aminoaciduria anormal. *Dermatologia Venezolana*, **15**, 43.

Salamon, T. & Schneyder, U.W. (1962) Über die Monilethrix. *Archiv für klinische und experimentelle Dermatologie*, **215**, 105.

Sfaello, Z. & Hariga, J. (1967) Monilethrix associé à la debilité mentale: étude d'une famille. *Archives Belges de Dermatologie et Syphiligraphie*, **23**, 363.

Smith, W.G. (1879) A rare nodose condition of the hair. *British Medical Journal*, **11**, 291.

Sobolawska, G. & Wilmanska, J. (1968) Monilethrix and argininosuccinuria. *Prezeglad Dermatologiczny*, **55**, 157.

Solomon, I.L. & Green, O.C. (1963) Monilethrix. *New England Journal of Medicine*, **269**, 1279.

Strandberg, J. (1922) A contribution to our knowledge of Aplasia moniliformis. *Acta Dermato-Venereologica*, **3**, 650.

Summerly, R. & Donaldson, E.M. (1962) Monilethrix. *British Journal of Dermatology*, **74**, 387.

Tamayo, L. (1983) Monilethrix-treated with the oral retinoid Ro-10-9359 (Tigason). *Clinical and Experimental Dermatology*, **8**, 393.

Tomkinson, J.G. (1932) Monilethrix: group of 22 cases. *British Medical Journal*, **ii**, 1009.

Thiel, E. (1959) Monilethrix und Frühstar. *Hautarzt*, **10**, 271.

Van Scott, E.J., Reinertson, R.P. & Steinmuller, R. (1957) The growing hair roots of the human scalp and morphologic changes therein following amethopterin therapy. *Journal of Investigative Dermatology*, **29**, 197.

Pseudomonilethrix (References p. 208)

It is uncommon to see patients who complain that their hair is of poor quality or brittle, and if the patient in question is a young child microscopy of the hair to exclude the classical shaft defects is a routine procedure. It should be a routine procedure also in the older child or adult. Bentley-Phillips & Bayles (1973, 1975) have found a syndrome which they named 'pseudomonilethrix' to be relatively frequent in South Africans of European or Indian descent. The status of the syndrome is uncertain; some of the shaft deformities may be artefactual.

The patients present with alopecia from the age of 8 onwards and their lack of hair can be shown to be the result of a defect, the inheritance of which is determined by an autosomal dominant gene, which renders the hair so fragile that it readily breaks with the trauma of brushing, combing or other hairdressing procedures.

On microscopy one, or occasionally two, of three abnormalities can be seen. There are (i) pseudomonilethrix—irregular nodes, which on electron microscopy prove to be the protruding edges of depressions in the shaft; (ii) irregular twists of 25–200° without flattening of the shaft; (iii) breaks with brush-like ends in apparently normal shaft. There is no keratosis pilaris. Most authorities now believe that pseudomonilethrix microscopic changes are artefactual; they can be produced by, in normal hairs, trauma from tweezers or forceps or compressing overlapping hairs between two glass slides when the indentation in one shaft caused by another overlying hair exactly mimics the appearance of pseudomonilethrix (Zitelli 1986).

The reduction of hairdressing trauma may be followed by a marked improvement in the condition.

References
Bentley-Phillips, B. & Bayles, M.A.H. (1973) A previously undescribed hereditary hair anomaly (pseudo-monilethrix). *British Journal of Dermatology*, **89**, 159.
Bentley-Phillips, B. & Bayles, M.A.H. (1975) Pseudomonilethrix. *British Journal of Dermatology*, **92**, 113.
Zitelli, J.A. (1986) Pseudomonilethrix: an artefact. *Archives of Dermatology*, **122**, 688.

Pili torti (References p. 214)

History and nomenclature
The first definite description of pili torti was given by Schütz in 1900, although earlier authors, notably Unna and Lassar, had referred to the condition. Schütz's paper was entitled 'Pili moniliformis', and reflects the confusion between twisting and beading of the hair shaft, which has still not been completely eliminated from the literature. In 1922 Rieche proposed the term trichokinesis which is still favoured by some German authors. Ormsby & Mitchell (1924, 1925) twice presented the same patient to the Chicago Dermatological Society. On the first occasion the diagnosis was 'atrophia pilorum'; monilethrix. Forster, in discussing the case, drew attention to the fact that the hairs were twisted and not beaded. On the second occasion the diagnosis was simply 'atrophia pilorum'. A very typical case of pili torti was described by Freund in 1925. In 1932 Galewsky suggested the term 'pili torti' which in the same year was adopted by Ronchese in America and has since been widely accepted.

In 'pili torti', the hairs are flattened and at irregular intervals completely rotated through 180° around their long axis (Hellier *et al.* 1940). This may be regarded as a definition of classical pili torti (Fig. 7.5). The increasing use of the scanning electron microscope (Fig. 7.6) is, however, making it clear that twisted hairs occur in many distinct forms, and that the twisting may be associated with a number of

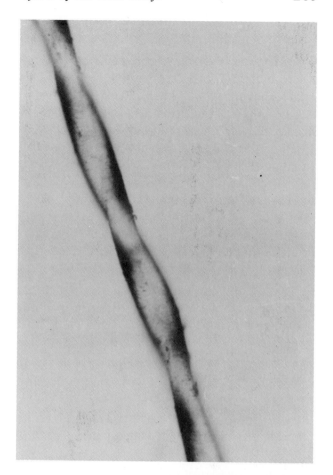

Fig. 7.5 Pili torti; light microscopic appearance.

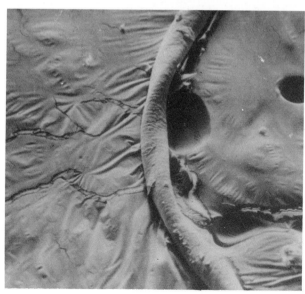

Fig. 7.6 Pili torti — scanning electron micrograph.

other shaft defects. Many more studies will be needed before the significance and specificity of minor variations can be established. As new syndromes are characterized a residue of cases remains in which twisted hair is apparently the sole defect; many reported cases cannot be classified retrospectively since even the known syndromes cannot be excluded on the inadequate data. Occasional twists of varying angle should not be taken to be this distinctive genetically 'fixed' abnormality of pili torti. Many dystrophies and distortions of the follicular zone of keratinization will vary the hair shaft 'bore', sometimes showing < 180° irregular twists.

Syndromes of which twisted hair is a feature

Menkes' syndrome: light-coloured twisted hair as a manifestation of a hereditary defect of intestinal copper transport: the inheritance is of sex-linked recessive type.

Björnstad's syndrome: twisted hair with sensorineural deafness: probable autosomal dominant inheritance.

Bazex syndrome: twisted hair, with basal carcinomas of the face and follicular atrophoderma.

Crandall's syndrome: twisted hair and deafness are associated with hypogonadism: probable sex-linked recessive inheritance.

Hypohidrotic ectodermal dysplasia: twisted hairs associated with characteristic facies and dental defects.

Pseudomonilethrix: twisted hair is associated in the individual or the family with apparently beaded hairs of autosomal dominant inheritance.
　　When patients with these syndromes are excluded, only pili torti remains, but there is evidence that they do not constitute a homogeneous entity; the hairs show considerable variation from patient to patient in their ability to withstand breaking and pulling forces: otherwise expressed the hairs in some patients weather badly, but in others they do not (Dawber 1977).
　　A syndrome has been reported (Pollitt *et al.* 1968) in which siblings with mental retardation had pili torti and trichorrhexis nodosa. Their hair keratin was deficient in cystine. However, dystrophic pili torti may occur with a normal cystine content (Lyon & Dawber 1977). This case developed less weathered hair after puberty but the twists remained—possibly due to hair sebum 'protecting' the hair shafts from weathering (Telfer *et al.* 1989).

Aetiology

In those cases in which classical pili torti of early onset appears to have occurred as an isolated defect, inheritance has usually been determined by an autosomal dominant gene (Appel & Messina 1942; Gedda & Cavalieri 1962). No explanation is available for the apparently high incidence in females. There are many reports of apparently sporadic cases (Laub *et al.* 1987). Some of these could be explained if one parent was affected so mildly that the diagnosis was overlooked. However, there are also cases in which the siblings of normal but consanguineous parents have been affected and in which recessive inheritance must be suspected (Pierini & Borda 1947). There is at present insufficient evidence to allow any dogmatic statements as to possible differences between the two phenotypes.

Pili torti of post-pubertal onset is genetically distinct (Beare 1952; Ullmo 1944). The inheritance of this form is apparently also of autosomal dominant type.

Local inflammatory processes which distort the follicles can result in distorted and twisted hairs, such as may be found around the edges of patches of cicatricial alopecia (Fig. 7.9) (Kurwa & Abdel-Aziz 1973); in these cases, the asymmetrical scarring of the inner root sheath leads to failure of the latter to control cell movement and hair shape; since these are local, twisting develops (Fig. 7.9). Localized pili torti has appeared to follow a scalp infection (Scott 1950). In another case (Schlammadinger 1938) permanent waving probably did no more than reveal the presence of a previously undetected defect. Acquired pili torti type changes were produced by synthetic retinoids (Hays & Camisa, 1985).

Pathology

The earlier reports emphasized that the affected hairs were flattened and twisted through 180° around their long axis; at irregular intervals along the shaft (Hellier *et al.* 1940). Electron microscopic studies have shown that structural defects other than flattening may accompany and indeed probably determine the development of twists. For example, ridging and fluting of the shafts has been described (Björnstad 1941). The X-ray diffraction pattern of hairs from one case (Hellier *et al.* 1940) was of normal α-keratin type, but there must be deviations from parallelism of the polypeptide chains. The load–extension curve resembled that of the wool of merino sheep; the hairs broke more easily than normal, but there was much variation between different hairs.

Histologically the only abnormality is some curvature of the hair follicles. With the scanning electron microscope the cuticle of the hair shaft appears normal (Dawber & Comaish 1970), though severe weathering changes and trichorrhexis nodes are not uncommon.

Clinical features

The hair is usually normal at birth, but is gradually replaced by abnormal hair which becomes clinically evident as early as the third month, or not until the second or third year. In one case a child was bald until 5 and then grew sparse twisted hairs (Clarke & Glicksberg 1941).

There is wide variation from case to case in the fragility of the hair, and hence in the clinical picture.

Affected hairs are brittle and may break off at a length of 5 cm or less, or grow longer in areas of the scalp least subject to trauma (Fig. 7.7). There may therefore

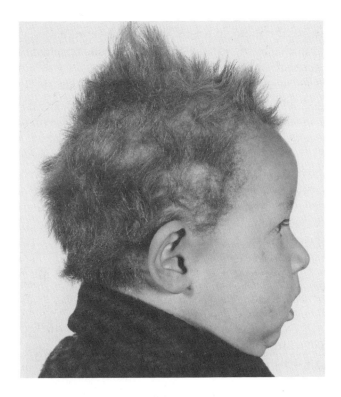

Fig. 7.7 Pili torti of dystrophic type.

be only a short coarse stubble over the whole scalp or there may be circumscribed baldness, irregularly patchy (Siskind 1947) or occipital (Nichamin 1958). Affected hairs have a spangled appearance in reflected light. In mild cases the abnormal hairs have to be carefully sought, for there may be few and the hair may appear grossly normal. Such is sometimes the case after puberty, as normal hairs may replace most of the pili torti during the later years of childhood. However, some patients remain severely affected throughout life. The case described by Lyon and Dawber (1977) continued to retain the pili torti microscopy into adolescence but the hair darkened, ceased to weather badly and grew to a cosmetically acceptable length (Telfer *et al.* 1989).

The involvement of sites other than the scalp has often been reported but is an inconstant feature, most often seen in the more severe cases. The eyebrows may be sparse and twisted (Freund 1925; Mitchell-Heggs & May 1947).

Other ectodermal defects may be associated with pili torti. Keratosis pilaris is the most frequent of them, but nail dystrophies, dental abnormalities, corneal opacities and mental retardation have all been reported, though not simultaneously. One girl aged 16 (Friederich & Seitz 1955) had sparse, twisted hair on the scalp, eyebrows, eyelids, axillae and pubis. She had dystrophic nails of thumbs and big toes, generalized hypohidrosis and a corneal dystrophy.

A boy aged 15 had soft blonde hair until the age of 3, when his hair became darker, coarse and brittle. The scalp hair was twisted and so were some of the sparse brittle vellus hairs on his limbs, and the eyebrows which appeared only at 13 and remained sparse. This may be the same syndrome described by Whiting *et al.* (1980) as corkscrew hair (Whiting 1987).

The post-pubertal type of pili torti presents as a patchy alopecia (Beare 1952; Kurwa & Abdel-Aziz 1973). Eyebrows and lashes, beard and body hair are sparse. The affected hairs are black.

Diagnosis
The diagnosis should be suspected if the hair is brittle and dry. The typical spangled appearance in reflected light (Fig. 7.8) is present only if the hair is at least moderately severely affected, yet is not so brittle that it breaks to leave only a sparse stubble.

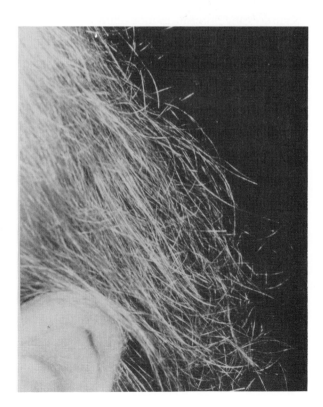

Fig. 7.8 Pili torti, showing 'spangling' effect.

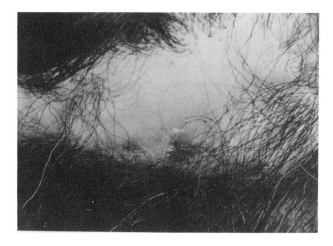

Fig. 7.9 Pili torti: acquired pili torti in cicatricial alopecia.

Microscopical examination of several hairs must be made to confirm the diagnosis. The associated defects of other syndromes with twisted hair should be sought.

Treatment

There is no effective treatment, but reduction of the physical and chemical trauma of hairdressing procedures may allow a considerable increase in length of the hair to take place.

References

Appel, B. & Messina, S.J. (1942) Pili torti hereditaria. *New England Journal of Medicine*, **226**, 912.

Beare, J.M. (1952) Congenital pilar defect showing features of pili torti. *British Journal of Dermatology*, **64**, 366.

Björnstad, R.T. (1941) Ein Fall von 'Pili Torti'. *Acta Dermato-Venereologica*, **22**, 242.

Clarke, G.E. & Glicksberg, E.L. (1941) Pili torti. *Archives of Dermatology and Syphilology*, **43**, 836.

Dawber, R.P.R. (1977) Weathering of hair in monilethrix and pili torti. *Clinical and Experimental Dermatology*, **2**, 271.

Dawber, R.P.R. & Comaish, S. (1970) Scanning electron microscopy of normal and abnormal hair shafts. *Archives of Dermatology*, **101**, 316.

Freund, E. (1925) Su un'anomalia congenita dei capelli finora non descritta. *Giornale Italiano de Dermatologia e Sifilografia*, **66**, 514.

Friederich, H.C. & Seitz, R. (1955) Über eine Forme der ektodermalen Dysplasie unter dem Bilde der Pili torti mit Augurbeteiligung und Störung der Schweisssekretion. *Dermatologische Wochenschrift*, **131**, 277.

Galewsky, E. (1932) Pili torti. *Archiv für Dermatologie und Syphilologie*, **167**, 659.

Gedda, L. & Cavalieri, R. (1962) Relievi genetici delle Distrofie congenita dei capelli. *Cronache dell'Istituto Dermopatico dell'Immacolata*, **17**, 3.

Hays, S.C. & Camisa, C. (1985) Acquired pili torti in 2 patients treated with synthetic retinoids. *Cutis*, **35**, 466.

Hellier, F.F., Astbury, W.J. & Bell, F.O. (1940) A case of pili torti. *British Journal of Dermatology*, **52**, 173.

Kurwa, A.R. & Abdel-Aziz, A.-H.M. (1973) Pili torti—congenital and acquired. *Acta Dermato-Venereologica*, **53**, 585.

Laub, D., Horan, R.F., & Yaffe, H. *et al.* (1987) A child with hair loss: pili torti, apparently unassociated with other abnormalities. *Archives of Dermatology*, **123** (8), 1071.

Lyon, J.B. & Dawber, R.P.R. (1977) A sporadic case of dystrophic pili torti. *British Journal of Dermatology*, **96**, 197.

Mitchell-Heggs, G.B. & May, W.R. (1947) Pili torti. *Proceedings of the Royal Society of Medicine*, **40**, 481.

Nichamin, S.J. (1958) Twisted hairs (pili torti). *American Journal of Diseases of Children*, **95**, 612.

Ormsby, O. & Mitchell, J.H. (1924) Atrophia pilorum. Monilethrix. *Archives of Dermatology and Syphilology*, **10**, 398.

Ormsby, O.S. & Mitchell, J.H. (1925) Atrophia pilorum. *Archives of Dermatology and Syphilology*, **12**, 146.

Pierini, L.E. & Borda, J.M.C. (1947) Pili torti. *Revista Argentina dje Dermatosifilogia*, **31**, 75.

Pollitt, R.J., Jenner, F.A. & Davies, M. (1968) Sibs with mental and physical retardation, with abnormal amino-acid composition of the hair. *Archives of Disease in Childhood*, **43**, 211.

Ronchese, F. (1932) Twisted hairs (pili torti). *Archives of Dermatology and Syphilology*, **26**, 98.

Schlammadinger, J. (1938) Pili torti. *Dermatologische Zeitschrift*, **78**, 206.

Schütz, J. (1900) Pili moniliformis. *Archiv für Dermatologie und Syphilologie*, **53**, 69.

Scott, O.L.S. (1950) Localised pili torti. *Proceedings of the Royal Society of Medicine*, **43**, 68.

Siskind, W.M. (1947) Pili torti. *Archives of Dermatology and Syphilology*, **56**, 540.

Telfer, N., Cutler, T.P. & Dawber, R.P.R. (1989) The natural history of pili torti. *British Journal of Dermatology*, **120**, 323.

Ullmo, A. (1944) Un nouveau type d'agnosie et du dystrophie pilaire familiale et héréditaire. *Dermatologica*, **90**, 74.

Whiting, D.A. (1987) Structural abnormalities of the hair shaft. *Journal of the American Academy of Dermatology*, **16**, 1.

Whiting, D.A., Jenkins, T. & Witcomb, M.J. (1980) Corkscrew hair—a unique type of congenital alopecia in pili torti. In *Hair, Trace Elements and Human Illness*, p. 238, ed. A.C. Brown & R.G. Crounse. Praeger, New York.

Björnstad's syndrome (Crandall's syndrome)

In 1935 Björnstad of Oslo reported five patients in whom pili torti was associated with sensorineural hearing loss. Four of the five were females; members of their families appear not to have been examined but the aunt of one patient is said to have had pili torti and hearing loss, and the brother of another probably had pili torti. A brother of the male patient had both pili torti and deafness. The loss of hair usually began in infancy but in one case it was not noticed until the age of 8. There was a correlation between the severity of the hair defect and the degree of hearing loss. On microscopy the hair shafts showed longitudinal ridging and irregular twisting. A further affected brother and sister suggests that the mode of inheritance is probably autosomal recessive (Voigtlander 1979).

Three brothers were reported with this same association of deafness and pili torti (Reed *et al.* 1967). Two of the brothers were re-investigated after they had reached puberty and were found to have secondary hypogonadism (Crandall *et al.* 1973) with deficiency of luteinizing and of growth hormones. The pedigree suggests that inheritance of this syndrome is determined by an autosomal recessive gene.

Other than that they share two features in common these syndromes must be regarded as distinct.

References

Björnstad, R.T. (1965) Pili torti and sensory neural loss of hearing. *Proceedings of the Fennoscandinavian Association of Dermatologists, Copenhagen*, p. 3.

Crandall, B.F., Samec, L., Sparkes, R.S. & Wright, S.W. (1973) A familial syndrome of deafness, alopecia and hypogonadism. *Journal of Pediatrics*, **82**, 461.

Reed, W.B., Stone, V.M., Boder, E. & Ziprkowski, L. (1967) Hereditary syndrome with auditory and dermatological manifestations. *Archives of Dermatology*, **95**, 456.

Voigtlander, V. (1979) Pili torti with deafness (Björnstad syndrome). *Dermatologica*, **159**, 50.

Menkes' kinky-hair syndrome (Trichopoliodystrophy) (References p. 217)

Aetiology

The inheritance of this syndrome is determined by a sex-linked recessive gene. Although the condition was not recognised until 1962 (Menkes *et al.* 1962) it is estimated to occur once in about 35,000 live births. The biochemical defect of Menkes' syndrome affects the skin, hair and central nervous system reflecting the fact that very many enzyme systems are copper dependent (Peltonen *et al.* 1983).

A partial block in the intestinal absorption of copper (Lott *et al.* 1975) leads to gross copper deficiency to which the pathological changes are believed to be attributable (Danks *et al.* 1972b).

Analysis of the abnormal hair showed a ninefold increase in the free sulphydryl content as compared with normal control subjects (Danks *et al.* 1972b). Similar but less marked changes have been found in the wool of copper-deficient sheep (Gillespie 1964).

Pathology (Menkes *et al.* 1962; Aguilar *et al.* 1966; Danks *et al.* 1971; Mollekaer 1974).

The internal elastic lamina of arteries is fragmented, resulting in tortuosity and wide variation in their calibre. The brain shows gliosis and cystic degeneration. The metaphyses of the long bones show changes resembling those of scurvy.

The serum levels of copper and of caeruloplasmin are low, as is the copper content of the hair (Singh & Bresnan 1973).

Study of the hairs shows several different patterns of hair twisting (Dupré & Enjobras 1980). There may be multiple loose twists in a single direction, or close twists in a single direction, or two or three twists in one direction, followed by two or three in the opposite direction or a single twist of 180° in one direction followed by a single twist in the other direction.

Clinical features

Hair. Hair present at birth is normal (Wesenberg *et al.* 1969; Danks *et al.* 1972a; Collie *et al.* 1980). As this is shed it is replaced by short, brittle, light-coloured, kinky hair, which on microscopy has the features of pili torti. During the early weeks only a few hairs are abnormal. Trichorrhexis nodosa has also been observed (Menkes *et al.* 1962) but this is a non-specific abnormality which occurs readily in structurally defective hair shafts. Monilethrix was mentioned in three case reports (Bray 1965; Billings & Degnan 1971; French *et al.* 1972), but the examination of a large number of specimens from several families showed only 'pili torti' (Danks *et al.* 1972a).

Skin. The skin generally is pale; the pallor was strikingly evident in an affected child of Negro parentage (Volpintesta 1974). The facies is recognizable; the cheeks are plump, the expression lacks emotive mobility, and the eyebrows are horizontal and twisted (Danks *et al.* 1972a).

Systemic. During the first 2 months the child may be apparently normal. There is progressive psychomotor retardation from the third month and the child is drowsy and lethargic. Temperature regulation is impaired and there is a high susceptibility to infection. Convulsions, usually myoclonic jerking movements, are frequent. Survival for more than a year or two is unusual.

Diagnosis
Before the characteristic hair changes appear at about 3 months the diagnosis may be suspected on the basis of the systemic symptoms and the facies. The suspicion may be strengthened by the radiological findings (Wesenberg *et al.* 1969) and confirmed by the estimation of the serum copper.

The heterozygote (Danks *et al.* 1972a)
The obligate heterozygote may have pili torti but her hair may be normal. The serum copper is normal. Skin fibroblasts from heterozygotes show metachromasia in primary culture, and this test may prove to be valuable in detecting carriers amongst the female relatives of a patient.

Treatment (Danks *et al.* 1972b; Bucknall *et al.* 1973; Lott *et al.* 1975)
Treatment with parenteral copper may become feasible as detailed knowledge of the metabolic defect accumulates.

References
Aguilar, M.J., Chadwick, D.L., Okuyama, K. & Kamoshita, S. (1966) Kinky-hair disease: I. Clinical and pathological features. *Journal of Neuropathology and Experimental Neurology*, **25**, 507.
Billings, D.M. & Degnan, M. (1971) Kinky hair syndrome. *American Journal of Diseases of Children*, **121**, 447.
Bray, P.F. (1965) Sex-linked neurodegenerative disease associated with monilethrix. *Pediatrics*, **36**, 417.
Bucknall, W.E., Haslam, R.H.A. & Holtzman, N.A. (1973) Kinky hair syndrome: response to copper therapy. *Pediatrics*, **52**, 653.
Collie, W.R., Goka, T.J., Moore, C.N. & Howell, R.R. (1980) Hair in Menkes' disease. A comprehensive review. In *Hair, Trace Elements and Human Illness*, p. 197, ed. A.C. Brown & R.C. Crounse. Praeger, New York.

Danks, D.M., Cartwright, E., Campbell, P.E. & Mayne, V. (1971) Menkes' kinky hair syndrome: a hereditable disorder of connective tissue. *Lancet*, **ii**. 1089.

Danks, D.M., Campbell, P.E., Stevens, B.J., Mayne, V. & Cartwright, E. (1972a) Menkes's kinky hair syndrome: an inherited defect in copper absorption with widespread effects. *Pediatrics*, **50**, 188.

Danks, D.M., Stevens, B.J., Campbell, P.E., Gillespie, J.M., Walker-Smith, J., Blomfield, J. & Turner, B. (1972b) Menkes' kinky-hair syndrome. *Lancet*, **i**, 1100.

Dupré, A. & Enjobras, O. (1980) Syndrom de Menkes an Pilotorten alternant. *Annales de Dermatologie et Vénéréologie (Paris)*, **102**, 269.

French, J.H., Sherard, E.S., Lubell, H., Brotz, M. & Moore, C.L. (1972) Trichopoliodystrophy. I. Report of a case and biochemical studies. *Archives of Neurology*, **26**, 229.

Gillespie, J.M. (1964) The isolation and properties of some soluble proteins from wool. VIII. The proteins of copper deficient wool. *Australian Journal of the Biological Sciences*. **17**, 282.

Lott, I.T., Di Paolo, R., Schwartz, D., Janonska, S. & Kaufer, J.N. (1975) Copper metabolism in the steely-hair syndrome. *New England Journal of Medicine*, **292**, 197.

Menkes, J.H., Alter, M., Steigleder, G.K., Weakley, D.R. & Sung, J.H. (1962) A sex-linked recessive disorder with retardation of growth, peculiar hair and focal cerebral and cerebellar degeneration. *Pediatrics*, **29**, 764.

Mollekaer, A.M. (1974) Kinky hair syndrome. *Acta Paediatrica Scandinavica*, **63**, 289.

Peltonen, L., Kuivaniemi, H., Palotie, A. *et al.* (1983) Alterations in copper and copper metabolism in Menkes' syndrome. *Biochemistry*, **22**, 6156.

Singh, S. & Bresnan, M.J. (1973) Menkes' kinky hair syndrome. *American Journal of Diseases of Children*, **125**, 572.

Volpintesta, E.J. (1974) Menkes' kinky hair syndrome in a black infant. *American Journal of Diseases of Children*, **128**, 244.

Wesenberg, R.L., Gwinn, J.L. & Barnes, G.R. (1969) Radiological findings in the kinky-hair syndrome. *Radiology*, **92**, 500.

Netherton's syndrome (bamboo hair) (References p. 220)

History and nomenclature

The hereditary association of an ichthyosiform erythroderma with hair shaft defects of 'trichorrhexis nodosa' type was noted by Touraine & Solente in 1937. In 1949 Comèl described and named ichthyosis linearis circumflexa, without referring to hair defects. The distinctive features of this ichthyosiform syndrome had in fact been recorded in 1922 by Rille (Frühwald 1964). Netherton (1958) observed the bamboo-like nodes in the fragile hairs of a girl 'with erythematous scaly dermatitis'. It has gradually become apparent that ichthyosis linearis circumflexa and 'bamboo hairs' (trichorrhexis invaginata) are two features of a single syndrome (Mevorah *et al.* 1974). Most cases of Netherton's syndrome have had ichthyosis linearis circumflexa (ILC) but some have ichthyosis vulgaris (Brodin & Porter 1980; Curban 1973), or both conditions (Schneider *et al.* 1962) or ichthyosiform erythroderma. All cases of ILC in which hair changes have been carefully sought have been found to show them. The syndrome is associated with the atopic state in about 75% of cases, which may explain the occasional association with ichthyosis vulgaris. In one pedigree ILC and ichthyosis vulgaris were found to segregate (Schneider *et al.* 1962).

ILC is thus an almost constant feature of the syndrome, with hair shaft defects of various types and degrees of severity. Until the nature of the underlying abnormality is fully understood the eponym Netherton's syndrome is acceptable. Some authorities (Hurwitz *et al.* 1971) question the variability of the syndrome.

Aetiology
The inheritance of Netherton's syndrome appears to be determined by an autosomal recessive gene of variable expressivity, but the apparent differences in the severity of the hair defect may be related to the trauma to which it is exposed. Girls are affected more often than boys.

Pathology (Ito *et al.* 1984)
The histological changes have until recently been considered not to be diagnostic, but it has now been shown by Mevorah & Frenk (1974) that in the figurate lesions there is eosinophilic degeneration of cells in the upper malpighian layers. The eosinophilic material, probably a glycolipoprotein, is seen also in the overlying parakeratotic horny layer. In the electron microscope the severity of the localized disturbance of keratinization is confirmed (Frenk & Mevorah 1972); the desmosome–tonafilament complex is reduced, membrane coating granules and keratolysation are lacking and dense round bodies are present. The horny layer has lost its lamellar structure.

Scanning electron microscopy of the hair shafts shows focal defects which produce the development of torsion nodules, invaginated nodules (trichorrhexis invaginata) (Fig. 7.10) and trichorrhexis nodosa (Orfanos *et al.* 1971; Murphy *et al.* 1989).

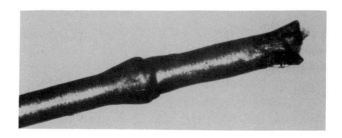

Fig. 7.10. Trichorrhexis invaginata in Netherton's syndrome.

Clinical features (Netherton 1958; Altman & Stroud 1969)
The patient may present primarily either with cutaneous changes or complaining of sparse and fragile hairs. Generalized scaling and erythema are present from birth or early infancy, but the degree, extent and persistence of the erythema are very variable. In some cases the erythema may be slight and transient. On the trunk and limbs the fine dry scales are associated with a polycyclic and serpiginous eruption, the horny margin of which slowly changes its pattern (Fig. 7.11). Rarely there may be small subcorneal bullae in this margin (Dimitrowa & Georgirwa 1961).

Atopic manifestations are superimposed in some patients (Porter & Starke

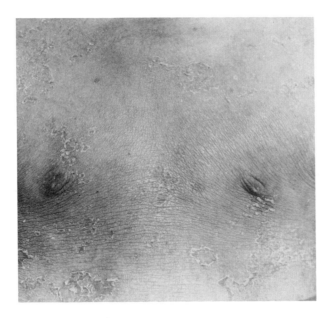

Fig. 7.11 Ichthyosis linearis circumflexa in Netherton's syndrome.

1968) when generalized dryness and flexural lichenification may be the predominant skin changes.

The hair defects may be detected only if deliberately sought, but in most cases are readily apparent clinically (Stevanović 1969; Randell & Wall 1972; Salamon *et al.* 1972). The hair is short, dry, lustreless and brittle, and the eyebrows and lashes are sparse or absent. Weathering and misguided 'treatment' and vigorous hairdressing may influence the severity of the cosmetic disability. Jones *et al.* (1986) described two cases in which neonatal hypernatraemia occurred.

Treatment
The protection of the hair from avoidable physical and chemical trauma may result in considerable cosmetic benefit. Nagata (1980) described response to some degree to photochemotherapy.

References
Altman, J. & Stroud, J. (1969) Netherton's syndrome and ichthyosis linearis circumflexa. *Archives of Dermatology*, **200**, 550.
Brodin, M.M.B. & Porter, P.S. (1980) Netherton's syndrome. *Cutis*, **26**, 185.
Curban, G.V. (1973) Ichthyosis linear circumflexa. *Anais Brasilieros de Dermatologia e Sifilografia*, **48**, 43.
Dimitrowa, J. & Georgirwa, S. (1961) Ichthyosis linearis circumflexa mit subkornealen Bläschen. *Dermatologische Wochenschrift*, **144**, 1041.
Frenk, E. & Mevorah, B. (1972) Ichthyosis linearis circumflexa Comèl with Trichorrhexis invaginata (Netherton's syndrome). *Archiv für dermatologische Forschung*, **245**, 42.
Frühwald, R. (1964) Zur Frage der Comelschen Krankheit. *Dermatologische Wochenschrift*, **150**, 289.
Hurwitz, S., Kirsch, N. & McGuire, J. (1971) Reevaluation of ichthyosis and hair shaft anomalies. *Archives of Dermatology*, **103**, 266.

Ito, M., Ito, K. & Hashimoto, K. (1984) Pathogenesis of trichorrhexis invaginata (bamboo hair). *Journal of Investigative Dermatology*, **83**, 1.

Jones, S.K., Thomason, L.M., Surbrugg, S.-K. & Weston, W.L. (1986) Neonatal hypernatraemia in 2 siblings with Netherton's syndrome. *British Journal of Dermatology*, **114**, 741.

Mevorah, B. & Frenk, E. (1974) Ichthyosis linearis circumflexa Comèl with trichorrhexis invaginata (Netherton's syndrome). *Dermatologica*, **149**, 193.

Mevorah, B., Frenk, E. & Brooke, E.M. (1974) Ichthyosis linearis circumflexa Comèl. *Dermatologica*, **149**, 201.

Murphy, G.M., Griffiths, W.A.D. & Grice, K. (1989) Netherton's syndrome. *Journal of the Royal Society of Medicine*, **82**, 683.

Nagata, T. (1980) Netherton's syndrome which responded to photochemotherapy. *Dermatologica*, **161**, 51.

Netherton, G.W. (1958) A unique case of trichorrhexis nodosa—'bamboo hairs'. *AMA Archives of Dermatology*, **78**, 483.

Orfanos, C.E., Mahrle, G. & Salamon, T. (1971) Netherton-Syndrom. *Hautarzt*, **22**, 397.

Porter, P.S. & Starke, J.C. (1968) Netherton's syndrome. *Archives of Disease in Childhood*, **43**, 319.

Randell, P.L. & Wall, L.M. (1972) Netherton's syndrome—case report. *Australian Journal of Dermatology*, **13**, 119.

Salamon, T., Lazovic, O. & Stenek, S. (1972) Über das Netherton-Syndrom. *Hautarzt*, **23**, 66.

Schneider, W., Coppenrath, R. & Bock, H.D. (1962) Ichthyosis linearis circumflexa bei familiären Auftreten von Ichthyosis vulgaris. *Archiv für klinische und experimentelle Dermatologie*, **215**, 79.

Stevanović, D.V. (1969) Multiple defects of the hair shaft in Netherton's disease. *British Journal of Dermatology*, **81**, 851.

Touraine, A. & Solente, D. (1937) Erythrokeratodermie du cuir chevelu et 'Trichorrhexis nodosa' familiales. *Bulletin de la Société française de Dermatologie et de Syphiligraphie*, **44**, 1011.

Trichorrhexis nodosa (References p. 224)

History and nomeclature

According to Jackson & McMurtry (1913) this defect of the hair shaft was first recognised by Samuel Wilks of Guy's Hospital in 1852, but his first published account of the condition appeared in his *Lectures on Pathological Anatomy* in 1857. Meanwhile Beigel of Vienna had published a description in 1855. A variety of terms have been proposed but trichorrhexis nodosa, suggested by Kaposi, has been generally favoured. Terms which have been frequently used more or less as synonyms are trichoclasis and fragilitas crinium, but both terms merely describe a consequence of the essential abnormality, the formation of nodes, through which rupture of the hair shaft readily occurs. Moreover, trichorrhexis nodosa is not the sole cause of fragile hair.

Aetiology

The literature of the past century has repeatedly revived the controversy as to whether trichorrhexis nodosa is a developmental defect, sometimes hereditary, the consequence of acquired nutritional or metabolic disturbance, or solely a response to trauma, physical or chemical (Chernosky 1974). Nor has there been any agreement concerning the incidence of trichorrhexis; some authors have considered it to be common, others rare. It is in fact the commonest defect of the hair shaft.

Trichorrhexis is best regarded as a distinctive response of the hair shaft to injury (Whiting 1987). If the degree or frequency of the injury be sufficient it can be induced in normal hair. The cuticular cells become disrupted allowing the cortical cells to splay out to form nodes (Dawber & Comaish 1970). If, however, the hair is abnormally fragile trichorrhexis may follow relatively trivial injury. The trauma of hairdressing procedures has often been incriminated (Cajkovac 1938; Chernosky & Owens 1966). Scratching may produce identical changes in the hairs in the genitocrural region (Chernosky & Owens 1966).

The severity of experimentally induced trichorrhexis nodosa was related to the degree of trauma, in patients with or without pre-existing trichorrhexis (Owens & Chernosky 1966). In one patient the cumulative effect of shampooing, brushing, sea bathing and sunlight led to seasonal recurrences each summer (Papa *et al.* 1972). In another the provocative trauma was a chemical hair staightener (Jolly & Carpenter, 1967).

Some authors have differentiated a generalized form from a much rarer localized form, often beginning early in life and sometimes genetically determined (Touraine & Clerfeuille 1938). In fact the distribution depends on the localization and nature of the trauma (Friederich 1950).

That congenital and hereditary defects of the hair shaft can predispose to trichorrhexis nodosa is well established. Some children have other characterized defects of hair shaft structure (Dorn 1956). Trichorrhexis nodosa may occur in pseudomonilethrix, in Netherton's syndrome or with pili annulati (Leider 1950).

Trichorrhexis nodosa is a feature of the rare metabolic defect argininosuccinic aciduria, in which it is associated with mental retardation (Allan *et al.* 1958). There is a deficiency of the enzyme argininosuccinase (Levin *et al.* 1961). Some 20 patients have been reported (Brenton *et al.* 1974). The patients can be classified in three groups, according to the age of the onset of the symptoms (Shih 1972). Where symptoms begin at birth early death is usual; gradual onset during the first months of life is characterized by physical and mental retardation and enlargement of the liver. Onset from the second year onwards is also characterized by psychomotor retardation and also by episodes of ataxia. The hair tends to be dry, brittle and lustreless and may show trichorrhexis nodosa (Rauschkolb *et al.* 1967) but not all patients with this metabolic disorder develop it (Cederbaum *et al.* 1973). As soon as the diagnosis is established a special diet should be provided (Shih 1972).

Trichorrhexis nodosa may occur in certain families as an apparently isolated defect of the hair; node formation and fracture are induced by minimal trauma and develop during the early months of life. Such a defect associated with abnormalities of teeth and nails was determined by an autosomal dominant gene in one family (Rousset 1952). Wolff *et al.* (1975) have described as trichorrhexis congenita the presence from birth of trichorrhexis nodosa confined to the scalp, in a boy with normal teeth and nails.

In a case of generalized trichorrhexis nodosa in a male adult (Leonard *et al.* 1980) electron histochemical study showed evidence of a disorder in the formation of α-keratin chains within the globular matrix of the hair cortex with respect to cystine. This cortical change together with vacuoles found in the endocuticle appear to be the defects which allow the formation of trichorrhexis nodosa in response to relatively trivial trauma.

Pathology

In simple trichorrhexis nodosa the shaft may appear normal with the light or electron microscope except at the nodes; or the shaft, apart from the proximal 1 cm, may show signs of abnormal wear and tear (Dawber & Comaish 1970). At the nodes the cortex bulges and is split by longitudinal fissures. If fracture occurs transversely through a node, i.e. trichoclasis, the end of the hair resembles a small paint brush (Figs. 7.12, 7.13).

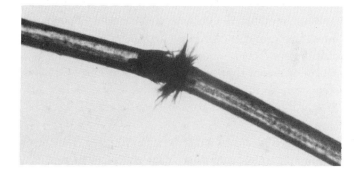

Fig. 7.12 Trichorrhexis nodosa; light microscopic appearance.

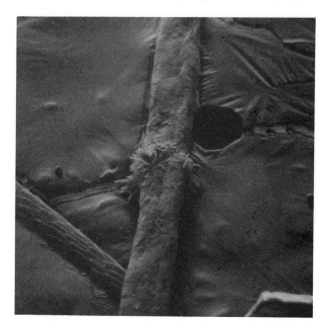

Fig. 7.13 Trichorrhexis nodosa — scanning electron micrograph.

Clinical features

In trichorrhexis nodosa complicating a congenital defect of the hair shafts the hair breaks so easily that large or small portions of the scalp show only broken stumps and alopecia may be quite gross.

In the much commoner conditions in which trauma plays a proportionately larger role and the predisposing inadequacy of the shaft a proportionately smaller one, there are three principal clinical presentations (Price 1975).

Proximal trichorrhexis nodosa occurs in Negroes. The hair is short in areas subjected to the greatest trauma, and trichorrhexis, trichoptilosis and trichoclasis are seen on microscopy.

Distal trichorrhexis nodosa occurs in other races. Often it is discovered incidentally and only a few whitish nodules are seen near the ends of scattered hairs. If many hairs are affected the patient may complain that the hair is dry, dull or brittle. On examination hairs with white nodules are seen among others which have fractured through the nodes.

The third clinical form was well described by Sabouraud (1921) but it appears now to be rare. In a localized area of scalp, moustache or beard, some hairs are broken, and others show from one to five or six nodules (Camacho-Martinez 1989). It is said that trauma of any sort can be excluded, and that spontaneous recovery eventually occurs.

Diagnosis

The congenital forms must be differentiated from other shaft defects. The distal acquired form may simulate dandruff or even pediculosis. In all cases diagnosis depends on careful microscopy and if possible scanning electron microscopy.

Treatment

The avoidance of all unnecessary trauma may be followed by marked improvement.

References

Allan, J.D, Cudsworth, D.C., Dent, C.E. & Wilson, V.K. (1958) A disease, probably hereditary, characterized by severe mental deficiency and a constant gross abnormality of amino acid metabolism. *Lancet,* i, 182.

Brenton, D.P., Cudsworth, D.C., Harthy, S., Lundy, S. & Kuzemko, J.A. (1974) Argininosuccinic-aciduria: clinical, metabolic and dietary study. *Journal of Mental Deficiency Research,* 18, 1.

Cajkovac, S. (1938) Ein Beitrag zur Frage der Schädigung des Haarschaftens. *Dermatologische Zeitschrift,* 77, 305.

Camacho-Martinez, F. (1989) Localised trichorrhexis nodosa. *Journal of the American Academy of Dermatology,* 20(4), 696.

Casals, D.A. & Castellanos, P.G. (1950) Trichorrexie noueuse circonscrite en plaque unique. *Annales de Dermatologie et de Syphiligraphie,* 10, 668.

Cederbaum S.D., Shaw, K.N.F., Valente, M. & Cotton, M.E. (1973) Argininosuccinic aciduria. *American Journal of Mental Deficiency,* 77, 395.

Chernosky, M.E. (1974) Acquired trichorrhexis nodosa. *The First Human Hair Symposium,* p. 36, ed. A.C. Brown. Medcom Press, New York.

Chernosky, M.E. & Owens, D.W. (1966) Trichorrhexis nodosa. *Archives of Dermatology,* 94, 577.

Dawber, R.P.R. & Comaish, S. (1970) Scanning electron microscopy of normal and abnormal hair shafts. *Archives of Dermatology*, **101**, 316.

Dochao, L. de A. & Vidal, A.Z. (1950) Tricoclasia idiopatica. *Actas Dermo-Sifilograficas*, **41**, 347.

Dorn, H. (1956) Dominant geschlechtschromosomengebundener Erbgang bei Trichoclasie. *Zeitschrift für Haut und Geschlectskrankheiten*, **20**, 129.

Friederich, H.C. (1950) Eine Beitrag zur Pathogenese der Trichorrhexis nodosa circumscripta. *Zeitschrift für Haut und Geschlectskrankheiten*, **8**, 163.

Jackson, G.T. & McMurtry, C.W. (1913) *A Treatise on the Diseases of the Hair*, p. 131. Kimpton, London.

Jolly, H.W. & Carpenter, C.L. (1967) Trichorrhexis nodosa following hair straightener. *Cutis*, **3**, 359.

Leider, M. (1950) Multiple simultaneous anomalies of the hair. *Archives of Dermatology and Syphilology*, **62**, 510.

Leonard, J.N., Gunner, C.L. & Dawber, R.P.R. (1980) Generalized trichorrhexis nodosa. *British Journal of Dermatology*, **103**, 85.

Levin, B., Mackay, H.R.M. & Oberholzer, V.G. (1961) Argininosuccinic aciduria, an inborn error of amino acid metabolism. *Archives of Disease in Childhood*, **36**, 622.

Owens, D.W. & Chernosky, M.E. (1966) Trichorrhexis nodosa. *Archives of Dermatology*, **94**, 568.

Papa, C.M., Mills, O.H. & Hanshaw, W. (1972) Seasonal trichorrhexis nodosa. *Archives of Dermatology*, **106**, 888.

Polemann, G. (1950) Zur Kenntnis der traumatischen Trichoklasie und der idiopatischen Trichoklasie Jackson–Sabouraud. *Archiv für Dermatologie und Syphilologie*, **190**, 535.

Price, V. (1975) Office diagnosis of structural hair anomalies. *Cutis*, **15**, 231.

Rauschkolb, E.W., Chernovsky, M.E., Knox, J.M. & Owens, D.W. (1967) Trichorrhexis nodosa—an error of amino acid metabolism. *Journal of Investigative Dermatology*, **48**, 260.

Rauschkolb, E.W., Freeman, R.G. & Farrell, G. (1968) Hair fragility. *Cutis*, **4**, 1315.

Rousset, M.J. (1952) Génodermatose difficilement classable (trichorrhexis nodosa) prédominant chez les mâles dans quatre générations. *Bulletin de la Société française de Dermatologie et de Syphiligraphie*, **59**, 298.

Sabouraud, R. (1921) Trichoclasie, trichorrhexie et trichophilose. *Annales de Dermatologie et de Syphiligraphie*, **2**, 445.

Shih, V.E. (1972) Early dietary management in an infant with argininosuccinase deficiency: preliminary report. *Journal of Pediatrics*, **80**, 645.

Touraine, A. & Clerfeuille, G. (1938) Les diverses variétés de trichorrhexie noueuse. *Bulletin de la Société française de Dermatologie et de Syphiligraphie*, **45**, 636.

Whiting, D.A. (1987) Structural abnormalities of the hair shaft. *Journal of the American Academy of Dermatology*, **16**, 1.

Wolff, H.H., Vigl, E. & Braun-Falco, O. (1975) Trichorrhexis congenita. *Hautarzt*, **26**, 576.

Trichothiodystrophy (References p. 228)

History and nomenclature

This term was coined (Price *et al.* 1980a,b) to describe brittle hair with an abnormally low sulphur content (Van Neste *et al.* 1989a). It is not yet certain whether the different syndromes of which it is a feature represent a single rather variable entity, or distinct entities sharing this feature (Van Neste *et al.* 1989b; Itin & Pittelknow 1990).

Pollitt's patients (Pollitt *et al.* 1968) were mentally and physically retarded. The Mexican family, whose origin in the town of Sabinos has led to this name being attached to the syndrome from which they suffer, have mental retardation, nail dysplasia, and reduced fertility (Arbisser *et al.* 1976; Howell *et al.* 1980). Members of the Amish community with trichothiodystrophy are mildly retarded mentally, and are of small stature (Watson *et al.* 1973; Jackson *et al.* 1974; Baden *et al.* 1976). One patient with this hair defect (Brown *et al.* 1970) was otherwise physically and mentally normal. Patients reported by Jorizzo *et al.* (1980) had lamellar ichthyosis, which has been a feature of other reported cases (e.g. Price *et al.* 1980).

Various syndrome complexes associated with brittle hair have been associated with trichothiodystrophy (Crovato *et al.* 1983):

1 Brittle hair – Intellectual impairment – Decreased fertility – Short stature (BIDS);
2 Ichthyosis and BIDS (IBIDS);
3 Photosensitivity and IBIDS—(Rebora *et al.* 1986) (PIBIDS). Van Neste *et al.* (1989b) described the association of TTD with xeroderma pigmentosa.

Where it has been possible to establish the mode of inheritance this has been of autosomal recessive type.

Pathology
The hair is brittle and weathers badly (Venning *et al.* 1986). With trauma it may break cleanly (trichoschisis) (Fig. 7.14) or may form nodes somewhat resembling trichorrhexis nodosa but without conspicuous release of individual spindle cells (Price *et al.* 1980). The hairs are flattened and can be twisted into various appearances—rather like a ribbon or shoe lace.

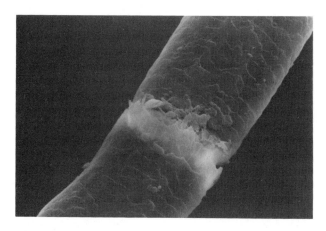

Fig. 7.14 Trichoschisis in trichothiodystrophy.

In the scanning electron microscope the hairs are seen to be flattened, and sometimes folded over themselves (ribbon-like). The shaft is irregular with ridging and fluting and the cuticular scales are patchily absent (Fig. 7.15).

With the polarizing microscope the hairs show alternating bright and dark zones (Fig. 7.16).

The sulphur content of the hair is much reduced.

Gummer and Dawber (1985), using transmission electron microscopic methods, showed a quantitative decrease in high-sulphur protein in the hair shaft and a failure of this protein to migrate to the exocuticular part of cuticle cells.

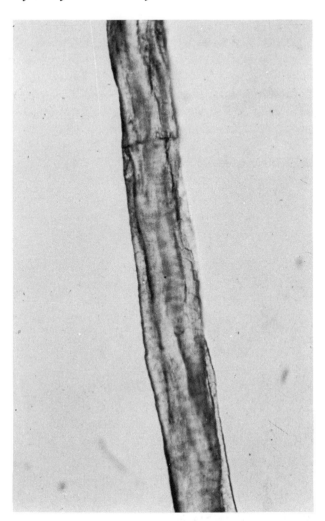

Fig. 7.15 Trichothiodystrophy. In the scanning electron microscope the hairs are seen to be flattened and irregularly ridged and fluted.

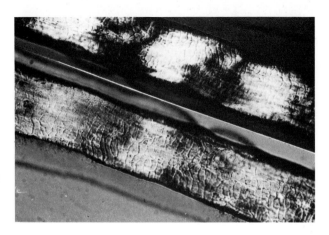

Fig. 7.16 Trichothiodystrophy: alternating bright and dark zones in the polarizing microscope.

Gillespie and Marshall (1983) showed that the low sulphur and cysteine were related to a decrease in high-sulphur protein.

Clinical features

The hair is sparse, short and brittle, but the degree of alopecia varies considerably (Fig. 7.17). In the Sabinos cases it is often almost total. There may be lamellar ichthyosis. The nails may be dystrophic.

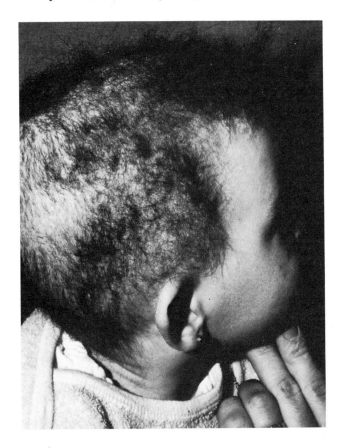

Fig. 7.17 Moderately severe alopecia in trichothiodystrophy.

Mental and physical development may be normal but one or both may be slightly, moderately or severely retarded.

Until further cases have been studied the relationship between the syndromes showing trichothiodystrophy is a matter for speculation.

References

Arbisser, A.I, Scott, C.I. Jr, Howell, R.R., Ong, P.S. & Cox, H.L. Jr (1976) A syndrome manifested by brittle hair with morphologic and biochemical abnormalities, developmental delay and normal stature. *Birth Defects, Original Article Series*, **12**, 219.

Baden, H.P., Jackson, C.E. & Weiss, L. (1976) The physico-chemical properties of hair in the BID syndrome. *American Journal of Human Genetics*, **28**, 514.

Brown, A.C., Belser, R.B. Crounse, R.G. & Wehr, B.F. (1970) A congenital hair defect: trichoschisis with alternating birefringence and low sulphur content. *Journal of Investigative Dermatology*, **54**, 496.

Crovato, F., Borrore, C. & Rebora, A. (1983) Trichothiodystrophy: BIDS, IBIDS & PIBIDS? *British Journal of Dermatology*, **108**, 247.

Gillespie, J.M. & Marshall, R.C. (1983) Comparison of the proteins of normal and trichothiodystrophic human hair. *Journal of Investigative Dermatology*, **80**, 195.

Gummer, C.L. & Dawber, R.P.R. (1985) Trichothiodystrophy: an ultrastructural study of the hair follicle. *British Journal of Dermatology*, **113**, 273.

Howell, R.R., Collie, W.R., Cavasos, O.I, Arbisser, A.I., Fraustadt, U., Marcks, S.N. & Parsons, D. (1980) The Sabinos brittle hair syndrome. In *Hair, Trace Elements and Human Illness*, p. 210, eds. A.C. Brown & R.G. Crounse. Praeger, New York.

Itin, P.H. & Pittelkow, M.R. (1990) Tricothiodystrophy: review of sulfur-deficient brittle hair syndromes and association with ectodermal dysplasias. *Journal of the American Academy of Dermatology*, **22**, 705.

Jackson, C.T., Weiss, J.L. & Watson, J.H.L. (1974) 'Brittle' hair with short stature, intellectual impairment and decreased fertility: an autosomal recessive syndrome in an Amish kindred. *Pediatrics*, **54**, 201.

Jorizzo, J.L., Crounse, R.G. & Winter, C.E. (1980) Lamellar ichthyosis, dwarfism, mental retardation and hair shaft abnormalities. *Journal of the American Schools of Dermatology*, **2**, 309.

Pollitt, R.J., Jenner, F.A. & Davies, M. (1968) Sibs with mental and physical retardation and trichorrhexis nodosa with associated abnormal composition of the hair. *Archives of Disease in Childhood*, **43**, 211.

Price, V.H., Odom, R.B., Jones, F.T. & Ward, W.H. (1980a) Trichothiodystrophy: sulfur-deficient brittle hair. In *Hair, Trace Elements and Human Illness*, p. 220, eds. A.C. Brown and R.G. Crounse. Praeger, New York.

Price, V.H., Odom, R.B., Ward, W.H. & Jones, F.T. (1980b) Trichothiodystrophy: sulfur-deficient brittle hair as a marker for a neuroectodermal symptom complex. *Archives of Dermatology*, **166**, 1375.

Rebora, A., Guarrera, M. & Crovato, F. (1986) Amino-acid analysis in hair from PIBI (D) S Syndrome. *Journal of the American Academy of Dermatology*, **15**, 109.

Van Neste, D., Degreef, H., Van Haute, N. *et al.* (1989a) High sulphur protein deficient hair. *Journal of the American Academy of Dermatology*, p. 195.

Van Neste, D., Miller, X. & Bohnert, E. (1989b) Clinical symptoms associated with trichothiodystropy. In *Trends in Human Hair Growth and Alopecia Research*, No. 19, p. 183. Kluwer Academic Publishing, Dortrecht.

Venning, V.A., Dawber, R.P.R., Ferguson, J.D.P. & Kanan, M.W. (1986) Weathering of hair in trichothiodystrophy. *British Journal of Dermatology*, **114**, 591.

Watson, J.H.L., Weiss, L. & Jackson, C.E. (1973) Scanning electron microscopy of human hair in a syndrome of trichoschisis with mental retardation. In *The First Human Hair Symposium*, p. 120, ed. A.C. Brown. Medcom Press, New York.

Marinesco–Sjögren syndrome

This rare syndrome, of autosomal recessive inheritance, has as its principal features (Norwood 1964) cerebellar ataxia, dysarthria, retarded physical and mental development and congenital cataracts. The teeth are abnormally formed and the lateral incisors may be absent. The nails are flat, thin and fragile.

The hair is sparse, fine, light in colour, short and brittle. On microscopy transverse fractures—trichoschisis—can be seen at the sites of impending fractures. In polarized light the hair is irregularly birefringent. Scalp biopsy shows normal anagen follicles, but with incomplete keratinization of the internal root sheath (Porter 1971).

References
Norwood, W.F. (1964) The Marinesco–Sjögren syndrome. *Journal of Pediatrics,* **65,** 431.
Porter, P.S. (1971) The genetics of human hair growth. *Birth Defects, Original Article Series,* **7,** 69.

Structural defects of the shaft without increased fragility

Pili annulati (ringed hair) (References p. 232)

History and nomenclature
The first description of ringed hair is often ascribed to Karsch of Münster (1846),
but the pigmentary defect in his patient was more complex, with rings of irregular
width as only one of several abnormal features. Erasmus Wilson in 1867 presented
to the Royal Society an account of the condition now known as ringed hair, or as
pili annulati or leucotrichia annularis.

Aetiology
The inheritance of ringed hair has been shown in many extensive pedigrees to be
determined by an autosomal dominant gene (Ehrhardt 1932; Reyn 1934; Juon
1942; Harris & Kalmus 1948; Ashley & Jacques 1950; Tomedei *et al.* 1987). One
pedigree (Ebbing 1957) is compatible with autosomal recessive inheritance, and
there are reports (e.g. McCleary & Montgomery 1955) of apparently sporadic cases
(Dini *et al.* 1988). However, the expressivity of the dominant gene is variable, and
mild cases without any great increase in hair fragility are easily overlooked. Blue
naevus and ringed hair were associated in some members of a family, but the two
conditions segregated (Dawber 1972).

Pathology and pathogenesis
With the light microscope abnormal dark bands alternate with normal, light bands
(Fig. 7.18); in reflected light the colours of normal and abnormal bands are
reversed. The light appearance of the abnormal bands in reflected light is due to air
spaces in the cortex (Cady & Trotter 1922). The rate of growth has been measured
in one case (Dawber 1972) and found to be 0.16 mm/day, which is less than half

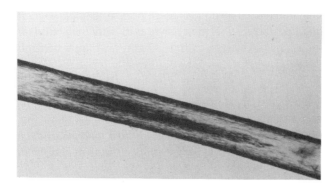

Fig. 7.18 Ringed hair:
alternating bright and
normal bands.

the average normal rate. Breaking stress analysis showed no significant abnormality in ringed hair, but fractures were always in the abnormal bands.

Electron microscopic studies (Price *et al.* 1968) showed that the clusters of air-filled cavities (Fig. 7.19), randomly distributed throughout the cortex in the

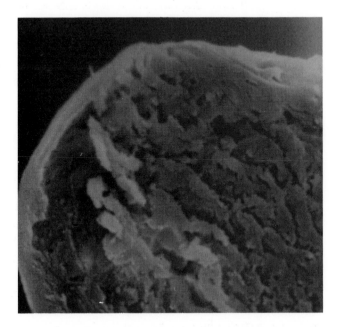

Fig. 7.19 Ringed hair: cortical spaces seen in the abnormal bands in the scanning electron microscope.

abnormal bands, lie partly within cortical cells and between macrofibrils, or in the case of larger cavities appear to replace cortical cells. There is perhaps a defect in the formation of the microfibril matrix complex (Musso 1970). Recent work has indicated that both these suggestions are correct. Hairs from the family described by Dawber (1972) showed an abnormal surface cuticle which appeared 'cobble-stoned' on scanning electron microscopy. The work of Gummer and Dawber (1981) using electron histochemical methods confirmed this; cuticular cells are thrown into folds.

On biochemical analysis (Dawber 1972) the cystine content of affected hair was low, but its sulphur content was normal. The pathogenesis of ringed hair remains uncertain. The abnormal bands appear to be produced at random and not cyclically in relation to specific periods of growth (Dawber 1972).

In Ebbing's (1957) patients in whom recessive inheritance of the trait seemed probable, the bands were regularly spaced. It remains to be seen whether this will prove to be a constant feature of a recessive form.

Clinical features
Ringed hair is associated with a very variable degree of fragility. When the fragility is slight and relatively few hairs are affected the condition may be discovered only

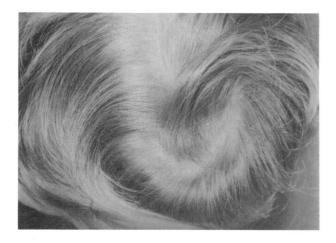

Fig. 7.20 Ringed hair.

when deliberately sought. If many hairs are affected and fragility is great then short hair may attract attention in early life and the spangled appearance of the shafts in reflected light can be readily detected (Fig. 7.20). The axillary hair is occasionally affected (Montgomery & Binder 1948). The fractures in some brittle hairs take the form of trichorrhexis nodosa (Leider 1950).

Diagnosis
The diagnosis is readily established on microscopy of affected hair. A defect in which partially twisted shafts have an elliptical cross section has been named pseudo pili annulati because such hair may give an impression of alternating light and dark bands (Price *et al.* 1970).

Prognosis and treatment
The prognosis is good in the sense that the severity of the defect does not increase with age, but the cosmetic appearance depends largely on restraint in the use of hairdressing procedures. If the hair can be spared chemical and physical trauma, including unnecessary brushing, it may grow to an acceptable length.

References
Ashley, L.M. & Jacques, R.S. (1950) Four generations of ringed hair. *Journal of Heredity*, **41**, 82.
Cady, L.O. & Trotter, M. (1922) Study of ringed hair. *Archives of Dermatology and Syphilology*, **6**, 301.
Dawber, R. (1972) Investigation of a family with pili annulati associated with blue naevus. *Transactions of the St John's Hospital Dermatological Society*, **58**, 51.
Dini, G., Casigliani, R., Rindi, L. *et al.* (1988) Pili annulati. *International Journal of Dermatology*, **27** (4), 256.
Ebbing, H.C. (1957) Gibt es auch bei Ringelhaaren (Pili annulati) einen einfach-rezessiven Erbgang? *Homo*, **8**, 35.
Ehrhardt, S. (1932) Ringelhaare in der Familie E. *Münchene medizinische Wochenschrift*, **79**, 949.
Gummer, C.L. & Dawber, R.P.R. (1981) Pili annulati: electron histochemical studies on affected hairs. *British Journal of Dermatology*, **105**, 303.

Harris, H. & Kalmus, H. (1948) On the manifestation of ringed hair in a mother and daughter. *Annals of Eugenics*, **14**, 209.

Juon, M. (1942) Eine Beobachtung familiären Auftretung von Pili annulati. *Dermatologica*, **86**, 117.

Karsch, A. (1846) De Capillitiri humani coloiebus quardan. Cit. by Landois (1866).

Landois, L. (1866) Das plötzliche Ergrauer der Haupthaare. *Archiv für pathologische Anatomie und Physiologie*, **35**, 575.

Leider, M. (1950) Multiple simultaneous anomalies of the hair. *Archives of Dermatology and Syphilology*, **62**, 510.

McCleary, J. & Montgomery, H. (1955) Ringed hair. Report of a case. *AMA Archives of Dermatology*, **71**, 526.

Montgomery, R.M. & Binder, A.I. (1948) Ringed hair. *Archives of Dermatology and Syphilology*, **58**, 177.

Musso, L.A. (1970) Pili annulati. *Australian Journal of Dermatology*, **11**, 67.

Price, V.H., Thomas, R.S. & Jones, F.T. (1968) Pili annulati. *Archives of Dermatology*, **98**, 640.

Price, V.H., Thomas, R.S. & Jones, F.T. (1970) Pseudo pili annulati. *Archives of Dermatology*, **102**, 54.

Reyn, A. (1934) Pili annulati occurring as a family disorder. *British Journal of Dermatology*, **46**, 168.

Tomedei, M., Ghetti, P., Puiatti, P. *et al.* (1987) Pili annulati: family study. *Giornale Italiano di Dermatologia e Venereologia*, **122** (9), 427.

Wilson, E. (1867) A remarkable alteration of appearance and structure of human hair. *Proceedings of the Royal Society*, **15**, 406.

Woolly hair (References p. 236)

History and nomenclature

Woolly hair is more or less tightly coiled hair occurring over the entire scalp or part of it, in an individual not of Negroid origin. The clinical syndromes of which woolly hair is a feature have been much confused by many authors. The investigation by Hutchinson *et al.* (1974) has done much to clarify the position; the classification proposed by these authors is followed here. It remains possible, however, that woolly hair is a feature also of other syndromes not yet characterized.

Classification and aetiology

1 Hereditary woolly hair. The inheritance of this disorder is determined by an autosomal dominant gene. It has been reported in six generations of a Rhineland family (Hoffmann 1953).

2 Familial woolly hair. The genetic evidence is inconclusive but the condition has occurred in siblings whose parents were normal. Autosomal recessive inheritance is probable (Furando *et al.* 1979).

3 Symmetrical circumscribed allotrichia appears to be a distinct syndrome (Knierer 1955).

4 Woolly hair naevus. This is a circumscribed developmental defect, present at birth, and apparently not genetically determined.

Hereditary woolly hair (Fig. 7.21)

Pathology. In some pedigrees the shaft diameter in affected individuals is reduced (Hutchinson *et al.* 1974); the hair is fragile and may show trichorrhexis nodosa. Pili

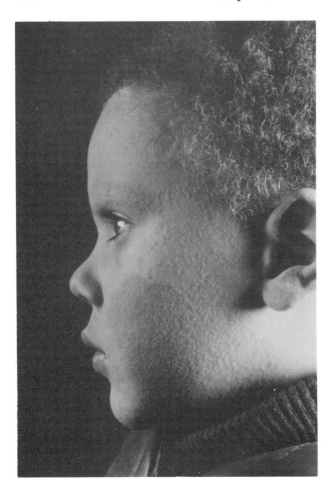

Fig. 7.21 Hereditary woolly hair associated with keratosis pilaris atrophicans (Neild *et al.* 1984).

torti and pili annulati have been reported as associated defects, but in different families.

Clinical features. Excessively curly hair is evident at birth or in early infancy; it has sometimes been described as Negroid in appearance (Mohr 1932; Hoffmann 1953), but tending to become less so in adult life (Schlaginhaufen 1945). Anderson (1936) considered that the hair, though tightly coiled, was not Negroid. The degree of variation in severity within a family is inconstant (Hutchinson *et al.* 1974). There is no consistent association with any hair colour (Schokking 1934). The hair shaft may be twisted (Verbov 1978).

In some cases the hair is brittle and breaks readily, probably as a result of trichorrhexis nodosa. The hair in sites other than the scalp is usually normal but Hoffmann (1953) found it to be sparse and thin.

Familial woolly hair

Pathology. There is a marked reduction in the diameter of hair shafts which may be poorly pigmented. The hair is brittle and on scanning electron microscopy shows signs of cuticular wear and tear (Hutchinson *et al.* 1974).

Clinical features. So few cases have been reported that generalizations are unwarranted. In three cases (Hutchinson *et al.* 1974) fine, tightly curled, poorly pigmented hair was present from birth; in two of them the hair never achieved a length of more than 2 or 3 cm. Eyebrows and body hair were sparse.

In.the case reports of Gottheil (1919) and of Sweitzer (1948) few details are given but the principal findings appear to have been essentially similar.

Salamon's (1963) patients had sparse dark brown, curly hair, and may have had the same condition, but the report again fails to give a sufficiently detailed description.

Symmetrical circumscribed allotrichia

History and nomenclature. Among cases reported as woolly hair naevus are some for which Norwood (1981) has proposed the term 'whisker hair' but which are identical with the cases reported by Knierer (1955) as symmetrical circumscribed allotrichia.

Clinical features. From adolescence onwards the hair in an irregular band extending around the edge of the scalp from above the ears towards the occipital region becomes coarse and whisker-like. A similar case was recorded by Bovenmyer (1979). Many people believe that whisker hair is synonymous with acquired progressive kinking.

Woolly hair naevus (Reda *et al.* 1990)

Pathology. The hair in the affected region of the scalp is finer than elsewhere. Electron microscopy of the abnormal hair showed the absence of cuticle; trichorrhexis nodosa was present (Crosti & Menni 1979).

Clinical features. The hair in a circumscribed area of the scalp is tightly curled from birth or from early infancy (Born 1957). The size of the affected areas usually increases only proportionately with general growth, but it may extend for 3 or 4 years (Post 1958). The abnormal hair may be slightly paler in colour than that of the rest of the scalp.

In over half of the reported cases a pigmented or epidermal naevus has been present but not in the same site. In Streitman's (1959) case, for example, a woolly hair naevus of the right occipital region was associated with a linear epidermal naevus of the left cheek, the left side of the neck and the left hand. A woolly hair naevus has been associated also with ocular defects (Jacobson & Lewis 1975).

Other cases have been reported by Wise (1927), Anderson (1943), Grant (1960) and Domonkos (1962).

References

Anderson, E. (1936) An American pedigree for woolly hair. *Journal of Heredity*, **27**, 444.
Anderson, N.P. (1943) Woolly-haired naevus of the scalp. *Archives of Dermatology and Syphilology*, **47**, 286.
Born, W. (1957) Über Umschriebene Kräuselnaevi innerhalb sonst glatten Kopfhaars. *Dermatologica*, **115**, 119.
Bovenmyer, D.A. (1979) Woolly hair naevus. *Cutis*, **24**, 322.
Crosti, C. & Menni, S. (1979) Woolly hair naevus. Osservazioni su tre casi clinici. *Giornale Italiano de Dermatologio/Minerva Dermatologica*, **114**, 45.
Domonkos, A.N. (1962) Woolly hair naevus. *Archives of Dermatology*, **85**, 568.
Furando, J., Gertalos, M.R. & Fontarnau, R. (1979) Woolly hair. Estudo histologica e ultrastructurale en quatro casos. *Actas Dermosiphiligraphicas*, **70**, 203.
Gottheil, W.S. (1919) Peculiar woolly hair. *Journal of Cutaneous Diseases*, **37**, 489.
Grant, P.W. (1960) A case of woolly hair naevus. *Archives of Disease in Childhood*, **35**, 512.
Hoffmann, E. (1953) Über einen Kräuselnaevus innerhalb sonst glatten Kopfhaares im Vergleich zum erblichen Kraushaar und zur Lockenbildung nach Röntgenepilation. *Dermatologica*, **197**, 281.
Hutchinson, P.E., Cairns, R.J. & Wells, R.S. (1974) Woolly hair. *Transactions of St John's Hospital Dermatological Society*, **60**, 160.
Jacobson, K.V. & Lewis, M. (1975) Woolly hair naevus with ocular involvement. *Dermatologica*, **151**, 249.
Knierer, W. (1955) Allotrichia circumscripta symmetrica capillitii. *Dermatologische Wochenschrift*, **132**, 794.
Mohr, O.L. (1932) Woolly hair, a dominant mutant character in man. *Journal of Heredity*, **23**, 345.
Neild, V.S., Pegun, J.S. & Wells, R.S. (1984) The association of keratosis pilaris atrophicans and woolly hair, with and without Noonan's syndrome. *British Journal of Dermatology*, **110**, 357.
Norwood, C.T. (1981) Whisker-hair—an update. *Cutis*, **27**, 651.
Post, C.F. (1958) Woolly hair nevus. *AMA Archives of Dermatology*, **78**, 488.
Reda, A.M., Rogers, R.S. & Peters, M.S. (1990) Woolly hair naevus. *Journal of the American Academy of Dermatology*, **22**, 377.
Salamon, T. (1963) Über eine Familie mit recessiver Kraushaarigkeit, Hypotrichose und anderen Anomalien. *Hautarzt*, **13**, 540.
Schaginhaufen, O. (1945) Helicotrichie in einem schweizerischen Stammbaum. *Archiv der Julius Klaus-Stiftung*, **20**, 201.
Schokking, C.P. (1934) Another woolly-hair mutation in man. *Journal of Heredity*, **25**, 337.
Streitman, B. (1959) Beitrag zur Kenntnis des Kräuselhaarnaevus. *Dermatologische Wochenschrift*, **139**, 185.
Sweitzer, S.E. (1948) Woolly hair naevus. *Archives of Dermatology and Syphilology*, **58**, 643.
Verbov, J. (1978) Woolly hair study of a family. *Dermatologica*, **157**, 42.
Wise, F. (1927) Woolly hair naevus: a peculiar form of birthmark of the hair of the scalp, hitherto undescribed, with a report of two cases. *Medical Journal and Record*, **125**, 545.

Acquired progressive kinking of hair (Fig. 7.22) (References p. 237)

History and nomenclature

Acquired progressive kinking (APK) of the scalp hair, described by Wise & Sulzberger in 1932, appears to be extremely rare, but many cases may not be

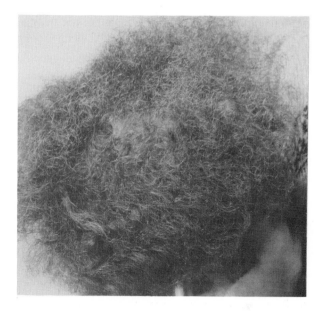

Fig. 7.22 Acquired progressive kinking of the hair in a man aged 28. The condition had been noticed at about the age of 15.

recorded. It is probably synonymous with whisker hair (Norwood 1979). Some have been confused with the woolly hair naevus, but APK is differentiated clinically by its onset in adolescence or adult life and its progressive extension over a period of years (Mortimer *et al.* 1985; Cullen & Fulghum 1989).

Aetiology and pathology
The aetiology of APK is unknown; there is as yet no evidence that it is genetically determined. The hairs in the affected region of the scalp show both structural and functional abnormalities (Coupe & Johnston 1969). They may be finer (Wise & Sulzberger 1932) or coarser than in the normal scalp, and they show irregularly distributed kinks and half-twists. The duration of anagen is reduced.

Clinical features
The patient gradually becomes aware that the hair in one region of the scalp is becoming kinky and that a progressive change in texture is accompanied by a decreased rate of growth, as a result of which he rarely requires a hair cut.

On examination the hair on one or more regions of the scalp is wiry, kinky and unruly, dry and lustreless. There are no sharply defined boundaries between normal and abnormal hair. In some of the cases described, the acquired kinking preceded the development of common male baldness (Mortimer *et al.* 1985).

References

Coupe, R.L. & Johnston, M.N. (1969) Acquired progressive kinking of the hair. *Archives of Dermatology*, **100**, 191.
Cullen, S.I. & Fulghum, D.D. (1989) Acquired progressive kinking of hair. *Archives of Dermatology*, **125**, 252.

Mortimer, P.S., Gummer, C.L., English, J. & Dawber, R.P.R. (1985) Acquired progressive kinking of hair. Report of 6 cases and review of the literature. *Archives of Dermatology*, **121**, 1031.

Norwood, O.T. (1979) Whisker hair. *Archives of Dermatology*, **115**, 930.

Wise, F. & Sulzberger, M.B. (1932) Acquired progressive kinking of the scalp hair accompanied by changes in its pigmentation. *Archives of Dermatology and Syphilology*, **25**, 99.

Uncombable hair syndrome (spun glass hair; cheveux incoiffables; pili trianguli et canaliculi)   (References p. 240)

Aetiology

This very distinctive hair shaft defect appears to have been first described by Dupré *et al.* (1973). Since then at least a dozen cases have been reported, some of them under the name of 'spun glass hair' (Stroud & Mehregan 1974). The mode of inheritance is probably autosomal dominant (Herbert *et al.* 1987); siblings were affected in two families (Grupper *et al.* 1974; Ferrándiz *et al.* 1980), in another it occurred in a father and his son (Yulzari *et al.* 1978).

Pathology

With the light microscope the hairs may appear more or less normal; very minor non-pathognomonic defects are mentioned by some authors (Grupper *et al.* 1974). Histological examination of the scalp, if the section cuts one or more follicles transversely, may show the shafts to be triangular. In the scanning electron microscope the triangular configuration of the shaft is clearly seen, and also a well-defined longitudinal depression (Ferrando *et al.* 1977; Dupré & Bonafé 1978) (Fig. 7.23). The terms 'pili trianguli et canaliculi' have been proposed for these defects. The pili canaliculi are present in all cases, pili trianguli in the majority and pili torti in a few (Ferrando *et al.* 1980). Van Neste *et al.* (1981) have suggested that the misshapen dermal papilli alters the shape of the internal root sheath which hardens (before the central forming hair) in a triangular cross-sectional shape; the hair shape then hardens into a shape complementing the root sheath. The defect

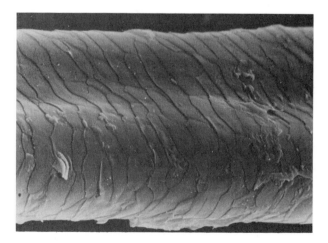

Fig. 7.23 Uncombable hair: longitudinal depression in hair shaft seen in the scanning electron microscope (Dr Van Neste, Dr Tennstedt and Dr J.-M. Lachapelle).

resembles the 'straight hair naevus' of which it may be a diffuse form. Personal observations of the authors, using electron histochemical studies, suggest that the 'rigidity' and difficulty in combing may be due to increased high-sulphur protein in the exocuticle—but this needs to be confirmed or refuted by studies on further cases.

Clinical features (Stroud & Mehregan 1974; Dupré *et al.* 1978)
The child's parents may become aware during the early months of infancy that its hair is abnormal, but more commonly the abnormality is first noticed at the age of about 3 years. On the other hand the onset, or at least awareness of the presence of the abnormality, may be as late as 12 years (Ferrando *et al.* 1980).

The hair is normal in quantity and sometimes also in length, but its wildly disorderly appearance totally resists all efforts to control it with brush or comb (Figs. 7.24, 7.25). In some cases these efforts lead to the hair breaking, but

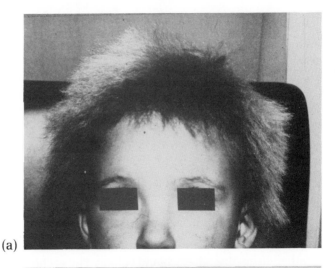

(a)

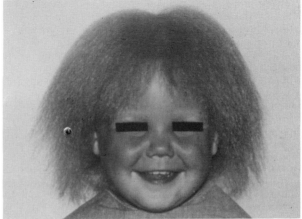

Fig. 7.24 Variations in the clinical appearance of uncombable hair:
(a) hair brittle and short (Dr J. Ferrando);
(b) longer unmanageable hair (Dr G. Holti).

(b)

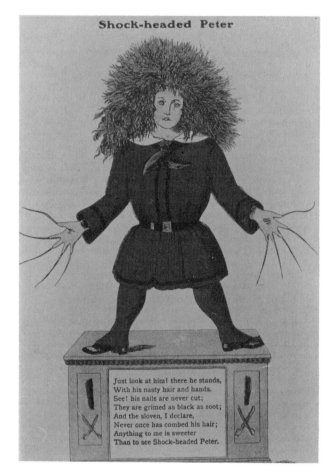

Shock-headed Peter

Just look at him! there he stands,
With his nasty hair and hands.
See! his nails are never cut;
They are grimed as black as soot;
And the sloven, I declare,
Never once has combed his hair;
Anything to me is sweeter
Than to see Shock-headed Peter.

Fig. 7.25 'Shock-headed Peter', a character in a traditional German nursery rhyme. It seems possible that this character was originally based on a case of uncombable hair.

increased fragility is not a constant feature (Baden *et al.* 1981). The hair is often a rather distinctive silvery blond colour. The eyebrows and eyelashes are normal.

During childhood a considerable degree of spontaneous improvement may occur.

Differential diagnosis
The clinical appearance is usually distinctive. With light microscopy the diagnosis cannot be reliably established unless triangular hairs are seen. The appearances in the electron microscope are distinctive. No treatment is known although oral biotin therapy has been suggested (Shelley & Shelley 1985).

References
Baden, H.P., Schoenfeld, R.J., Stroud, J.D. & Happle, R (1981) Physicochemical properties of spunglass hair. *Acta Dermato-Venereologica*, **61**, 441.

Dupré, A., Rochiccidi, P. & Bonafé, J.-L. (1973) 'Cheveux incoiffables': anomalie congénitale des cheveux. *Bulletin de la Société française de Dermatologie et de Syphiligraphie*, **80**, 111.

Dupré, A. & Bonafé, J.-L. (1978) A new type of pilar dysplasia. The uncombable hair syndrome with pili trianguli et canaliculi. *Archives of Dermatological Research*, **261**, 217.

Dupré, A., Bonafé, J.-L., Litoux, F. & Victor, M. (1978) Le syndrome des cheveux incoiffables. Pili trianguli et canaliculi, *Annales de Dermatologie et de Vénéréologie (Paris)*, **105**, 627.

Dupré, A. & Bonafé, J.-L. (1979) A propos du syndrome des cheveux incoiffables. *Annales de Dermatologie et de Vénéréologie (Paris)*, **106**, 617.

Ferrándiz, C., Peyrí, J., Henkes, J., Ferrando, J. & Fontarnáu, R. (1980) 'Pili canaliculi' familiar. *Actas Dermo-sifiliograficas*, **71**, 227.

Ferrando, J., Gratacos, M.R., Fontarnau, R. & Castells Rodellas, A. (1977) Síndrome de los cabellos 'impeinables'. *Medicina cutanea Ibero-Latino-Americana*, **5**, 39.

Ferrando, J., Fontarnau, R., Gratacos, M.R. & Mascaro, J.M. (1980) Pili canaliculi ('Cheveux incoiffables' ou 'Cheveux en fibre de verre'). Dix nouveaux cas avec étude au microscope électronique á balayage. *Annales de Dermatologie et de Vénéréologie (Paris)*, **107**, 243.

Grupper, C., Attal, C. & Gougne, B. (1974) Syndrome des cheveux incoiffables. *Bulletin de la Société française de Dermatologie et de Syphiligraphie*, **81**, 299.

Herbert, A.A., Charrow, J., Esterly, N.B. & Fretzin, D.F. (1987) Uncombable hair (pili trianguli et canaliculi); evidence for dominant inheritance with complete penetrance. *American Journal of Medical Genetics*, **28** (1), 185.

Shelley, W.B. &. Shelley, E.D. (1985) Uncombable hair syndrome: observations on response to biotin. *Journal of the American Academy of Dermatology*, **13**, 97.

Stroud, J.D. & Mehregan, A.H. (1974) 'Spun-glass' hair, a clinico-pathological study of an unusual hair defect. *First Human Hair Symposium*, p. 43, ed. A.C. Brown. Medcom Press, New York.

Van Neste, D., Armijo-Subieta, F., Tennstedt, D. *et al.* (1981) The uncombable hair syndrome: four non-familial cases. *Archives of Dermatological Research*, **217**, 223.

Yulzari, M., Laurent, R., Makki, S. & Agache, P. (1978) Syndromes des cheveux incoiffables. Deux nouveaux cas familiaux avec étude au microscope électronique à balayage. *Annales de Dermatologie et de Vénéréologie (Paris)*, **105**, 633.

Straight hair naevus

In the straight hair naevus the hairs in a circumscribed area of a Negro scalp are straight, and are round in cross-section. The abnormal hair may be associated with an epidermal naevus (Day 1967; Gibbs & Berger 1970), but in one case (Downham *et al.* 1976) hair was shed at the age of 5–6 months from a circumscribed patch of apparently normal scalp and regrew straight and was still doing so when the patient was 15. In the scanning electron microscope the cuticular scales were small and their pattern was disorganized. This has been suggested as a localized form of cheveux incoiffables.

References

Day, T.L. (1967) Straight-hair nevus, ichthyosis hystrix, leucokeratosis of the tongue. *Archives of Dermatology*, **96**, 606.

Downham, T.F., Chapel, T.A. & Lupulescu, A.P. (1976) Straight-hair nevus syndrome: a case report with scanning electron microscope findings of hair morphology. *International Journal of Dermatology*, **15**, 498.

Gibbs, R.L. & Berger, R.A. (1970) The straight-hair nevus. *International Journal of Dermatology*, **9**, 47.

Loose anagen syndrome

This distinctive, newly described condition (Price & Gummer 1989; Hamm & Traupe 1989) features anagen hairs that are loosely anchored and easily pulled from the scalp; 29 cases have been described. The majority are children, aged 2–9 years, mostly girls. The hairs pulled out were misshapen without an external root sheath. Histology revealed premature keratinization of the inner root sheath layers of Huxley and Henle. Trichograms show 98–100% anagen hairs with no telogen hairs. Generally, length and density increase with age.

References

Hamm, H. & Traupe, H. (1989) Loose anagen hair of children. *Journal of the American Academy of Dermatology,* **20,** 242.

Price, V.H. & Gummer, C.L. (1989) Loose anagen syndrome. *Journal of the American Academy of Dermatology,* **20,** 249.

Other abnormalities of the shaft

Trichoclasis

Trichoclasis is the common 'greenstick' fracture of the hair shaft. Transverse fractures of the shaft occur, partly splinted by intact cuticle; cuticle, cortex and sulphur content are normal. This sign may be seen in a variety of congenital and acquired 'fragile' hair states.

The condition termed trichorrhexis blastysis (Stankler *et al.* 1982)—unusual facies, failure to thrive, unexplained diarrhoea and abnormal hairs—showed scanning electron micrographs resembling trichoclasis.

Reference

Stankler, L., Lloyd, D., Pollitt, R.J. *et al.* (1982) Unexplained diarrhoea and failure to thrive in 2 siblings with unusual hair. *Archives of Disease in Childhood,* **57,** 212.

Trichoptilosis (References p. 243)

History and nomenclature

The term trichoptilosis was suggested by Devergie in 1872 to describe longitudinal splitting of the hair shaft. The patient will often refer to the condition as 'split ends'.

Aetiology

Trichoptilosis is the commonest macroscopic response of the hair shaft to the cumulative effects of chemical and physical trauma (Friederich & Fröb 1949). It can readily be produced experimentally by vigorous brushing of normal hair, and it occurs in the nodes of pili torti. It is one component of the 'weathering' process particularly, seen in long hair in normal individuals and any congenital 'brittle hair' syndrome.

Pathology
The distal end of the hair shaft is split longitudinally into two or several divisions. The split commonly extends 2 or 3 cm along the shaft, but may be more prolonged. Other microscopic evidence of hair damage may be present.

Clinical features
Trichoptilosis is often an incidental finding in a woman who complains that her hair is dry and brittle. Sometimes self-examination, prompted by cosmetic advertisements, has led her to make her own diagnosis. Trichorrhexis nodosa and trichoclasis are often present in the same patient. Central trichoptilosis, a longitudinal split in the hair shaft without involvement of the tip sometimes occurs (Burkhart *et al.* 1981).

Treatment
Careful explanation is necessary to encourage the patient to avoid further chemical trauma, for unless she does so the condition will inevitably recur. If the split ends are unsightly they may be cut.

References
Friederich, H.C. & Fröb, G. (1949) Zur Pathogenese der Trichoptilosis. *Dermatologische Wochenschrift*, 120, 674.
Burkhart, C.G., Huttner, J.J. & Bruner, J. (1981) Central trichoptilosis. *Journal of the American Academy of Dermatology*, 5, 703.

Circle hairs

Circle and spiral hairs occur in middle-aged men on the back, abdomen and thighs as small, dark circles next to hair follicles. They are an unusual form of ingrown hair lying in a coiled track just below the stratum corneum and can be easily extracted. Keratin follicular plugging is not associated cf. scurvy of keratosis pilaris rolled and 'corkscrew' hairs.

Reference
Levit, F. & Scott, M.J.J.R. (1983) Circle hairs. *Journal of the American Academy of Dermatology*, 8, 423.

Trichomalacia (References p. 244)

History and nomenclature
In 1942 Miescher of Zurich described as trichomalacia a patchy alopecia in which some follicles are plugged and contain soft, deformed, swollen hairs. Miescher & Schmuziger (1957) and Haensch & Blaich (1960) attributed the changes to the repeated trauma resulting from a hair-pulling tic, and subsequent histological studies in trichotillomania confirm this opinion. However, in one case in a mentally

retarded child, Nuller & Girardet (1957) thought trauma could be excluded as a cause.

The condition described by Pinkus (1965) in a strain of mice appears not to be identical, although there are many points of histological similarity.

Pathology
Above the bulb the cells of the hair shaft appear to be disconnected and the hair is shapeless or partially disintegrated. High in the follicle the shaft is thin and may be coiled. Birefringence of affected hairs is reduced or absent (Pinkus 1965). In any affected area of scalp a proportion of hairs remain normal. Whiting (1987) describes biopsy specimens as showing partially avulsed hair roots which are deformed and twisted; clefting occurs between matrix cells and between hair bulb and outer connective tissue sheath. There is no inflammatory reaction; these changes are said to be pathognomonic of trichotillomania.

Clinical features
These are those of trichotillomania. If a non-traumatic form of trichotillomania occurs in man, it has not yet been reliably reported.

References
Haensch, R. & Blaich, W. (1960) Trichomalacia und Trichotillomania. *Archiv für klinische und experimentelle Dermatologie*, **210**, 447.
Miescher, G. (1942) Trichomalacie. *Archiv für Dermatologie und Syphilologie*, **183**, 117.
Miescher, G. & Schmuziger, P. (1957) Trichomalacie und Trichotillomanie. *Dermatologica*, **114**, 199.
Nuller, R. & Girardet, P. (1957) Contribution à l'etiologie de la trichomalacie. *Dermatologica*, **115**, 717.
Pinkus, H. (1965) Transient alopecia in weanling BD mice (trichomalacia). In *Biology of the Skin and Hair Growth*, p. 747, eds. A.G. Lyne & B.F. Shaw, Angus & Robertson, Sydney.
Whiting, D.A. (1987) Structural abnormalities of the hair shaft. *Journal of the American Academy of Dermatology*, **16**, 1.

Trichoschisis

Trichoschisis is a clean, transverse fracture across the hair shaft through cuticle and cortex; the fracture is associated with localized absence (loss) of cuticular cells. It is said to be a characteristic microscopic finding of the many syndromes associated with trichothiodystrophy. It probably represents a clean fracture through hair with decreased high-sulphur matrix protein content and particularly a similar decrease in the exocuticle and A-layer of cuticular cells. It may be prominent in the sulphur deficiency syndromes but it should not be seen as specific or pathognomonic.

Reference
Brown, A.C., Belsher, R.B., Crounse, R.G. & Wehr, R.F. (1970) A congenital hair defect: trichoschisis and alternating birefringence and low-sulphur content. *Journal of Investigative Dermatology*, **54**, 496.

Pohl–Pinkus constriction

In some individuals a zone of decreased shaft diameter coincides in time with a surgical operation or an illness, or the administration of folic acid antagonists, or other drugs which inhibit mitosis; it was first described by Pohl in 1894—he later changed his name to Pinkus. The proportion of hairs so affected is variable and it seems probable that hairs in early anagen are most susceptible to a period of hypoproteinaemia or disturbed protein synthesis. This phenomenon was present in 21 of 100 patients (Sims 1967); whether the illness or operation had been associated with pyrexia was not a relevant factor. The most marked changes were seen after haemorrhage from peptic ulcers. The lower incidence of the phenomenon that in an earlier study in Berlin (Pinkus 1971) may be attributable to the generally improved nutritional status of the patients.

These constrictions in the hair shaft have been considered to be analogous to the transverse furrows in the nails (Beau's lines) which also coincide with episodes of ill-health. However, in a patient in whom regularly recurring changes were present in nails and hair shafts (Fabry 1965) the latter showed an increase in diameter, and not a constriction corresponding to each furrow in the nails. Longer narrowings, resembling monilethrix, may occur with 'bolus' doses of cytotoxic drugs that do not lead to anagen effluvium.

References

Fabry, H. (1965) Gleichzeitiges rhythmisches Auftreten von Querfurchen der Nägel und gruppierten Knotenbildungen der Haare. *Zeitschrift für Haut und Geschlectskrankheiten*, **39**, 336.

Pinkus, F. (1971) *Die Einwirkung von Krankheiten auf das Kopfhaar des Menschen.* Karger, Berlin.

Sims, R.T. (1967) Reduction of hair shaft diameter associated with illness. *British Journal of Dermatology*, **79**, 43.

Tapered hairs

Tapered hairs may occur in association with many other structural abnormalities of the hair shaft. They may arise in association with any process inhibiting cell division in the hair matrix; severe inhibition may lead to fracture if the narrowing of the fibre is marked. If the matrix inhibitory influence is temporary the shaft may widen again, giving a local 'dumbbell-like' appearance in the emerging shaft, for example, due to cytotoxic drugs not leading to complete anagen effluvium. An alternative type of tapered hair is the so-called 'embryonic' anagen hair—short hairs with tapered pointed tips seen in trichotillomania but also in acquired progressive kinking (Coupe & Johnston 1969) and regrowing hair in alopecia areata.

Reference

Coupe, R.L. & Johnston, M.M (1969) Acquired progressive kinking of hair: structural changes and growth dynamics. *Archives of Dermatology*, **100**, 191.

Bayonet hairs are characterized by a 2–3 mm spindle-shaped, hyperpigmented expansion of the hair cortex just proximal to a tapered tip and may be associated with hyperkeratinization of the upper third of the follicle. It is probably related to the first type of tapered hair described above.

Trichonodosis (References p. 247)

History and nomenclature
The first description of knotting of the hair is said (McCarthy 1940) to have been given by Duncan Bulkley of New York in 1881. Michelson (1884) proposed the term noduli laqueati, and noted that naturally curly hair was most frequently affected. Galewsky (1906) coined the term trichonodosis, which is now generally employed; his patients were a father and son, and he therefore suggested that a genetic factor might be implicated. However, Kren (1907) found the condition in 35 of 64 consecutively examined patients with skin disease.

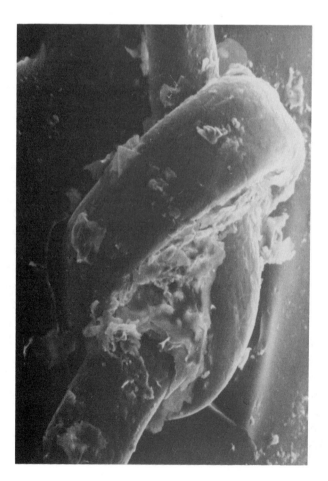

Fig. 7.26 Trichonodosis — scanning electron micrograph, showing knotting of scalp hair.

Aetiology

The knotting of the hair shafts is induced by trauma. Short curly hair of relatively flat diameter is most readily affected (Dawber 1974). Knots were found most frequently in Negroid hair and in short, curly Caucasoid hair; none was seen in long, straight hair. In another investigation (English & Jones 1973) trichonodosis was found in 36 of 134 normal subjects; all those, male and female, with long kinky hair, over 50% of men with short kinky hair and 30% of males or females with long curly hair.

Pathology

The only abnormalities are secondary to the knotting and are localized to that part of the shaft which forms the knot (Dawber 1974). In the scanning electron microscope the cuticle shows longitudinal fissuring and fractures, and cuticular scales are lost (Fig. 7.26).

Clinical features (McCarthy 1940; Pratt 1947)

Trichonodosis is usually an incidental finding, for it is inconspicuous and must be deliberately sought. One or a few hairs only are affected. The trauma of brushing or combing may cause the shaft to break at the site of the knot.

Pubic and other body hair may show knotting, as a result of rubbing and scratching in the presence of pediculosis (Scott 1951).

References

Dawber, R.P.R. (1974) Knotting of scalp hair. *British Journal of Dermatology*, **91**, 169.

English, D.T. & Jones, H.E. (1973) Trichonodosis. *Archives of Dermatology*, **107**, 77.

Galewsky, E. (1906) Über eine noch nicht beschreibene Haarerkrankung (Trichonodosis). *Archive für Dermatologie und Syphilologie*, **81**, 195.

Kren, O. (1907) Trichonodosis. *Wiener klinische Wochenschrift*, **20**, 916.

McCarthy, L. (1940) *Diagnosis and Treatment of Diseases of the Hair*, p. 213. Kimpton, London.

Michelson, P. (1884) Anomalien des Haarwachstums und der Haarfärbung in Handbuch der speziellen. *Pathologie und Therapie*, **14**, 89.

Pratt, A.G. (1947) Trichonodosis. *Archives of Dermatology and Syphilology*, **56**, 262.

Scott, M.J. (1951) Trichonodosis. Report of a case. *Archives of Dermatology and Syphilology*, **63**, 769.

Trichostasis spinulosa (References p. 248)

History and nomenclature

Galewski in 1911 appears to have been the first to describe this condition. In 1912 Franke proposed the term 'pinselhaar' (thysanothrix) and further cases were described the following year. Hochstetter (1913) and Nobl (1913) reported cases and the latter suggested the term trichostasis spinulosa, which most authors now favour. The condition was thought to be uncommon until Mitchell (1925) and Burgess (1932) showed that it is of frequent occurrence, but easily overlooked. When it was specifically sought 51 cases were seen in 1 month in Madras (Kailasam *et al.* 1979).

Aetiology
The aetiology of trichostasis spinulosa has aroused much speculation, seldom supported by investigation. A suggested failure to expel normally formed vellus hairs (Hochstetter 1913), perhaps the result of follicular hyperkeratosis induced by exogenous chemicals (Poschacher 1925) has not been confirmed, and many authors have supported Burgess' (1932) belief that the defect is of developmental origin. Ladany (1954) thought trichostasis was no more than a variant of the comedo, and pointed out that 85% of comedones contain from one to ten or more vellus hairs. Trichostasis is now regarded as a normal age-related process with retention of telogen hairs in large sebaceous follicles (Goldschmidt *et al.* 1974).

Trichostasis is found most commonly in the middle-aged or elderly and is said by most authors to occur particularly on the nose and face (Ladany 1954). Other sites were perhaps not always examined, for others have found it to be not uncommon on the trunk and limbs (Young *et al.* 1985), and in young as well as older adults (Sarkany & Gaylarde 1971). Cases have been reported from most European countries, from North America, from India and from Japan (Ishikawa 1969).

Pathology
The affected follicles contain up to 50 vellus hairs embedded in a keratinous plug. A mild perifolliculitis is often present. The condition must be differentiated from the 'multiple hairs' of Flemming–Giovannini in which up to seven hairs grow from a composite papilla with a common outer root sheath (Pinkus 1951).

Clinical features (Frain-Bell 1956; Ishikawa 1969)
Those reported to be affected have ranged in age from 17 to over 60. The lesions, which closely resemble comedones, may occur predominantly on the nose, forehead and cheeks, or the face may be spared and the nape, the back, shoulders, upper arms and chest may be affected. The lesions vary greatly in number. On inspection with a hand lens the 'comedones' seem to be unusually prominent and in some cases a tuft of hairs may be seen projecting through the horny plug. They have been observed in solar elastosis of the nape of the neck (Braun-Falco and Vakilzadeh 1967).

Treatment
Keratolytic preparations have often been recommended but we have found them to be of little value. The most effective treatment is topical retinoic acid (Mills & Kligman 1973) which should be used as in the treatment of acne. Depilatory wax has also been successfully employed (Sarkany & Gaylarde 1971).

References
Braun-Falco, O. & Vakilzadeh, F. (1967) Trichostasis spinulosa. *Hautarzt*, **18**, 501.
Burgess, J.F. (1932) Trichostasis spinulosa. *Archives of Dermatology and Syphilology*, **25**, 40.

Frain-Bell, W. (1956) Trichostasis spinulosa. *Transactions of St John's Hospital Dermatological Society*, **36**, 41.

Franke, F. (1912) Das Pinselhaar; Thysanothrix. *Dermatologische Wochenschrift*, **55**, 1269.

Galewski, K. (1911) Über eine eigenartige Verhorungsanomalie der Follikel und deren Haare. *Archiv für Dermatologie und Syphilologie*, **106**, 215.

Goldschmidt, H., Hajyo-Tomoka, M.J. & Kligman, A.M. (1974) Trichostasis spinulosa: a common inapparent follicular disorder of the aged. *First Human Hair Symposium*, p. 50, ed. A.C. Brown. Medcom Press, New York.

Hochstetter, B. (1913) Über eine seltene anomalie des Haarwechsels. *Dermatologische Zeitschrift*, **20**, 316.

Ishikawa, K. (1969) Trichostasis spinulosa. *Hautarzt*, **20**, 367.

Kailasam, V., Kailasam, A. & Thambiah, A.S. (1979) Trichostasis spinulosa. *International Journal of Dermatology*, **18**, 297.

Ladany, E. (1954) Trichostasis spinulosa. *Journal of Investigative Dermatology*, **23**, 33.

Mills, O.H. & Kligman, A.M. (1973) Topically applied tretinoin in the treatment of trichostasis spinulosa. *Archives of Dermatology*, **108**, 378.

Mitchell, J.H. (1925) Trichostasis spinulosa or pinselhaar. *Archives of Dermatology*, **11**, 80.

Nobl, G. (1913) Trichostasis spinulosa. *Archiv für Dermatologie und Syphilologie*, **114**, 611.

Pinkus, H. (1951) Multiple hairs (Flemming–Giovannini). *Journal of Investigative Dermatology*, **17**, 291.

Poschacher, A. (1925) Über trichostasis spinulosa. *Acta Dermato-Venereologica*, **6**, 107.

Sarkany, I. & Gaylarde, P.M. (1971) Trichostasis spinulosa and its management. *British Journal of Dermatology*, **84**, 311.

Young, M.C., Jorizzo, J.L., Sanchez, R.L. *et al.* (1985) Trichostasis spinulosa. *International Journal of Dermatology*, **24**, 575.

Pili multigemini (pili bifurcati) (References p. 250)

History and nomenclature

The term pili multigemini describes an uncommon developmental defect of hair follicles as a result of which multiple matrices and papillae form hairs which emerge through a single pilosebaceous canal. The condition was described by Flemming in 1883 and named and studied by Giovannini in a series of papers from 1907 to 1910 (Giovannini 1910). It then attracted little notice until Pinkus drew attention to it in 1951.

The incidence of multigeminate hairs in the general population is unknown. Numerous follicles showing this defect have been seen in a patient with cleidocranial dysostosis (Mehregan & Thompson 1979).

Pathology

From two to eight matrices and papillae, each with its internal root sheath, form hairs which are often flattened, ovoid or triangular in configuration and may be grooved. In the follicular canal contiguous hairs may adhere, bifurcate and then re-adhere. This abnormality has been separately described as pili bifurcati (Weary *et al.* 1973) and may also occur as an isolated defect in otherwise normal follicles.

Clinical features

Multigeminate follicles occur mainly on the face, especially along the lines of the jaw. Tufts of hair may be seen emerging from a few or many follicles. Their discovery is often a matter of chance but the patient may complain of recurrent inflammatory nodules, leaving scars.

Treatment
Treatment is unsatisfactory. If the hairs are plucked, they regrow (Mehregan & Thompson 1979).

References
Flemming, W. (1883) Ein Drillingshaar mit gemeinsamer innerer Wurzelscheide. *Monatshefte für praktische Dermatologie*, **2**, 163.
Giovannini, S. (1910) I peli con papilla composita. *Anatomischer Anzeiger*, **37**, 39.
Mehregan, A.H. & Thompson, W.S. (1979) Pili multigemini. Report of a case in association with cleidocranial dysostosis. *British Journal of Dermatology*, **100**, 315.
Pinkus, H. (1951) Multiple hairs (Flemming–Giovannini). *Journal of Investigative Dermatology*, **17**, 291.
Weary, P.E., Hendricks, A.A., Wawner, F. & Ajgaonkar, G. (1973) Pili bifurcati. A new anomaly of hair growth. *Archives of Dermatology*, **108**, 403.

Peripilar keratin casts (pseudonits)

Peripilar casts are tubular masses of amorphous (keratinous) material of varied size that surround the hair shaft. They are cast from within the hair follicle infundibulum and before they separate may bulge out from the follicular openings, the so-called parakeratotic comedones.

Weathering of the hair shaft (References p. 254)

All hair fibres undergo some degree of cuticular and secondary cortical breakdown from root to tip before being shed during the telogen or early anagen phase of the hair cycle. The term weathering of hair has been limited by some authorities to structural changes in the hair shaft due to cosmetic procedures; indeed, both *in vivo* and *in vitro* studies carried out by cosmetic scientists have shown the type of damage that factors such as combing, brushing, bleaching and permanent waving can cause (Swift & Brown 1972; Brown & Swift 1975; Robinson 1976). However, in considering the degeneration of hair fibres, cosmetic and other influences such as natural friction, wetting and ultraviolet radiation are so interwoven that it is more useful in practice to define weathering as the progressive degeneration of hair from root to tip due to a variety of environmental and cosmetic factors. Scalp hair, having a long anagen phase and being subject to more frictional damage and cosmetic treatment, shows more deep cuticular and cortical degeneration than fibres from other sites.

Weathering of scalp hair has been studied in greater detail than hair from other sites. The progressive changes from root to tip are shown in Figs 7. 27–7.33. At the root end surface cuticle cells are closely apposed to deeper layers (Fig. 7.27). Within a few centimetres of the scalp, the free margin of these cells lifts up and breaks irregularly (Fig. 7.28) (Garcia *et al.* 1978). Increasing scale loss leads to surface

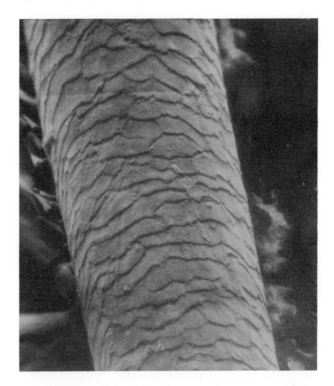

Fig. 7.27 Normal cuticle, near the scalp surface.

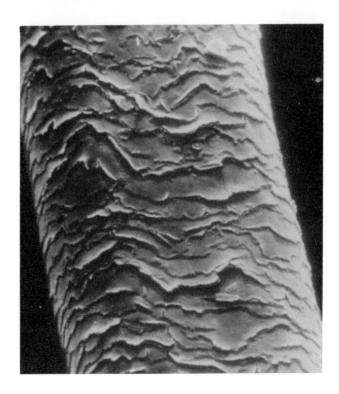

Fig. 7.28 Weathering, lifting and breaking of the free edges of cuticular cells a few centimetres from the scalp surface.

areas denuded of cuticle (Fig. 7.29). Many fibres show complete loss of overlapping scales well proximal to the tip (Fig. 7.30). This is particularly common on long hair shafts which frequently also have a frayed tip. Proximal to terminal fraying, longitudinal fissures may be present between exposed cortical cells (Figs 7.31 & 7.32). Hairs subjected to considerable friction damage may show transverse fissures and some nodes of the type seen in trichorrhexis nodosa (Dawber

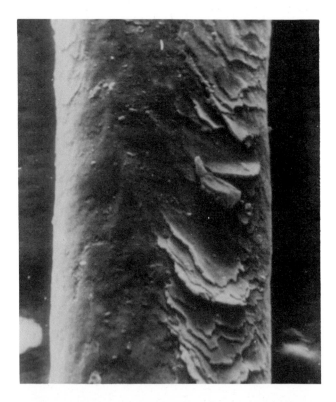

Fig. 7.29 Weathering: areas denuded of cuticle.

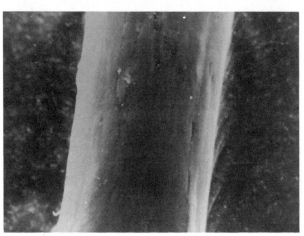

Fig. 7.30 Weathering: complete loss of cuticular scales.

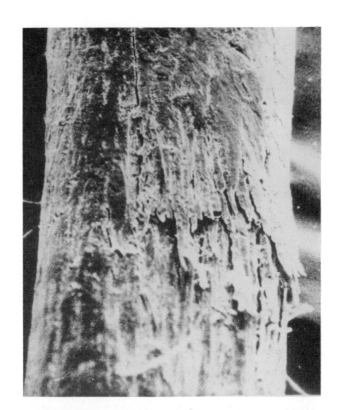

Fig. 7.31 Weathering: fissures between exposed cortical cells.

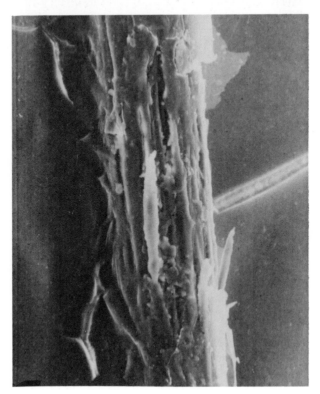

Fig. 7.32 Weathering: more advanced longitudinal fissuring.

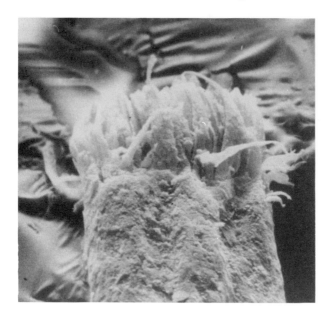

Fig. 7.33 Weathering: breakage of a severely distorted shaft.

& Comaish 1970; Chernosky 1974). Hair that has been bleached or permanently waved may show shaft distortion (Fig. 7.33); apart from the biochemical weakening of such fibres, the altered shape increases the propensity for friction damage to occur. The changes seen in Figs 7.29–7.31 are mostly seen near the distal part of the hair shaft in normal scalp hair.

Trichorrhexis nodosa is the severest form of weathering. Many of the changes seen in normal hair towards the tip are visible more proximally in congenitally weakened hair (Rauschkolb *et al.* 1967; Pollitt *et al.* 1968; Lyon & Dawber 1977) and in trichorrhexis nodosa caused by over-use of cosmetic treatments (Camacho-Martinez 1989).

In some hair structural abnormalities such as monilethrix and pili torti, specific weathering patterns may be seen (Dawber 1980).

References

Brown, A.G. & Swift, J.A. (1975) Hair breakage; the scanning electron microscope as a diagnostic tool. *Journal of the Society of Cosmetic Chemists*, **26**, 289.

Camacho-Martinez, F. (1989) Localised trichorrhexis nodosa. *Journal of the American Academy of Dermatology*, **20**, 696.

Chernosky, M.E. (1974) Acquired trichorrhexis nodosa. In *The First Human Hair Symposium*, ed. A.C. Brown. Medcom Press, New York.

Dawber, R.P.R. & Comaish, S. (1970) Scanning electron microscopy of normal and abnormal hair shafts. *Archives of Dermatology*, **101**, 316.

Dawber, R.P.R. (1980) Weathering of hair in some genetic hair dystrophies. In *Hair, Trace Elements and Human Illness*, eds. A.C. Brown & R.G. Crounse. Praeger, New York.

Garcia, M.L., Epps, J.H. & Yare, R.S. (1978) Normal cuticle wear patterns in human hair. *Journal of the Society of Cosmetic Chemists*, **29**, 155.

Lyon, J.B. & Dawber, R.P.R. (1977) A sporadic case of dystrophic pili torti. *British Journal of Dermatology*, **96**, 197.

Pollitt, R.J., Jenner, F.A. & Davies, M. (1968) Sibs with mental and physical retardation and trichorrhexis nodosa with abnormal amino-acid composition of the hair. *Archives of Disease in Childhood*, **42**, 211.

Rauschkolb, E.W., Chernosky, M.E. & Knox, J.M. (1967) Trichorrhexis nodosa, an error of amino-acid metabolism. *Journal of Investigative Dermatology*, **48**, 260.

Robinson, V.N.E. (1976) A study of damaged hair. *Journal of the Society of Cosmetic Chemists*, **27**, 155.

Swift, J.A. & Brown, A.G. (1972) The critical determination of fine changes in the surface architecture of human hair due to cosmetic treatment. *Journal of the Society of Cosmetic Chemists*, **23**, 695.

Longitudinal ridging and grooving

One or several longitudinal grooves and ridges can occur along the hair shaft; the overlying cuticle is usually intact in the absence of severe weathering influences. It is a microscopic sign that may occur in many different forms in Marie-Unna syndrome, uncombable hair syndrome, the narrow internodes of monilethrix and many other hereditary and congenital abnormalities, and may represent altered moulding of hair by misshapen internal root sheath.

Bubble hair

Brown *et al.* (1986) reported an unusual, apparently unique, case of an acquired localized reversible hair shaft defect with intrinsic 'bubbles' within hairs, thought to be due to repeated cosmetic trauma.

Reference

Brown, V.M., Crounse, R.G. & Abele, D.C. (1986) An unusual new hair shaft abnormality, 'bubble hair'. *Journal of the American Academy of Dermatology*, **15**, 1113.

Chapter 8
Hypertrichosis

Introduction

Hypertrichosis is the term used to describe all forms of hair growth that are excessive for the site and age of an individual and which do not conform to the pattern of androgen-mediated hirsutism.

Hypertrichosis may occur as a manifestation of, or a sequel to, a wide range of circumstances. In some cases, the hair growth is conspicuous and persistant; in others it may be feint and transitory and included only in the most complete descriptions of the disorder.

There are a number of difficulties in establishing a classification for the conditions associated with hypertrichosis. Firstly, clinical descriptions of the pattern of hair growth are often complete and vague. Secondly, the terms hirsuties and hypertrichosis are often used interchangeably and thirdly, our understanding of the mechanisms controlling hair growth are still poorly understood.

Congenital hypertrichosis
(References p. 261)

There exists much confusion in the literature concerning the congenital generalized hypertrichoses due to the plethora of names which have been contributed to this state; Felgenhauer reviewed the literature in 1969 and found no fewer than 29 names such as apeman, bearman, dogman, manlion and wildman etc. Many of these unfortunate subjects were paraded in circuses and showgrounds as techniques for hair removal were either not available or not considered. It is probable that many of these conditions would now be diagnosed as the following congenital and metabolic disorders or as androgen-mediated hirsuties.

Hypertrichosis lanuginosa

Hypertrichosis lanuginosa (HL) is a rare disorder characterized by the retention and continued growth of foetal lanugo hair (Flesch 1954). There have, however, been no studies to determine whether there are differences in lanugo compared to vellus or terminal hair nor has there been any confirmation that the hair roots are synchronized (as *in utero*).

It is transmitted by an autosomal dominant gene but about a third of cases are sporadic (Felgenhauer 1969) and there has been a single pedigree reported with a possible autosomal recessive inheritance (Janssen & de Lange 1946).

Clinical features. The infants are born with a thick coat of fine, silky hair which may be as long as 5 cm covering the entire non-glabrous surface (see Fig. 8.1).

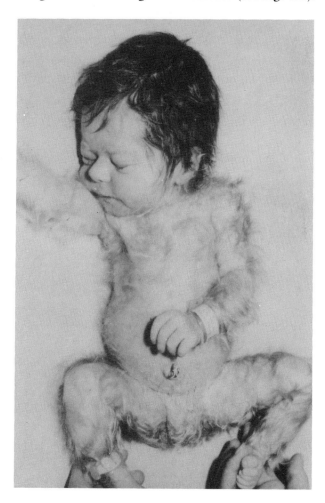

Fig. 8.1 Hypertrichosis lanuginosa acquisita in a girl aged 4 days (courtesy of Dr J.W. Partridge, Leamington Spa and *Archives of Disease in Childhood*).

The scalp hair may be easily distinguished from the body hair. The degree of hair growth may increase in severity during infancy but in some cases tends to decrease during early childhood (Gardner 1964; Berres & Nitschke 1968; Beighton 1970; Partridge 1987). At the age of 3–4 years, the cheeks, back and the proximal aspects of the limbs are most prominently affected. A heavy growth on the eyebrows may occur (Knowles 1921; Beighton 1970). Profuse growth in the ear may lead to difficulty with hearing and the external auditory canal may need to be surgically cleared. At puberty there is the usual growth of sexual hair but without the usual conversion to terminal hair and therefore long, fine lanugo hairs grow in the beard and the pubic and axillary regions.

There may be an associated delay or a deficiency in dental development (Danforth 1925) or retention of the deciduous teeth (Freire-Maia *et al.* 1976). Individuals are otherwise entirely healthy and have a normal intellect.

There is presumably a degree of variability in the overall course; many of the cases reported from the 18th to the present century remained hairy throughout their lives (Danforth 1925; Mense 1921). We have examined the 28-year-old father of a case of HL recently reported (Partridge 1987). He carries the gene and was extremely hypertrichotic as a child but now has only sparse body and facial hair. Individual pedigrees exhibit variations from the norm, such as bushy eyebrows (Beighton 1970) or neonatal teeth and pyloric stenosis (case and her twin sisters reported by Partridge 1987).

Hypertrichosis with gingival fibromatosis

Hypertrichosis may develop in association with gingival fibromatosis and epilepsy. This association was recognised before the introduction of the hydantoins and therefore the side effect of these drugs represents a phenocopy. Most cases (80%) are familial and the condition has only been reported in Caucasian and mongoloid races (Witkop 1971).

Hypertrichosis is noted at or soon after birth; the face, upper limbs and the middle of the back are most prominently affected (Winter & Simpkiss 1974). The gingival abnormality usually presents after 10 years; however, in the more severe cases in which epilepsy is associated there is gingival enlargement in infancy.

Hypertrichosis with gingival fibromatosis may be associated with multiple hamartomata and peri- or post-pubertal giant fibroadenomata of the breasts (Cowden's disease) (Witkop & Gentry 1979). The hypertrichosis is usually present at birth but may be delayed until 4 or 5 years and it may increase in severity at the menarche. The hair may be uncharacteristically coarse and pigmented for the family.

Hypertrichosis with osteochondrodysplasia

An association of congenital hypertrichosis with a distinct abnormality of the skeleton has been described (see Fig. 8.2) (Cantu *et al.* 1982). The physical

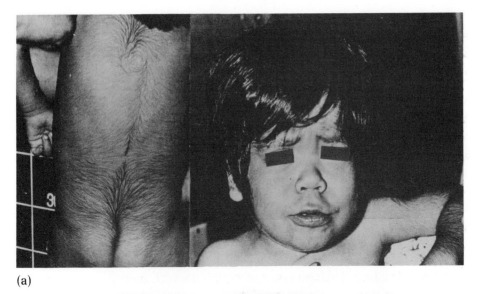

(a)

(b)

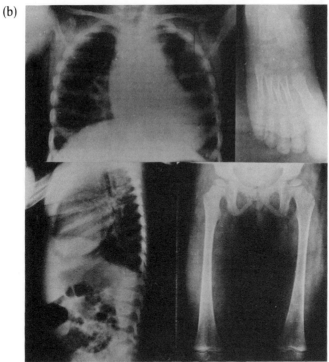

Fig. 8.2 Osteochondrodysplasia with hypertrichosis:
(a) clinical appearance of a girl aged $4\frac{1}{4}$ years;
(b) X-rays of the same girl demonstrating a narrow thorax and cardiomegaly, platyspondyly and ovoid vertebral bodies, hypoplastic ischiopubic rami, small abdurator foramina, enlarged medulla of Erlenmeyer flask-shaped femora which show bands of growth arrest (courtesy of Professor J.M. Cantu, Guadelajara).

characteristics include a narrow thorax and cardiomegaly, and radiological abnormalities of the ribs, vertebrae, ischiopubic rami and generalized osteopenia. The mode of inheritance is thought to be autosomal recessive.

X-linked hypertrichosis

A pedigree with an apparent X-linked dominant mode of transmission has been described (Macias-Flores *et al.* 1984). There is generalized hypertrichosis at birth which increases in severity during the first year. The hair growth is generalized but is particularly dense over the face, back, upper chest and pubic area. The facial growth obscures the eyebrow margins; only the eyes and lips may be visible beneath the dense growth of hair (see Fig. 8.3). There is a mild reduction in hair growth on the trunk and limbs after puberty.

Prepubertal hypertrichosis

We have recently described a series of healthy children with generalized hypertrichosis which had been noted at birth but which increased in severity in

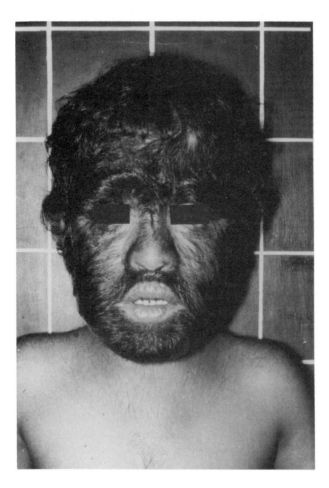

Fig. 8.3 Facial appearance of the X-linked dominant hypertrichosis in a boy aged $8\frac{1}{2}$ years (courtesy of Professor J.M. Cantu, Guadelajara).

early childhood (Barth *et al.* 1988). It occurs in both Asian and European children and in none of the cases was there a family history of hypertrichosis.

There is hair growth on the temples spreading across the forehead, bushy eyebrows, and marked growth on the upper back and proximal limbs (see Fig. 8.4). This form of hypertrichosis differs from hypertrichosis lanuginosa as the hair is terminal and root studies have revealed asynchronous growth whereas lanugo hair roots are synchronized.

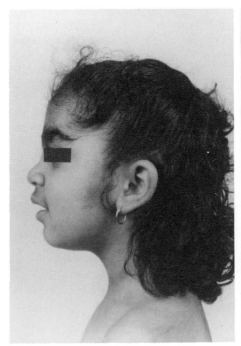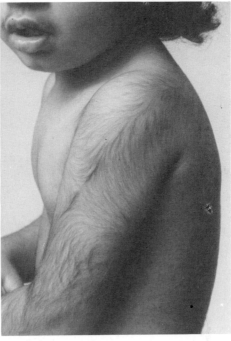

Fig. 8.4 Hypertrichosis in an otherwise healthy $2\frac{1}{2}$-year-old girl:
(a) the face reveals fine pigmented hair on the forehead, temples and cheeks;
(b) shoulders, upper arms and lateral trunk (courtesy of *Archives of Disease in Childhood*).

This hypertrichosis may represent the condition often described as 'racial hirsuties'. We believe that this latter nomenclature is misleading as this form of hypertrichosis is not limited to a specific race nor is it androgen mediated (suggested by the term 'hirsuties'). However, it may be a form of hypertrichosis which is seen in post-pubertal females that is assumed to be androgen dependent but which does not respond to anti-androgen therapy.

References

Barth, J.H., Wilkinson, J.D. & Dawber, R.P.R. (1988) Prepubertlal hypertrichosis: normal or abnormal? *Archives of Disease in Childhood*, **63**, 666.
Beighton, P. (1970) Congenital hypertrichosis lanuginosa. *Archives of Dermatology*, **101**, 669.

Berres, H.H. & Nitschke, R. (1968) Vergleichende klinische und morphologische Untersuchungen zwischen einem Neugeborenen mit Hypertrichosis universalis und gleichaltrigen hautgesunden Kindern. *Zeitschrift für Kinderheilkunde*, **102**, 327.

Cantu, J.M., Garcia-Cruz, D., Sanchez-Corona, J., Hernandez, A. & Nazara, Z. (1982) A distinct osteochondrodysplasia with hypertricosis—individualisation of a probable autosomal recessive entity. *Human Genetics*, **60**, 36.

Danforth, C.H. (1925) Studies on hair with special reference to hypertrichosis. VII. Hypertrichosis. *Archives of Dermatology and Syphilology*, **12**, 381.

Felgenhauer, W.-R. (1969) Hypertrichosis lanuginosa universalis. *Journal de Génétique Humaine*, **17**, 1.

Flesch, P. (1954) Hair growth. In *Physiology and Biochemistry of the Skin*, p. 619, ed. S. Rothman. University of Chicago Press, Chicago.

Freire-Maia, M., Felizali, J. & Figueredo, A.C. (1976) Hypertrichosis lanuginosa in a mother and son. *Clinical Genetics (Copenhagen)*, **10**, 303.

Gardner, A.L.K. (1964) A case of hypertrichosis universalis. *East African Medical Journal*, **41**, 345.

Janssen, T.A.E. & de Lange, C. (1946) Hypertrichosis (trichostasis) lanuginosa. *Nederlandschische Tijdschrift voor Geneeskunde*, **90**, 198.

Knowles, F.C. (1921) Hypertrichiasis in childhood: the so-called 'dog-faced' boy. *Pennsylvania Medical Journal*, **24**, 401.

Macias-Flores, M.A., Garcia-Cruz, D., Rivera, H., Escobar-Lujan, M., Melendrez-Vega, A., Rivas-Campos, D., Rodriguez-Collazo, F., Moreno-Arellano, I. & Cantu, J.M. (1984) A new form of hypertrichosis inherited as an X-linked dominant trait. *Human Genetics*, **66**, 66.

Mense, K. (1921) Über hypertrichosis lanuginensis, s. primaria. *Beitrage zur Pathologie und Anatomie*, **68**, 486.

Partridge, J.W. (1987) Congenital hypertrichosis lanuginosa: neonatal shaving. *Archives of Disease in Childhood*, **62**, 623.

Winter, G.B. & Simpkiss, M.J. (1974) Hypertrichosis with hereditary gingival hyperplasia. *Archives of Disease in Childhood*, **49**, 394.

Witkop, C.J. Jr. (1971) Heterogeneity in gingival fibromatosis. *Birth Defects: Original Article Series*, *VIII*, p. 210.

Witkop, C.J. Jr. & Gentry, W.C. Jr. (1979) Gingival fibromatosis, Cowden type. In *Birth Defects Compendium*, 2nd edn., p. 464, ed. D. Bergasma. Macmillan Press, London.

Congenital circumscribed hypertrichosis
(References p. 267)

Congenital melanocyte naevi

Coarse hair often accompanies melanocytic naevi present at birth. Such naevi may be extensive and grossly disfiguring. The German term 'Tierfellnevus' (animal skin naevus) is graphically descriptive (Fig. 8.5). The naevus may be flat with a more-or-less dense covering of hair, but is often raised and is sometimes irregularly nodular. Nodule formation is not necessarily evidence of malignant change (Krinitz & Wozniak 1972) but should raise this suspicion, for malignant melanoma develops in a significant proportion of these lesions. Early excision, if necessary in stages, is advisable on both prophylactic and cosmetic grounds, if it is technically practicable.

Becker's naevus

Becker's naevus, as originally described (1939), is a localized unilateral area of hyperpigmentation and hypertrichosis. It has subsequently been widely reported

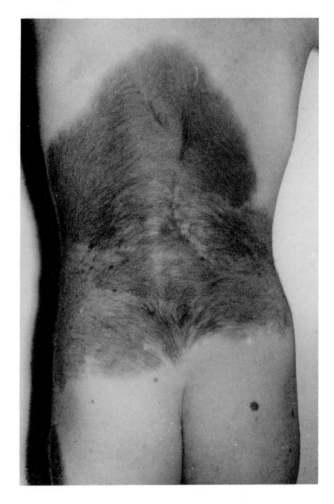

Fig. 8.5 Congenital melanocytic naevus with hypertrichosis.

and an incidence of 0.5% has been reported in French army recruits (Tymen *et al.* 1981). It occurs predominantly in males and has been described in families (Pannizon & Schnyder 1988; Jain & Fisher 1989) and most races (Copeman & Wilson-Jones 1965).

Histopathology. Histologically there may be little to differentiate lesional from peri-lesional skin. There are no naevus cells (Copeman & Wilson-Jones 1965). There may be increased basal pigmentation of a somewhat acanthotic epidermis. The dermis may be thickened and contain bundles of smooth muscle (Haneke 1979). Ultrastructure reveals giant melanosomes and multiple layers of basement membrane surrounding the dermal venules (Bharvan & Chang 1979). There are increased numbers of melanin-laden melanophores in the dermis (Frenk & Delacrétaz 1970).

Aetiology. The aetiology of this naevus is unclear. The original cases and others described by Tymen *et al.* (1981), Copeman and Wilson-Jones (1965) and Ruffli (1972) followed sun exposure. However, we believe that it represents a functional androgen-dependent naevus for the following reasons. Firstly, the occurrence of this disorder in males to females is in a ratio of 10:1 (Copeman & Wilson-Jones 1965). Secondly, the lesion develops at puberty. Thirdly, acneiform lesions and terminal hairs are present within the lesion and both are considered to occur in the skin in response to androgen stimulation and fourthly, affected skin contains androgen receptors (Person *et al.* 1984).

Clinical features (Copeman & Wilson-Jones 1965; Tymen *et al.* 1981). Most cases of Becker's naevus probably develop about the time of puberty although most series have defined the onset by age. The appearance of the naevus is characterized by variable pigmentation, hypertrichosis and acneiform papules and pustules. The lesion is usually a well-defined though irregularly shaped patch of brown pigmentation often with smaller islands of pigmentation beyond its margin. Hypertrichosis which develops in only 50%, occurs after puberty but is often not uniformly distributed over the pigmented area and some hairs may grow on normal skin. Both pigmentation and hypertrichosis extend irregularly for several years, but do not cross the midline. The pigmentation is said slowly to decrease in some cases (Entwistle & Nurse 1967).

Becker's naevus is unilateral. About half (30–50%) occur on the shoulder, most of the remainder on the trunk and a few on the limbs or face (Fig. 8.6).

Many associated abnormalities have been described with Becker's naevus: hypoplasia of the ipsilateral breast and/or arm; bony abnormalities of the spine and thoracic cage; enlargement of the ipsilateral foot and morphoea (Ruffli 1972; Glinick *et al.* 1983).

Diagnosis. Hypertrichosis extending onto the face beyond the edge of the pigmented areas may cause diagnostic problems unless the characteristic pattern of the pigmentation is recognized.

Treatment. Either the hypertrichosis or the pigmentation may present the greater cosmetic problem. We have seen a good result from electrolysis in unilateral facial hypertrichosis. The pigmentation is very difficult to treat.

Lumbosacral hypertrichosis in spinal dysraphism. Dysraphism—failure of spinal fusion—occurs four times more frequently in girls than in boys. Transfixation of the cord by a bony spicule—diastematomyelia—or tethering of cord or cauda by fibrous cords, may result in serious damage to the cord as differential growth of vertebra and cord exerts traction on the latter. The defect is usually in the sacral region but may be lumbar, thoracic or cervical. There may be no overlying cutaneous abnormality but usually there is a tuft of long soft silky hair—*a fauntail*—a capillary naevus, a lipoma or a dimple or sinus. In the presence of

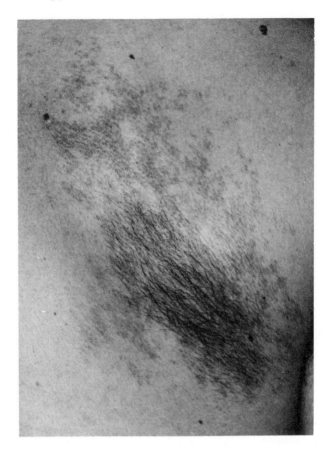

Fig. 8.6 Becker's naevus of the right scapular region.

cord traction progressive neurological signs develop from early childhood; weakness of the legs, sensory loss and a sphincter impairment.

In every case full neurological and radiological investigation is essential. Diastematomyelia is an indication for surgical intervention. In the absence of conclusive radiological findings prolonged observation is essential so that surgery may be undertaken at the first sign of cord damage.

Underlying kyphoscoliosis may be associated with focal hypertrichosis (Reed *et al.* 1989).

Naevoid hypertrichosis
Hypertrichosis of limited extent may occur as a developmental defect in the absence of any other cutaneous abnormality (Figs 8.7, 8.8).

Hypertrichosis overlying benign tumours
Plexiform neurofibromata in Von Recklinghausen's disease may be covered by an area of hypertrichosis and hyperpigmentation. When these occur over the spine abnormal hair whorls may be seen (Riccardi 1987).

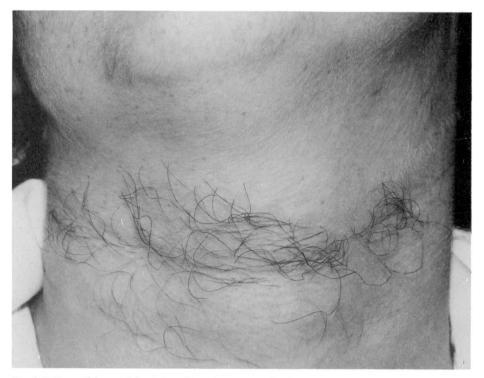

Fig. 8.7 Naevoid hypertrichosis in a linear pattern on the front of the neck in a young woman who did not have androgenetic hirsutism.

Congenital smooth muscle hamartomata usually present as asymptomatic swellings. They normally occur on the trunk. The majority of lesions are associated with overlying hypertrichosis and hyperpigmentation (Berberian & Burnett 1986; Goldman *et al.* 1987). Transient piloerection may be induced by stroking the skin if there are associated smooth muscle elements (Gvosden *et al.* 1987).

Congenital hemihypertrophy with hypertrichosis
Hemihypertrophy is usually present at birth but may become more noticeable at puberty. It is often associated with mental retardation and cutaneous abnormalities. These may include naevi, telangiectases and hypertrichosis (Hurwitz & Klaus 1971). Seemingly appropriate increases in the activity of the adnexal secretory glands have not been apparent to clinical observation (Scott 1935). There may be associated internal abnormalities and tumours; children with this disorder should therefore be carefully evaluated.

Transient thickening of the skin with hypertrichosis
Unexplained hypertrichosis was present on the limbs at birth in a full-term male infant. The hairy skin appeared somewhat thickened and parchment-like. The

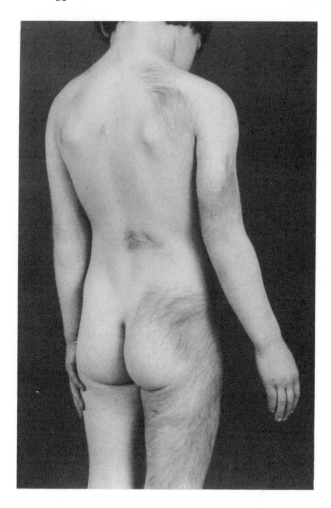

Fig. 8.8 Multifocal naevoid hypertrichosis affecting the right side of the body in an apparently dermatomal distribution. This case has been reported by Cox *et al.* (1989) (illustrated courtesy of Dr R.A. Hardie, Ayr, Scotland).

hair had been shed after 4 months and the texture of the skin had returned to normal (Van der Meiren *et al.* 1960).

References

Becker, W.S. (1949) Concurrent melanosis and hypertrichosis in the distribution of nevus unius lateris. *Archives of Dermatology and Syphilology*, **60**, 155.

Berberian, B.J. & Burnett, J.W. (1986) Congenital smooth muscle hamartoma: a case report. *British Journal of Dermatology*, **115**, 711.

Bharvan, J. & Chang, W.H. (1979) Becker's melanosis: an ultrastructural study. *Dermatologica*, **159**, 221.

Copeman, P.C.M. & Wilson-Jones, E. (1965) Pigmented epidermal hairy naevus (Becker). *Archives of Dermatology*, **92**, 249.

Cox, N.H., McClure, J.P. & Hardie, R.A. (1989) Naevoid hypertrichosis—report of a patient with multiple lesions. *Clinical and Experimental Dermatology*, **14**, 62.

Entwistle, B.R. & Nurse, D.S. (1967) Becker's melanosis and hypertrichosis. *Australasian Journal of Dermatology*, **9**, 198.

Frenk, E. & Delacrétaz, J. (1970) Zur ultrastructur der Beckerschen melanom. *Hautartz*, 21, 397.

Glinick, S.E., Alper, J.C., Bogaars, H. & Brown, J.A. (1983) Becker's melanosis: associated abnormalities. *Journal of the American Academy of Dermatology*, 9, 509.

Goldman, M.P., Kaplan, R.P. & Heng, M.C.Y. (1987) Congenital smooth-muscle hamartoma. *International Journal of Dermatology*, 26, 448.

Gvosden, A.B., Barnett, N.K. & Schron, D.S. (1987) Congenital pilar and smooth muscle nevus. *Pediatrics*, 79, 1021.

Haneke, E. (1979) The dermal component in melanosis neviformis Becker. *Journal of Cutaneous Pathology*, 6, 53.

Harris, H.W. & Miller, O.F. (1976) Midline cutaneous and spinal defects. *Archives of Dermatology*, 112, 1724.

Hurwitz, S. & Klaus, S.N. (1971) Congenital hemihypertrophy with hypertrichosis. *Archives of Dermatology*, 103, 98.

Jain, H.C. & Fisher, B.K. (1989) Familial Becker's naevus. *International Journal of Dermatology*, 28(4), 263.

James, C.C.M. & Lassman, L.P. (1960) Spinal dysraphism. *Archives of Disease in Childhood*, 35, 315.

Krinitz, K. & Wozniak, K.D. (1972) Malignes Melanom und Tierfellnaevus. *Dermatologische Medizinschrift*, 158, 130.

Pannizon, R. & Schnyder, U.W. (1988). Familial Becker's naevus. *Dermatologica*, 176, 275.

Person, J.R. & Longcope, C. (1984) Becker's nevus: an androgen-mediated hyperplasia with increased androgen receptors. *Journal of the American Academy of Dermatology*, 10, 235.

Reed, O.M., Mellette, J.R. & Fitzpatrick, J.E. (1989) Familial cervical hypertrichosis with underlying kyphoscoliosis. *Journal of the American Academy of Dermatology*, 20, 1069.

Riccardi, V.M. (1987) Neurofibromatosis and Albright's disease. *Dermatologic Clinics*, 5, 193.

Ruffli, T. (1972) Melanosis Becker mit lokalisierter sklerodermie. *Dermatologica*, 145, 222.

Scott, A.J. (1935) Hemihypertrophy. *Journal of Pediatrics*, 6, 650.

Tymen, R., Forestier, J.-F., Boutet, B. & Colomb, D. (1981) Naevus tardif de Becker. *Annales de Dermatologie et de Vénéreologie (Paris)*, 108, 41.

Van der Meiren, L., Achten, G. & Pierard, P. (1960) Hypertrichose chez un nouveau-né. *Archives Belges de Dermatologie et Syphiligraphie*, 16, 206.

Congenital syndromes of hypertrichosis and mental retardation
(References p. 270)

Coffin–Siris syndrome

This syndrome is characterized by profound mental and growth retardation with congenital absence of the distal phalanges and nails of the fifth fingers and toes. There is usually a generalized hypertrichosis with bushy eybrows and eyelashes but paradoxically the scalp hair is often sparse (Coffin & Siris 1970; Carey & Hall 1978).

Cornelia de Lange syndrome

Hypertrichosis is a constant and distinctive feature of this rare syndrome. The cause is unknown and most cases are sporadic. In some cases siblings have been affected and some features of the syndrome have been identified in other relatives (Daniel & Higgins 1971; Beck 1974).

The birthweight is low and there is both physical and mental retardation. There is a mild generalized hypertrichosis and abundant head hair with low frontal and nuchal hair lines. The eyebrows are bushy and confluent and the eyelashes are long and curved. The palpebral fissure has an anti-mongoloid slant. Marbling of the skin is conspicuous and often persistent. One or more fingers may be short. The nose is upturned, but downturned labial commissures result in a 'carp' mouth.

There is a variable range of other defects which may occur in addition to the above abnormalities. These are predominantly ocular (Milot & Demay 1972) and skeletal, but may involve other systems (Noe & Hammond 1967; Soderquist & Reed 1968; Pashayan *et al.* 1969; Jaqueti *et al.* 1973).

Gorlin–Chaudhry–Moss

This collection of abnormalities has been reported in only two siblings; marked generalized hypertrichosis with mid-facial flattening, patent ductus arteriosus and hypoplasia of the teeth, eyes and labia majora (Gorlin *et al.* 1960).

Leprechaunism

Leprechaunism is an entity characterized by a grotesque elfin-like face with thick lips, large, low-set ears, breast enlargement and prominent genitalia. Absence of subcutaneous tissue gives rise to excessive folding of the skin. Generalized hypertrichosis occurs in three-quarters of cases (Summitt 1979).

Lissencephaly

This is a form of arrested brain development in which no sulci or gyri develop, rendering the surface of the brain smooth. There is severe mental and growth retardation and affected children rarely survive more than 1 year. Hypertrichosis may be localized to the face or back but may be extensive (Dieker 1969).

Rubinstein–Taybi syndrome

The broad thumbs syndrome, as its original describers modestly prefer to call it, is also a collection of many clinical signs. Hypertrichosis occurs in 64% of cases and affects the trunk, limbs and face. The more important diagnostic features are growth and mental retardation, beaked nose with a low septum, high arched palate, hypertelorism, broad first (and other) digits and cryptorchidism (Rubinstein 1969).

Schinzel–Giedion syndrome

This syndrome has been described in two reports of unrelated children. The cutaneous features are generalized hypertrichosis and abundant folds of skin overlying a short neck. The face is characterized by mid-face retraction. The nose is short with a saddle, a short bridge and upturned tip. There are also club feet, hypoplasia of dermal ridges and radiological bony abnormalities which particularly affect the skull, ribs and terminal phalanges (Donnai & Harris 1979; Schinzel & Giedion 1978).

References

Beck, B. (1974) Familial occurrence of Cornelia de Lange's syndrome. *Acta Pediatrica*, **63**, 225.

Carey, J.C. & Hall, B.D. (1978) The Coffin—Siris syndrome. *American Journal of Diseases of Children*, **132**, 667.

Coffin, G.S. & Siris, E. (1970) Mental retardation with absent fifth fingernail and terminal phalanx. *American Journal of Diseases of Children*, **119**, 433.

Daniel, W.L. & Higgins, J.V. (1971) Biochemical and genetic investigation of the de Lange syndrome. *American Journal of Diseases of Children*, **121**, 401.

Dieker, H., Edwards, R.H., Zu Rhein, G., Chou, S.M. Hartman, H.A. & Opitz, J.M. (1969) The lissencephaly syndrome. *Birth Defects: Original Article Series*, V, No. 2, p. 53.

Donnai, D. & Harris, R. (1979) A further case of a new syndrome including midface retraction, hypertrichosis, and skeletal anomalies. *Journal of Medical Genetics*, **16**, 483.

Gorlin, R.J., Chaudhry, A.P. & Moss, M.I. (1960) Craniofacial dysostosis, patent ductus arteriosus, hypertrichosis, hypoplasia of the labia majora, dental and eye anomalies—a new syndrome? *Journal of Pediatrics*, **56**, 778.

Jaquetti, G., Ledo, A., Gay, C., Gallego, J.R., Gonzalez, P. & Corripio, F. (1973) Syndrome de Cornelia Lange. *Hospital General*, **13**, 359.

Milot, J. & Demay, F. (1972) Ocular anomalies in de Lange syndrome. *American Journal of Ophthalmology*, **74**, 394.

Noe, O. & Hammond, J. (1967) de Lange's Amsterdam dwarfism: case report and etiological considerations. *American Journal of Mental Deficiency*, **71**, 991.

Pashayan, H., Whelan, D., Guttman, S. & Fraser, F.C. (1969) Variability of the de Lange syndrome: report of 3 cases and genetic analysis of 54 families. *Journal of Pediatrics*, **75**, 853.

Rubinstein, J.H. (1969) The broad thumbs syndrome—progress report 1968. *Birth Defects: Original Article Series*, V, No. 2, p. 25.

Schinzel, A. & Giedeon, A. (1978) A syndrome of severe midface retraction, multiple skull anomalies, clubfeet and cardiac and renal malformations in sibs. *American Journal of Medical Genetics*, **1**, 361.

Soderquist, N.A. & Reed, W.B. (1968) Cornelia de Lange syndrome. *Cutis*, **4**, 1335.

Summitt, R.L. (1979) Leprechaunism. In *Birth Defects Compendium*, 2nd edn, p. 644, ed. D. Bergasma. Macmillan Press, London.

Hypertrichosis associated with metabolic disorders
(References p. 273)

Lipoatrophic diabetes (Berardinelli syndrome; Lawrence–Seip syndrome)
Loss of subcutaneous fat may be evident at birth. Physical growth is rapid until puberty. The sunken cheeks, broad nasal root and large ears produce a distinctive facies. The liver and spleen may be large. There may be some degree of mental retardation. The penis or clitoris is enlarged and polycystic ovaries are common.

Hypertrichosis of face, neck, arms and legs increases from birth onwards. The head hair is abundant and curly. Acanthosis nigricans of the axillae, wrists and ankles is common (Berardinelli 1954; Janaki *et al.* 1980). The pattern of hair growth in this condition is poorly described and it may represent a similar state to the HAIR-AN syndome.

Insulin-resistant diabetes begins in childhood or adolescence. There may at first be no glycosuria. Hyperlipaemia is constant.

Mucopolysaccharidoses

Six distinct genetically determined disorders of mucopolysaccharide metabolism are now recognised (McKusick & Neufeld 1983). The syndromes show some features in common but differ in many ways both clinically and biochemically.

These conditions variably result in physical abnormalities, mental retardation and early death. Increased body hair growth is a secondary feature which occurs in most forms but is most prominent in the Sanfilippo variant (McKusick & Neufeld 1983). Hypertrichosis typically develops at different ages in the three main forms: in Hurler's at 18–24 months, in Hunter's at 2–4 years and in the Sanfilippo form at 4–6 years (Leroy & Crocker 1966). The hair has been described as covering the trunk and extremities and being dense and lanugo in appearance (Hambrick & Scheie 1962).

Winchester syndrome

This disorder is characterized by dwarfism, joint and bony abnormalities, peripheral corneal opacities and coarse facial features (Winchester *et al.* 1969). The cutaneous features are thickened localized plaques of leathery skin which gradually become hyperpigmented and hypertrichotic (Cohen *et al.* 1975). It was originally thought to be a mucopolysaccharidosis but more recent investigation has classified it as a non-lysosomal connective tissue disease (Hollister *et al.* 1974).

The porphyrias

Hypertrichosis is a feature, sometimes a conspicuous one, in several of the forms of porphyria. The development of hypertrichosis would appear to follow the occurrence of photosensitivity reactions and, therefore, there is excess hair only on those exposed sites such as the face and hands. Indeed, the photosensitivity is often so severe as to ensure minimum exposure of the skin.

Hypertrichosis is a particular feature of congenital or erythropoietic porphyria (Gunther's disease). Hypertrichosis of face and limbs is usually present (Caruso & Previti 1959) and is occasionally extensive, particularly on the face (Fig. 8.9) (Handa 1965).

Hypertrichosis has also been reported in cases of erythropoietic proto-porphyria (Bhutani *et al.* 1972), porphyria variegata and porphyria cutanea tarda (PCT) (Pinol Aguade *et al.* 1973). Hypertrichosis may be a particularly important sign of PCT in American blacks in whom blistering is unusual (Zeligman 1963). In the form of hepatic PCT induced by exposure to chemicals such as hexachlorobenzene, hypertrichosis may be very gross. Many of those affected in the Turkish epidemic of 1954–5 were known as 'monkey children' (Cam & Nigogosyan 1963).

The association, particularly in a child, of hypertrichosis with light sensitivity should suggest the need for a full investigation of the patient's porphyrin metabolism and a careful study of the family histories (Rimington *et al.* 1967).

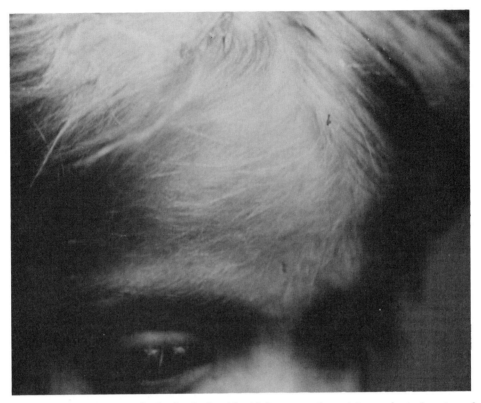

Fig. 8.9 Hypertrichosis on the forehead of a girl with hepato-erythropoietic porphyria (courtesy of Dr A. Massa. Portugal).

Malnutrition

Malnutrition is normally considered to be a cause of scalp hair loss; however, hypertrichosis of the limbs and trunk has been observed in previously well-fed children receiving a grossly deficient diet (Castellani 1938). It has also been recorded in coeliac disease (Holzel 1951).

Anorexia nervosa

The patient is usually a young woman who restricts her diet, excluding carbohydrates in particular. Severe emaciation may result. In some patients downy hypertrichosis of the trunk and arms is a striking feature; it was present in 12 of 33 women aged 15–29 (Ryle 1936). More recent studies record a much lower incidence of hypertrichosis (Bartels 1946) or fail to mention this symptom (Williams 1958).

Juvenile hypothyroidism

Children with primary hypothyroidism may have generalized hypertrichosis. There is a diffuse pattern of hair growth affecting the temples, back, shoulders and limbs. In all the published cases there have been other manifestations of hypothyroidism; dry skin, constipation, short stature or sluggish nature. Replacement therapy with thyroxine has been reported to give dramatic improvement (Perloff 1955; Stern & Kelnar 1985). In a further case tight curls of the body hair was a prominent feature (Maekawa *et al.* 1983).

Pretibial myxoedema

Localized plaques of myxoedema of the lower legs occur in about 4% of patients with hyperthyroidism (Gimllett 1960) and in about 40% of those with malignant exophthalmos. Most have elevated levels of long-acting thyroid stimulator. In some cases lesions first appear only after the start of anti-thyroid treatment.

Flesh-coloured nodules appear on the shins; sometimes the firm non-pitting oedema of the shins and ankles is more diffuse. Hypertrichosis over the lesions is frequent. Clubbing and other features of thyroid acropachy may be associated.

References

Bartels, E.D. (1946) Studies on hypometabolism: I. Anorexia nervosa. *Acta Medica Scandinavica*, **124**, 185.

Berardinelli, W. (1954) An undiagnosed endocrine-metabolic syndrome. *Journal of Endocrinology*, 14, 193.

Bhutani, L.K., Deshpande, S.G. & Sood, S.K. (1972) Erythropoietic protoporphyria: first report in an Indian. *British Medical Journal*, ii, 741.

Cam, C. & Nigogosyan, G. (1963) Acquired toxic porphyria cuyanea tarda due to hexachloroben-zene. *Journal of the American Medical Association*, **183**, 88.

Caruso, P. & Previti, A. (1960) Contributo allo studio de la porfiria eritropoietica: due casi con anemia emolitica, splenomegalia, ipofunzionlita surrenalica. *Minerva Pediatrica*, **12**, 250.

Castellani, A. (1938) Note on some little known conditions of the lanugo hair. *Journal of Tropical Medicine and Hygiene*, **41**, 400.

Cohen, A.H., Hollister, D.W. & Reed, W.B. (1975) The skin in the Winchester syndrome. *Archives of Dermatology*, **111**, 230.

Gimllett, T.N.D. (1960) Pretibial myxoedema. *British Medical Journal*, ii, 398.

Hambrick, G.W. Jr. & Scheie, H.G. (1962) Studies of the skin in Hurler's syndrome. *Archives of Dermatology*, **85**, 455.

Handa, F. (1965) Congenital porphyria. *Archives of Dermatology*, **91**, 130.

Hollister, D.W., Rimoin, D.L., Lachman, R.S., Cohen, A.H., Reed, W.B. & Westin, G.W. (1974) The Winchester syndrome: a nonlysosomal connective tissue disease. *Journal of Pediatrics*, **84**, 701.

Holzel, A. (1951) Hypertrichosis in childhood. *Acta Paediatrica Scandinavica*, **40**, 59.

Janaki, V.P., Premalantha, S., Raghuvarta Rao, N. & Thambiah, A.S. (1980) Lawrence–Seip syndrome. *British Journal of Dermatology*, **103**, 693.

Leroy, J.G. & Crocker, A.C. (1966) Clinical definition of the Hurler–Hunter phenotype. *American Journal of Diseases of Children*, **112**, 518.

Maekawa, Y., Kito, M. & Hiramatsu, R. (1983) Rolled hair and hypertrichosis: a manifestation of juvenile hypothyroidism. *The Journal of Dermatology (Japan)* 10, 157.

McKusick, V.A. & Neufeld, E.F. (1983) The mucopolysaccharide storage diseases. In *The Metabolic Basis of Inherited Disease*, 5th edn, p. 751, eds. JB Stanbury, JB Wyngaarden, DS Fredrickson, JL Goldstein, MS Brown. McGraw-Hill, New York.

Perloff, W.H. (1955) Hirsutism: a manifestation of juvenile hypothyroidism. *Journal of the American Medical Association*, **157**, 651.

Pinol Aguade, J., Lecha, M., Almeida, J., Herrero, C. & Gaby de Mascaro, C. (1973) Porfiria cutanea tarda en ninos. *Medicina cutanea*, 7, 37.

Rimington, C., Magnus, I.A., Ryan, E.A. & Cripps, D.J. (1967) Porphyria and photosensitivity. *Quarterly Journal of Medicine*, 36, 29.

Ryle, J.A. (1936) Anorexia nervosa. *Lancet*, ii, 190.

Stern, S.R. & Kelnar, C.J.H. (1985) Hypertrichosis due to hypothyroidism. *Archives of Disease in Childhood*, 60, 763.

Williams, E. (1958) Anorexia nervosa: a somatic disorder. *British Medical Journal*, ii, 19.

Winchester, P., Grossman, H., Lim, W.N. & Danes, B.S. (1969) A new acid mucopolysaccharidosis with skeletal deformities simulating rheumatoid arthritis. *American Journal of Roentgenology*, 106, 121.

Zeligman, I. (1963) Patterns of porphyria in the American Negro. *Archives of Dermatology*, 88, 616.

Hypertrichosis in teratogenic syndromes

Fetal alcohol syndrome

The fetal alcohol syndrome is not uncommon. The infants (60%) of chronic alcoholic women are either stillborn or severely diseased (Jones & Smith 1975).

Such infants are small and microcephalic with mental and physical retardation and defects of the heart and of the joints. The facies is unusual and may be distinctive with short palpebral fissures, a prominent nose and maxillary hypoplasia. Numerous other defects may include hypertrichosis, which may be very conspicuous, and capillary haemangiomatosis (Hanson *et al.* 1976).

References

Hanson, J.W., Jones, K.L. & Smith, D.W. (1976) Fetal alcohol syndrome experience with 41 patients. *Journal of the American Medical Association*, 235, 1458.

Jones, K.L. & Smith, D.W. (1975) The fetal alcohol syndrome. *Teratology*, 12, 1.

Iatrogenic hypertrichosis
(References p. 276)

Definition

A clear distinction should be drawn between iatrogenic hirsutism, in which hair growth is increased in part or all of the male sexual pattern, and iatrogenic hypertrichosis, in which there is a uniform growth of fine hair increased over extensive areas of the trunk, hands and face.

Aetiology

The mode of action of the offending drugs on hair follicles is not known; the same mechanism is not involved in all cases. Cortisone, diphenylhydantoin and penicillamine are all known to affect collagen, but in different ways. Psoralens presumably induce hypertrichosis in predisposed subjects by accentuating the tendency of sunlight to induce this temporary change. The stimulation of hair growth on sun-exposed sites by benoxaprofen may have a similar mechanism.

Clinical features

Existing vellus hairs increase in length and less so in diameter. The hairs are seldom more than 3 cm in length and are considerably finer than terminal hair. The hair growth is often first noticed on the back and the extensor aspect of the limbs but later the rest of the trunk and the face are seen to be involved. The hair usually reverts to the normal for the sex, age and site within a year after the drug is discontinued.

It is not clear whether possible differences in the pattern of hypertrichosis are significantly related to any particular drug, since racial and other genetic factors must be taken into account.

Diphenylhydantoin induces hypertrichosis after 2–3 months, more in girls than in boys. It affects the extensor aspects of the limbs, then the face and trunk and clears within a year of cessation of therapy (Livingstone *et al.* 1955).

Diazoxide produces hypertrichosis in all children but it seems to be a cosmetic problem in only one-half. The increased growth is apparent after 3–6 weeks therapy and is entirely lost 4 months after cessation of therapy in children (Koblenzer & Baker 1968; Prigent *et al.* 1988); in adults the hair growth may last longer (Burton *et al.* 1975). Histological examination of the skin demonstrates that the majority of hair roots are in the anagen phase (compared to control subjects in whom the roots are predominantly telogen) and that the anagen predominance remains throughout therapy. There are no associated changes in the sebaceous glands (Koblenzer & Baker 1968).

Minoxidil commonly induces hypertrichosis (Burton & Marshall 1979). It is apparent after a few weeks therapy and the hair falls 2 months after stopping therapy (Lorette & Nivet 1985).

Hypertrichosis of some degree (Fig. 8.10) develops in 60% of patients treated with cyclosporin within the first 6 months of therapy (Bencini *et al.* 1986a; Griffiths *et al.* 1986). Keratosis pilaris may precede the appearance of thick pigmented hair on the face, trunk and limbs. Severe hypertrichosis appears to be more common in dark-skinned subjects. Involvement of other parts of the pilosebaceous unit occurs; keratosis pilaris (21%), sebaceous hyperplasia (10%) and acne (15%) even in the absence of other acneigenic immunosuppressive therapy (Bencini *et al.* 1986b).

Benoxaprofen induces a fine downy growth of hair on the face and exposed extremities after only a few weeks. In all the described patients hypertrichosis followed the development of photosensitivity (Fenton *et al.* 1982).

Streptomycin caused hypertrichosis in 22 of 27 children who had received 1 g daily for miliary tuberculosis meningitis (Fono 1950). Buffoni (1951) observed hypertrichosis in about 66% of cases of meningitis so treated, and postulated that the streptomycin did not act directly on the follicles.

Prolonged administration of cortisone may induce hypertrichosis, most marked on the forehead, the temples and the sides of the cheeks, but also on the back and the extensor aspects of the limbs.

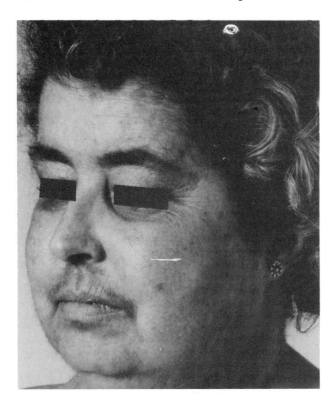

Fig. 8.10 Fine downy facial hypertrichosis due to cyclosporin therapy used for immunosuppression after renal transplant.

Penicillamine appears to cause lengthening and coarsening of hair on the trunk and limbs.

Psoralens, used in the treatment of vitiligo and psoriasis, may induce temporary hypertrichosis of light-exposed skin (Singh & Lal 1967).

References

Bencini, P.L., Montagnino, G., Sala, F., De Vecchi, A., Crosti, C. & Parantino, A. (1986a) Cutaneous lesions in 67 cyclosporin-treated renal transplant recipients. *Dermatologica*, **172**, 24.

Bencini, P.L., Montagnino, G., Crosti, C., Sala, F. & De Vecchi, A. (1986b) Acne in a kidney transplant patient treated with cyclosporin A. *British Journal of Dermatology*, **114**, 396.

Buffoni, L. (1951) Streptomicina e ipertricosi. *Minerva Paediatrica*, **3**, 710.

Burton, J.L. & Marshall, A. (1979) Hypertrichosis due to minoxidil. *British Journal of Dermatology*, **101**, 593.

Burton, J.L., Schutt, W.H. & Caldwell, I.W. (1975) Hypertrichosis due to diazoxide. *British Journal of Dermatology*, **93**, 707.

Fenton, D.A., English, J.S. & Wilkinson, J.D. (1982) Reversal of male pattern baldness, hypertrichosis, and accelerated hair and nail growth in patients receiving benoxaprofen. *British Medical Journal*, **248**, 1228.

Fono, R. (1950) Appearance of hypertrichosis during streptomycin treatment. *Annali Paediatrici*, **174**, 389.

Griffiths, C.E.M., Powles, A.V., Leonard, J.N., Fry, L., Baker, B.S. & Valdimarsson, H. (1986) Clearance of psoriasis with low dose cyclosporin. *British Medical Journal*, **293**, 731.

Koblenzer, P.J. & Baker, L. (1968) Hypertrichosis lanuginosa associated with diazoxide therapy in prepubertal children: a clinicopathological study. *Annals of the New York Academy of Sciences,* **150**, 373.

Livingstone, S., Peterson, D. & Bohs, L.L. (1955) Hypertrichosis occurring in association with dilantin therapy. *Journal of Pediatrics,* **47**, 351.

Lorette, G. & Nivet, H. (1985) Hypertrichose diffuse au minoxidil chez un enfant de deux ans et demi. *Annales de Dermatologie et Vénéréologie (Paris)* **112**, 527.

Prigent, F., Gantzer, A., Romain, O., Massonaud, M., Auffrant, C. & Bompard, Y. (1988) Hypertrichose diffuse acquise au cours d'un traitement par diazoxide chez un nouveau-ne. *Annales de Dermatologie et Vénéréologie (Paris)* **115**, 191.

Singh, G. & Lal, S. (1967) Hypertrichosis and hyperpigmentation with systemic psoralen treatment. *British Journal of Dermatology,* **79**, 501.

Acquired generalized hypertrichosis

Hypertrichosis lanuginosa acquisita (References p. 279)

History and nomenclature

The rapid growth of long, fine, downy hair over a large area of the body, replacing not only normal terminal hair but also the primary vellus of forehead and cheeks and the secondary vellus of the bald scalp, is a dramatic event. The illustrated account of an elderly Italian who exhibited this phenomenon after a serious illness (Le Double & Houssay 1912) is an example of the extreme and certainly very rare form. It is now becoming clear that the less conspicuous growth of lanugo, particularly on the face of patients with malignant diseases is not so uncommon; Fretzin (1967) called it 'malignant down'. Since in all cases the characteristic abnormality is the replacement of hair of other types by hair with the characteristics of foetal lanugo, the term acquired hypertrichosis lanuginosa is appropriate, even though in one patient (Le Marquand & Bohn 1951) the growth of hair on the previously bald scalp was apparently of terminal type.

Aetiology

In one reported case (Ormsby 1930) the patient is said to have been otherwise healthy, but no follow up was published. The patients referred to by Le Double & Houssay (1912) were said to have had influenza. A diffuse form of hypertrichosis may develop in Cushing's disease and lanugo-like hypertrichosis developing in pregnancy and falling in the early postnatal months has been described.

With these exceptions all patients with acquired hypertrichosis lanuginosa have had malignant disease, the nature of which is shown in Table 8.1. The ages of the patients range from 19 to 69 years and females outnumber males by 3:1. No paediatric cases have been described. Endocrine investigations, wherever performed, have shown no consistent or apparently relevant abnormalities.

Histopathology

The abnormal hair is fine, poorly pigmented or unpigmented, long and straight (Fig. 8.11). In one case, papillomatosis of the skin of the trunk, with histological

Table 8.1 Malignancies associated with hypertrichosis lanuginosa acquisata (Jemec 1986)

	No. cases	Sex	Age
Bladder	1	F	35
Breast	1	F	54
Colon	7	F	39–60
Gallbladder	1	M	65
Liver	1	F	32
Lungs	3	F	43–69
	6	M	44–69
Lymphoma	3	F	28–48
Myeloma	1	F	53
Ovary	1	F	56
Pancreas	1	F	19
Uterus	3	F	46–66

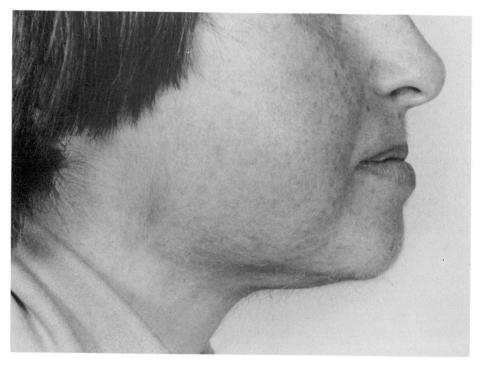

Fig. 8.11 Acquired hypertrichosis of the face associated with carcinoma of the uterus.

features somewhat similar to acanthosis nigricans, was described (Hensley & Glynn 1969). Histological studies in another case (Hegedus & Schorr 1972) showed the lanugo follicles lying almost parallel to the surface, and apparently derived from 'mantle' hair follicles.

Clinical features

All accounts emphasize the rapidity with which the hypertrichosis develops. Dense fine white or red-black hairs replace the normal vellus hairs. The hairs are finest on the face, where they grow on forehead, eyelids, nose and ears, giving the patient a simian appearance. Terminal hair on the scalp, beard and pubes tends not to be replaced but lanugo up to 15 cm long may densely cover all other surfaces except the genitalia and the palms and soles. Long-bald scalp may show an equally dense growth, its lighter colour and firm texture contrasting with the remaining darker and coarser terminal hair. In one case the rate of growth of the lanugo on trunk and limbs was found to be about 2.5 cm/week (Le Marquand & Bohn 1951).

The extent and degree of the lanuginous transformation varies considerably. In early cases the growth of down on the forehead and temples may be the only abnormality.

The lanugo may develop a few weeks or up to 2 years before a carcinoma is diagnosed (Goodfellow *et al.* 1980).

A number of other cutaneous abnormalities have been described in patients with hypertrichosis lanuginosa acquisata. Keratotic lesions have developed on the palms and soles (Fretzin 1967) and limbs (Wadskov *et al.* 1976). Glossitis has been reported in several cases (Fretzin 1967; Wadskov *et al.* 1976; Knowling *et al.* 1982; Jemec 1986). Hegedus & Schorr (1972) reported prominent, discrete red papules on the distal two-thirds of the tongue.

Other well-recognised cutaneous markers of internal malignancy have been noted in these patients. Acquired ichthyosis was reported in a woman with lymphatic leukaemia (Ricken 1979). Acanthosis nigricans and palmar hyper-keratosis was reported in two further cases (Dingley & Marten 1957; Goodfellow *et al.* 1980).

References

Dingley, E. & Marten, R.H. (1957) Adenocarcinoma of the ovary presenting as acanthosis nigricans. *Journal of Obstetrics and Gynaecology of the British Commonwealth*, **64**, 898.

Fretzin, D.F. (1967) Malignant down. *Archives of Dermatology*, **95**, 294.

Goodfellow, A., Calvert, H. & Bohn, G. (1980) Hypertrichosis lanuginosa acquisata. *British Journal of Dermatology*, **103**, 431.

Hegedus, S.I. & Schorr, W.F. (1972) Acquired hypertrichosis lanuginosa and malignancy. *Archives of Dermatology*, **106**, 84.

Hensley, G.T. & Glynn, K.P. (1969) Hypertrichosis lanuginosa as a sign of internal malignancy. *Cancer*, **24**, 1051.

Jemec, G.B.E. (1986) Hypertrichosis lanuginosa acquisata: report of a case review of the literature. *Archives of Dermatology*, **122**, 805.

Knowling, M.A., Meakin, J.W., Hradsky, N.S. & Pringle, J.F. (1982) Hypertrichosis lanuginosa acquisata associated with adenocarcinoma of the lung. *Canadian Medical Association Journal* **126**, 1308.

Le Double, A.-F. & Houssay, F. (1912) *Les Velus*, p. 28. Vigot, Paris.

Le Marquand, H.S. & Bohn, G.L. (1951) Recurrent peptic ulcer with generalised hypertrichosis including growth of hair on the bald scalp and later development of signs suggesting adrenal failure. *Proceedings of the Royal Society of Medicine (London)*, **44**, 155.

Ormsby, O. (1930) Acute hypertrichosis. *Archives of Dermatology and Syphilology*, **21**, 663.

Ricken, K.H. (1979) Hypertrichosis lanuginosa et terminalis acquisata und pseudoichthyosisals para neoplastische Syndrom bei chronisch lymphatische leukämie. *Zeitschrift für Hautkrankheiten*, **54**, 819.

Wadskov, S., Bro-Jorgensen, A. & Sondergaard, J. (1976) Acquired hypertrichosis lanuginosa. *Archives of Dermatology*, **112**, 1442.

Hypertrichosis with head injuries and other cerebral disturbances

The development of hypertrichosis some 1–4 months after a head injury is a well-recognised phenomenon, especially in children, but occasionally reported in adults. The head injury has usually been severe but the precise localization of the lesion responsible for the hair growth has not been ascertained, although in one case compression injury of the mid-brain leading to adrenal over-activity was suspected (Epstein 1947).

A typical case (Bartuska 1963) was a 7-year-old Negro boy; 6 weeks after a severe head injury he developed long silky hair on the forehead, cheeks, trunk and limbs, but no pubic or axillary hair. A young German woman aged 17, in the third month after a severe head injury, showed a strong growth of fine hair on her face, shoulders, chest and abdomen. Her eyebrows merged and vibrissae projected from her nostrils. The pattern of her pubic hair changed from horizontal to accuminate. Four months later she had regained her previous hair pattern at all sites (Tarnow 1957, 1971). Another case (Tarnow 1971) was a German boy aged 7 who developed a dense growth of fine hair on his limbs during the fourth month after a head injury, and also some pubic hair. All the excess hair had been lost 15 months later. A girl aged 14 (Robinson 1955) developed generalized hypertrichosis 3 months after receiving multiple injuries in a motor accident; the excess hair, which was mainly on the extensor aspects of the limbs, was lost within 6 months. These and other similar case reports make it clear that a head injury, and perhaps severe shock without physical injury, can induce either hypertrichosis or hirsutism, or both. Spontaneous recovery is the rule. The mechanism for the extensive growth of hair is unknown. However, it is unlikely to be hyperandrogenic hirsuties as head injuries are sometimes associated with hypogonadotrophic hypogonadism (Woolf *et al.* 1986).

Rarely cerebral damage of infective origin can cause hypertrichosis; it followed encephalitis in a child aged two and a half (Stegagno & Vignetti 1955).

The rare hereditary globoid leucodystrophy, also known as Krabbe's disease, is usually fatal before the age of 2. Hypertrichosis has been present in some cases (Tavri *et al.* 1970).

References

Bartuska, D.G. (1963) Hypertrichosis in a brain-damaged child. *Journal of the American Medical Women's Association*, **18**, 711.

Epstein, E. (1947) Posttraumatisch zentragener Hirsutismus nach Commotio cerebri. *Weiner klinische Wochenschrift*, **47**, 520.

Robinson, R.L.V. (1955) Temporary acquired hypertrichosis following traumatic shock. *AMA Archives of Dermatology*, **17**, 401.

Stegagno, G. & Vignetti, P. (1955) Considerazioni su di ipertricosi con cerebropatia in una bambina di $2\frac{1}{2}$ anni. *Archivo Italiano di pediatria e puericolture*, **17**, 421.

Tarnow, G. (1957) Vorübergehender Hirsutismus nach Contusio cerebri. *Nervenarzt*, **28**, 327.

Tarnow, G. (1971) Haarkleidstörungen nach schweren Hirntraumen. *Journal of Neurovisceral Relations*, (Suppl), **10**, 549.

Tavri, G.M., Shalini, K.C.M., Martin, K.B., Bhaktavizian, A. & Backharvat, B.K. (1970) Globoid leucodystrophy (Krabbe's disease). *Indian Journal of Medical Research*, **58**, 993.

Woolf, P.D., Hamill, R.W., McDonald, J.V., Lee, L.A. & Kelly, M. (1986) Transient hypogonadotrophic hypogonadism after head injury: effects on steroid precursors and correlation with sympathetic nervous system activity. *Clinical Endocrinology*, **25**, 265.

Acquired circumscribed hypertrichosis
(References p. 282)

Cutting or shaving the hair influences neither its rate of growth nor the calibre of the hair shaft. However, repeated or long-continued inflammatory changes involved the dermis, whether or not clinically evident scarring is produced, may result in the growth of long and coarse hair at this site. Although rarely reported, the phenomenon is of common occurrence. The cause of the hair growth is usually obvious but may be overlooked when the trauma is occupational; for example, circumscribed patches of hypertrichosis on the left shoulder in men frequently carrying heavy sacks (Csillag 1921). A patch of hypertrichosis on one forearm is sometimes seen in mental defectives who have acquired the habit of chewing this site (Ressmann & Butterworth 1952). Sometimes the hypertrichosis, which may involve too few follicles to have attracted the patient's attention, develops at the site of an accidental wound or a vaccination scar (Linser 1926). It has developed on the back of the hand and fingers 3 months after the excision of warts; the coarse dark hairs 3–5 cm in length were shed after 2 months (Friederich & Gloor 1970). We have seen it surrounding a meniscectomy scar. It has been reported also in irregular pattern on the legs in chronic venous insufficiency (Schraibman 1967), around the edges of a burn (Shafir & Tsur 1979), and at the site of multiple clusters of excoriated insect bites (Tisocco *et al.* 1981).

Long-continued cutaneous hyperaemia without permanent dermal change can also induce increased hair growth which is usually reversible. Hypertrichosis of this type may occur near inflamed joints and has been reported particularly in association with gonococcal arthritis (Heidemann 1934) and in the skin overlying chronic osteomyelitis of the tibia (Schuller & Frost 1956). Very exceptionally, inflammatory dermatoses, especially in children, may induce a temporary overgrowth of hair. It has been observed after eczema (Edel 1938), and after varicella (Naveh & Friedman 1972). A linear pattern of hypertrichosis on the leg has been described after recurrent thrombophlebitis which persisted for a year (Soyuer *et al.* 1988). Hypertrichosis may occur in the indurated skin in melorheostotic scleroderma. The diagnosis is established by radiological examination when the skin has completely healed. The damaged skin in epidermolysis bullosa may also become hypertrichotic (Cofano 1955).

Children have developed itching eczema and local hypertrichosis at the site of injection of diphtheria/tetanus vaccine adsorbed on aluminium chloride (Pembroke & Marten 1979). We have observed similar changes at the site of BCG vaccination.

Hypertrichosis of one leg after a prolonged period of occlusion by plaster of Paris is a phenomenon well-known to orthopaedic surgeons. It occurs mainly in children. The hypertrichosis may be attributed either to protection of the skin by the plaster from normal weathering or due to increased skin temperature. The hair returns to normal within a few weeks of removal of the plaster.

References

Cofano, A.R. (1955) Su un caso di epidermolisi bollosa distrofica con accentuada ipertricosi. *Annali Italiani di Dermatologia*, **10**, 195.

Csillag, J. (1921) Über Berufshypertricose. *Archiv für Dermatologie und Syphilologie*, **134**, 147.

Edel, K. (1938) Hypertrichosis als verwikkeling bij eczeem. *Nederlandische Tijdschrift voor Geneeskunde*, **82**, 2466.

Friederich, H.C. & Gloor, M. (1970) Postoperativ 'irrative' Hypertrichose. *Zeitschrift für Haut und Geschlechtskrankheiten*, **45**, 10.

Heidemann, H. (1934) Et tifaelde af hypertrichjose opstaalt i tilknytning til en gonorrhoisk ledaffektasjon. *Ugeskrift for Laeger*, **96**, 553.

Linser, A. (1926) Demonstrationen: Patient mit einer hypertrichosis irritativa. *Klinische Wochenschrift*, **115**, 149.

Miyachi, Y., Hori, T. Yamada, A. & Ueo, T. (1979) Linear melorheostotic scleroderma and hypertrichosis. *Archives of Dermatology*, **115**, 1233.

Naveh, Y. & Friedman, A. (1972) Transient circumscribed hypertrichosis following chickenpox. *Pediatrics*, **50**, 487.

Pembroke, H.C. & Marten, R.H. (1979) Unusual cutaneous reactions following diphtheria and tetanus immunization. *Clinical and Experimental Dermatology*, **4**, 345.

Ressmann, A.C. & Butterworth, T. (1952) Localized acquired hypertrichosis (as a result of biting in mentally deficient). *Archives of Dermatology and Syphilology*, **65**, 458.

Schraibman, I.G. (1967) Localized hirsutism. *Postgraduate Medical Journal*, **43**, 545.

Schuller, P.A. & Frost, J.A. (1956) Osteomilitis cronica de perone e hipertrichosis localizada. *Medicina* (Madrid), **24**, 360.

Shafir, R. & Tsur H. (1979) Local hirsutism at the periphery of burned skin. *British Journal of Plastic Surgery*, **32**, 93.

Soyuer, U., Aktas, E. & Ozesmi, M. (1988) Post phlebitic localized hypertrichosis. *Archives of Dermatology*, **124**, 30.

Tisocco, L.A., Del Campo, D.V., Bennin, B. & Barsky, S. (1981) Acquired localised hypertrichosis. *Archives of Dermatology*, **117**, 129.

Chapter 9
Traumatic Alopecia

Introduction
Trichotillomania
Cosmetic traumatic alopecia
Accidental traumatic alopecia

Introduction

The term traumatic alopecia is applied to alopecia induced by physical trauma. These cases fall into three main categories:

1 Alopecia resulting from the deliberate, though at times unconscious, efforts of the patient, who is under tension or is psychologically disturbed—trichotillomania.

2 Alopecia resulting from cosmetic procedures applied incorrectly or with misguided and excessive vigour or frequency—cosmetic alopecia.

3 Alopecia resulting from accidental trauma—accidental alopecia.

Trichotillomania
(References p. 289)

History and nomenclature

The term trichotillomania was suggested by Hallopeau in 1889 for the compulsive habit which induces an individual repeatedly to pluck his own hair. There are obvious objections to this overdramatic term for what is often a trivial problem, but its use has been generally preferred to 'trichomania' proposed by Besnier, or to 'autodépilation', proposed by Coppola (cit. Galewsky 1928). The term 'tic d'épilation', used by Raymond, is particularly appropriate for the condition commonly seen in young children, but has not found favour.

Pathology (Lachapelle & Pierard 1977) (Figs 9.1, 9.2)

The histological changes vary according to the severity and duration of the hair plucking. Numerous empty hair canals are the most consistent feature. Some follicles are severely damaged; there are clefts in the hair matrix, the follicular epithelium is separated from the connective tissue sheath, and there are intra-epithelial and perifollicular haemorrhages (Mehregan 1970). Injured follicles may form only soft, twisted hairs—a process which has been described as a separate entity under the name of trichomalacia (Mehregan 1970; Sanderson & Hall-Smith 1970). Many follicles are in catagen and some in early anagen. There are few or no follicles in telogen (Steck 1979). Some dilated follicular infundibula contain horny plugs (Muller & Winkelmann 1972).

283

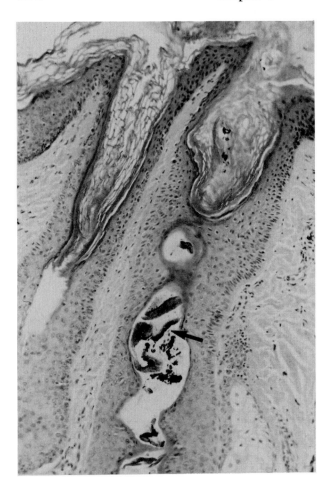

Fig. 9.1 Trichotillomania; biopsy of scalp, showing empty hair follicles. The empty follicle assumes a corkscrew shape and contains melanin casts (arrow) (Professor J.M. Lachapelle).

Experimental studies in sheep showed that tension on the wool fibres leads to an increase in growth rate, but a decrease in diameter and in overall volume. The surrounding epidermis becomes thickened, with a well-defined granular layer.

Aetiology and psychopathology

Trichotillomania occurs more than twice as frequently in females as in males but below the age of 6 boys outnumber girls by 3:2, and the peak incidence in boys is in the 2–6 age group (Muller 1980). It is seven times more frequent in children than adults (Mehregan 1970). The child develops the habit of twisting hair round its fingers and pulling it whilst in bed, in class or watching television. The act is only partially conscious and may replace the habit of thumb-sucking. Various psychiatric studies (Schachter 1961; Monroe & Abse 1963; Greenberg & Sarner 1965; Oranje *et al.* 1986) are not in complete agreement but emotional deprivation in the maternal relationship is considered important in initiating the habit. Others

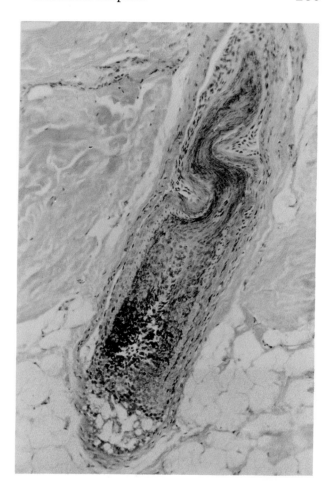

Fig. 9.2 A hair bulb has been partially plucked. Serous exudate fills the space between bulbar cells and the surrounding connective tissue sheaths. Clefts have formed between the cells of the hair matrix. Trichomalacia, the distortion of a fully developed anagen hair, is diagnostic of trichotillomania. Note the absence of inflammatory reaction.

believe that the habit develops in the presence of repressed aggression (Cossidente and Sarti 1984; Oranje *et al.* 1986). The habit is perhaps more common in children of low intelligence, but also occurs in those of average or high intelligence (Bartsch 1956; Oranje *et al.* 1986).

The rarer and more severe form occurs predominantly in females of any age from early adolescence onwards, and most are aged 11–40; the peak incidence in females is between 11 and 17 (Muller 1980). The hair pulling begins in a provocative social situation in a subject who is often greatly disturbed psychologically (Sanderson & Hall-Smith 1970). Exceptionally severe forms may be seen in young patients and the minor forms in older patients.

Clinical features
In the younger patients the hair pulling tic develops gradually and unconsciously but is not usually denied by the patient. Hair is plucked most frequently from one

frontoparietal region. There results an ill-defined patch on which the hairs are twisted and broken at various distances from the clinically normal scalp (Figs 9.3–9.6). The texture and colour of the broken hairs are of course unaffected. Sometimes other parts of the scalp are attacked. More than one member of a family may be found to have acquired the habit, or even several members of a community such as a school (Davis 1922). One young child plucked the hair of her contemporaries as well as her own (Reuter 1951).

In the more severe form the patient usually consistently denies that she is touching her hair, but in a few cases admits it and complains that uncomfortable sensations, described in bizarre terms, are relieved by plucking the hair (Blaisdell 1916). The patient presents with an extensive area of scalp on which the hair has been reduced to a coarse stubble uniformly 2.5–3 mm long; the length is dictated by the impossibility of manually plucking shorter hairs. Most characteristically the plucked area covers the entire scalp apart from the margin, hence the validity of the term 'tonsure alopecia' (Sanderson & Hall-Smith 1970). The hair plucking may be continued for years and the disfiguring baldness is held by the patient to be responsible for her psychological problems. A mother and daughter have been affected at the same time (Hall-Smith 1966).

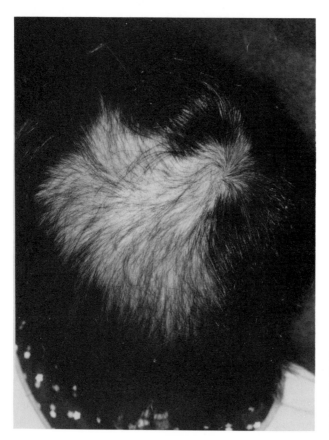

Fig. 9.3 Trichotillomania. Circumscribed but irregular pattern of alopecia, with numerous twisted and broken hairs (Professor J.M. Lachapelle, Louvain).

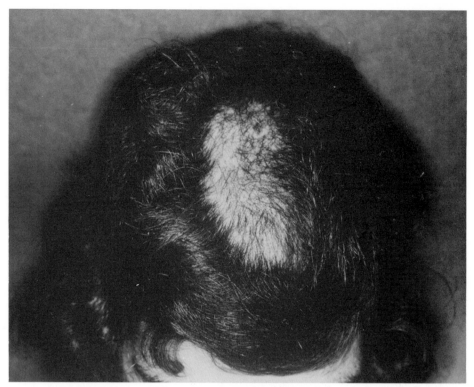

Fig. 9.4 Trichotillomania (Professor J.M. Lachapelle, Louvain).

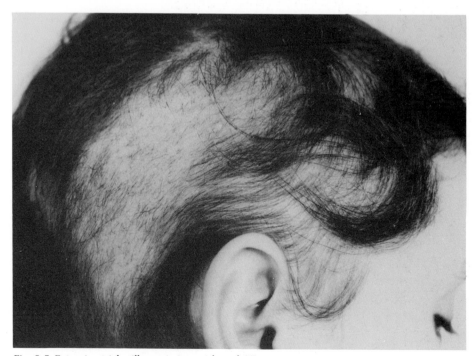

Fig. 9.5 Extensive trichotillomania in a girl aged 17.

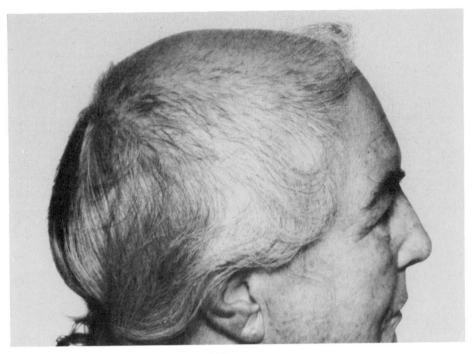

Fig. 9.6 Trichotillomania in a woman aged 72.

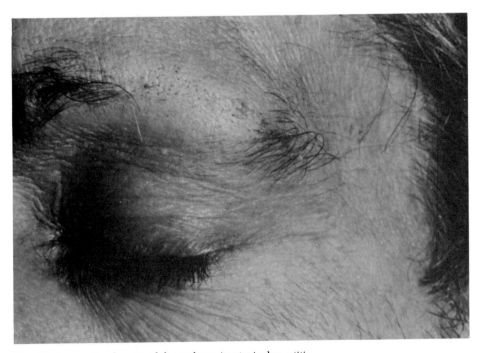

Fig. 9.7 Traumatic alopecia of the eyebrow in atopic dermatitis.

Much more unusual is the habit of plucking the eyelashes, eyebrows and beard (Fig. 9.7) (Sonck 1958; Rohrback 1963; Mehregan 1970; Jillson 1983).

Very exceptionally the patient may pluck hair also, or only, from other regions of the body, such as the mons pubis and perianal region (Galewsky 1928). Rare cases are reported in which the hair is cut with scissors; the term trichotemnomania has been proposed for this activity.

The child may also suck and even eat the hair (trichophagy). In such cases examination of the mouth may reveal hairs (Cossidente & Sarti 1984; Oranje *et al.* 1986) and enquiry should be made for systemic symptoms related to the presence of a hairball, e.g. dysphagia, vomiting, anaemia, abdominal pain or constipation. This symptom was present in 10% of children with trichotillomania (Oranje *et al.* 1986). Nail biting and rarely other forms of self-mutilation may co-exist in 14% of children (Oranje *et al.* 1986).

Differential diagnosis

The minor form in young children is often confused with ringworm or with alopecia areata. In ringworm the texture of the infected hairs is abnormal and the scalp surface may be scaly. It is wise to examine all cases under Wood's light and also to examine broken hairs under the microscope. Alopecia areata may be difficult to exclude with certainty at the first examination, but the course of the condition soon establishes the correct diagnosis. We have known the hair-pulling tic develop in a child recovering from typical alopecia areata.

The severe form presents no real problem if the diagnosis is once considered. In the face of the patient's persistent denials biopsy may be useful and conclusive. The almost complete lack of telogen hairs may provide a helpful clue.

Treatment and prognosis

The habit tic in young children is usually readily eradicated, except in the mentally retarded. The child's problem should be discussed with them and their parents. The diagnosis is often rejected by the parents who have not observed the child pulling the hair and find it unacceptable to believe that the problem is self-inflicted. In a recent series over 50% required psychiatric referral (Oranje *et al.* 1986). Usually support from the dermatologist is sufficient and a soft, woolly, whiskery toy is often advocated; behaviour therapy is also suggested to be helpful.

Tonsure trichotillomania is a very different proposition. Some patients recover, but many fail to do so, despite skilled psychiatric care which may involve the use of major or minor tranquillizers and psychotherapy (Cossidente & Sarti 1984).

References

Bartsch, E. (1956) Beitrag zur Ätiologie der Trichotillomanie im Kindesalter. *Psychiatrie, Neurologie und Medizinische Psychologie*, **8**, 173.
Blaisdell, J.H. (1916) Trichotillomania: a report of two cases of this rare neurodermatosis. *Journal of Cutaneous and Genitourinary Diseases*, **34**, 363.

Cossidente, A. & Sarti, M.G. (1984) Psychiatric syndromes with dermatologic expression. In *Stress and Skin Diseases: Psychosomatic Dermatology*, p. 201, ed. E. Panconesi. Lippincott, J.B., Philadelphia.

Davis, H. (1922) Pseudo-alopecia areata. *British Journal of Dermatology*, **34**, 162.

Galewsky, E. (1928) Über Trichotillomania. *Dermatologische Zeitschrift*, **53**, 208.

Greenberg, H. & Sarner, C.A. (1965) Trichotillomania. *Archives of General Psychiatry*, **12**, 482.

Hallopeau, H. (1889) Alopécie par grattage (Trichomanie ou Trichotillomanie). *Annales de Dermatologie et de Syphiligraphie*, **10**, 440.

Hall-Smith, S.P. (1966) Familial trichotillomania. *Transactions of the St John's Hospital Dermatological Society*, **52**, 135.

Jillson, O.F. (1983) Alopecia. II. Trichotillomania (Trichotillohabitus). *Cutis*, **31**, 383.

Lachapelle, J.-M. & Pierard, G.E. (1977) Traumatic alopecia in trichotillomania: a pathologic interpretation of histologic lesions in the pilosebaceous unit. *Journal of Cutaneous Pathology*, **4**, 57.

Mehregan, A.H. (1970) Trichotillomania: a clinicopathologic study. *Archives of Dermatology*, **102**, 129.

Monroe, J.T., Jr. & Abse, D.W. (1963) The psychopathology of trichotillomania and trichophagy. *Psychiatry*, **26**, 95.

Muller, S.A. (1980) Trichotillomania. In *Hair, Trace Elements and Human Illness*, p. 306, eds. A.C. Brown & R.G. Crounse. Praeger, New York.

Muller, S.A. & Winkelmann, R.K. (1972) Trichotillomania. *Archives of Dermatology*, **105**, 535.

Oranje, A.P., Peereboom-Wynia, J.D.R. & De Raeymaecker, D.M.J. (1986) Trichotillomania in childhood. *Journal of the American Academy of Dermatology*, **15**, 614.

Reuter, K. (1951) Ein besonderer Fall von Trichotillomanie. *Zeitschrift für Haut und Geschlechtskrankheiten*, **10**, 287.

Rohrbach, D. (1963) Zwei Fälle von Trichotillomanie im Bereich der Cilien. *Hautarzt*, **114**, 122.

Sanderson, K.V. & Hall-Smith, P. (1970) Tonsure trichotillomania. *British Journal of Dermatology*, **82**, 343.

Schachter, M. (1961) Zum Problem der kindlichen Trichotillomanie. *Praxis der Kinderpsychologie*, **10**, 120.

Sonck, C.E. (1958) Ein seltene Abart von Trichotillomanie. *Hautarzt*, **9**, 183.

Steck, W.D. (1979) The clinical evaluation of pathologic hair loss with a diagnostic sign of trichotillomania. *Cutis*, **24**, 293.

Cosmetic traumatic alopecia
(References p. 294)

History and nomenclature

The dictates of religion, of custom and of fashion have imposed an immense variety of physical stresses on human hair. The nomenclature of the resulting patterns of baldness inevitably lacks any consistency. It is possible only to list the clinical syndromes most widely reported; any new hairdressing technique may give rise to new patterns. The 'chignon alopecia' of our grandmothers' days may yet return.

Pathology

Two processes are responsible for most of the pathological changes observed. Hair, sometimes already weakened by chemical applications, may be broken by friction or by tension. Prolonged tension may induce follicular inflammatory changes which may eventually lead to scarring. Traction alopecia is induced particularly readily in subjects with incipient common baldness, for the telogen hairs, which make up a higher proportion of the total, are more readily extracted than anagen hairs (Ikeda & Yamada 1967).

Clinical features

Traumatic marginal alopecia. The essential changes in the many variants of this syndrome are the presence of short broken hairs, folliculitis and some scarring in circumscribed patches at the scalp margins.

In one form which is caused by the tension imposed by procedures intended to straighten kinky hair (Costa 1946) alopecia commonly begins in triangular areas in front of and above the ears, but may involve other parts of the scalp margin, or even linear areas in other parts of the scalp (Fig. 9.8). Sabouraud (1931) had described as alopecia linearis frontalis (Fig. 9.9) a similar process in young French girls, beginning with inflammatory papules and broken hairs in front of the ears, and extending anteriorly as a band 1–3 cm wide. Itching and crusting were sometimes severe. The so-called 'pony-tail' hair style, traditional in the women of Greenland but enjoying intermittent popularity elsewhere, may cause similar changes in the frontal hair margin (Hjorth 1957; Slepyan 1958). Keratin cylinders—'hair casts'—may surround many hairs just above the scalp surface (Rollins 1961).

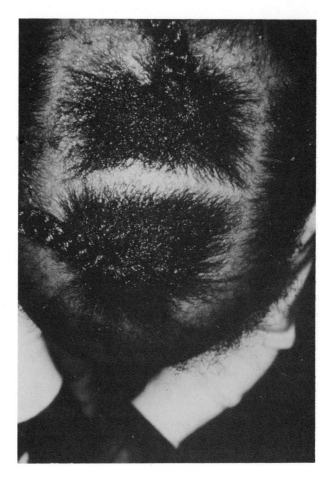

Fig. 9.8 Traction alopecia.

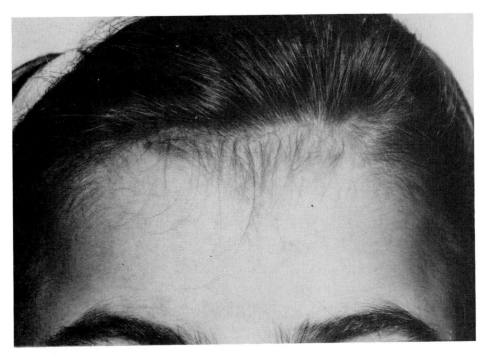

Fig. 9.9 Traumatic alopecia; mild alopecia linearis frontalis.

Frontal and parietal traction alopecia may occur in young Sikh boys as a result of twisting their uncut hair tightly on top of the head (Singh 1975), and tight braiding and wooden combs produce traction alopecia in the Sudan (Morgan 1960); frontal loss is reported in Libyan women as a result of traction from a tight scarf (Malhotra & Kanwar 1980). Parietal patches have been produced by the traction exerted by clips holding a nurse's cap in place (Renna & Freedberg 1973).

Afro-Caribbean hair styles with tight braiding of the hair into rows known variously as corn or cane rows or braids and Cain rows may cause marginal alopecia and central alopecia with widening of the partings (Fig. 9.8).

Brush roller alopecia. The popular brush rollers, if applied frequently and with too much vigour, may cause irregular patches of more or less complete alopecia, surrounded by a zone of erythema with broken hairs (Lipnik 1961).

Hot-comb alopecia. Negro women who use hot combs to straighten the hair (Fig. 9.10) may develop a progressive cicatricial alopecia, slowly, extending centrifugally from the vertex (Lo Presti *et al.* 1968).

Massage alopecia. The over-enthusiastic application of medication to the scalp, with firm massage, may cause baldness (Bowers 1950); one of these six patients had trichorrhexis nodosa.

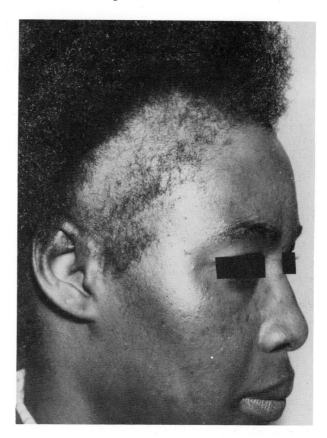

Fig. 9.10 Traumatic alopecia
from the use of hair
straighteners.

Brush alopecia. Vigorous brushing may cause significant damage to hair that is
already fragile as the result of a developmental defect. The 'bristles' with square or
otherwise angular tips, present in some brushes made of synthetic fibres, may prove
particularly traumatic (Saville 1958).

Alopecia secondary to hair weaving. Patchy traction alopecia has been reported to
result from the cosmetic procedure of weaving additional hair into persistent
terminal hair in order to camouflage common baldness (Perlstein 1969).

Deliberate alopecia. We have seen a family from Pakistan in which three sisters
during childhood were subjected to tight plaiting and traction of the central V of the
frontal hair. The resulting V of alopecia was considered desirable (Fig. 9.11).

Diagnosis
The traumatic cosmetic alopecias do not present any diagnostic difficulties,
provided the possibility is considered. Their cause is rarely recognized by the patient
and is often accepted with suspicion.

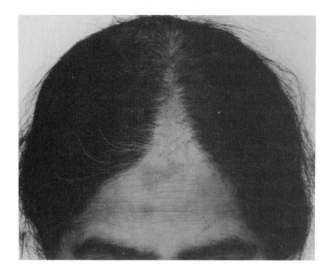

Fig. 9.11 Deliberate traction alopecia induced by plaiting.

References

Bowers, R.E. (1950) Massage alopecia. *British Journal of Dermatology*, **62**, 262.

Costa, O.C. (1946) Traumatic Negroid alopecia. *British Journal of Dermatology*, **58**, 280.

Hjorth, N. (1957) Traumatic marginal alopecia. A special-type—alopecia Greenlandica. *British Journal of Dermatology*, **69**, 317.

Ikeda, T. & Yamada, M. (1967) Both telogen effluvium and traction alopecia mainly occur in patients with a condition of alopecia prematura. *Acta Dermatologica (Kyoto)*, **62**, 47.

Lipnik, M.J. (1961) Traction alopecia from brush rollers. *Archives of Dermatology*, **84**, 493.

Lo Presti, P., Papa, C.M. & Kligman, A.M. (1968) Hot comb alopecia. *Archives of Dermatology*, **98**, 234.

Malhotra, Y.K. & Kanwar, A.J. (1980) Traumatic alopecia among Libyan women. *Archives of Dermatology*, **116**, 987.

Morgan, H.V. (1960) Traction alopecia. *British Medical Journal*, **ii**, 115.

Perlstein, H.H. (1969) Traction alopecia due to hair weaving. *Cutis*, **5**, 440.

Renna, F.G. & Freedberg, I.M. (1973) Traction alopecia in nurses. *Archives of Dermatology*, **108**, 684.

Rollins, T.G. (1961) Traction folliculitis with hair casts and alopecia. *American Journal of Diseases of Children*, **101**, 609.

Sabouraud, R. (1931) De l'alopécie liminaire frontale. *Annales de Dermatologie et de Syphiligraphie*, **2**, 446.

Saville, A. (1958) The nylon brush. *British Journal of Dermatology*, **70**, 296.

Singh, G. (1975) Traction alopecia in Sikh boys. *British Journal of Dermatology*, **92**, 232.

Slepyan, A.H. (1958) Traction alopecia. *Archives of Dermatology*, **78**, 395.

Accidental traumatic alopecia

(References p. 295)

Alopecia secondary to accidental mechanical trauma to the scalp is usually no diagnostic problem (Friederich 1950) but in some circumstances the trauma may be unperceived and the cause of the hair loss undetected.

Women who had undergone prolonged pelvic operations in the Trendelenburg position, developed 12 to 26 days later a vertical patch of alopecia, which was preceded by oedema, exudation and crusting. Pressure ichaemia during the operation was considered to be the cause of the alopecia (Abel & Lewis 1960; Abel 1964).

In one large clinic 60 cases of occipital pressure alopecia were observed after open-heart surgery over a period of 3 years (Lawson *et al.* 1976). In 29 of these cases the hair loss was permanent. To prevent the development of alopecia under these conditions prolonged pressure ischaemia must be avoided.

Temporary alopecia followed prolonged pressure on the scalp of a foam rubber ring, used to prevent such an occurrence (Patel & Henschel 1980).

Permanent alopecia followed constant pressure during more than 6 hours of an operation by the head strap securing a face mask (Gormley & Sokoll 1967).

References

Abel, R.R. & Lewis, G.M. (1960) Postoperative (pressure) alopecia. *Archives of Dermatology*, **81**, 34.
Abel, R.R. (1964) Postoperative (pressure) alopecia. *Anesthesiology*, **25**, 870.
Friederich, H.-C. (1950) Ein Beitrag zu dem mechanischen Schädigungen des Haares und des Haarbodens. *Dermatologische Wochenschrift*, **121**, 344.
Gormley, T. & Sokoll, M.D. (1967) Permanent alopecia from pressure of headstrap. *Journal of the American Medical Association*, **199**, 157.
Lawson, N.W., Mills, N.L. & Ochsner, N.L. (1976) Occipital alopecia following cardiopulmonary bypass. *Journal of Thoracic and Cardiovascular Surgery*, **71**, 342.
Patel, K.D. & Henschel, E.O. (1980) Postoperative alopecia. *Anaesthesia and Analgesia*, **59**, 311.

Chapter 10
Alopecia Areata

History and nomenclature
(References p. 297)

Cornelius Celsus, (*c.* 30 AD) has been credited with the first description of alopecia areata (AA), which even now is sometimes referred to as 'area celsi'. The term 'alopecia areata' was first used by Sauvages (1706–67) in his *Nosologia medica* published in Lyons in 1760. Robert Willan gave a fuller description of the condition but named it 'porrigo decalvans', and Thomas Bateman used the same term in his atlas. Alibert, however, considered 'porrigo tonsurans' to be the same as 'porrigo decalvans'. It was therefore inevitable that when Gruby in 1843 found a fungus in 'porrigo decalvans' the parasitic theory of AA was firmly launched on its misleading course. In 1851 Hebra clearly separated AA from herpes tonsurans, but at first still accepted that AA was of fungal origin. He later revised his opinion (Hebra & Kaposi 1874).

The period from 1850 to 1900 saw the rapid development of microbiology, at a time when the need for controls in clinical and laboratory investigations had yet to be appreciated. Even after sound diagnostic criteria were established a battle raged between the 'parasitic' school, which included both Hutchinson and Radcliffe Crocker (1903) in Britain and Bazin in France, and their opponents, most of whom favoured the fashionable 'trophoneurotic' hypothesis put forward originally by von Barensprung of Berlin in 1858. The dictatorial Erasmus Wilson held this view, but before he is given credit for denying the parasitic origin of AA it must be recalled that he also denied that ringworm was an infection. The earlier protagonists of the origin of AA believed that a fungus was the organism concerned. Later bacteria were suspected. A paper by the dermatologist George Thin, presented by Thomas Huxley, described to the Royal Society his *Bacterium decalvans* (Thin 1882). Many other bacteria were incriminated for a time; Sabouraud in 1896 blamed the microbacillus which he held responsible also for seborrhoea but later admitted his error. These claims may seem fanciful, but as late as 1913 Jackson and McMurtry of New York felt that the parasitic theory 'cannot be wholly rejected'. However, outbreaks of AA in closed communities are still unexplained.

The trophoneurotic theory, with some modifications in emphasis, is still held by some authorities. The theory is highly adaptable and, if it cannot be proved, is difficult to disprove. The alleged production of AA in cats by nerve section (Joseph 1886) and the many clinical observations relating the onset of alopecia to emotional stress or to head injury could be taken to support this rather vaguely formulated hypothesis. Vitiligo, scleroderma and thyroid disease, which were known to be significantly associated with AA, were considered to be 'trophic' or 'nervous disorders'. The trophoneurotic hypothesis could be modified and elaborated to admit the concept of 'irritation'. Some dozens of papers claimed significant associations between AA and dental defects or errors of refraction. The most extravagant claims were those of the 'dystrophic theory' of Jacquet (1902) of Paris who found a dental 'cause' in almost every case; he appears not to have been disconcerted when his countryman Bailly of Lyons (Bailly 1910) showed dental defects were equally common in those without AA.

With the development of endocrinology late in the 19th century another tangled strand had to be woven into the working hypothesis. AA was known to be associated with disorders of endocrine glands, notably the thyroid. These disorders, themselves 'trophic', were treated and the fortuitous regrowth of the bald patches was accepted as proof that the disorder had 'caused' the alopecia. By the 1920s most dermatologists had abandoned the parasitic theory of AA and had put forward hypotheses which blended the trophoneurotic and the endocrine theories appropriate to each national temperament. Then came the ogre of 'focal sepsis', which found favour in many countries since it offered and justified a vigorous therapeutic approach. Even the most conservative of clinicians claimed that focal sepsis, usually of teeth or upper respiratory tract, but occasionally gastrointestinal, was the cause of almost all cases of alopecia areata.

The past 25 yars has produced a growing volume of reliable clinical, microscopical and immunological observations (Perret *et al.* 1990). New hypotheses have been advanced but conflict and controversy remain. This chapter endeavours, by examining the evidence, to separate fact from speculation.

References

Bailly (1910) *L'Origine Gingivodentaire de la Pelade*. Lyons, publisher unknown.
Hebra, F. & Kaposi, M. (1874) *On Diseases of the Skin*, vol. 3, p. 209 trans. and ed. W. Tay. New Sydenham Society, London.
Jackson, G.T. & McMurtry, C.W. (1913) *A Treatise on Diseases of the Hair*, p. 107. Kimpton, London.
Jacquet, L. (1902) Nature et traitement de la pelade—la pelade d'origine dentaire. *Annales de Dermatologie et de Syphiligraphie*, **3**, 97, 180.

Joseph, M. (1886) Experimentelle Untersuchungen über die Ätiologie der Alopecia areata. *Monatshefte für praktischer Dermatologie*, **5**, 483.

Perret, C.M., Steijten, P.M. & Happle, R. (1990) Alopecia areata: pathogenesis and treatment. *International Journal of Dermatology*, **29**(2), 83.

Radcliffe Crocker, H. (1903) *Diseases of the Skin*, 3rd edn., p. 1138. Lewis, London.

Thin, G. (1882) On bacterium decalvans, an organism associated with the destruction of the hair in alopecia areata. *Proceedings of the Royal Society*, **33**, 247.

Aetiology
(References p. 304)

It is not at present possible to attribute all or indeed any case of AA to a single cause. Among the many factors which appear to be implicated in at least a proportion of cases are the patient's genetic constitution, the atopic state, non-specific immune and organ-specific autoimmune reactions, and emotional stress. The process can be reversed to a variable extent by several very different therapeutic measures; corticosteroids, local irritants, photochemotherapy, induction of contact dermatitis or by the drugs minoxidil and cyclosporin A. The different chemistries and modes of action of these therapies have opened new channels of research. However, the subsequent studies have done little more than reinforce the generally held belief that both genetic predisposition and the atopic state influence prognosis but the triggering mechanisms remain obscure.

Genetic factors

The incidence of a family history of AA has been reported as 27% in Cleveland, USA (Sander *et al.* 1980), 24% in England (Friedmann 1981b), 22% in France (Sabouraud 1929), 18% in the Netherlands (De-Waard-Van der Spek *et al.* 1989), 6.3% in Poland (Bastos Araujo & Poiares Baptista 1967) and 4% in Italy (Olivetti & Bubola 1965). However, Saenz (1963) could find no evidence of hereditary factors in Spaniards. These figures are so varied that they suggest a difference in the diligence with which the family history was sought and reported. The mode of inheritance is thought to be autosomal dominant with variable penetrance (Sander *et al.* 1980). Racial factors may also be important as Arnold (1952) found AA disproportionately common among Japanese in Hawaii.

There have been several studies of AA in twins, with some pairs showing concurrent onset (Omens & Omens 1946; Hendren 1949; Weidmann *et al.* 1956). HLA studies have shown conflicting results. Kianto *et al.* (1977) found an increased prevalence of HLA-B12 in a series of Finnish patients with AA but this was not confirmed by Kuntz *et al.* (1977) or Orecchia *et al.* (1987). Hacham-Zadeh *et al.* (1981) found an increased prevalence of HLA-B18 in 46 patients independent of clinical features. However, Orecchia *et al.* (1987) showed increased prevalence of HLA-DR5 which was linked to disease severity in 127 patients but these workers failed to demonstrate any difference in class I HLA markers when compared with a control population.

The atopic state

The association between AA and the atopic state was noted by Robinson and Tasker (1948) but was thought to be linked to common emotional factors. In a Danish study the incidence of atopic dermatitis in association with AA was only 1% (Gip *et al.*1969). In a large North American series eczema or asthma or both were present in 18% of children and in 9% of adults with AA; 23% of children with alopecia totalis were found to be atopic (Muller & Winkelmann 1963). In Japan, Ikeda (1965) found a 10% incidence of atopy in all AA patients. More recent assessments using controlled studies and prick test positivity to common allergens to identify atopy has shown a higher association of up to 52.4% (Penders 1968; Young *et al.* 1978). There is clearly an association between the two conditions which is worthy of more detailed epidemiological study.

Down's syndrome (Scherbenske *et al.* 1990)

Wunderlich and Braun-Falco (1965) found 13 cases of AA among 100 Down's syndrome patients and Du Vivier and Munro (1975) found 60 cases among 1000 patients with Down's syndrome but only 1 in 1000 mentally-retarded controls. In 25 of the 60 cases the alopecia was total or universal.

Down's syndrome is a chromosomal defect. Thyroid antibodies occur more frequently than in normal subjects and this increased incidence has been reported in two other chromosomal defects, Klinefelter's syndrome and Turner's syndrome. The incidence of anti-thyroid antibodies in Down's syndrome patients with AA is significantly higher than in Down's syndrome without AA and in normal subjects. Brown *et al.* (1977) found depressed total lymphocyte levels in 18 of 19 patients with Down's syndrome and AA. Fialkow (1966) found that Down's sufferers and their mothers are abnormally susceptible to thyroid disease, but the incidence of AA in the parents of Down's syndrome patients has not been studied. These interesting findings cannot yet be reliably interpreted due to the small numbers involved but the area is worthy of further study.

Autoimmunity

The suggestion that AA is an autoimmune disease was first proposed in 1958 by Rothman in discussion of a paper by Van Scott (1958). There is widespread agreement with this hypothesis despite the fact that the evidence is at best circumstantial. Support has come from three main areas of research; association with autoimmune diseases, humoral immunity and cell-mediated immunity.

Association with autoimmune diseases
Thyroid disease is the most frequently described disease in association with AA but the published figures are contradictory. Muller and Winkelmann (1963) in the largest study reported to date found evidence of thyroid disease in 8% of 736

cases compared with less than 2% in the control population in North America. In England Cunliffe *et al.* (1969) found thyroid disease in 19 of 58 females with alopecia areata and 2 of 18 males, and this was a significantly higher incidence than in their control subjects who had psoriasis. Milgraum *et al.* (1987) found 24% of 45 children under 16 years with AA to have abnormal thyroid function tests and/or elevation of thyroid microsomal antibody levels. However, Salamon *et al.* (1971) in Yugoslavia and Main *et al.* (1975) in Scotland found no evidence of thyroid dysfunction in patients with AA. Reliable statistics based on the prospective study of large numbers of patients are lacking, but there are reports of cases (e.g. Klein *et al.* 1974) in which Hashimoto's thyroiditis and AA have co-existed and Kern (1974) has found a statistically significant association between AA and Hashimoto's disease, pernicious anaemia and Addison's disease. Brown (1980) and Brown *et al.* (1982) have suggested an increased incidence of autoimmune gonadal disease in male AA patients, but these findings remain unconfirmed. The association of vitiligo with AA is accepted by most authors (Fig. 10.1). Anderson (1950) and Muller and Winkelmann (1963) reported an

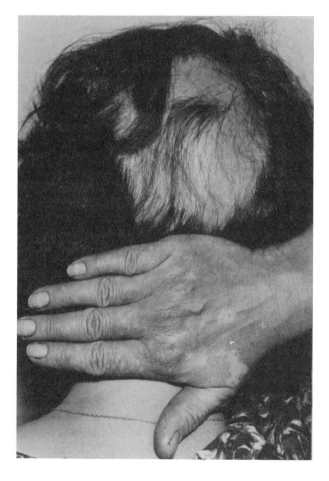

Fig. 10.1 Alopecia areata and vitiligo in the same patient.

incidence of 4%. Main *et al.* (1975) found vitiligo in 9%. Perinaevoid alopecia similar to perinaevoid vitiligo (Sutton's halo naevus) has been reported (Pecoraro 1963).

The following disorders, all of a possible immunological nature, have also been reported in association with AA; pernicious anaemia (Cunliffe *et al.* 1968), systemic lupus erythematosus and rheumatoid arthritis (Muller & Winkelmann 1963), polymyalgia rheumatica (Faergemann 1979), myasthenia gravis (Tan 1974), ulcerative colitis (Allen & Moschella 1974), lichen planus (Tan 1974) and the candida–endocrinopathy syndrome (Stankler & Bewscher 1972).

Humoral immunity

Studies of organ-specific antibodies in AA have given conflicting results, perhaps due to small groups of patients and controls and differing methodology (Friedmann 1985). Cunliffe *et al.* (1969), Klaber and Munro (1978), Betterle *et al.* (1975) and Cochran *et al.* (1976) found no associations. However, Main *et al.* (1975) showed increased anti-smooth muscle antibodies. Du Vivier and Munro (1975) found that Down's syndrome sufferers with AA had an increased frequency of anti-thyroid antibodies. Galbraith *et al.* (1984) also found an increase in thyroid autoantibodies. Kern *et al.* (1973) and Friedmann (1981b and 1985) in a controlled study of 229 cases reported increased frequencies of thyroid antibodies in 30% of females and 10% of males and an increased frequency of gastric parietal cell antibodies which tended to be more common in males. In 45 children with AA under 16 years of age Milgraum *et al.* (1987) found detectable antibody levels to thyroid microsomal function (11%), smooth muscle (16%) and parietal cells (4%).

Cell-mediated immunity

Studies of cell-mediated immunity in AA also yield an inconsistent picture; again small studies have led to conflicting results. Circulating total T-cell numbers have been reported to be reduced (Brown *et al.* 1977; Giannetti *et al.* 1978; D'Ovidio *et al.* 1981; Friedmann 1981a) or normal (Herzer *et al.* 1979; Thestrup-Pederson *et al.* 1982; Hordinsky *et al.* 1984). Suppressor T-cell numbers have been variously reported as reduced (D'Ovidio *et al.* 1981; Ledesma & York 1982), normal (Gu *et al.* 1983) or increased (Gu *et al.* 1981a; Filipovitch *et al.* 1982; Hordinsky *et al.* 1984). Gu *et al.* (1981a,b) also reported an increase in non-antigen-specific spontaneous and antibody-dependent cell-mediated cytotoxic responses of peripheral blood lymphocytes. Friedmann (1985) attempted to resolve this conflict by suggesting that while there is general agreement that a reduction in numbers of circulating T-cells occurs in AA, the level of reduction is related to disease severity. Similarly, the impairment of helper T-cell function and the change in suppressor T-cell numbers may also reflect changes in disease activity. Fiedler-Weiss (1987) and Fiedler-Weiss and Buys (1987) have reported that patients with AA responding to topical minoxidil treatment showed an increase in peripheral blood lymphocyte levels and that mitogen-induced blastogenesis in lymphocytes was reduced after therapy. Galbraith *et al.* (1987) showed an increase in T-cell rosetting in patients responding to treatment with the immunomodulator inosiplex when compared with controls. Prospective longitudinal studies are therefore necessary to establish the natural history of the disease to resolve these problems.

Immunohistology
The strongest direct evidence for autoimmunity comes from the consistent finding of a lymphocytic infiltrate in and around hair follicles. Monoclonal antibody studies have shown the infiltrate to be predominantly of T-cells. Todes-Taylor *et al.* (1984) showed a predominance of helper T-cells but Perret *et al.* (1984) and Ranki *et al.* (1984) found an increase in T-suppressor cells in the peribulbar infiltrate. Langerhan's cells have also been seen in the peribulbar region (Wiesner-Menzel & Happle 1984). Biopsies from scalps of patients treated with the contact allergen diphencyprone (Happle *et al.* 1986), oral and topical cyclosporin (Gupta *et al.* 1990; de Prost *et al.* 1986) and oral and topical minoxidil (Fiedler-Weiss & Buys 1987; Fiedler & Buys 1987) have shown a reduction in the peribulbar T-cell population in regrowing AA but no change in the absence of regrowth. No such changes were found in biopsies of patients responding to treatment with squaric acid dibutylester (Johansson *et al.* 1986). Direct immunofluorescent examination has failed to demonstrate anti-follicle antibodies in affected scalps (Klaber & Munro 1978; Herzer *et al.* 1979; Muller *et al.* 1980; Igarashi *et al.* 1980). Deposition of complement at the hair follicle basement membrane has been reported by Bystryn *et al.* (1979), but was also seen in normal scalp and male pattern alopecia. Nunzi *et al.* (1980) demonstrated an elutable antibody in lymphocytes from eight patients with AA. This antibody reacted with the endothelia of perifollicular capillaries but this work has yet to be confirmed. Friedmann (1981a) was unable to demonstrate a response of lymphocytes from patients with AA to crude scalp extract *in vitro*. Messenger *et al.* (1984) and Messenger and Bleehen (1985) reported ectopic expression of MHC type II antigen HLA-DR by epithelial cells in the presumptive cortex and root sheaths of hair follicles in active lesions of AA. A similar situation has been demonstrated in the thyroid gland (Hanafusa 1983) and is thought to represent a mechanism through which cells may present their own specific surface antigens to sensitized MHC-restricted T-inducer cells. However, Bröcker *et al.* (1987) and Khoury *et al.* (1988) have shown that the expression of HLA-DR on hair follicle keratinocytes is secondary to the lymphoid infiltration rather than a primary initiating event. Studies with γ-interferon, which is known to induce MHC type II antigen expression, are awaited.

AA appears to belong to the group of organ-specific autoimmune diseases. There is a shared hereditary susceptibility, organ-specific antibodies occur with increased frequency in patients with AA and there is altered T-cell regulation of the immune response. However, unlike most organ-specific autoimmune diseases direct activity against hair follicle components has yet to be demonstrated. The other organ-specific autoimmune diseases involve destructive processes which lead to cessation of function. Since hair follicle activity is only switched off, rather than destroyed, any autoimmune mechanism would have to be directed against a controlling growth factor or its receptor as occurs in Graves' disease. Further research in this area is obviously required. Prospective long-term studies and the relationship between lymphocyte and disease activity (Friedmann 1985) are worthy of further attention.

Emotional stress

A wealth of case-lore suggests that stress may be an important precipitating factor in some cases of AA. Attempts at objective evaluation using standard psychiatric procedures such as the Rorschach test showed over 90% of patients with AA to be psychologically abnormal (Panconesi & Mantellassi 1955, 1956) and up to 29% to have psychological factors and family situations that may have affected the onset or course of the disease (De-Waard-Van der Spek *et al.* 1989). Macalpine (1958), a psychiatrist, studied 125 patients with AA and came to the conclusion that emotional factors did not play a significant role in this disorder. There are many reports of individual cases in which emotional stress appeared to precipitate the initial attack of AA, or subsequent recurrences (Peck 1948; Kaplan & Reisch 1952; Ledo-Dunipe 1952; Reinhold 1960; Swift 1961; Degossely 1965; Feldman & Rondón Lugo 1973). Experienced clinicians (e.g. Obermayer & Bowen 1956) wrote 'the perpetuating role of emotional tension states ... is well authenticated'. Alleged cures by suggestion (Bonjour 1932) or sleep therapy (Martin *et al.*1959) have been claimed to support the stress hypothesis. A very prolonged and intensive investigation of twins with AA was, however, inconclusive (Hommes & Prick 1968).

Stress is an important precipitating factor in some cases of AA. In many cases it appears to play no part, except when it arises secondarily as a result of the cosmetic disfigurement (Lubowe 1959), when it may be important in perpetuating the condition. The findings of Ferraro (1979) using the Bernereuter personality index showed 'feelings of inferiority, introspection and a need for encouragement'.

The role of organic nervous disease in AA is unknown. Parisis *et al.* (1968) have shown apparent association between EEG abnormalities and AA particularly in acute forms in post-menopausal women. A study showing EEG abnormalities in the region of the brain stem in 70% of 50 patients awaits confirmation (Haas & Lehnert 1971).

The 'reflex-irritation' extension of the trophoneurotic theory is revived from time to time either in association with errors of refraction (Haynes & Parry 1949) with intra-ocular foreign bodies (McGrath 1951) or with dental lesions (Grace 1942). No evidence suggesting that such occurrences are more than fortuitous has been reported. The significance of the observation that 67% of 428 bald patches in 134 patients were within the distribution of C2 is uncertain (Hönemann & Höfer 1970). The radiological examination of the cervical region of the spine showed no relevant abnormalities (Höfer *et al.* 1969).

References

Allen, H.B. & Moschella, S.L. (1974) Ulcerative colitis associated with skin and hair changes *Cutis,*14,85.

Anderson, I. (1950) Alopecia areata: a clinical study. *British Medical Journal,* **ii**, 1250.

Arnold, H.L. (1952) Alopecia areata: prevalence in Japanese and prognosis after reassurance. *AMA Archives of Dermatology and Syphilology,* **66**, 191.

Bastos Araujo, A. & Poiares Baptista, A. (1967) Algunas consideracions sobre 300 casos de pelada. *Traballos da Sociedad Portuguesa de Dermatologia e Venereologia,* **25**, 135.

Bereston, E.S. & Robinson, H.M. (1951) Alopecia areata in two brothers and two sisters. *AMA Archives of Dermatology and Syphilology,* **64**, 204.

Betterle, C., Peserico, A., Dal Prete, G. & Trisotto, A. (1975) Autoantibodies in alopecia areata. *Archives of Dermatology,* **111**, 927.

Bonjour, J. (1932) Observations on alopecia areata. *Urological and Cutaneous Review,* **36**, 674.

Brenner, W., Diem, E. & Gschnait, F. (1979) Coincidence of vitiligo, alopecia areata, onychodystrophy, localised scleroderma and lichen planus. *Dermatologica,* **159**, 356.

Bröcker, E.B., Echternacht-Happle, K., Hamm, H. & Happle, R. (1987) Abnormal expression of Class I and Class II major histocompatibility antigens in alopecia areata: modulation by topical immunotherapy. *Journal of Investigative Dermatology,* **88**, 564.

Brown, A.C. (1980) Autoimmune gonadal disease. In *Trace Elements, Hair and Human Illness,* p. 313, eds. A.C. Brown & R.G. Crounse. Praeger, New York.

Brown, A.C., Olkowski, Z.L., McLaren, J.R. & Kutner, M.H. (1971) Alopecia areata and vitiligo associated with Down's syndrome. *Archives of Dermatology,* **113**, 1296.

Brown, A.C., Olkowski, Z.L. & McLaren, J.R. (1977) Thymus lymphocytes of the peripheral blood in patients with alopecia areata. *Archives of Dermatology,* **113**, 688.

Brown, A.C., Follard, Z.F. & Jarrett, W.H. (1982) Ocular and testicular abnormalities in alopecia areata. *Archives of Dermatology,* **118**, 546.

Bystryn, J.C., Orentreich, N. & Shezel, F. (1979) Direct immunofluorescence studies in alopecia areata and male pattern alopecia. *Journal of Investigative Dermatology,* **73**, 317.

Cochran, R.E.I., Thomson, J. & MacSween, R.N.M. (1976) An autoantibody profile in alopecia totalis and diffuse alopecia. *British Journal of Dermatology,* **95**, 61.

Cunliffe, W.J., Hall, R., Newell, D.J. & Stevenson, C.J. (1968) Vitiligo, thyroid disease and autoimmunity. *British Journal of Dermatology,* **80**, 135.

Cunliffe, W.J., Hall, R., Stevenson, C.F. & Weightman, D. (1969) Alopecia areata, thyroid disease and autoimmunity. *British Journal of Dermatology,* **81**, 879.

Degossely, M. (1965) L'Interêt de l'étude psychomatique dans quelques cas de pelade totale. *Archives Belges de Dermatologie et Syphiligraphie,* **21**, 257.

De Prost, Y., Teillac, D., Paquez, F., Carrugi, L., Bachelez, H. & Touraine, R. (1986) Placebo-controlled trial of topical cyclosporin in severe alopecia areata. *Lancet,* **ii**, 803.

De-Waard-Van der Spek, F.B., Oranje, A.P., De Raeymaecker, D.M. & Peereboom-Wynia, J.D.R. (1989) Juvenile versus maturity-onset alopecia areata—a comparative retrospective clinical study. *Clinical and Experimental Dermatology,* **14**, 429.

D'Ovidio, R., Vena, G.A., & Angelini, G. (1981) Cell-mediated immunity in alopecia areata. *Archives of Dermatological Research,* **271**, 265.

Du Vivier, A. & Munro, D.D. (1975) Alopecia areata, autoimmunity and Down's syndrome. *British Medical Journal,* **i**, 191.

Faergemann, J. (1979) Lichen sclerosus et atropicus generalisata, alopecia and polymyalgia rheumatica found in the same patient. *Cutis,* **23**, 757.

Feldman, M. & Rondón Lugo, A.J. (1973) Consideracions psicosomatics en la alopecia areata. *Medicina Cutanea,* **7**, 95.

Ferraro, S. (1979) Il Bernereuter Personality Inventory in ammelati di area Celsi. *Clinica Dermatologica,* **10**, 51.

Fialkow, P.J. (1966) Autoimmunity and chromosomal aberrations. *American Journal of Human Genetics,* **18**, 93.

Fiedler, V.C. & Buys, C.M. (1987) Immunohistochemical characterisation of the cellular infiltrate in severe alopecia areata before and after minoxidil treatment. *Dermatologica*, **17** (Suppl. 2), 29.

Fiedler-Weiss, V.C. (1987) Potential mechanisms of minoxidil-induced hair growth in alopecia areata. *Journal of the American Academy of Dermatology*, **16**, 653.

Fiedler-Weiss, V.C. & Buys, C.M. (1987) Response to minoxidil in severe alopecia areata correlates with T lymphocyte stimulation. *British Journal of Dermatology*, **117**, 759.

Filipovich, A.H., Hordinsky-Kramarczuk, M., Nelson, D. & Hollgren H. (1982) The correlation between inducer/suppressor ratios, generation of concanavalin A-activated suppressor cells and mitogen-stimulated proliferation of peripheral blood lymphocytes in patients with alopecia areata and normal controls. *Clinical Immunology and Immunopathology*, **25**, 21.

Fischer, H.R. (1953) Alopecia areata bei eneigen Zwillingen. *Zeitschrift für Haut und Geschlechtskrankheiten*, **15**, 178.

Friedmann, P.S. (1981a) Decreased lymphocyte reactivity and autoimmunity in alopecia areata. *British Journal of Dermatology*, **105**, 145.

Friedmann, P.S. (1981b) Alopecia areata and autoimmunity. *British Journal of Dermatology*, **105**, 153.

Friedmann, P.S. (1985) Clinical and immunologic associations of alopecia areata. *Seminars in Dermatology*, **4**, 9.

Galbraith, G.M.P., Thiers, B.H., Vasaly, D.V. & Fudenberg, H.H. (1984) Immunological profiles in alopecia areata. *British Journal of Dermatology*, **110**, 163.

Galbraith, G.M.P., Thiers, B.H., Jensen, J. & Hoehler, F. (1987) A randomised double-blind study of inosiplex (isoprinosine) therapy in patients with alopecia totalis. *Journal of the American Academy of Dermatology*, **16**, 977.

Giannetti, A., Disilverio, A., Castallazzi, A.N. & Maccario, R. (1978) Evidence for defective T-cell function in patients with alopecia areata. *British Journal of Dermatology*, **98**, 361.

Gip, L., Lodin, A. & Molin, L. (1969) Alopecia areata. *Acta Dermato-Venereologica*, **49**, 180.

Grace, J.D. (1942) Extensive alopecia areata of dental origin. *Archives of Dermatology and Syphilology*, **45**, 349.

Gu, S.-Q., Ros, A.-M., Thyresson, N. & Wasserman, J. (1981a) Blood lymphocyte subpopulations and antibody-dependent cell-mediated cytotoxicity (ADCC) in alopecia areata and universalis. *Acta Dermato-Venereologica*, **61**, 125.

Gu, S.-Q., Ros, A.-M., Thyresson, N. & Wasserman, J. (1981b) Spontaneous cell-mediated cytotoxicity (SCMC) in patients with alopecia universalis. *Acta Dermato-Venereologica*, **61**, 434.

Gu, S.-Q., Petrini, B., Ros, A.-M., Thyresson, M. & Wasserman, J. (1983) T-lymphocyte subpopulations in alopecia areata and psoriasis: identification with monoclonal antibodies and Fc receptors. *Acta Dermato-Venereologica*, **63**, 244.

Gupta, A.K., Ellis, C.N., Cooper, K.D., Nickoloff, B.J., Ho, V.C., Chan, L.S., Hamilton, T.A., Tellner, D.C., Griffiths, E.M. & Voorhees, J.J. (1990) Oral cyclosporine for the treatment of alopecia areata. A clinical and immunohistochemical analysis. *Journal of the American Academy of Dermatology*, **22**, 242.

Haas, W. & Lehnert, W. (1971) Elektroenzephalographisch nachgewissene Funktionstörungen des oralen Hirnstammes bei der Alopecia areata. *Dermatologische Wochenschrift*, **157**, 855.

Hacham-Zadeh, S., Brautbar, C., Cohen, C.A. & Cohen, T. (1981) HLA and alopecia areata in Jerusalem. *Tissue Antigens*, **18**, 71.

Hanafusa, T., Pujol-Borrell, R., Chiovato, L., Russell, R.C.G., Doniach, D. & Bottazzo, G.F. (1983) Aberrant expression of HLA-DR antigen on thymocytes in Graves' disease: relevance for auto-immunity. *Lancet*, **ii**, 1111.

Happle, R., Klein, H.M. & Macher, E. (1986) Topical immunotherapy changes the composition of the peribulbar infiltrate in alopecia areata. *Archives of Dermatological Research*, **278**, 214.

Haynes, J.A. Jr. & Parry, T.L. (1949) Alopecia areata associated with refractive errors. *Archives of Dermatology and Syphilology*, **59**, 340.

Hendren, O.S. (1949) Identical alopecia areata in identical twins. *Archives of Dermatology and Syphilology*, **60**, 793.

Herzer, P., Czarnetzki, B.M., Holzmann, H. & Lemmel, E. (1979) Immunological studies in patients with alopecia areata. *International Archives of Allergy and Applied Immunology*, **58**, 212.

Höfer, W., Hönemann, W. & Sierke, M.L. (1969) Haufigkeit und Bedeutung degenerativer Veränderungen der Halswirbelsäule bei der Alopecia areata. *Hautarzt*, **20**, 276.

Hommes, O.P. & Prick, J.J.G. (1968) *Alopecia Maligna*. North-Holland Publishing Company, Amsterdam.

Hönemann, W. & Höfer, W. (1970) Bestehen Beziehungen zwischen der Lokalisation der Alopecia-areata-Herde und der nervalen Versorgung des Kopfes? *Dermatologische Monatschrift*, **156**, 683.

Hordinsky, M.K., Hollgren, H., Nelson, D. & Filipovitch, A.H. (1984) Suppressor cell number and function in alopecia areata. *Archives of Dermatology*, **12**, 188.

Igarashi, A., Takeuchi, S. & Seto, Y. (1980) Immunofluorescence studies of complement C_3 in hair follicles of normal scalp and of scalp affected by alopecia areata. *Acta Dermatologica Venereologica*, **60**, 33.

Ikeda, T. (1965) A new classification of alopecia areata. *Dermatologica*, **131**, 421.

Johansson, E., Ranki, A., Reunala, T., Kianto, L. & Niemi, K.M. (1986) Immunohistological evaluation of alopecia areata treated with squaric acid dibutylester (SADBE). *Acta Dermato-Venereologica*, **66**, 485.

Kaplan, H. & Reisch, M. (1952) Universal alopecia: a psychosomatic appraisal. *New York State Journal of Medicine*, **52**, 1144.

Kern, F. (1974) Laboratory evaluation of patients with alopecia areata. *First Human Hair Symposium*, p. 222, ed. A.C. Brown. Medcom, New York.

Kern, F., Hoffmann, W.H., Hambrick, G.W. & Blizzard, R.M. (1973) Alopecia areata: immunologic studies and treatment with prednisone. *Archives of Dermatology*, **107**, 407.

Khoury, E.L., Price, V.P. & Greenspan, J.S. (1988) HLA-DR expression by hair follicle keratinocytes in alopecia areata: evidence that it is secondary to the lymphoid infiltration. *Journal of Investigative Dermatology*, **90**, 193.

Kianto, U., Reunala, T., Karvonen, J., Lassus, A. & Tiilikainen, A. (1977) HLA-B_{12} in alopecia areata. *Archives of Dermatology*, **113**, 1716.

Klaber, M.R. & Munro, D.D. (1978) Alopecia areata: immunofluorescence and other studies. *British Journal of Dermatology*, **99**, 383.

Klein, V., Weissheimer, B. & Zaun, H. (1974) Simultaneous occurrence of alopecia areata and immunothyroiditis. *International Journal of Dermatology*, **13**, 116.

Kuntz, B.M., Selzle, D., Braun-Falco, O., Scholz, S. & Albert, E.D. (1977) HLA antigens in alopecia areata. *Archives of Dermatology*, **113**, 1716.

Ledesma, G.N. & York, K.K. (1982) Suppressor cell decrease in alopecia areata. *Archives of Dermatological Research*, **274**, 1.

Ledo-Dunipe, E. (1952) Emocion y alopecias en areas. *Acta Dermo-Sifiliograficas*, **44**, 139.

Lerchin, E. & Schwimmer, B. (1975) Alopecia areata associated with discoid lupus erythematosus. *Cutis*, **15**, 87.

Lubowe, I.I. (1959) The clinical aspects of alopecia areata, totalis and universalis. *Annals of the New York Academy of Science*, **83**, 458.

Macalpine, I. (1958) Is alopecia areata psychosomatic? *British Journal of Dermatology*, **70**, 117.

Main, R.A., Robbie, R.B., Gray, E.S., Donald, D. & Horne, C.H.W. (1975) Smooth muscle antibodies and alopecia areata. *British Journal of Dermatology*, **92**, 389.

McGrath, H. (1951) Alopecia associated with an intraocular foreign body. *Archives of Ophthalmology*, **46**, 319.

Martin, P., Levy, A., Minvielle, J., Risacher, D. & Birouste, M.-J. (1959) Application de la médecine psychosomatique à la dermatologie. *Presse Médicale*, **67**, 461.

Messenger, A.G. & Bleehen, S.S. (1985) Expression of HLA-DR by anagen hair follicles in alopecia areata. *Journal of Investigative Dermatology*, **85**, 569.

Messenger, A.G., Bleehen, S.S., Slater, D.N. & Rooney, N. (1984) Expressions of HLA-DR in hair follicles in alopecia areata. *Lancet*, **ii**, 287.

Milgraum, S.S., Mitchell, A.J., Bacon, G.E. & Rasussen, J.E. (1987) Alopecia areata, endocrine function and autoantibodies in patients 16 years of age or younger. *Journal of the American Academy of Dermatology,* **17**, 57.

Muller, H.K., Rook, A.J. & Kubba, R. (1980) Immunohistology and autoantibody studies in alopecia areata. *British Journal of Dermatology,* **102**, 609.

Muller, S.A. & Winkelmann, R.K. (1963) Alopecia areata. *Archives of Dermatology,* **88**, 290.

Noble, G. (1933) Familiäre universelle Alopecie: Spontanheilung nach fünf Jahren. *Weiner klinische Wochenschrift,* **46**, 90.

Nunzi, E., Hamarlinck, F. & Cormane, R.H. (1980) Immunopathological studies in alopecia areata. *Archives of Dermatological Research,* **269**, 1.

Obermayer, M.E. & Bowen, E.T. (1956) Trichotillomania and alopecia areata. *Pediatric Clinics of North America,* **3**, 639.

Olivetti, L. & Bubola, D. (1965) Osservazioni cliniche su 160 casi de area Celsi. *Giornale Italiano de Dermatologia,* **106**, 376.

Omens, D.V. & Omens, H.D. (1946) Alopecia areata in twins. *Archives of Dermatology and Syphilology,* **53**, 193.

Orecchia, G., Belvedere, M.C., Martinetti, M., Capelli, E. & Rabbiosi, G. (1987) Human leukocyte antigen region involvement in the genetic predisposition to alopecia areata. *Dermatologica,* **175**, 10.

Panconesi, E. & Mantellassi, G. (1955) Fattori psichici nella etiopatogenesi dess' area celsi. *Rassegna di Dermatologia e Sifilografia,* **8**, 121.

Panconesi, E. & Mantellassi, G. (1956) Ulteriori risultati di indageni psicodiagnostiche nella alopecia areata. *Rassegna di Dermatologia e Sifilografia,* **8**, 205.

Parisis, N.G., Fabry, H. & Muller, E. (1968) Neue Aspekte der Pathogenese des Alopecia areata in Zusammenhang mit elektroencephalographische Untersuchungen. *Aesthetische Medizin,* **17**, 277.

Peck, R.E. (1948) Alopecia [*sic*] areata as conversion symptom. *Journal of the Medical Association of Georgia,* **37**, 226.

Pecoraro, V. (1963) Relaciones etiologicas entre la pelada y el vitiligo. *Archivos Argentinos de Dermatologia,* **13**, 297.

Penders, A.J.M. (1968) Alopecia areata and atopy. *Dermatologica,* **136**, 395.

Perret, C., Wiesner-Menzel, L. & Happle, R. (1984) Immunohistochemical analysis of T-cell subsets in the peribulbar and intrabulbar infiltrates of alopecia areata. *Acta Dermato-Venereologica,* **64**, 26.

Ranki, A., Kianto, U., Kanerva, L., Tolvanen, E. & Johansson, E. (1984) Immunohistochemical and electron microscopic characterization of the cellular infiltrate in alopecia (Areata, Totalis and Universalis). *Journal of Investigative Dermatology,* **83**, 7.

Reinhold, M. (1960) Relationship of stress to the development of symptoms in alopecia areata and chronic urticaria. *British Medical Journal,* **i**, 846.

Robinson, S.S. & Tasker, S. (1948) Alopecia areata associated with neurodermatitis. *Urological and Cutaneous Reviews,* **52**, 468.

Sabouraud, R. (1929) Sur l'étiologie de la pelade. *Archives de Dermato-Syphiligraphiques de la Clinique de l'Hôpital Saint-Louis,* **1**, 31

Saenz, H. (1963) Nuevo contribución al estudio de la alopecia areata en España. *Actas Dermo-Sifiliograficas,* **54**, 357.

Salamon, T., Musafija, A. & Miliceric, M. (1971) Alopecia Areata und Erkrankungen der Thyreoidea. *Dermatologica,* **142**, 62.

Sander, D.N., Bergfield, W.F. & Krakauer, R.S. (1980) Alopecia areata: an inherited autoimmune disease. In *Hair, Trace Elements and Human Illness,* p. 434, eds. A.C. Brown & R.G. Crounse. Praeger, New York.

Schenk, E.A., Schneider, P. & Brown, A.C. (1980) Autoantibodies in alopecia and vitiligo. In *Hair Trace Elements and Human Illness,* p. 334, eds. A.C. Brown & R.G. Crounse. Praeger, New York.

Scherbenske, J.M., Benson, P.M., Rotchford, J.P. & James, W.D. (1990) Cutaneous and ocular manifestations of Down's syndrome. *Journal of the American Academy of Dermatology,* **22**, 933.

Stankler, L. & Bewscher, P.D. (1972) Chronic mucocutaneous candidiasis, endocrine deficiency and alopecia areata. *British Journal of Dermatology*, **86**, 238.

Swift, S. (1961) Folie à deux. *Archives of Dermatology*, **84**, 932.

Tan, R.S.-H. (1974) Ulcerative colitis, myasthenia gravis, atypical lichen planus, alopecia areata, vitiligo. *Proceedings of the Royal Society of Medicine*, **67**, 195.

Thestrup-Pederson, K., Bisballe, S., Jensen, J.R. & Zachariae, H. (1982) Immunological studies in patients with alopecia areata receiving dinitrochlorbenzene and cimetidine therapy. *Archives of Dermatological Research*, **273**, 261.

Todes-Taylor, N., Turner, R., Wood, G.S., Stratte, P.T. & Morhenn, V.B. (1984) T-cell subpopulation in alopecia areata. *Journal of the American Academy of Dermatology*, **11**, 216.

Torok, M., Kincses, E. & Bohatka, L. (1977) Common incidence of the alopecia totalis maligna and Sjögren syndrome. *Szemeszet*, **114**, 49.

Walker, S.A. & Rothmann, S. (1950) Alopecia areata: a statistical study and consideration of endocrine influences. *Journal of Investigative Dermatology*, **14**, 403.

Weidmann, A.I., Zion, L.S. & Mamelok, A.E. (1956) Alopecia areata occurring simultaneously in identical twins. *AMA Archives of Dermatology*, **74**, 424.

Wiesner-Menzel, L. & Happle, R. (1984) Intrabulbar and peribulbar accumulation of dendritic OKT 6-positive cells in alopecia areata. *Archives of Dermatological Research*, **276**, 333.

Wunderlich, C. & Braun-Falco, O. (1965) Mongolism and alopecia areata. *Medizinische Wochenschrift*, **10**, 477.

Young, E., Bruns, H.M. & Berrens, L. (1978) Alopecia areata and atopy (Proceedings). *Dermatologica*, **156**, 308.

Experimental induction of alopecia areata

There have been many unsuccessful attempts to induce experimentally patches of alopecia areata (Joseph 1886; Ikeda 1967; Thiers & Klaschka 1970). Friedmann (1985) proposed that the athymic nude mouse might be a useful model in which to study alopecia areata. Sawada *et al.* (1987) showed that cyclosporin A, a potent modulator of T-cell activity, stimulated hair growth of nude mice. Gilhar and Kreuger (1987) and Gilhar *et al.* (1988) reported that hair grafts from patients with alopecia areata and alopecia universalis were transplanted successfully onto athymic nude mice and that hair growth within the grafts could be stimulated by cyclosporin A. Interesting work in progress (but reported only in abstract so far) includes the alopecic (DEBRA) rat (Horne *et al.* 1987) which loses hair in association with a marked peri- and intra-follicular lymphocytic infiltrate.

References

Friedmann, P.S. (1985) Clinical and immunologic associations of alopecia areata. *Seminars in Dermatology*, **4**, 9.

Gilhar, A. & Kreuger, G.G. (1987) Hair growth in scalp grafts from patients with alopecia areata and alopecia universalis grafted onto mude mice. *Archives of Dermatology*, **123**, 44.

Gilhar, A., Pillar, T. & Etzioni, A. (1988) The effect of topical cyclosporin on the immediate shedding of human scalp hair grafted onto nude mice. *British Journal of Dermatology*, **119**, 767.

Horne, K.A., Jahoda, C.A.B., Johnson, B.E., Michie, H.J. & Oliver, R.F. (1987) An animal model for alopecia (Abstract). *Journal of Investigative Dermatology*, **89**, 316.

Ikeda, T. (1967) Produced alopecia areata based on the focal infection theory and mental motion theory. *Dermatologica*, **134**, 1.

Joseph, M. (1886) Experimentele Untersuchungen über die Ätiologie der Alopecia areata. *Monatshefte für praktischer Dermatologie*, **5**, 483.

Sawada, M., Terada, N., Taniguchi, H., Tateishi, R. & Mori, Y. (1987) Cyclosporin A stimulates hair growth in nude mice. *Laboratory Investigations*, **56**, 684.

Thiers, W. & Klaschka, F. (1970) Tierexperimentelle Sensibilisingsstudien als Beitrag zur Pathogenese der Alopecia areata. *Archiv für klinische und experimentelle Dermatologie*, **237**, 51.

Pathology and pathodynamics
(References p. 311)

Eckert *et al.*(1968) proposed that AA progresses as a wave of follicles which enter telogen prematurely and this has become the generally accepted view. Van Scott (1958) found up to 75% of follicles in anagen and suggested that re-entry into anagen takes place. Anagen/telogen ratios vary considerably with the stage and duration of the disease process. Biopsy specimens taken early in the course of the disease show the majority of follicles in telogen or late catagen. Some anagen hair bulbs are situated at a higher level in the dermis than normal (Van Scott & Ekel 1958). A peribulbar lymphocytic infiltrate is seen around follicles, this being more dense in early lesions. Van Scott (1959) found that the peribulbar lymphocytic infiltrate may involve the inner root sheath but did not involve the dermal papilla. The infiltrate consists predominantly of T-cells (Perret *et al.*1982) with increased numbers of Langerhans cells (Bröcker *et al.* 1987). The infiltrate disappears during regrowth but the sequence of events is unknown. Established lesions show no decrease in follicle number and the anagen/telogen ratio is variable. Anagen development is halted when the inner root sheath has assumed a conical shape with evidence of early cortical differentiation but no cortical keratinization. This stage is equivalent to anagen III. Van Scott (1958) stated that growth was halted in anagen IV, but at that stage cortical keratinization should have commenced and this conflicts with the findings of more recent observers. Characteristic abnormalities of the hair shaft in AA have been recognised for over a century. Pathognomonic are the exclamation-mark hairs (Fig.10.2) which are, however, not invariably present. These hairs average about 3 mm in length (Eckert *et al.* 1968). They are thought to be club hairs of normal calibre and pigmentation but the distal ends are ragged and frayed (Jackson *et al.* 1971; Peereboom-Wynia 1988). Below their broken tips they taper towards a small but otherwise normal club. Dystrophic anagen hairs are several centimetres long, of reduced calibre and often misshapen. In the areas showing early regrowth, some follicles contain multiple fine hair shafts. The single consistent histological feature is the presence of a dense peribulbar and intra-follicular lymphocytic infiltrate. This infiltrate is invariably present in the disease process. The upper, permanent portion of the hair follicle may also be involved in the infiltrate either in anagen or telogen. Atrophy of sebaceous glands is rare but the secretory activity of the glands declines with the duration of the disease (Schweikert 1967). Messenger and Bleehen (1984) found that lesional anagen follicles demonstrated injury which was confined to keratinocytes in the presumptive cortex. In an extension of this work Messenger and colleagues (1986) proposed a hypothetical model which satisfied the histo-

Fig. 10.2 Exclamation-mark
hair.

logical evidence to explain the formation of exclamation-mark hairs and the
non-destructive nature of the disease.

   In an electron microscopic study of AA Messenger and Bleehen (1984) showed
that lesional anagen follicles had evidence of non-specific injury to matrix cells
around the upper pole of the dermal papilla and to cells of the presumptive cortex.
Cell injury was not seen in the lower bulb matrix nor in other differentiating
compartments such as the inner root sheath. These workers also confirmed the
presence of degenerative changes in the suprapapillary matrix. Messenger and
Bleehan (1985) demonstrated aberrant expression of HLA-DR in cells of the
precortical matrix and presumptive cortex. Such aberrant expression of HLA-DR
antigen has been described in a number of disorders in which cell-mediated
immune reactions are implicated. Messenger and his colleagues suggested that
the presence of HLA-DR antigen in cells of the precortical matrix provided evidence
that this site could be of fundamental importance in the pathogenesis of AA and
may be the primary target for the disease process. These findings have been

confirmed by Bröcker *et al.* (1987) and Khoury *et al.* (1988) but both of these groups suggested that HLA-DR expression by keratinocytes was secondary to the lymphoid infiltration.

The concept of fundamental damage occurring in the cells of the precortical matrix and the presumptive cortex does permit explanation of the alterations in the hair cycle. Alopecia areata affects the follicle in anagen but does not cause an abrupt cessation of mitotic activity in the matrix. Once in telogen the follicle is thought to be 'safe' but when re-entry into anagen takes place the attack is resumed, anagen development can go no further, and the follicle returns prematurely to telogen. There is therefore a cyclical process which may explain why follicles are not destroyed permanently. The variations observed in the number of normal telogen hairs, dystrophic hairs and exclamation-mark hairs were interpreted by Messenger *et al.* (1986) who postulated that the follicle can respond in three different ways to pathological trauma depending on the severity of the insult. At its most severe the process damages and weakens the hair in the keratogenous zone and at the same time precipitates the follicle into catagen and then telogen. Such hairs break when the keratogenous zone reaches the surface of the scalp; these are later extruded as exclamation-mark hairs. Alternatively a follicle may simply be precipitated into normal catagen and subsequently be shed as a club hair. Such follicles may then produce dystrophic anagen hairs. Finally, it is possible that some follicles are injured just sufficiently to induce dystrophic changes, whilst they continue to grow in the anagen phase.

The change in pigmentary activity has yet to be explained for while exclamation-mark hairs are usually pigmented, dystrophic anagen hairs show variable pigmentation. AA halts anagen in anagen III. In the human hair bulb melanin pigment is transferred exclusively to cortical keratinocytes and this activity and the activation of hair bulb melanocytes also takes place in anagen III (Kukita 1957). Galbraith *et al.* (1988) demonstrated autoreactivity of sera to pigmented cells but this has not been confirmed.

References

Bröcker, E.B. Echternacht-Happle, K., Hamm, H. & Happle, R. (1987) Abnormal expression of Class I and Class II major histocompatibility antigens in alopecia areata: modulation to topical immunotherapy. *Journal of Investigative Dermatology*, **88**, 564.

Eckert, J., Church, R.E. & Ebling, F.J. (1968) The pathogenesis of alopecia areata. *British Journal of Dermatology*, **80**, 203.

Galbraith, G.M., Miller, D. & Emerson, D.L. (1988) Western blot analysis of serum antibody reactivity with human melanoma cell antigens in alopecia areata and vitiligo. *Clinical Immunology and Immunopathology*, **48**, 317.

Jackson, D., Church, R.E. & Ebling, F.J. (1971) Alopecia areata hairs. A scanning electron microscopic study. *British Journal of Dermatology*, **85**, 242.

Khoury, E.L., Price, V.P. & Greenspan, J.S. (1988) HLA-DR expression by hair follicle keratinocytes in alopecia areata: evidence that it is secondary to the lymphoid infiltration. *Journal of Investigative Dermatology*, **90**, 193.

Kukita, A. (1957) Changes in tyrosinase activity during melanocyte proliferation in the hair growth cycle. *Journal of Investigative Dermatology*, **28**, 273.

Messenger, A.G. & Bleehen, S.S. (1984) Alopecia areata: light and electron microscopic pathology of the regrowing white hair. *British Journal of Dermatology*, **110**, 155.

Messenger, A.G. & Bleehen, S.S. (1985) Expression of HLA-DR by anagen hair follicles in alopecia areata. *Journal of Investigative Dermatology*, **85**, 569.

Messenger, A.G., Slater, D.N. & Bleehen, S.S. (1986) Alopecia areata: alterations in the hair growth cycle and correlation with the follicular pathology. *British Journal of Dermatology*, **114**, 337.

Peereboom-Wynia, J.D.R., Koerten, H.K., Van Joost, Th. & Stolz, E. (1989) Scanning electron microscopy comparing exclamation mark hairs in alopecia areata with normal hair fibres, mechanically broken by traction. *Cinical and Experimental Dermatology*, **14**, 47.

Perret, C.H., Bröcker, E.B., Wiesner-Menzel, L. & Happle, R. (1982) *In situ* demonstration of T-cells in alopecia areata. *Archives of Dermatology*, **273**, 155.

Schweikert, H.U. (1967) Quantitative Untersuchungen über die Talgdrüsenfunktion bei Alopecia areata. *Archiv für klinische und experimentelle Dermatologie*, **230**, 96.

Van Scott, E.J. (1958) Morphologic changes in pilosebaceous units and anagen hairs in alopecia areata. *Journal of Investigative Dermatology*, **31**, 35.

Van Scott, E.J. (1959) Evaluation of disturbed hair growth in alopecia areata and in other alopecias. *Annals of the New York Academy of Science*, **83**, 480.

Van Scott, E.J. & Ekel, T.M. (1958) Geometric relationships between the matrix of the hair bulb and its dermal papilla in normal and alopecic scalp. *Journal of Investigative Dermatology*, **31**, 281.

Heterogeneity
(References p. 313)

Most authorities have regarded AA as a clinicopathological entity but the bewildering variety of its associated diseases and the unpredictability of its course would be more readily explained if AA was a heterogeneous clinical syndrome. This view was shared by Mitchell and Krull (1984). Ikeda (1965) proposed a classification which took into account other clinical features in addition to the alopecia itself. Studies in the Netherlands (Penders 1967; Mali 1975; De-Waard-Van der Spek *et al.* 1989) and in the U.K. (Rook 1977) have supported Ikeda's hypothesis and suggested that there may be considerable geographical variation in the relative incidence of the various types of AA.

Ikeda's four types may be categorized as follows—the incidence figures are those she recorded in Japan.

Type I. The common type accounted for 83% of patients. It occurred mainly between the ages of 20 and 40, and usually ran a total course of less than 3 years. Individual patches tended to regrow in less than 6 months, and alopecia totalis developed in only 6%.

Type II. The atopic type accounted for 10% of patients. The onset was usually in childhood and the disease ran a lengthy course in excess of 10 years. Individual patches tended to persist for over a year and alopecia totalis developed in 75%.

Type III. The prehypertensive type (4%) occurred mainly in young adults and ran a rapid course with an incidence of alopecia totalis in 39%.

Type IV. The 'combined' type (5%) occurred mainly in patients over 40 and ran a prolonged course, but resulted in alopecia totalis in only 10%.

There has been little support for Ikeda's prehypertensive type, but most authors agree that the presence of atopy confers a poor prognosis and slow rate of remission. Almost all the published work on AA has been based on the assumption that AA is a single entity. The clinical description below follows this convention since Ikeda's approach to the disease has not yet been applied sufficiently widely for its validity to be established.

References

De-Waard-Van der Spek, F.B., Oranje, A.P., De Raeymaecker, D.M. & Peereboom-Wynia, J.D.R. (1989) Juvenile versus maturity-onset alopecia areata—a comparative retrospective clinical study. *Clinical and Experimental Dermatology*, **14**, 429.

Ikeda, T. (1965) A new classification of alopecia areata. *Dermatologica*, **113**, 421.

Mali, J.W.H. (1975) Alopecia areata. *British Journal of Dermatology*, **93**, 605.

Mitchell, A.J. & Krull, E.A. (1984) Alopecia areata: pathogenesis and treatment. *Journal of American Academy of Dermatology*, **11**, 763.

Penders, A.J.M. (1967) Alopecia areata and atopy. *Dermatologica*, **136**, 395.

Rook, A.J. (1977) Common baldness and alopecia areata. In *Recent Advances in Dermatology*, vol. 4, p. 223, ed. A.J. Rook. Churchill Livingstone, Edinburgh.

Age and sex incidence
(References p. 314)

The available statistics are all based on hospital attendance figures and therefore do not reflect the true incidence of AA. It is certain that financial status, accessibility and customs influence outpatient attendance in different ways in different countries and therefore that apparent geographical differences cannot be accepted without further evidence. Table 10.1 shows a summary of the approximate age of onset of AA in five countries. The reported sex incidence has varied widely from males outnumbering females by 3 to 1 (Bastos Araujo & Poiares Baptista 1967) through equality (Walker & Rothman 1950; Muller & Winkelmann 1963) to twice as common in females (Friedmann 1985). Onset in the first year is unusual, but it has been recorded in the fourth month of life (Switzer 1947). In an investigation in Italy confined to children with AA (Bessone 1965) less than 1% of 213 cases began in the first year, and the peak incidence was in the fourth and fifth years. Onset before the age of 2 was recorded in under 2% of 736 cases in North America (Muller & Winkelmann 1963).

Table 10.1 Age-associated occurrence (%) of onset of alopecia areata in 5 countries

	Country				
Age of onset	UK[1]	Spain[2]	USA[3]	Portugal[4]	Sweden[5]
Before 21	44	35	27	32.5	35
After 40	19.5	20	30	20	25

[1]Anderson (1950); [2]Lopez (1951); [3]Muller & Winkelmann (1963); [4]Bastos Araujo & Poiares Baptista (1967); [5]Gip *et al.* (1969).

In summary, if all clinical variants of AA are grouped together the hospital statistics of most countries show the sexes to be approximately equally affected, and the onset to occur at any age with peak decade lying at some point between the ages of 20 and 50.

References

Anderson, I. (1950) Alopecia areata: a clinical study. *British Medical Journal*, **ii**, 1250.
Bastos Araujo, A. & Poiares Baptista, A. (1967) Algunas consideracons sobre 300 casos de pelada. *Traballos da Sociedade Portugesa de Dermatologia e Venereologia*, **15**, 135.
Bessone, L. (1965) Rilievi statistici sull'alopecia areata nell'infanzia. *Aggiornamento Pediatrico*. **16**, 1.
Friedmann, P.S. (1985) Clinical and immunologic associations of alopecia areata. *Seminars in Dermatology*, **4**, 9.
Gip, L., Lodin, A. & Molin, L. (1969) Alopecia areata. *Acta Dermato-Venereologica*, **49**, 180.
Lopez, B. (1951) Contribución al conocimiento de la etiopatogenia y tratamiento de la pelada. *Actas Dermo-Sifiliograficas*, **42**, 589.
Muller, S.A. & Winkelmann, R.K. (1963) Alopecia areata. *Archives of Dermatology*, **88**, 290.
Switzer, S.E. (1947) Alopecia areata in an infant. *Archives of Dermatology and Syphilology*, **55**, 143.
Walker, S.A. & Rothman, S. (1950) Alopecia areata. A statistical study and consideration of endocrine influences. *Journal of Investigative Dermatology*, **14**, 403.

Clinical features
(References p. 322)

The characteristic initial lesion of AA is commonly a circumscribed totally bald, smooth patch; it is often noticed by chance by a parent, hairdresser or friend (Fig. 10.3). Exclamation-mark hairs (Fig. 10.4) may be present at its margin, where hairs which appear normal may also be very readily extracted (Peereboom-Wynia *et al.* 1989). A few patients complain of irritation, tenderness or

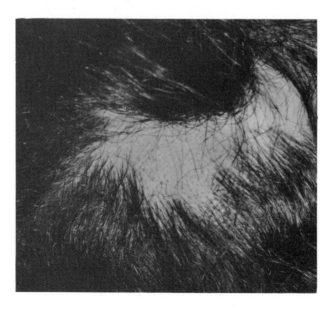

Fig. 10.3 Alopecia areata: circumscribed patches in a man aged 20.

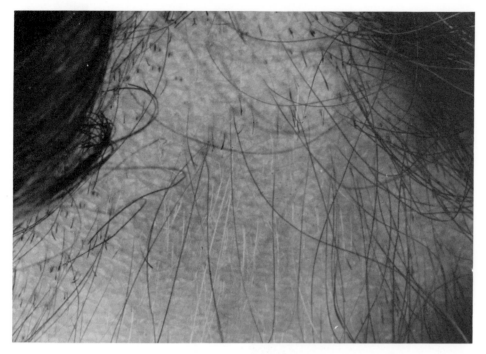

Fig. 10.4 Alopecia areata with numerous exclamation-mark hairs.

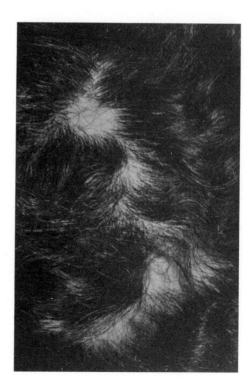

Fig. 10.5 The reticular pattern of alopecia areata at an early stage; often seen in atopic subjects.

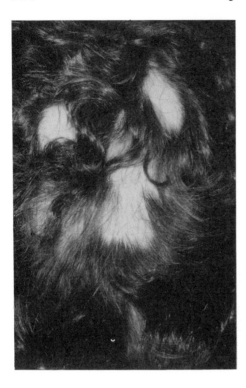

Fig. 10.6 A more advanced
stage of alopecia areata. This
form, in which there is a network of irregularly linked
patches, has a poorer prognosis
than the commoner form with
multiple discrete patches.

paraesthesiae immediately preceding the development of a new patch. Subsequent
progress is very varied; the initial patch may regrow within a few months, or
further patches may appear after an interval of 3–6 weeks and then in a cyclical
fashion (Figs 10.5 & 10.6). These intervals are of varying duration. A succession
of discrete patches may rapidly become confluent by the diffuse loss of remaining
hair (Fig. 10.7). In some cases the initial hair loss is diffuse and total denudation
of the scalp has been reported within 48 hours. However, a diffuse hair loss may
occur over part or the whole of the scalp without the development of bald areas.
Regrowth is often at first fine and unpigmented, but usually the hairs gradually
resume their normal calibre and colour. Regrowth in one region of the scalp may
occur whilst the alopecia is extending in others (Fig. 10.8).

It has been claimed that the scalp is the first affected site in over 60% of cases.
However, this figure could be wildly inaccurate because patches on the face and
limbs of children and fair-haired people are very difficult to identify even when
sought deliberately. In dark-haired men patches in the beard are conspicuous
and in such individuals are often the first to be noticed. The eyebrows and
eyelashes are lost in many cases of AA and may be the only sites affected (Fig.
10.9) The term alopecia totalis is applied to total or almost total loss of scalp hair
(Fig. 10.10) and alopecia universalis is the loss of all body hair. The extension
of alopecia along the scalp margin is known as ophiasis (Fig. 10.11). Several
investigators have recorded the site of the initial patch in the scalp. Anderson

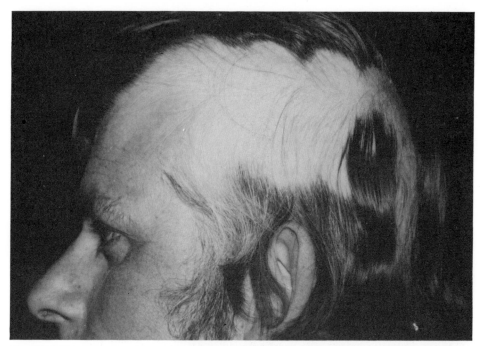

Fig. 10.7 Alopecia areata in a man aged 43: confluence of patches to form extensive areas of baldness.

Fig. 10.8 Alopecia areata in a male adolescent. Hair of normal calibre regrows but further patches develop simultaneously and the pattern changes over a period of weeks. This variant of the reticular pattern of alopecia areata tends to run a long course.

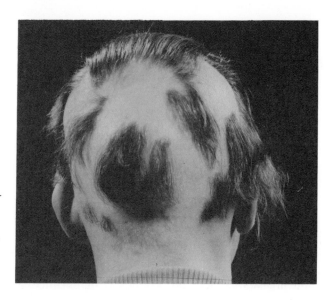

(1950) found the occipital area to feature in 35% of males and 15% of females whereas the frontovertical region was found in 31% of females and only 15% of males. AA strictly confined to one-half of the body has been reported after a head injury (Klingmüller 1958). The site of the initial patch, whether in the scalp or

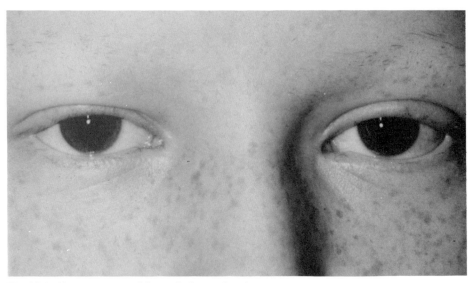

Fig. 10.9 Alopecia areata of the eyelashes and eyebrows.

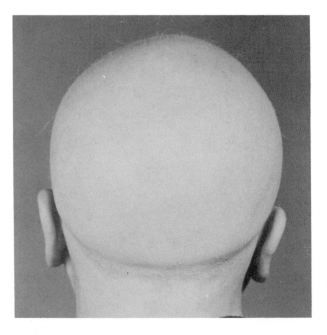

Fig. 10.10 Alopecia totalis.
There is a sparse regrowth of
unpigmented vellus hair.

not, appears to have no prognostic significance. Alopecia areata may remain
confined to a single patch at any body site (Kile 1960). Equally, however, the
onset at any site does not preclude subsequent involvement elsewhere on the body.

Progress
Rook (1977) highlighted the gloomy outlook for the sufferer of AA. Further
evidence of heterogeneity in AA is provided by the difference in prognosis reported

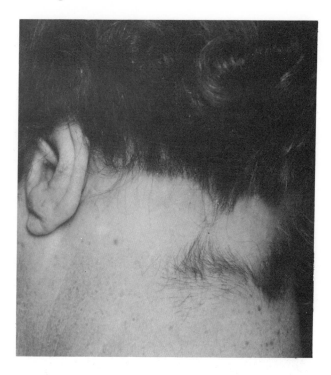

Fig. 10.11 Alopecia areata: ophiasic form. This patient also had extensive vitiligo of which one small patch can be seen here.

from various countries. In Chicago (Walker & Rothman 1950) the duration of the initial attack was less than 6 months in 33%, and less than 1 year in 50%, but 33% never recovered from the initial attack. The incidence or relapse in the whole of this series of 230 patients was 86% but in those followed up for 20 years it was 100%. Of those patients developing AA before puberty 50% became totally bald and none recovered. In contrast only 25% of those developing AA after puberty became totally bald and 5.3% recovered. Muller and Winkelmann (1963) from the Mayo Clinic reported that only 1% of the children and 10% of adults with alopecia totalis showed complete regrowth. Gómez Orbaneja (1963) reported a less favourable course in 140 cases from Madrid in which AA ran a short course in 49% and became total in 34% and universal in 6.7%. In Sweden, Gip *et al.* (1969) found recovery in 34% of males and 37% of females within a 10–15 year follow-up with a tendency for earlier regrowth in females (54% within 6 months) than in males (35% within 6 months). Schmitt (1953) showed complete recovery of alopecia universalis in only 10 of 50 patients; the poorer prognosis being in cases of prepubertal onset. Pregnancy is sometimes associated with the regrowth of longstanding severe AA but the recovery is usually temporary (Sulen *et al.* 1956). In no case of alopecia areata is a completely confident prognosis justifiable; one woman lost all her hair at 16, failed to regrow it despite eight pregnancies, but recovered it almost completely at the age of 50 (Freeman 1952).

These diverse and not strictly comparable findings are difficult to interpret. Alopecia areata in the atopic state undoubtedly has a poor prognosis, and if hair loss is total before puberty it is unlikely to regrow permanently. Alopecia areata

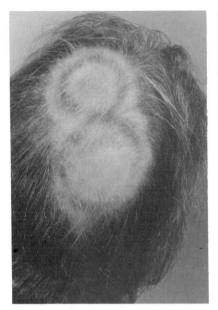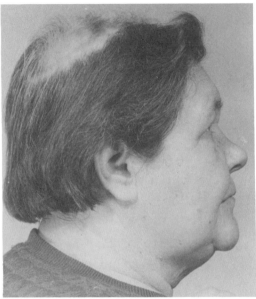

Figs 10.12 and 10.13 Alopecia areata in a patient with myxoedema. The annular pattern of regrowth is occasionally seen in any patient with alopecia areata treated with topical corticosteroids.

at any age, in a non-atopic subject, may be given a reasonably good prognosis, providing it has remained circumscribed for over 6 months. Family history of atopy does not seem to affect the prognosis. The ophiasic pattern of AA deserves its bad reputation whether associated with atopy (De-Waard-Van der Spek *et al.* 1989) or sickle-cell anaemia (El Nasr & Roaiyah 1954). Annular regrowth may occur with myxoedema or spontaneously during treatment (Figs. 10.12 & 10.13).

White hair in alopecia areata

Klingmüller (1958a) showed that white hairs were spared initially by the disease process. Patients with sudden diffuse onset of AA would appear to 'go white' over the course of a few days (Helm & Milgrom 1970). This has been reported in several famous historical personalities (Jellinek 1972).

Associated clinical changes

Nails. Nail involvement in AA (Fig. 10.14) has been reviewed by Baran and Dawber (1984). The reported incidence of nail dystrophy (Fig. 10.15) in AA ranges from 7 to 66%. The nail involvement varies from marked alteration of the nails to diffuse, fine pitting (Fig. 10.16). It may involve the majority of nails but solitary nail involvement may also occur. Gross nail dystrophy is said to be proportional to the degree of hair loss (De-Waard-Van der Spek *et al.* 1989). Onychodystrophy may precede or follow resolution of the AA (Horn & Odom 1980). Nail changes include

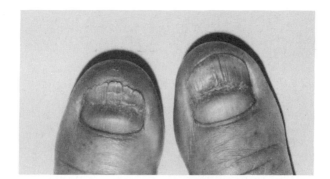

Fig. 10.14 Severe nail involvement in alopecia areata in a woman aged 62.

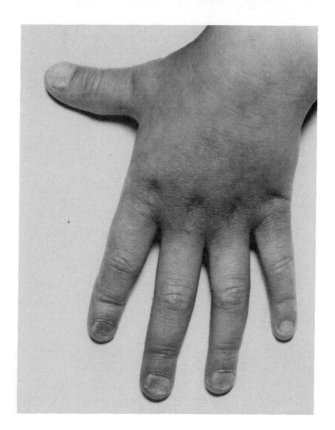

Fig. 10.15 Alopecia areata: severe dystrophy of all finger nails in a girl aged 5.

thinning (commonest) or thickening. Surface modifications include ridging with frequent onychorrhexis, cross fissures, Beau's lines or transverse lines of uniform pits which are similar to those seen in psoriasis.

Eyes. There are many reports of cataracts in association with alopecia totalis (Muller & Brunsting 1963) and in two of five adults so affected, rapid impairment of vision coincided with episodes of sudden and widespread hair loss. However, Summerly *et al.* (1966) found symptomless punctate lens opacities with equal

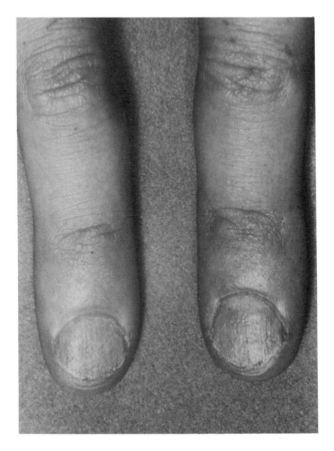

Fig. 10.16 Alopecia areata: nail pitting and longitudinal striation.

frequency in 58 patients with AA and normal controls. Horner's syndrome, ectopia of the pupil, iris atrophy or tortuosity of the fundal vessels were reported by Langhof & Lenke (1962) but these findings require confirmation.

References

Anderson, I. (1950) Alopecia areata: a clinical study. *British Medical Journal*, **i**, 1250.

Baran, R. & Dawber, R.P.R. (1984) In *Diseases of the Nails and Their Management*, p. 192, eds. R. Baran & R.P.R. Dawber. Blackwell Scientific Publications, Oxford.

De-Waard-Van der Spek, F.B., Oranje, A.P., De Raeymaecker, D.M. & Peereboom-Wynia, J.D.R. (1989) Juvenile versus maturity-onset alopecia areata—a comparative retrospective clinical study. *Clinical and Experimental Dermatology*, **14**, 429.

El Nasr, H.S. & Roaiyah, M.F.A. (1954) Prognosis of alopecia areata. *Journal of the Egyptian Medical Association*, **37**, 476.

Freeman, K.I. (1952) Alopecia areata. *Canadian Medical Association Journal*, **67**, 6.

Gip, L., Lodin, A. & Molin, L. (1969) Alopecia areata. *Acta Dermato-Venereologica*, **49**, 180.

Gómez Orbaneja, J. (1963) Modalidades clínicas evolutivas de la alopecia areata. *Actas Dermo-Sifiliográficas*, **54**, 353.

Helm, F. & Milgrom H. (1970) Can scalp hair suddenly turn white? *AMA Archives of Dermatology*, **102**, 162.

Horn, R.T. & Odom, R.E. (1980) Twenty-nail dystrophy of alopecia areata. *Archives of Dermatoloy*, **116**, 573.

Jellinek, J.E. (1972) Sudden whitening of the hair. *Bulletin of the New York Academy of Medicine*, **48**, 1003.

Kile, R.L. (1960) Alopecia of the eyelashes. *AMA Archives of Dermatology*, **81**, 959.

Klingmüller, G. (1958a) Über 'plötzliches Weissworden' und psychische Traumen bei der Alopecia areata. *Dermatologica*, **117**, 84.

Klingmüller, G. (1958b) Alopecia areata—Alopecia traumatica diffusa. *Dermatologische Wochenschrift*, **138**, 1053.

Langhof, H. & Lenke, L. (1962) Ophthalmologische Befunde bei Alopecia areata. *Dermatologische Wochenschrift*, **146**, 585.

Muller, S.A. & Brunsting, L.A. (1963) Cataracts in alopecia areata. *AMA Archives of Dermatology*, **88**, 202.

Muller, S.A. & Winkelmann, R.K. (1963) Alopecia areata. *AMA Archives of Dermatology*, **88**, 290.

Peereboom-Wynia, J.D.R., Koerten, H.K., Van Joost, T. & Stolz, E. (1989) Scanning E.M. comparing exclamation mark hairs in alopecia areata with normal hair fibres mechanically broken by traction. *Clinical and Experimental Dermatology*, **14**, 47.

Rook, A.J. (1977) Common baldness and alopecia areata. In *Recent Advances in Dermatology*, vol. 4, p. 236, ed. A.J. Rook. Blackwell Scientific Publications, Oxford.

Schmitt, C.L. (1953) Trauma as a factor in the production of alopecia universalis. (Preliminary report). *Pennsylvania Medical Journal*, **56**, 975.

Sulen, J.C., Stolte, L.A.M., Bakker, J.A.J. & Verboom, E. (1956) Alopecia areata. *Acta Endocrinologica*, **23**, 60.

Summerly, R., Watson, D.M. & Copeman, P.W.M. (1966) Alopecia areata and cataracts. *AMA Archives of Dermatology*, **93**, 411.

Walker, S.A. & Rothman, S. (1950) Alopecia areata. A statistical study and consideration of endocrine influences. *Journal of Investigative Dermatology*, **14**, 403.

Diagnosis
(Reference p. 324)

The diagnosis of AA in the typical circumscribed form usually presents no difficulties, and can be confirmed microscopically by the presence of exclamation-mark and dystrophic hairs. Occasionally lupus erythematosus may simulate AA, and must be differentiated by biopsy (Borda *et al.* 1965). In the absence of exclamation-mark hairs or in the presence of scaling, ringworm must be excluded by examination under Wood's lamp, and by microscopy and culture. A traumatic alopecia, self-inflicted as a result of a hair pulling tic, may cause difficulties and can indeed be associated with AA which has drawn a child's attention to the scalp. The presence of numerous small irregular patches should suggest the possibility of secondary syphilis; other clinical evidence of this disease should be sought and serological tests for syphilis should be carried out. Such tests are advisable in all cases of apparently atypical AA in which the diagnosis is in some doubt. The diffuse onset of AA cannot be differentiated clinically from post-febrile and other disturbances of the hair cycle, but dystrophic hairs should be sought since they are readily distinguished from the normal club hairs of the latter. In chronic circumscribed lesions it is sometimes difficult to exclude scarring with certainty. After a period of observation a biopsy may be desirable if doubt still remains.

The rare congenital triangular alopecia (see Chapter 3) is often not noted until the age of 5 or 6 or even later. It is diagnosed by its characteristic shape and site.

Reference

Borda, J.M., Abulafia, J. & Brechsbaum, E. (1965) Lupus eritematoso peladoide de cuero canelludo. *Archives Argentinos de Dermatologia*, **15**, 129.

Treatment
(References p. 330)

The variable and uncertain natural history of AA accounts for the multiplicity of uncritical claims for a large variety of therapeutic procedures. In order to overcome this problem workers have tended to choose patients with alopecia totalis or alopecia universalis because these conditions tend to run a more stable course and are traditionally more difficult to treat. Although there is an undoubted relationship between AA and alopecia totalis or alopecia universalis the latter conditions are not necessarily good models in which to test for therapeutic efficacy in AA because they represent only a small proportion of the population suffering from AA. However, it would seem reasonable to propose that a therapy which was successful on alopecia totalis and alopecia universalis might also find success in AA. This approach treats AA as a homogeneous entity, which may not be justified as at least three authors (Ikeda 1965; Penders 1967; Rook 1977) agree that Ikeda's type I might be expected to run a relatively benign course with a high natural remission and only 6% developing alopecia totalis, whereas Ikeda's original type II (atopic) group were much less fortunate with 75% developing alopecia totalis. It seems reasonable, therefore, that future clinical trial design should, at least, separate the atopic subjects before randomization rather than during analysis.

The sad fact that there is no universally proven treatment for AA is evident from the multiplicity of claims for therapeutic success. Many claims are anecdotal but the analysable evidence can be divided into four main areas:
1 non-specific irritants, e.g. dithranol and phenol;
2 'immune inhibitors', e.g. systemic steroids and PUVA;
3 'immune enhancers', e.g. contact dermatitis induction, cyclosporin A and inosiplex; and
4 of unknown action, e.g. minoxidil.

Many counter-irritants have been employed in AA but most studies predate the modern era of clinical trials; therefore, claims of effectiveness for phenol (Bechet 1941; Robinson & Robinson 1954), benzoyl benzoate (Robinson & Robinson 1954), and UVB in erythema doses (Krook 1961; Frentz 1977) cannot be substantiated. However, claims for dithranol have some scientific support. Goodman (1939) suggested the use of dithranol but modern interest was stimulated by Schmoeckel *et al.* (1979). Mitchell and Krull (1984) in a review article comment that in those occasional responsive patients clinical irritation is not an absolute requirement for success. However, Nelson and Spielvogel (1985) produced very little irritation in their subjects and failed to see a response but Fiedler-Weiss and Buys (1987a) reported a good cosmetic response in 25% of their patients with severe AA but all experienced pruritus, local erythema and scaling.

Systemic corticosteroids

Systemic corticosteroids will restore normal hair growth in many cases of AA. The hairs show abrupt repigmentation and thickening without discontinuity of the shaft (Berger & Orentreich 1960). Controversy remains, however, as to the justification for prescribing these potentially hazardous drugs because most cases relapse at some stage during or after withdrawal of treatment. The efficacy of cortisone in all but a few cases of long duration and early onset was reported by Dillaha and Rothman (1952a,b) who emphasized that hair was lost when the steroid was discontinued and that treatment could not be recommended for general use. Reports of dramatic success in long standing alopecia universalis have been made (Lubowe 1959; Shelley *et al.* 1959). Very high doses up to 100 mg prednisolone daily (Winter *et al.* 1976) have been recommended but universal side effects due to the steroids were noted and in this clinical trial more than two-thirds of the patients experienced significant hair loss after stopping treatment. These problems have prompted other dermatologists to try mixed regimes of systemic, topical and intra-lesional steroids (Unger & Schemmer 1978).

Topical and intra-lesional steroids

Attempts to reduce the hazard of systemic steroids have included both topical and intra-lesional administration. There have been a number of claims for the effectiveness of topical application using fluocinolone (Gill & Baxter 1963; Pascher *et al.* 1970) and halcinonide (Montes 1977). However, the only double-blind study was that by Pascher *et al.* (1970). At best, persistent regrowth occurs in those cases in which it might have been expected to occur spontaneously. In some cases a troublesome folliculitis may result.

Intra-lesional steroids have proved more helpful but the positive indications for their use remain limited. Rony and Cohen (1955) first reported success with hydrocortisone injections. Intra-lesional triamcinolone suspension is now preferred either by needle injection (Porter & Burton 1971) or by jet injection (Abell & Munro 1973). Porter and Burton (1971) reported that the response to either triamcinolone acetonide or hexacetonide was 'all or nothing' and if it occurred it was maintained for about 9 months. Intra-lesional corticosteroids have a small but useful role in the mangement of AA. They can be used to accelerate regrowth in a circumscribed patch of AA which is cosmetically disfiguring or difficult to conceal and can be useful for maintaining regrowth of the eyebrows in alopecia totalis (Berger 1961) but great care must be exercised to avoid steroid side effects in the eye. Atrophy may be an unsightly complication of intra-lesional corticosteroids (Fig. 10.17) and is usually confined to the injection site but has been reported in a linear pattern following the direction of lymphatic flow over the forehead (Kikuchi & Horikawa 1975; Gupta & Rasmussen 1987).

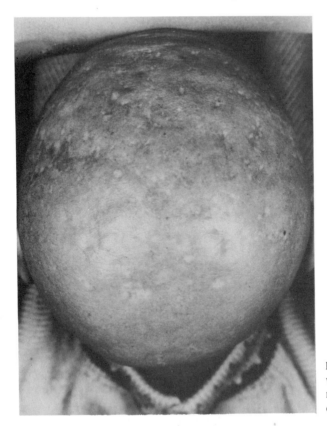

Fig. 10.17 Total alopecia areata with extensive scarring, the result of intra-lesional injection of corticosteroids.

Topical immunotherapy

The use of potent sensitizing chemicals to induce and maintain contact dermatitis of the scalp has produced regrowth of hair in some sufferers of AA with both localized and severe forms. Variable success has been attributed to dinitrochloro-benzene (DNCB), squaric acid dibutyl ester (SADBE) and diphencyprone (DCP) with sporadic reports of success with the plant *Primula obconica*. The first report of regrowth after DNCB is attributed to Rosenberg and Drake (1976). Sensitization was induced by painting the skin with a 2% solution of DNCB. The application 10 days later of a 0.1% solution provoked a dermatitis reaction in those patients (the majority) who became sensitized. Weekly applications were then made to the bald areas using the minimum concentration to induce mild inflammatory changes (often as low as 0.0001%).

Many clinical trials followed and reported variable success with this drug from 10% up to 78%, the effect being greatest in localized AA and least effective in alopecia totalis and alopecia universalis (Frentz & Eriksen 1977; Happle & Echternacht 1977; Breuillard 1978; Daman *et al.* 1978; Happle *et al.* 1978; De Prost *et al.* 1979; Hehir & du Vivier 1979; Warin *et al.* 1979; Friedmann 1981; Swanson *et al.* 1981; De Prost *et al.* 1982; Temmerman *et al.* 1984;

Valsecchi *et al.* 1986). Patients with a family history of AA (Happle 1980), a personal or family history of atopy (De Prost *et al.* 1982) and those who failed to produce a dermatitis reaction all failed to produce good regrowth. Friedmann (1981) in a more critical analysis found that the features which correlated with disease activity—the presence of autoantibodies, reduced total T-cells and T-cell reactivity—reduced the response to DNCB. Reports of mutagenicity and carcinogenicity of DNCB (Krakta *et al.* 1979; Summer & Göggelmann 1980; Strobel & Röhrborn 1980) led to the search for other potential sensitizing chemicals. SADBE and DCP are potent sensitizers and free from mutagenic activity but, unlike DNCB, are encountered rarely in everyday life or in the workplace. Most authors have used a 2% solution of SADBE in acetone as the sensitizing dose followed by application of the minimum dose to achieve contact dermatitis. Happle and colleagues (1979, 1980) have been the leading advocates for SADBE with good results in up to 70% of patients. Flowers *et al.* (1982), Case *et al.* (1984) and Johansson *et al.* (1986) all claimed good results in approximately half the patients treated. Giannetti and Orecchia (1983), Valsecchi *et al.* (1986) and Caserio (1987) produced lower success rates. Tosti *et al.* (1986) found SADBE no better than placebo in patchy AA. Caserio (1987) found that the reasons for failure to respond were more than 2 years' duration of disease, extent of hair loss, inability to obtain good sensitization and patients less than 16 years old. Happle *et al.* (1983) have also reported encouraging results with diphencyclopropenone (DCP) and their enthusiasm was echoed by Kietzmann *et al.* (1985) who reported an 85% success rate. However, Orecchia and Rabbiosi (1985), Oschendorf *et al.* (1988) and Ashworth *et al.* (1989) were less successful. MacDonald-Hull and Norris (1988) found a 50% overall response rate but only 29% of their patients were satisfied with the result. Tosti *et al.* (1986) found no difference in the response rate between DCP and a placebo. Success may be related to the exclusion of light after application as DCP is photo-degraded rapidly on exposure to ultraviolet and visible light. Alternative contact sensitizers have been suggested: Rhodes *et al.* (1981) found success in AA with *Primula obconica*; Mitchell and Krull (1984) failed to produce regrowth with 2% poison ivy/oak antigen but reported difficulty in sensitizing their patients.

In recent years topical diphencyprone has been used as a sensitizer with much promise in the short term; its limitations are similar to those of other sensitizers (Naldi *et al.* 1990).

The mechanism of action of contact sensitization in AA remains speculative. DNCB was significantly more effective than an irritant (croton oil) (Swanson *et al.* 1981). Two concepts of local immune modulation have been advanced. Daman *et al.* (1978) proposed that effector T-cells were attracted into the area; Happle (1980) suggested the occurrence of localized antigen competition and Bröcker *et al.* (1987) extended this theory to claim that repeated application activated non-specific suppressor mechanisms to suppress the effector cells responsible for AA.

The rôle for topical contact sensitization in the treatment of AA is limited. Side effects include pruritus, blistering, secondary infection and urticaria. Acquired tolerance may be reduced by cimetidine 300 mg three times daily for 3–4 weeks (Daman *et al.* 1978; De Prost *et al.* 1982). The rate of response of alopecia totalis seems to be so disappointing that the risks of uncomfortable side effects probably outweigh any benefits. These methods may be worth trying in patients with tufted, almost total, alopecia and longstanding patchy alopecia.

Photochemotherapy

Rollier and Warcewski (1974) reported induction of hair regrowth in AA with 8-methoxypsoralen (8-MOP) and sunlight. Further reports using 8-MOP plus UVA (PUVA) have claimed success for up to 60% of patients (Claudy & Gagnaire 1980, 1983; Lassus *et al.* 1980, 1984). Lassus *et al.* (1980) found equal success with oral or topical 8-MOP but favoured topical administration. Claudy and Gagnaire (1983) reported good responses only when total body irradiation was employed. Lassus *et al.* (1984), Mitchell & Douglass (1985), Van der Schaar and Sillevis-Smith (1984) also reported good results in 30% of patients but 20–40 treatment exposures were necessary to achieve benefit and all series reported a high relapse rate of 50–90% on stopping therapy. There is a poor response in alopecia totalis; Lassus *et al.* (1984) found that while the ophiasic type responded better than alopecia totalis, patients with atopy responded less well than non-atopics. The mechanism of action is unknown as PUVA may be acting as a primary irritant. However, PUVA has many effects on the local immune response within skin, and these may be important in the action of PUVA in AA. One report of successful treatment with topical haematoporphyrin plus UVA (Monfrecola *et al.* 1987) has yet to be confirmed. Total body PUVA is probably more effective than local irradiation but since the dose may need to exceed several hundred joules the treatment is probably rarely justified.

Minoxidil

Minoxidil (2,4-diamino-6-piperidinopyrimide-3-oxide) is a potent vasodilator used for the treatment of severe hypertension. Its oral use is limited because of a reversible but cosmetically unacceptable hypertrichosis of the face, arms and legs (Linas & Nies 1981). Preliminary reports of a high success rate with topical minoxidil in AA (Weiss *et al.* 1981; Fenton & Wilkinson 1982) have been followed by double-blind and dose–response studies which were less encouraging. Topical 1% minoxidil in an open study of a mixed AA/alopecia totalis population (Weiss *et al.* 1984) produced cosmetically acceptable regrowth in 20%. Tosti *et al.*(1986), however, found no difference between a 3% solution of monixidil and placebo in moderate patchy AA. Price (1987a,b) in a double-blind study of 3% topical solution showed cosmetically acceptable regrowth in three of 11 patients on minoxidil and one of 14 on placebo. In a continuation study a better response was seen at 64 weeks and Price (1987b) commented that the outcome was dependent on initial severity. The highest response rate has been obtained by 5% topical minoxidil solution (Fiedler-Weiss *et al.* 1986; Fiedler-Weiss 1987b) with demonstrable regrowth in 85% of 47 patients with severe AA but this was not cosmetically acceptable in the majority. In a comparative study Fiedler-Weiss (1987b) found a 5% solution to produce hair regrowth in a significantly higher number of cases than a 1% solution, but two of 66 patients using the 5% solution developed contact dermatitis to minoxidil. In an attempt to increase tissue minoxidil levels Fiedler-Weiss *et al.* (1987) used oral minoxidil 5 mg 12-hourly—the result was a faster response rate than with the 5% topical solution but in only 18% was the regrowth cosmetically acceptable. Neither serum nor tissue minoxidil levels correlated with regrowth which would suggest that occlusion of the treated scalp or improvement in vehicle or topical minoxidil application would be unlikely to improve the response rate.

The mechanism of action of minoxidil in AA is also unknown. Evidence points towards an effect on circulating and tissue lymphocytes and hair follicle keratinocytes. Fiedler-Weiss (1987a) and Fiedler-Weiss and Buys (1987b) looked at scalp biopsies of responders to 1% and 5% topical minoxidil and found dose related changes in increased hair follicle length, a decreased total T-lymphocyte count and decreased helper and suppressor T-cell numbers in the infiltrate. These workers also found that the responders showed increased T-cell blastogenesis before treatment which returned to the level of controls after treatment—this effect was not seen in the non-responders. Oral 5 mg minoxidil 12-hourly produced the same effect as the topical 5% solution but, in addition, produced a significant reduction in perifollicular Langerhans cell numbers (Fiedler & Buys 1987). Fiedler-Weiss (1987a) reported increased proliferation of keratinocytes and lymphocytes in tissue culture following the addition of minoxidil. Katsuoka *et al.* (1987) however, failed to demonstrate an effect on dermal papilla cells in culture. Thus the exact site of action of minoxidil in patients appearing to respond to treatment with AA is unclear.

Topical minoxidil is yet another therapy whose initial promising reports have not been substantiated. Clearly, further multicentre clinical trials are needed with stratification prior to randomization to take account of poor prognostic factors such as atopy before the true picture will emerge.

Immune modulation

Drugs which alter the immune state might be expected to shed some light on the pathogenesis of AA and may also be of therapeutic benefit. Oral cyclosporin A, a powerful modulator of T-cell function, apparently produced regrowth in two cases of alopecia totalis (Gebhart *et al.* 1986; Gupta *et al.* 1988; Gupta *et al.* 1990). However, oral cyclosporin A causes a generalized hypertrichosis and is both nephro- and hepato-toxic. Topical cyclosporin A has been tried in concentrations from 5–10% (w/v) in various oily excipients and produces sporadic patchy regrowth which was better than placebo (de Prost *et al.* 1986; Thomson *et al.* 1986). Lowy *et al.* (1985) and Galbraith *et al.* (1984) reported success with oral inosiplex but the effect was lost within 2–3 weeks of cessation. A further double-blind placebo-controlled study showed a better response than placebo;

however only partial regrowth was seen but growth was maintained in the majority after crossover to placebo (Galbraith *et al.* 1987). This work remains to be confirmed.

Summary

The decision whether or not to treat AA should be made at an early stage. Nothing can justify the prolonged use of expensive placebos. If the prognosis is poor, for example, in a prepubertal atopic with total alopecia, a full explanation and help in adjusting to the problems of wearing a wig will be of far greater value to the child than the false raising of unwarranted hopes. However, in the majority of cases in which the prognosis is good, reassurance, aided if necessary by topical or intra-lesional corticosteroids, can be advised. Systemic corticosteroids are justifiable only in exceptional circumstances. Of the newer therapies, topical diphencyprone seems to show the most promise.

References

Abell, E. & Munro, D.D. (1973) Intralesional treatment of alopecia areata with triamcinolone acetonide by jet injection. *British Journal of Dermatology*, **88**, 55.

Ashworth, J., Tuyp, E. & Mackie, R. (1989) Allergic and irritant contact dermatitis compared in the treatment of alopecia totalis and universalis. A comparison of the value of topical diphencyprone and tretinoin gel. *British Journal of Dermatology*, **120**, 397.

Bechet, P.E. (1941) Extensive alopecia areata. Result of treatment. (Society Proceedings). *AMA Archives of Dermatology*, **44**, 512.

Berger, R.A. (1961) Alopecia areata of eyebrows—corticosteroids. *AMA Archives of Dermatology*, **83**, 151.

Berger, R.A. & Orentreich, N. (1960) Abrupt changes in hair morphology following corticosteroid therapy in alopecia areata. *AMA Archives of Dermatology*, **82**, 408.

Breuillard, F. (1978) Dinitrochlorobenzene in alopecia areata. *Lancet*, **ii**, 1304.

Bröker, E.B., Echernacht-Happle, K., Hamm, H. & Happle, R. (1987) Abnormal expression of class I and class II major histocompatibility antigens in alopecia areata: modulation by topical immuno-therapy. *Journal of Investigative Dermatology*, **88**, 564.

Case, P.C., Mitchell, A.J., Swanson, N.A., Vaderveen, E.E., Ellis, C.N. & Headington, J.T. (1984) Topical therapy of alopecia areata with squaric acid dibutylester. *Journal of the American Academy of Dermatology*, **10**, 447.

Caserio, R.J. (1987) Treatment of alopecia areata with squaric acid dibutylester. *AMA Archives of Dermatology*, **123**, 1036.

Claudy, A.L. & Gagnaire, D. (1980) Photochemotherapy of alopecia areata. *Acta Dermato-Venereo-logica*, **60**, 171.

Claudy, A.L. & Gagnaire, D. (1983) PUVA treatment of alopecia areata. *AMA Archives of Dermatology*, **119**, 975.

Daman, L.A., Rosenberg, E.W. & Drake, L. (1978) Treatment of alopecia areata with dinitrochloro-benzene. *Archives of Dermatology*, **114**, 1036.

De Prost, Y., Plaquez, F.-R. & Touraine, R. (1979) Traitement de la pelade par application locale de DNCB. *Annales de Dermatologie et de Vénéréologie*, **106**, 437.

De Prost, Y., Plaquez, F.-R. & Touraine, R. (1982) Dinitrochlorobenzene treatment of alopecia areata. *AMA Archives of Dermatology*, **118**, 542.

De Prost, Y., Teillac, D., Plaquez, F., Carrugi, L., Bachelez, H. & Touraine, R. (1986) Placebo-controlled trial of topical cyclosporin in severe alopecia areata (corresp.). *Lancet*, **ii**, 803.

Dillaha, C.J. & Rothman, S. (1952a) Therapeutic experiments in alopecia areata with orally administered cortisone. *Journal of the American Medical Association*, **150**, 546.

Dillaha, C.J. & Rothman, S. (1952b) Treatment of alopecia areata totalis and universalis with cortisone acetate. *Journal of Investigative Dermatology*, **18**, 5.

Fenton, D.A. & Wilkinson, J.D. (1982) Alopecia areata treated with topical minoxidil. *Journal of the Royal Society of Medicine*, **75**, 963.

Fiedler, V.C. & Buys, C.M. (1987) Immunohistochemical characterization of the cellular infiltrate in severe alopecia areata before and after minoxidil treatment. *Dermatologica*, **175** (Suppl.), 29.

Fiedler-Weiss, V.C. (1987a) Potential mechanisms of minoxidil-induced hair growth in alopecia areata. *Journal of the American Academy of Dermatology*, **16**, 653.

Fiedler-Weiss, V.C. (1987b) Topical minoxidil solution (1% and 5%) in the treatment of alopecia areata. *Journal of the American Academy of Dermatology*, **16**, 745.

Fiedler-Weiss, V.C. & Buys, C.M. (1987a) Evaluation of anthralin in the treatment of alopecia areata. *AMA Archives of Dermatology*, **123**, 1491.

Fiedler-Weiss, V.C. & Buys, C.M. (1987b) Response to minoxidil in severe alopecia areata correlates with T-lymphocyte stimulation. *British Journal of Dermatology*, **117**, 759.

Fiedler-Weiss, V.C., West, D.P., Buys, C.M. & Rumsfield, J.A. (1986) Topical minoxidil dose–response effect in alopecia areata. *American Archives of Dermatology*, **122**, 180.

Fiedler-Weiss, V.C., Rumsfield, J.A., Buys, C.M., West, D.P. & Wendrow, A. (1987) Evaluation of oral minoxidil in the treatment of alopecia areata. *American Archives of Dermatology*, **123**, 1488.

Flowers, F.P., Slazinski, L., Fenske, N.A. & Pullara, T.J. (1982) Topical squaric acid dibutylester therapy for alopecia areata. *Cutis*, **70**, 733.

Frentz, G. (1977) Topical treatment of extended alopecia. *Dermatologica*, **155**, 147.

Frentz, G. & Eriksen, K. (1977) Treatment of alopecia areata with DNCB—an immunostimulation? *Acta Dermato-Venereologica*, **57**, 370.

Friedmann, P.S. (1981) Response of alopecia areata to DNCB—influence of autoantibodies and route of sensitisation. *British Journal of Dermatology*, **105**, 285.

Galbraith, G.M.P., Thiers, B.H. & Fudenberg, H.H. (1984) An open-label trial of immunomodulation therapy with inosiplex (Isoprinosine) in patients with alopecia totalis and cell-mediated immunodeficiency. *Journal of the American Academy of Dermatology*, **11**, 224.

Galbraith, G.M.P., Thiers, B.H., Jensen, J. & Hoehler, F. (1987) A randomised double-blind study of inosiplex (Isoprinosine) therapy in patients with alopecia totalis. *Journal of the American Academy of Dermatology*, **16**, 977.

Gebhart, W., Schmidt, J.N., Schemper, M., Spona, J., Kaposa, H. & Zazgornik, J. (1986) Cyclosporin-A induced hair growth in human renal allograft recipients and alopecia areata. *Archives of Dermatological Research*, **278**, 238.

Giannetti, A. & Orecchia, G. (1983) Clinical experience on the treatment of alopecia areata with squaric acid dibutylester. *Dermatologica*, **167**, 280.

Gill, K.A. & Baxter, D.L. (1963) Alopecia totalis—treatment with fluocinolone acetonide. *AMA Archives of Dermatology*, **87**, 384.

Goodman, M.H. (1939) Relation between pigmentation and growth of hair. *AMA Archives of Dermatology*, **40**, 76.

Gupta, A.K. & Rasmussen, J.E. (1987) Perilesional linear atrophic streaks associated with intralesional corticosteroid injections in a psoriatic plaque. *Pediatric Dermatology*, **4**, 259.

Gupta, A.K., Ellis, C.N., Tellner, D.C. & Voorhees, J.J. (1988) Cyclosporin A in the treatment of severe alopecia areata. *Transplantation Proceedings*, **XX** (Suppl. 4), 105.

Gupta, A.K., Ellis, C.N., Cooper, K.D., Nickoloff, B.J. & Griffiths, C.E.M. (1990) Oral cyclosporin for the treatment of alopecia areata. *Journal of the American Academy of Dermatology*, **22**, 242.

Happle, R. (1980) Antigenic competition as a therapeutic concept for alopecia areata. *Archives of Dermatological Research*, **267**, 109.

Happle, R. & Echternacht, K. (1977) Alopecia areata: erfolgreich Halbseitenbehandlung mit DNCB. *Zeitschrift für Haukrankheiten*, **52**, 1129.

Happle, R., Cebulla, K. & Echternacht-Happle, K. (1978) Dinitrochlorobenzene therapy for alopecia areata. *AMA Archives of Dermatology*, **114**, 1629.

Happle, R., Büchner, U., Kalvaran, K.J. & Echternacht-Happle, K. (1979) Contact allergy as a therapeutic tool for alopecia areata: application of squaric acid dibutylester. *Archives of Dermatological Research*, **264**, 101.

Happle, R., Kalvaran, K.J., Büchner, U., Echternacht-Happle, K., Göggelmann, W. & Summer, J.H. (1980) Contact allergy as a therapeutic tool for alopecia areata: application of squaric acid dibutylester. *Dermatologica*, **161**, 289.

Happle, R., Hausen, B.M. & Wiesner-Menzel, L. (1983) Diphencyprone in the treatment of alopecia areata. *Acta Dermato-Venereologica*, **63**, 49.

Hehir, M.E. & Du Vivier, A. (1979) Alopecia areata treated with DNCB. *Clinical and Experimental Dermatology*, **4**, 385.

Ikeda, T. (1965) A new classification of alopecia areata. *Dermatologica*, **131**, 421.

Johansson, E., Ranki, A., Reunala, T., Kianto, U. & Niemi, K.M. (1986) Immunohistological evaluation of alopecia areata treated with squaric acid dibutylester (SADBE). *Acta Dermato-Venereologica*, **66**, 485.

Katsuoka, K., Shell, H., Wessel, B. & Hornstein, O.P. (1987) Effects of epidermal growth factor, fibroblast growth factor, minoxidil and hydrocortisone on growth kinetics in human hair bulb papilla cells and root sheath fibroblasts cultured *in vitro*. *Archives of Dermatological Research*, **279**, 247.

Kietzmann, H., Hardung, H. & Christophers, E. (1985) Therapie der Alopecia areata mit Diphenyl-cyclopropenone. *Hautarzt*, **36**, 331.

Kikuchi, I. & Horikawa, S. (1975) Perilymphatic atrophy of the skin. *Archives of Dermatology*, **111**, 795.

Krakta, J., Goerz, G., Vizethum, W. & Stroebel, R. (1979) Dinitrochlorobenzene: influence on the cytochrome P-450 system and mutagenic effects. *Archives of Dermatological Research*, **266**, 315.

Krook, G. (1961) Treatment of alopecia areata with Kromayer's ultra-violet lamp. *Acta Dermato-Venereologica*, **41**, 178.

Lassus, A., Kianto, W., Johansson, E. & Juvakoski, T. (1980) PUVA treatment for alopecia areata. *Dermatologica*, **161**, 298.

Lassus, A., Eskelinen, A. & Johansson, E. (1984) Treatment of alopecia areata with three different PUVA modalities. *Photodermatology*, **1**, 141.

Linas, S.L. & Nies, A.S. (1981) Minoxidil. *Annals of Internal Medicine*, **94**, 61.

Lowy, M., Ledoux-Corbusier, M., Achten, G. & Wybran, J. (1985) Clinical and immunologic response to Isoprinosine in alopecia areata and alopecia universalis: association with auto-antibodies. *Journal of the American Academy of Dermatology*, **12**, 78.

Lubowe, I.I. (1959) The treatment of alopecia universalis with methyl prednisolone (Medrol) associated with vitiligo, involving arms, forearms, neck and thigh. *AMA Archives of Dermatology*, **79**, 665.

MacDonald Hull, S. & Norris, J.F. (1988) Diphencyprone in the treatment of long-standing alopecia areata. *British Journal of Dermatology*, **119**, 367.

Mitchell, A.J. & Krull, E.A. (1984) Alopecia areata: pathogenesis and treatment. *Journal of the American Academy of Dermatology*, **11**, 763.

Mitchell, A.J. & Douglass, M.C. (1985) Topical photochemotherapy for alopecia areata. *Journal of the American Academy of Dermatology*, **12**, 644.

Monfrecola, G., D'Anna, F. & Delfino, M. (1987) Topical hematoporphyrin plus UVA for treatment of alopecia areata. *Photodermatology*, **4**, 305.

Montes, L.F. (1977) Topical halcinonide in alopecia areata and in alopecia totalis. *Journal of Cutaneous Pathology*, **4**, 47.

Naldi, L., Parazzini, F. & Cainelli, T. (1990) Role of topical immunotherapy in the treatment of alopecia areata. *Journal of the American Academy of Dermatology*, **22**, 654.

Nelson, D.A. & Spielvogel, R.L. (1985) Anthralin therapy for alopecia areata. *International Journal of Dermatology*, **24**, 606.

Orecchia, G. & Rabbiosi, G. (1985) Treatment of alopecia areata with diphencyprone. *Dermatologica*, **171**, 193.

Oschendorf, F.R., Mitrou, G. & Milbradt, R. (1988) Therapie der Alopecia areata mit Diphenylcyclo-propenon. *Zeitschrift für Hautkrankheiten*, **63**, 94.

Pascher, F., Curtin, S. & Andrade, E. (1970) Assay of 0.2% fluocinolone acetonide cream for alopecia areata and totalis. *Dermatologica*, **141**, 193.

Penders, A.J.M. (1967) Alopecia areata and atopy. *Dermatologica*, **136**, 395.

Porter, D. & Burton, J.L. (1971) A comparison of intra-lesional triamcinolone hexacetonide and triamcinolone acetonide in alopecia areata. *British Journal of Dermatology*, **85**, 272.

Price, V.H. (1987a) Topical minoxidil in extensive alopecia areata, including 3-year follow-up. *Dermatologica*, **175** (Suppl. 2), 36.

Price, V.H. (1987b) Topical minoxidil (3%) in extensive alopecia areata, including long-term efficacy. *Journal of the American Academy of Dermatology*, **16**, 737.

Rhodes, E.L., Dolman, W., Kennedy, C. & Taylor, R.R. (1981) Alopecia areata regrowth induced by *Primula obconica. British Journal of Dermatology*, **104**, 339.

Robinson, H.M. & Robinson, R. (1954) A new approach to the local treatment of alopecia areata. *Southern Medical Journal*, **47**, 894.

Rollier, R. & Warcewski, Z. (1974) Le traitement de la pelade par la méladinine. *Bulletin de la Société Française de Dermatologie et de Syphiligraphie*, Paris, **81**, 97.

Rony, H.R. & Cohen, D.M. (1955) The effect of cortisone in alopecia areata. *Journal of Investigative Dermatology*, **25**, 285.

Rook, A.J. (1977) Common baldness and alopecia areata. In *Recent Advances in Dermatology*, Vol. 4, p. 223, ed. A.J. Rook. Churchill Livingstone, Edinburgh.

Rosenberg, E.W. & Drake, L. (1976) In Discussion of Dunaway, D.A.: Alopecia areata. *AMA Archives of Dermatology*, **112**, 256.

Schmoeckel, C., Weissmann, I., Plewig, G. & Braun-Falco, O. (1979) Treatment of alopecia areata by anthralin induced dermatitis. *Archives of Dermatology*, **115**, 1254.

Shelley, W.B., Harun, J.S. & Lehmann, J.M. (1959) Long-term triamcinolone therapy of alopecia universalis. *AMA Archives of Dermatology*, **80**, 433.

Strobel, R. & Röhrborn, G. (1980) Mutagenic and cell transforming activities of 1-chlor-2, 4-dinitrobenzene (DNCB) and squaric-acid-dibutylester (SADBE). *Archives of Toxicology*, **45**, 307.

Summer, K.-H. & Göggelmann, W. (1980) 1-Chloro-2,4-dinitrobenzene depletes glutathione in rat skin and is mutagenic in *Salmonella typhimurium. Mutation Research*, **77**, 91.

Swanson, N.A., Mitchell, A.J., Leahy, M.S., Haddington, J.T. & Diaz, L.A. (1981) Topical treatment of Alopecia Areata. *Archives of Dermatology*, **117**, 384.

Temmerman, L., de Weert, J., de Keyser, L. & Kint, A. (1984) Treatment of alopecia areata with dinitrochlorobenzene. *Acta Dermato-Venereologica*, **64**, 441.

Thomson, A.W., Aldridge, R.D. & Sewell, H.F. (1986) Topical cyclosporin in alopecia areata and nickel contact dermatitis (corresp.). *Lancet*, **ii**, 971.

Tosti, A., De Padova, M.P., Minghetti, G. & Veronesi, S. (1986) Therapies versus placebo in the treatment of patchy alopecia areata. *Journal of the American Academy of Dermatology*, **15**, 209.

Unger, W.P. & Schemmer, R.J. (1978) Corticosteroids in the treatment of alopecia totalis. *AMA Archives of Dermatology*, **114**, 1486.

Valsecchi, R., Cainelli, T., Foiadelli, L. & Rossi, A. (1986) Topical immunotherapy of alopecia areata. A follow-up study. *Acta Dermato-Venereologica*, **66**, 269.

Van der Schaar, W.W. & Sillevis-Smith, J.H. (1984) An evaluation of PUVA-therapy for alopecia areata. *Dermatologica*, **168**, 250.

Warin, A.P., Hehir, M.E. & Du Vivier, A. (1979) Alopecia areata treated with DNCB. *Clinical and Experimental Dermatology*, **4**, 385.

Weiss, V.C., West, D.P. & Mueller, C.E. (1981) Topical minoxidil in alopecia areata (corresp.). *Journal of the American Academy of Dermatology*, **5**, 224.

Weiss, V.C., West, D.P., Fu, T.S., Robinson, L.A., Cook, B., Cohen, R.L. & Chambers, D.A. (1984) Alopecia areata treated with topical minoxidil. *AMA Archives of Dermatology*, **120**, 457.

Winter, R.J., Kern, F. & Blizzard, E.M. (1976) Prednisone therapy for alopecia areata. *AMA Archives of Dermatology*, **122**, 1549.

Chapter 11
Cicatricial Alopecia

Introduction

Cicatricial alopecia is the generic term applied to alopecia which accompanies or follows the destruction of hair follicles, whether by a disease affecting the follicles themselves or by some process external to them. The follicles may be absent as the result of a developmental defect or may be irretrievably injured by trauma, as in burns of radiodermatitis. They may be destroyed by a specific and identifiable infection—favus, tuberculosis or syphilis, for example—or by the encroachment of a benign or malignant tumour. In other cases their destruction can be reliably attributed to a named, though still mysterious, disease process such as lichen planus or lupus erythematosus or sarcoidosis. When all the clinically and histologically acceptable causes have been eliminated, two named syndromes of cutaneous origin remain, pseudopelade and the less well-defined folliculitis decalvans. Once these too have been excluded, there still remain cases in which any greater precision of diagnosis than 'cicatricial alopecia' may be unwarranted.

The clinical recognition of an area of scarring in the scalp should initiate detailed investigations. Scarring is not always easy to identify with complete confidence, even with a hand lens if the scarred area is small, and it may be desirable to re-examine the patient after an interval, or to take a biopsy. Once the preliminary diagnosis of cicatricial alopecia has been made, the scalp should be searched for other changes—folliculitis, follicular plugging, telangiectasia or broken hairs—and hairs, even if grossly normal in appearance, should be extracted from the edge of the bald area for microscopy and culture. If no firm diagnosis is achieved then general skin examination and systemic studies should be carried out where appropriate.

If the decision is made to take a biopsy, its site must be carefully selected and an early lesion should be preferred; late lesions may have lost all evidence of their origin. Several punch biopsies are preferable to a single elliptical biopsy—in this way the biopsies can be oriented along follicles and different stages of the disease process can be investigated.

Classification of causes
(Reference p. 337)

The causes of cicatricial alopecia are classified here into broad groups, and the individual causes are then considered in greater detail (classification modified from Ebling and Rook 1968).

1 *Developmental defects and hereditary disorder*
   Aplasia cutis
   Facial hemiatrophy (Romberg's syndrome)
   Epidermal naevi
   Hair follicle hamartomas
   Incontinentia pigmenti
   Focal dermal hypoplasia of Goltz
   Porokeratosis of Mibelli
   Scarring follicular keratosis
   Ichthyosis
   Darier's disease
   Epidermolysis bullosa
   Polyostotic fibrous dysplasia
   Conradi's syndrome (chondro-dystrophia calcificans)

2 *Physical injuries*
   Mechanical trauma
   Scalp necrosis after embolization surgery

   Burns
   Radiodermatitis

3 *Medicaments*

4 *Fungal infections*
   Kerion
   Trichophyton violaceum
   T. sulphureum
   Favus (Fig. 11.1)

5 *Bacterial infections*
   Tuberculosis
   Syphilis

6 *Pyogenic infections*
   Carbuncle
   Furuncle
   Folliculitis
   Acne necrotica

7 *Protozoal infections*
   Leishmaniasis

8 *Virus infections*
   Herpes zoster

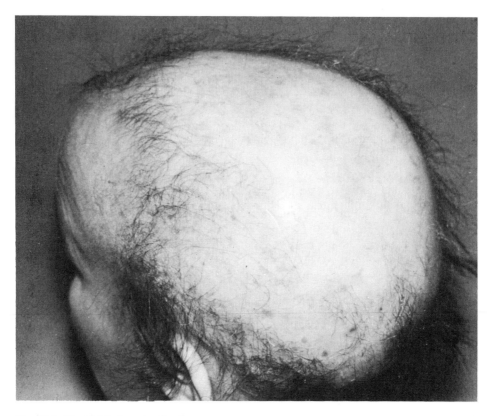

Fig. 11.1 Cicatricial alopecia after favus.

Varicella
AIDS—secondary infections
  (various)
9 *Tumours*
  Basal cell epithelioma
  Squamous cell epithelioma
  Syringoma
  Metastatic tumours
  Reticuloses
  Adnexal tumours
10 *Dermatoses of uncertain aetiology*
  Lichen planus
  Graham-Little syndrome
  Tufted folliculitis
  Dermatomyositis
  Lupus erythematosus

Scleroderma morphoea
Necrobiosis lipoidica
Pyoderma gangrenosa
Lichen sclerosus
Mastocytosis
Sarcoidosis
Cicatricial pemphigoid
Follicular mucinosis
Temporal arteritis
Erosive pustular dermatosis
Eosinophilic cellulitis
11 *Clinical syndromes*
  Dissecting cellulitis of the scalp
  Pseudopelade
  Folliculitis decalvans
  Alopecia parvimacularis

Small irregular areas of scarring, together with broken and weathered hairs, may occur as the only defects as the result of the continued abuse of hair dyes and other cosmetics. However, such changes may complicate other forms of alopecia as a result of the patient's misguided efforts to improve her appearance.

Reference

Ebling, F.J. & Rook, A.J. (1968) In *Textbook of Dermatology*, eds. A.J. Rook, D.S. Wilkinson & F.J. Ebling. Blackwell Scientific Publications, Oxford.

The clinical syndromes

History and nomenclature (References p. 338)

In the literature of the 19th century and earlier there are descriptions of cases of cicatricial alopecia probably conforming to these three clinical syndromes, but although the cause of favus was discovered in the fifth decade of the last century such influential authorities as Erasmus Wilson continued for several decades to deny that the structures observed were anything other than 'phytiform degeneration'. The routine exclusion of bacterial and fungal infection in all cases of scarring alopecia was certainly not widely practised until the turn of the century. The earlier case reports cannot, therefore, be assessed with any confidence.

In 1885 Brocq of Paris described what later became known as *pseudopelade*, but as he himself subsequently admitted (Brocq 1907) it continues to confuse the nomenclature. Pseudopelade, studied in detail by Photinos (1930), is now regarded as a syndrome in which destruction of follicles leading to permanent patchy baldness is not accompanied by any clinically evident inflammatory pathology.

Quinquaud (1888–9) described a form of scarring alopecia in which pustular folliculitis of the advancing margin was a conspicuous feature. To this condition the term *folliculitis devalvans* is now commonly applied. Unfortunately Lailler described similar cases as acne decalvans. Folliculitis decalvans affecting areas other than the scalp has been separately described by Arnozan (1892). Differing in degree from folliculitis decalvans is lupoid sycosis, so called by Milton (1865) and by Brocq *et al.* (1905). The follicles are destroyed by a granulomatous inflammatory process simulating lupus vulgaris. Unna (1889) applied the term ulerythema sycosiforme to the same condition.

Alopecia parvimaculata as described by Dreuw (1910) is a questionable entity. It has been regarded as pseudopelade occurring in childhood, but it differs from that syndrome in several respects.

Pinkus (1978), using acid alcoholic orcein stain, studied the distribution of elastic fibres around the hair follicles in many sections from biopsies in cicatricial alopecia of a variety of types. He found that the fibrous strands which replaced destroyed follicles in lichen planus and lupus erythematosus consist of collagen without elastic-like bodies or elastic fibres. In lupus erythematosus there is, in addition, widespread destruction of elastic fibres in the interfollicular dermis. The cases included 180 which satisfied the diagnostic criteria of pseudopelade: absence of sebaceous glands, more or less normal epidermis, no significant follicular plugging, small areas of subepidermal loss of elastic fibres, collagenous and elastic fibrosis at sites of destroyed follicles. Of these 180 cases, 106 showed additional features, which led Pinkus to differentiate them provisionally as 'fibrosing alopecia'. The most striking of these features is the development of elastic fibres around the lower part of the follicle, even at an early stage in the process. The features of fibrosing alopecia were a general hyperplasia of elastic fibres in the interfollicular dermis and the presence of less perifollicular cellular infiltrate than in pseudopelade. The age and sex incidence of the two conditions did not differ significantly. It remains to be established whether there are clinical differences.

Whatever the type of scarring alopecia, once the process has been shown to have become arrested, or in a static phase, surgical removal of the affected area should be considered. This has become more relevant in recent times because of the ability to remove even large areas with good cosmetic results (Roenigk & Wheeland 1987).

References

Arnozan, H. (1892) Folliculites dépilantes des parties glabres. *Annales de Dermatologie et de Syphiligraphie*, **3**, 491.

Brocq, L. (1885) Alopecia. *Journal of Cutaneous and Venereal Diseases*, **3**, 49.

Brocq, L., Lenglet, E. & Ayrignac, J. (1905) Recherches sur l'alopécie atrophiante, variété pseudopelade. *Annales de Dermatologie et de Syphiligraphie*, **6**, 1, 97, 209.

Brocq, L. (1907) Pseudopelade. In *Traité Élémentaire de Dermatologie Pratique*, vol. 2, p. 648. Doin, Paris.

Dreuw, H. (1910) Über epidemische Alopecie. *Monatshefte für praktische Dermatologie*, **51**, 18.

Milton, J.L. (1865) cit. Jackson, G.T. & McMurtry, C.W. (1913) *A Treatise of Diseases of the Hair*, p. 182. Kimpton, London.

Photinos, P. (1930) *La Pseudopelade de Brocq*. Maloine, Paris.

Pinkus, H. (1978) Differential patterns of elastic fibres in scarring and non-scarring alopecias. *Journal of Cutaneous Pathology*, **5**, 93.

Quinquaud, E. (1888) Folliculite destructive des regions vélues. *Bulletin et Mémoires de la Société médicale des Hôpitaux de Paris*, **5**, 395.

Quinquaud, E. (1889) Folliculite épilante décalvante. *Annales de Dermatologie et de Syphiligraphie*, **10**, 99.

Roenigk, R.K. & Wheeland, R.G. (1987) Tissue expansion in cicatricial alopecia. *Archives of Dermatology*, **123**, 641.

Unna, P.G. (1889) Über Ulerythema sycosiforme. *Monatshefte für praktische Dermatologie*, **9**, 134.

Pseudopelade (References p. 341)

Nomenclature and aetiology. The term pseudopelade is used here to designate a slowly progressive cicatricial alopecia, without clinically evident folliculitis. There is no doubt that lichen planus can produce a very similar clinical picture and there are some authorities who maintain on the basis of associated skin lesions and histopathological findings that 90% of cases of 'pseudopelade' are caused by lichen planus (Kaminsky *et al.* 1967). In another series of 35 cases lichen planus was diagnosed in only about 15% (Gay Prieto 1955). At a later stage lupus erythematosus also can cause similar changes. However, some patients with pseudopelade never show any clinical or histological evidence of lichen planus (Ronchese 1960; Braun-Falco *et al.* 1986). Pseudopelade is therefore generally regarded as a clinical syndrome which may be the end result of any one of a number of different pathological processes (known and unknown) (Degos *et al.* 1954).

Pathology (Laymon 1947; Lopez & Cardenas 1948; Degos *et al.* 1954). If clinically normal scalp at the edge of a plaque of pseudopelade is examined, numerous lymphocytes are seen around the upper two-thirds of the follicles. Later the follicles are destroyed and the epidermis becomes thin and atrophic, and the dermis densely sclerotic.

Clinical features (Van der Meiren 1933; Laymon 1947; Degos *et al.* 1954). Although both sexes may be affected, and the condition has occurred in childhood (Reinertson 1958), the patient is usually a woman and usually over 40. She may complain of slight irritation at first, but more often a small bald patch, discovered by chance by the patient or by her hairdresser, is the first evidence of the disease. The initial patch is most often on the vertex, but may occur anywhere on the scalp. The course thereafter is extremely variable. In a majority of cases extension of the process takes place only very slowly; indeed after 15 or 20 years the patient may still be able to arrange her hair to conceal the patches effectively. In some cases extension occurs more rapidly, and exceptionally there may be almost total baldness after 2 or 3 years.

On examination the affected patches are smooth, soft and slightly depressed. At an early stage in the development of any individual patch there may be some erythema, diffuse or perifollicular (Miescher & Lenggenhager 1947). The patches tend to be small and round or oval, but irregular bald patches may be formed by confluence of many lesions. The hair in uninvolved scalp is normal, but if the process is active the hairs at the edges of each patch are very easily extracted (Figs. 11.2, 11.3). Detailed studies by Braun-Falco *et al.* (1986) strongly support support the idea that pseudopelade is a distinct entity with the clinical criteria shown in Table 11.1.

Diagnosis. The characteristic feature is the development of small patches of cicatricial alopecia in the absence of any clinical change other than transient erythema.

Treatment. If the scarring alopecia can be shown to be secondary to lichen planus

Chapter 11

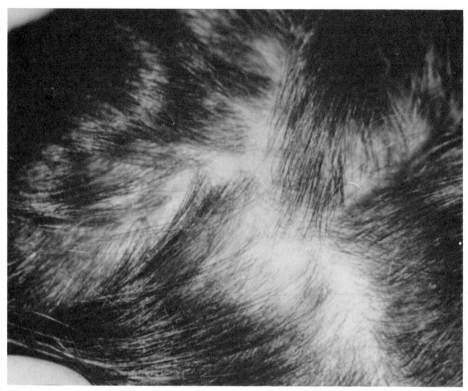

Fig. 11.2 Pseudopelade—early lesions.

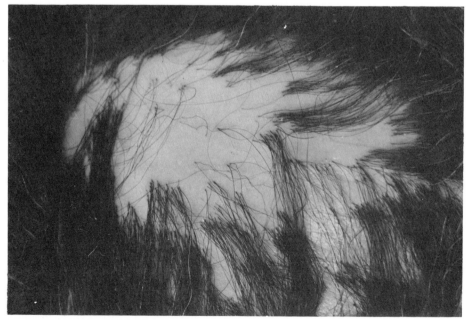

Fig. 11.3 Pseudopelade—advanced.

Table 11.1 Diagnostic criteria for pseudopelade (Braun-Falco *et al.* 1986)

Clinical criteria
  Irregularly defined and confluent patches of alopecia
  Moderate atrophy (late stage)
  Mild perifollicular erythema (early stage)
  Female:male = 3 : 1
  Long course (more than 2 years)
  Slow progression with spontaneous termination possible

Direct immunofluorescence
  Negative or at least only IgM (Pincelli *et al.* 1987)

Histological criteria
  Absence of marked inflammation
  Absence of widespread scarring
  Absence of significant follicular plugging
  Absence, or at least decrease, of sebaceous glands
  Presence of normal epidermis (only occasionally atrophy)
  Fibrotic streams into subcutis

or lupus erythematosus, then the treatment appropriate for these conditions may be prescribed. However, whether the baldness is of known or unknown origin it is irreversible. If the disfigurement is considerable and no active inflammatory changes are present, autografting from unaffected to scarred scalp may be considered (Stough *et al.* 1968; Curban & Gollman 1973), or surgical 'expansion' techniques in severe cases.

The intra-dermal injection of corticosteroids has seemed not to influence the extension of the disease process in cases of unknown origin.

References

Braun-Falco, Imei, S., Schmoeckel, C. *et al.* (1986) Pseudotelede of Brocq. *Dermatologica,* **172**, 18.
Curban, G.V. & Gollman, B. (1973) Pseudopelade de Brocq. *Medicina Cutanea,* **7**, 65.
Degos, R., Rabut, R., Duperrat, B. & Leclerq, R. (1954) L'état pseudopeladique. *Annales de Dermatologie et de Syphiligraphie,* **81**, 5.
Gay Prieto, J. (1955) Pseudopelade of Brocq: its relationship to some forms of cicatricial alopecia and to lichen planus. *Journal of Investigative Dermatology,* **24**, 323.
Kaminsky, A., Kaminsky, C.A., de Kaminsky, A.R. & Abulafia, J. (1967) Liquen folicular alopeciante. *Medicina Cutanea,* **2**, 135.
Laymon, C.W. (1947) The cicatricial alopecias. *Journal of Investigative Dermatology,* **8**, 99.
Lopez, B. & Cardenas, M. (1948) Contribución al estudio de la pseudopelade de Brocq. *Actas Dermosifiliograficas,* **39**, 478.
Miescher, G. & Lenggenhager, R. (1947) Über Pseudopelade, Brocq. *Dermatologica,* **94**, 122.
Pincelli, C., Girolomoni, G. & Benassi, L. (1987) Pseudopelade of Brocq: an immunologically mediated disease? *Dermatologica,* **176**, 49.
Reinertson, R.P. (1958) Pseudopelade with nail dystrophy. *Archives of Dermatology,* **78**, 282.
Ronchese, F. (1960) Pseudopelade. *Archives of Dermatology,* **82**, 336.
Stough, D.B., Berger, R.A. & Orentreich, N. (1968) Surgical improvement of cicatricial alopecia of diverse etiology. *Archives of Dermatology,* **97**, 331.
Van der Meiren, L. (1933) Contribution à l'étude de la pseudopelade. *Annales de Dermatologie et de Syphiligraphie,* **4**, 928.

Folliculitis decalvans (References p. 343)

History and nomenclature. The history of the complex cicatricial alopecia syndromes has been briefly summarized above. Under the general term folliculitis decalvans we group together the various syndromes in which clinically evident chronic folliculitis leads to progressive scarring. The 'foliculite dépilante' of Arnozan differs from Quinquaud's folliculitis decalvans in that the latter affects the scalp, and the former other regions of the body, but they may co-exist. Similarly lupoid sycosis, with its many synonyms, is a scarring folliculitis affecting predominantly the beard.

Aetiology. The cause of folliculitis decalvans is still uncertain. *Staphylococcus aureus* may be grown from the pustules but, more often, only ordinarily non-pathogenic organisms are isolated. Some abnormality of the host must be postulated. Some authors have emphasized the possible role of the seborrhoeic state and some have used the term 'cicatrizing seborrhoeic eczema' (Laymon 1947), but folliculitis decalvans is rare and the seborrhoeic state is common, so the association probably has no special significance.

Shitara *et al.* (1947) reported severe folliculitis decalvans in two siblings who also had chronic oral candidiasis; defective cell-mediated immunity was demonstrated. It seems probable that a failure in the immune response or in leucocyte function may be the essential abnormality in most cases, perhaps in all.

Folliculitis decalvans of the scalp occurs in both sexes. It affects women aged 30–60 and men from adolescence onwards; rarely it may be present from infancy (Loewenthal 1957). In other sites it affects mainly adult males.

Pathology. Follicular abscesses with a polymorphonuclear infiltrate are directly succeeded by scarring, or there may be a prolonged intermediate stage of granulomatous folliculitis with numerous lymphocytes, and some plasma cells and giant cells. Eventually only the remains of follicles can be detected in areas of scar tissue.

Clinical features. Any or all hairy regions may be involved, and in the syndrome sometimes referred to as 'atrophic folliculitis in seborrhoeic dermatitis' as described by Hallopeau, the beard, pubes, axillae and inner thighs may be involved, and less often the scalp as well. The severity of the inflammatory changes fluctuates, but the course is prolonged.

The scalp alone may be involved or the scalp together with pubes and axillae. There are multiple rounded or oval patches each surrounded by crops of follicular pustules. There may be no other changes, but successive crops of pustules, each followed by destruction of the affected follicles, produce slow extension of the alopecia. In some cases the folliculitis spreads along the scalp margin in a coronal distribution (Bogg 1963).

When the face is affected the area in front of the ears is often the first to be involved. Large pustules or reddish-brown lupoid papules are succeeded by dense scarring. The process tends to remain unilateral and if it spreads to the scalp, is usually confined to the temple, although it may extend along the frontal hair line (Binazzi 1954).

In the clinical syndrome in which the so-called 'glabrous' skin is principally involved (Miller 1961) the lesions, on thighs, legs and arms, tend to be symmetrical.

Tufted folliculitis (Tong & Baden 1989; Dalziel *et al.* 1990) may be a variant in subtype of this entity—an upper follicular acute inflammatory polymorphonuclear infiltrate is clinically associated with close grouping or 'tufting' of hairs.

Treatment. All patients should be investigated for underlying defects of immune response and of leucocyte function, as a possible guide to effective treatment.

Systematic antibiotics will often prevent further extension of the disease, but only for as long as they are administered. Brozena *et al.* (1988) reported a single case, which after only minimal benefit from a variety of oral antibiotics, resolved after 10 weeks of rifampicin therapy and had no new lesions up to 1 year later.

References

Binazzi, M. (1954) In tema di folliculiti decalvanti. *Annali Italiani di Dermatologia e di Sifiligrafi*, **9**, 325.

Bogg, A. (1963) Folliculitis decalvans. *Acta Dermato-Venereologica*, **43**, 14.

Brozena, S.J., Cohen, L.E. & Fenske, N.A. (1988) Folliculitis decalvans—response to rifampicin. *Cutis*, **42**, 512.

Dalziel, K., Telfer, N. & Dawber, R.P.R. (1990) Tufted folliculitis. *American Journal of Dermatopathology* (in press).

Laymon, C.W. (1947) The cicatricial alopecias. *Journal of Investigative Dermatology*, **8**, 99.

Loewenthal, L.J.A. (1957) A case of lupoid sycosis or ulerythema sycosiforme, beginning in infancy. *British Journal of Dermatology*, **69**, 443.

Miller, R.F. (1961) Epilating folliculitis of the glabrous skin. *Archives of Dermatology*, **83**, 115.

Shitara, A., Igareshi, R. & Morohashi, M. (1974) Folliculitis decalvans and cellular immunity—two brothers with oral candidiasis. (In Japanese.) *Japanese Journal of Dermatology*, **28**, 133.

Tong, A.K.F. & Baden, H. (1989) Tufted folliculitis. *Journal of the American Academy of Dermatology*, **21**, 1096.

Alopecia parvimaculata (References p. 344)

History and nomenclature. Dreuw in Germany in 1910 reported an outbreak of alopecia affecting 60 of the 85 boys in two schools. The patches of alopecia were small, irregularly round or angular, and appeared atrophic, but in 90% the hair regrew satisfactorily, permanent scarring alopecia developing in the remaining 10%. There were no inflammatory changes and no fungus or other organisms could be discovered.

Bowen (1899) of Boston, USA, had reported two outbreaks of a similar clinical entity. Four of 26 girls affected in the second outbreak had some residual atrophy. Bowen later (1915) expressed the opinion that his cases had been similar to those reported by Dreuw, and not alopecia areata.

At intervals other outbreaks have been reported. Each report arouses the same heated controversy as have earlier publications on epidemic alopecia areata. Some critics insist that a fungus infection must have been overlooked; other critics are more concerned in establishing whether or not the condition is 'true' alopecia areata. The mystery is at present unresolved, but there is sufficient evidence that outbreaks of alopecia, distinct from alopecia areata and not of mycotic origin, do occur. It is not yet clear whether they constitute a single aetiological entity (Davis 1914).

Pathology. Few histological studies have been recorded. Sabouraud (1932) mentions non-specific inflammatory changes involving some follicles, whilst sparing others. The degree of scarring depends on the number of contiguous follicles destroyed. In some cases the pathological changes eventually resemble those of pseudopelade (Loewenthal & Lurie 1956).

Clinical features (Semon 1923; Hoffmann & Martin 1925; Heermann 1930; Höfer 1964). All reported cases have been children. The patches of alopecia are of rapid onset, quickly reaching their greatest extent, and are usually numerous. They seldom exceed 1–2 cm in diameter, and are characteristically irregularly angular in shape. Over the course of a few weeks the hair regrows in most cases, to leave no clinically evident alopecia, but in some patches in some patients cicatricial alopecia results.

Diagnosis. Mycotic infection must be excluded by microscopy and by culture. The multiple bites of insects, scratched and secondarily infected, can give rise to small patches of alopecia, but the history should exclude this diagnosis.

References

Bowen, J.T. (1899) Two epidemics of alopecia areata in an asylum for girls. *Journal of Cutaneous Diseases*, **17**, 1899.
Bowen, J.T. (1915) Epidemic alopecia in small areas. *Journal of Cutaneous Diseases*, **33**, 343.
Davis, H. (1914) Epidemic alopecia areata. *British Journal of Dermatology*, **26**, 207.
Dreuw, H. (1910) Klinische Beobachtungen bei 101 haarkrankten Schulknaber. *Monatsheft für praktische Dermatologie*, **51**, 103.
Heermann (1930) Über Alopecia parvimaculata. *Zentralblatt für Dermatologie*, **32**, 174.
Höfer, W. (1964) Sporadisches Auftreten von Alopecia parvimacularis. *Dermatologische Wochenschrift*, **149**, 381.
Hofmann, E. & Martin, H. (1925) Ueber epidemisch auftretenden klein-fleckigen Haarausfall (Alopecia parvimaculata) *Deutsche medizinsche Wochenschrift*, **51**, 1153.
Loewenthal, L.J.A. & Lurie, H.I. (1956) An outbreak of linear scarring alopecia. *British Journal of Dermatology*, **68**, 88.
Sabouraud, R. (1932) *Diagnostic et Traitement des Affections du Cuir Chevelu*, p. 404. Masson, Paris.

Semon, H.C. (1923) Epidemic alopecia in small areas. *Archives of Dermatology and Syphilology*, **8**, 785.

Lichen planus
(References p. 349)

Aetiology

Lichen planus is a disease or, more probably, a 'reaction pattern', of unknown origin. It accounts for about 1% of new cases referred to departments of dermatology in Europe. It occurs throughout the world, but there are marked regional variations in its incidence and in its clinical manifestations. These variations probably result from relative differences in the importance of various aetiological agents.

A lichenoid eruption with all or most of the pathological and clinical features of lichen planus can be induced by a wide range of drugs (Almeyda & Levantine 1971), including gold, mepacrine (atabrine), para-aminosalicylic acid, aminophenazole, and phenothiazine derivatives. Since only a small proportion of individuals exposed to any of these drugs develop a reaction of this type, it has been suggested that the afflicted are predisposed, perhaps by a congenital deficiency in the epidermis of glucose-6-phosphate dehydrogenase (Cotton *et al.* 1972). The familial incidence of ordinary lichen planus, though unusual, is well recognized (Jadassohn 1953; Depaoli 1970). It is possible that immunological mechanisms will prove to be implicated in some of the many cases without discoverable cause; claims that a virus has been incriminated have not been confirmed. The eruption shows too many clinical, histological and associated disease relationships to be classified as an organ-specific autoimmune disease.

Pathology

The initial abnormality is in the epidermis; fibrillar changes in the basal cells lead to the formation of colloid bodies, and at an early stage these, and macrophages containing pigment, may be seen in the dermis. By immunofluorescence fibrin and IgM may be detected in the upper dermis, and various components of complement in the basement zone (Baart de la Faille Kuyper & Baart de la Faille 1974). The wounded basal cells are continually replaced by the migration of cells from neighbouring normal epidermis (Presbury & Marks 1974).

In the established lesion (Ellis 1967) the horny layer and granular layer are thickened and there is irregular acanthosis. Flattening of the rete pegs gives rise to a saw-tooth configuration. There is liquefaction degeneration of the basal cells. Close up against the epidermis is a dense infiltrate of lymphocytes and some histiocytes. In many sections some colloid bodies can be seen. If the process involves hair follicles the infiltrate extends around them and the hairs are replaced by keratin plugs. The follicles may ultimately be totally destroyed.

Clinical features

Lichen planus occurs at any age, but in over 80% of cases the onset is between 30 and 70 (Altman & Perry 1961). Significant involvement of the scalp is relatively infrequent—only 10 of 807 patients in one series (Altman and Perry 1961)—but the incidence is probably rather higher than such figures suggest since they tend to exclude those patients in whom alopecia, classified as pseudopelade, was the only manifestation of the disease. Scalp involvement occurs in over 40% of patients with either of two unusual variants of lichen planus, the bullous or erosive form and lichen planopilaris (Fig. 11.4). Most patients seen with scalp lesions are middle-aged women, but a girl aged 13 with scarring and follicular keratosis has been reported (Borda *et al.* 1961). The authors have seen eight cases of scarring lichen planus during the years 1981–89; seven were in individuals of Indian extraction, the other being white Caucasoid in type.

Recent scalp lesions may show violaceous papules, erythema and scaling (Borda *et al.* 1961; Sannicandro 1954), but before long, follicular plugs become

Fig. 11.4 Lichen planopilaris. Alopecia occurs in 40% of cases of this unusual form of lichen planus.

conspicuous and scarring replaces all other changes (Figs 11.5, 11.6). Eventually the plugs are shed from the scarred areas which remain white and smooth. If the patch is extending horny plugs may still be present in follicles around its margins.

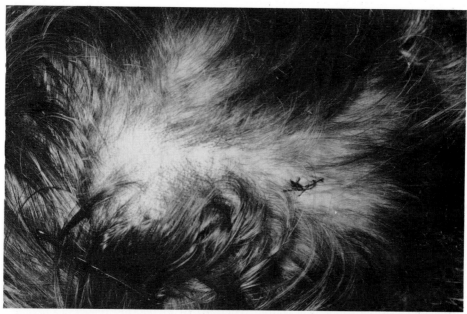

Fig. 11.5 Lichen planus. The conspicuous follicular plugging is a distinctive but inconstant feature.

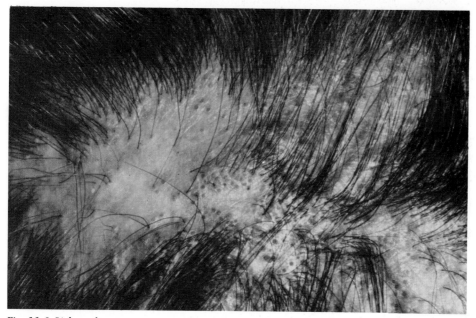

Fig. 11.6 Lichen planus.

More often the scalp lesions are well established by the time the patient attends hospital and the irregular white patches are not clinically diagnostic and may indeed not show any distinctive histological features. This is the clinical picture known as pseudopelade. The diagnosis of lichen planus can be made only in the presence of unquestionable lesions elsewhere and lichen planus histology. These may take the form of bullous lichen planus with shedding of nails (Cram *et al.* 1966), of bullous lesions associated with typical lichen planus of the skin and mucous membranes (Ebner 1973) or of lichen planus of very limited extent involving for example only the nails (Corsi 1937). In some cases of lichen planus of the scalp a presumptive diagnosis has to be based on a history of lichen planus in other sites.

In a clinical syndrome which has caused much controversy (see Graham-Little syndrome) groups of horny follicular papules on the trunk and limbs either precede or follow the development of scarring alopecia. The evidence that this syndrome is at least in many cases a manifestation of lichen planus is based on its occasional association with typical lichen planus (Sachs & de Oreo 1942; Silver *et al.* 1953) and the presence in early lesions of histological changes acceptable as lichen planus (Ellis & Kirby-Smith 1941; Sachs & de Oreo 1942; Spier & Keilig 1953; Waldorf 1966).

The scalp may be involved also in lichenoid eruptions of chemical origin. For example when the hypertrophic plaques of a lichenoid reaction to gold involve the scalp, they are liable to leave permanent scars (Woods 1968) and the scalp is affected in a proportion of lichenoid reactions to mepacrine (Feder 1949).

Prognosis
In some patients the course of lichen planus of the scalp is slow and only a few inconspicuous patches are present after many years. However, particularly if the skin lesions are of bullous or planopilaris type, they may rapidly result in extensive and permanent baldness.

Diagnosis
Except in the rare cases in which classical papular lesions occur in the scalp, the diagnosis is based on the presence of typical lichen planus elsewhere. It follows that in all cases of cicatricial alopecia the whole skin surface and the oral mucosa must be examined. Histological examination may provide confirmatory evidence if the lesions are not of long duration.

Treatment
Drugs or other chemicals causing the reaction must be diligently sought and excluded, with greater hope of success in 'atypical' lichenoid eruptions. In such cases a short course of systemic treatment with a corticosteroid may be desirable. In other cases intra-lesional corticosteroids are helpful but only at a stage when

active inflammatory changes are still present. Potent topical steroids such as clobetasol propionate ointment twice daily may slightly inhibit the process.

References

Almeyda, J. & Levantine, A. (1971) Drug reactions. XVI. Lichenoid drug eruptions. *British Journal of Dermatology*, **85**, 604.

Altman, J. & Perry, H.O. (1961) The variations and course of lichen planus. *Archives of Dermatology*, **84**, 179.

Baart de la Faille Kuyper, E.H. & Baart de la Faille, H. (1974) An immunofluorescence study of lichen planus. *British Journal of Dermatology*, **90**, 365.

Black, M.M. & Wilson Jones, E. (1972) The role of the epidermis in the histopathogenesis of lichen planus. *Archives of Dermatology*, **105**, 81.

Borda, J.M. Mazzini, R.H.E. & Ruiz, D.A. (1961) Liquen del cuero cabelludo. *Archivos argentinos de Dermatologia*, **11**, 257.

Corsi, H. (1937) Atrophy of hair follicle and nail matrix in lichen planus. *British Journal of Dermatology*, **49**, 376.

Cotton, D.W.K. Van den Hurk, J.J.M.A. & Van der Staak, W.B.J.M. (1972) Lichen planus: an inborn error of metabolism. *British Journal of Dermatology*, **87**, 341.

Cram, D.L., Kierland, R.R. & Winkelmann, R.K. (1966) Ulcerative lichen planus of the feet. *Archives of Dermatology*, **93**, 692.

Depaoli, M. (1970) Lichen ruber planus familiare. *Giornale italiano di Dermatologia*, **45**, 1.

Ebner, H. (1973) Lichen ruber planus mit Onychatrophie und narbiger Alopezie. *Dermatologica*, **147**, 219.

Ellis, F.A. & Kirby-Smith, H. (1941) Lichen planus et acuminatus atrophicans (Feldman). *Archives of Dermatology and Syphilology*, **43**, 628.

Ellis, F.A. (1967) Histopathology of lichen planus based on analysis of one hundred biopsy specimens. *Journal of Investigative Dermatology*, **48**, 143.

Feder, A. (1949) Clinical observations on atypical lichen planus and related dermatoses presumably due to atabrine toxicity. *Annals of Internal Medicine*, **31**, 1078.

Jadassohn, W. (1953) Lichen ruber planus familiaris. *Journal de Génétique humaine*, **2**, 153.

Presbury, D.G.C. & Marks, R. (1974) The epidermal disorder in lichen planus: an *in vitro* study. *British Journal of Dermatology*, **90**, 373.

Sachs, W. & de Oreo, W. (1942) Lichen planopilaris. *Archives of Dermatology and Syphilology*, **45**, 1081.

Sannicandro, G. (1954) Études sur le lichen ruber planus typique et atypique ulcéro-érosif, ulcero-hémorragique, scléro-cicatriciel, alopécique et sur ses rapports avec les modifications de la protidopoièse. *Annales de Dermatologie et de Syphiligraphie*, **81**, 380.

Silver, H., Chargin, L. & Sachs, P.M. (1953) Follicular lichen planus (lichen planopilaris). *Archives of Dermatology and Syphilology*, **67**, 346.

Spier, H.W. & Keilig, W. (1953) Lichen ruber follicularis decalvans (Graham-Little Syndrom) und seine Beziehungen zur Pseudopelade Brocq. *Hautarzt*, **4**, 457.

Waldorf, D.S. (1966) Lichen planopilaris. *Archives of Dermatology*, **93**, 684.

Woods, B. (1968) Lichen post-aurique. *Transactions of the St John's Hospital Dermatological Society*, **54**, 118.

Graham-Little syndrome
(References p. 351)

History and nomenclature

In 1915 Graham-Little of London reported the case of a woman aged 55, who had been referred to him by Lassueur of Lausanne. She had suffered for 10 years from slowly progressive cicatricial alopecia and for 5 months from groups of horny papules. Piccardi (1914) had reported a similar case the previous year. Since then many further cases have been reported but the discussion as to whether or not this syndrome is or is not a form of lichen planus is still unresolved after 60 years, although the immunofluorescent findings in typical cases strongly suggested lichen planus (Horn *et al.* 1982). However, whatever its cause or causes the syndrome is distinctive. It is known eponymously and variously as the Graham-Little, Lassueur–Graham-Little, or Piccardi–Lassueur–Little syndrome.

Pathology
In the scalp the mouths of affected follicles are filled by large horny plugs. The underlying follicle is progressively destroyed and eventually an atrophic epidermis covers sclerotic dermis. In the axillae and pubic region the follicles are likewise destroyed, although the skin does not appear clinically to be atrophic.

Clinical features
Most patients have been women between the ages of 30 and 70. The essential features of the syndrome are progressive cicatricial alopecia of the scalp, loss of pubic and axillary hair without clinically evident scarring, and the rapid development of keratosis pilaris (Rongioletti *et al.* 1990). The sequence of events and their relative severity differ widely from case to case.

In most patients the earliest change has been patchy cicatricial alopecia of the scalp. In Graham-Little's (1915) patient, aged 55, the scalp had been affected for about 10 years by what is described as 'an inflammatory process' resulting in bald patches, before she suddenly developed a widespread irritable eruption consisting of horny papules with spine-like projections grouped in well defined plaques on trunk and limbs. In several other patients (e.g. Dore 1915; Beatty & Speares 1915; Pagès *et al.* 1961; McCafferty 1928) the scalp alopecia has preceded the widespread keratosis pilaris by months or years. In Senear's (1920) patient alopecia was present from the age of 9; grouped horny papules of the back and arms developed at 22, then cleared, but recurred at 30. In some patients however (e.g. Reiss *et al.* 1958; Valentino *et al.* 1974) the alopecia and the keratosis pilaris appear to have developed more or less simultaneously, or the keratosis pilaris has preceded the discovery of the alopecia (e.g. Alessi & Dal Pozzo 1968).

The scalp changes are commonly described simply as patches of cicatricial alopecia. Some authors specifically mention associated follicular plugging of the scalp (Reiss *et al.* 1958) and others refer to 'scaly red patches' (Alessi & Dal Pozzo 1968).

The keratosis pilaris is referred to in early case reports of lichen spinulosus, which emphasize that the horny papules are prolonged into conspicuous spines.

In most cases they have developed progressively over a period of weeks or months and have been grouped into plaques, often on the trunk, or on the trunk and limbs, but occasionally involving the eyebrows and the sides of the face. Such a distribution has been noted in a woman aged 69 (Reiss *et al.* 1958), in a man aged 46 (Ormsby 1920) and also in a man aged 22, in whom cicatricial alopecia had been present since the age of 10 (Pagès *et al.* 1961). Pruritus is an inconstant symptom; it was noted in several reported cases and was troublesome in a patient under the author's care (Kubba & Rook 1975).

Thinning and ultimately total loss of pubic and axillary hair has been noted in many cases; other reports fail to mention it.

Treatment

None is known. Surgical treatment may be considered as in other cicatricial alopecias.

References

Alessi, E. & Dal Pozzo, V. (1968) Sindrome di Piccardi–Little–Lassueur. *Giornale Italiano di Dermatologia*, **109**, 493.

Arnozan, X. (1892) Folliculite dépilantes des partier glabres. *Bulletin de la Société Français de Dermatologie et Syphiligraphie*, **3**, 187.

Beatty, W. & Speares, J. (1915) A case of Folliculosis (? Folliculitis) decalvans and lichen spinulosus. *British Journal of Dermatology*, **27**, 331.

Brocq, L., Langlet, E. & Agrinac, J. (1905) Recherches sur alopécie atrophisante, variété pseudopelade. *Annales de Dermatologie et de Syphiligraphie*, **6**, 1, 97, 209.

Dore, S.E. (1915) Lichen spinulosus and folliculitis decalvans. *British Journal of Dermatology*, **27**, 295.

Graham-Little, E.G. (1915) Folliculitis decalvans et atrophicans. *British Journal of Dermatology*, **27**, 183.

Horn, R.T., Goette, D.K., Odom, R.B. *et al.* (1982) Immunofluorescent findings and clinical changes in two cases of follicular lichen planus. *Journal of the American Academy of Dermatology*, **7**, 203.

Kubba, R. & Rook, A. (1975) The Graham-Little syndrome. *British Journal of Dermatology*, **93**, (Suppl. 11), 53.

McCafferty, L.K. (1928) Folliculitis decalvans et atrophicans (Little). *Archives of Dermatology and Syphilology*, **18**, 514.

Ormsby, O. (1920) Folliculitis decalvans and lichen spinulosus. *Archives of Dermatology and Syphilology*, **1**, 471.

Pagès, F., Lapeyre, J. & Misson, R. (1961) Syndrome de Lassueur-Graham-Little. *Annales de Dermatologie et de Syphiligraphie*, **88**, 272.

Piccardi, G. (1914) Cheratosi spinulosa del capillizio a suoi rapporti con al pseudo-pelade di Brocq. *Giornale Italiano della Malattie Veneree e della Pelle*, **49**, 416.

Reiss, F., Reisch, M. & Buncke, C.M. (1958) Keratodermatitis folliculitis decalvans. *Archives of Dermatology*, **78**, 616.

Rongioletti, F., Ghigliotti, G., Gambina, C. & Rebora, A. (1990) Agminate lichen follicularis with cysts and comedones. *British Journal of Dermatology*, **122**, 844.

Senear, F.E. (1920) Folliculitis decalvans and lichen spinulosus. *Archives of Dermatology and Syphilology*, **2**, 198.

Valentino, A., Andreassi, L. & Sbano, E. (1974) Sindrome de Piccardi–Little–Lassueur. *Giornale e Minerva Dermatologica*, **109**, 588.

Scarring follicular keratosis
(References p. 354)

History and nomenclature
Numerous syndromes have been described and elaborately named, all of them characterized by keratosis pilaris, associated with some degree of inflammatory change leading to destruction of the affected follicles (Rand & Arndt 1987).

Only detailed clinical and genetic studies can provide the essential facts to allow reliable differentiation of syndromes which some authorities regard as forms of degrees of a single state and others accept as distinct entities. The reported cases can be temporarily but conveniently classified in three groups, in addition to which certain apparently well-defined entities can be recognized:

1 Atrophoderma vermiculata (acne vermiculata, folliculitis ulerythematosa reticulata): there is honeycomb atrophy of the cheeks. Scarring alopecia may occur, but rarely.

2 Keratosis pilaris atrophicans faciei (ulerythema oophryogenes): the process is more or less confined to the eyebrow region.

3 Keratosis pilaris decalvans (keratosis follicularis spinulosa decalvans, follicular ichthyosis). Keratosis pilaris of variable extent is associated with cicatricial alopecia (Rand & Baden 1983).

Aetiology
All these conditions are assumed to be genetically determined although many cases occur sporadically. Such genetic data as are available are considered under the individual forms.

Pathology
The follicles are initially distended by horny plugs, the dermis is oedematous and there is some lymphocytic infiltration around follicles and vessels. Later the follicles are destroyed. Small epithelial cysts may be numerous, particularly in keratosis pilaris atrophicans faciei.

Clinical features
Atrophoderma vermiculata usually begins in childhood. Follicular plugs, often in the pre-auricular regions, are gradually shed to leave reticulate atrophy. The extent of the process on the face is variable. Exceptionally cicatricial alopecia of the scalp may be associated (Fisher 1957).

Keratosis pilaris atrophicans faciei is present from early infancy. Erythema and horny plugs begin in the outer halves of the eyebrows which they eventually destroy, and then advance medially and to a variable extent on to the cheeks. Involvement of the scalp has apparently not been reported in cases in which the eyebrows are predominantly involved, but there are case histories to which this diagnosis has been applied but which appear to be more rationally classified in one of the other categories in which alopecia has occurred. Such cases emphasize the need for improved diagnostic criteria.

Autosomal dominant inheritance has been reported on several occasions (e.g. Mertens 1968).

Keratosis pilaris decalvans is also such a variable syndrome that several genotypes must be considered. Keratosis pilaris begins in infancy or childhood, often on the face. Its ultimate extent may be confined to the face or to face and limbs, or be more or less universal. It is often succeeded by atrophy on the face, but rarely on the limbs or trunk. Cicatricial alopecia is noted from early childhood or later, and may be localized or extensive.

A brother and sister (Barber 1928) had follicular scars on cheeks and temples, numerous epithelial cysts, keratosis pilaris of limbs and trunk with atrophy in some sites, and cicatricial alopecia of the vertex.

A girl aged 17 with cicatricial alopecia since 3 (Degos & Delzant 1961) had extensive keratosis pilaris of limbs and trunk.

Three members of one family developed keratosis pilaris of the face in early childhood (MacLeod 1909) and then extensively on the back and limbs, and on the scalp where horny papules replaced hairs. Somewhat similar changes were noted in two boys by Zeligman & Fleisher (1959). A similar syndrome was reported (Kubba *et al.* 1975) in a young man who had keratosis pilaris and severe cicatricial alopecia; recurrent attacks of folliculitis of the scalp were controlled by systemic antibiotics. Cockayne (1938) in his notable review of the existing literature attempted to impose some order on the incomplete published case reports. The occurrence of cases similar to those reported by MacLeod (1909) in other siblings, born of normal parents, suggested recessive inheritance but the evidence was incomplete. Other case reports with several of these features are those of Oliver & Gilbert (1926) and of Hadida (1948). The former described two American boys with sparse hair and keratosis pilaris of the scalp. Hadida's patient was an Algerian girl who lost all her hair at the age of 2 months and then grew sparse black, short, brittle hair; she had keratosis pilaris of face, scalp, trunk and limbs. Her eyebrows and eyelashes were normal.

The pattern of hair loss in the family reported by Ullmo (1944) was in the distribution of the Marie-Unna type of congenital alopecia apart from the presence of keratosis pilaris on the face, and mildly on the back and limbs.

Five individuals in three generations of a Finnish family (Kuokkanen 1971) showed in varying degree keratosis pilaris of face, trunk and limbs, cicatricial alopecia, keratoderma of the distal third of palms and soles and corneal dystrophy. The full syndrome was present only in one of the two affected males. In a pedigree reported by Lamaris (cit. Cockayne 1938) in which keratosis follicularis decalvans was associated with corneal dystrophy, sex-linked recessive inheritance was demonstrated. Franceschetti *et al.* (1956) reported a sporadic instance of this association, also in a boy. In a pedigree (Greither 1960) 7 of 13 females in three generations had scalp alopecia progressing from puberty to menopause, complete loss of axillary and pubic hair, prominent keratosis pilaris of scalp and axillae, slight palmoplantar keratoderma, brittle small nails, centrofacial lentiginosis and reduced sweat gland function.

What may be another distinct syndrome associates extremely severe keratosis pilaris—'closely woven keratotic bristles'—with almost complete alopecia, reduced sweating and deafness (Morris *et al.* 1969). An infant which died on the seventh day had the same syndrome (Myers *et al.* 1971).

Also distinct is a sex-linked recessive syndrome (Cantu *et al.* 1974) reported from Mexico in which almost complete absence of hair, eyebrows and eyelashes, and generalized keratosis pilaris are associated with congenital proportionate dwarfism, microcephaly and cerebral atrophy.

Diagnosis

Although the scalp may be involved in Darier's disease, gross loss of hair is exceptional. The Graham-Little syndrome commonly affects middle-aged women. Cicatricial alopecia is associated with follicular horny papules which are usually in well-defined groups and do not develop until after the alopecia has become established. The histological findings will exclude the rare generalized follicular hamartoma.

Treatment

Only symptomatic measures are available. Retinoic acid deserves a trial. The status of oral retinoids remains controversial, though anecdotal response has been noted.

References

Barber, H.W. (1928) Folliculitis erythematosa reticulata combined with lichen spinulosus, epidermal cysts and folliculitis decalvans. *British Journal of Dermatology*, **40**, 24.

Cantu, J.-M., Hernandez, A., Larracilla, J., Trejo, A. & Macotela-Ruiz, E. (1974) A new X-linked recessive disorder with dwarfism, cerebral atrophy, and generalized keratosis follicularis. *Journal of Pediatrics*, **84**, 564.

Cockayne, E.A. (1938) *Inherited Abnormalities of the Skin and its Appendages*, p. 140. Oxford University Press, Oxford.

Degos, R. & Delzant, O. (1961) Keratose pilaire rouge avec large plaque d'alopécie atrophiante. *Bulletin de la Société française de Dermatologie et de Syphiligraphie*, **68**, 688.

Fisher, A.A. (1957) Keratosis pilaris rubra atrophicans faciei with diffuse alopecia of the scalp. *Archives of Dermatology*, **75**, 283.

Franceschetti, A., Rossano, R., Jadassohn, W. & Paillard, R. (1956) Keratosis follicularis spinulosa decalvans. *Dermatologica*, **112**, 512.

Greither, A. (1960) Über drei Generationen vererbte, auf Frauen beschränkte Keratosis follicularis mit Alopecie, Hypidrose und abortiven Palmar-Plantar-Keratosen in ihren Beziehungen zur Hypotrichosis congenita hereditaria. *Archiv für klinische und experimentelle Dermatologie*, **210**, 123.

Hadida, E. (1948) Hypoplasie congénitale des cheveux. *L'Algérie médicale*, **51**, 115.

Kubba, R., Mitchell, J.N.S. & Rook, A. (1975) Keratosis pilaris with recurrent folliculitis decalvans. *British Journal of Dermatology*, **93** (Suppl. 11), 55.

Kuokkanen, K. (1971) Keratosis follicularis spinulosa decalvans, in a family from northern Finland. *Acta Dermato-Venereologica*, **51**, 146.

MacLeod, J.M.H. (1909) Three cases of 'Ichthyosis follicularis' associated with baldness. *British Journal of Dermatology*, **21**, 165.

Mertens, R.L.J. (1968) Ulerythema ophryogenes and atopy. *Archives of Dermatology*, **97**, 662.

Morris, J., Ackerman, A.B. & Koblenzer, P.J. (1969) Generalized spiny hyperkeratosis, universal alopecia and deafness. *Archives of Dermatology*, **100**, 692.

Myers, E.N., Stool, S.E. & Koblenzer, P.J. (1971) Congenital deafness, spiny hyperkeratosis and universal alopecia. *Archives of Otolaryngology (Chicago)*, **93**, 68.

Oliver, E.A. & Gilbert, N.C. (1962) Congenital alopecia. *Archives of Dermatology and Syphilology*, **13**, 359.

Rand, R.E. & Arndt, K.A. (1987) Follicular syndromes with inflammation and atrophy. In *Dermatology in General Medicine*, 3rd edn., p. 717. McGraw-Hill, New York.

Rand, R.E. & Baden, H. (1983) Keratosis follicularis spinulosa decalvans: report of two cases and review of the literature. *Archives of Dermatology*, **119**, 22.

Ullmo, A. (1944) Un nouveau type d'agénésie et de dystrophie pilaire familiale et héréditaire. *Dermatologica*, **90**, 74.

Zeligman, I. & Fleisher, T.C. (1959) Ichthyosis follicularis. *AMA Archives of Dermatology*, **80**, 413.

Cicatricial pemphigoid (benign mucosal pemphigoid/ocular pemphigus)
(References p. 356)

Aetiology
Cicatricial pemphigoid affects predominantly the elderly, and women more than men (Pearson 1977).

Pathology
Bullae are formed beneath the intact epidermis (Susi & Sklar 1971). Direct immunocytochemical studies show linear deposits of IgG, IgA, C_3 and C_4 may be found in the basement membrane zone, but circulating basement membrane zone antibodies (IgG or IgA) are not always demonstrable (Bean & Michel 1973; Holubar *et al.* 1973).

Clinical features (Leenutaphong *et al.* 1989)
The skin is involved in 40–50% of cases, and the disease affects predominantly the ocular and/or genital mucous membrane. However, the skin lesions may precede the mucosal lesions by months or years.

The skin lesions are usually confined to a limited area within which bullae repeatedly recur, leaving a dense scar. The favoured sites are the face, and in particular the scalp (Slepyan *et al.* 1961; Honeyman *et al.* 1980). Skin lesions, predominantly on the head and neck, are the major feature of the Brunsting–Perry variant.

Diagnosis
The bullae and the frequently associated mucosal lesions differentiate the scalp lesions from other forms of cicatricial alopecia. Immunofluorescence histology is helpful.

Treatment

Management will often be dictated by the need to control mucosal lesions. If recurrent bullae in a localized area of skin are troublesome, excision and grafting may be successful (Slepyan *et al.* 1961); whether to prescribe oral corticosteroids or immunosuppressive drugs for skin lesions alone is controversial but topical clobetasol propionate cream may inhibit the process to some degree.

References

Bean, S.F. & Michel, B. (1973) Cicatricial pemphigoid. In *Immunopathology of the Skin. Labeled Antibody Studies*, p. 55, eds. E.H. Beutner, T.P. Chorzelski, S.F. Bean & R.G. Jordon. Dowde Hutchings & Rees, Stroudsburg.

Holubar, K., Hönigsmann, H. & Wolff, K. (1973) Cicatricial pemphigoid. *Archives of Dermatology*, **108**, 50.

Honeyman, J., Navarrette, W., De le Parra, M.A. & Pinto, A. (1980) Pemfigoid cicatricial cutaneo localizado en cabeza y cuello (Brunsting-Perez). *Archivos Argentinos de Dermatologia*, **30**, 135.

Leenutaphong, V., vonKries, R. & Plewig, G. (1989) Localised cicatricial pemphigoid (Brunsting–Perry): electron microscopic study. *Journal of the American Academy of Dermatology*, **21**, 1089.

Pearson, R.W. (1977) Advances in the diagnosis and treatment of blistering diseases: a selective review. In *Year Book of Dermatology*, p. 7, eds. F. Malkinson & R.W. Pearson. Year Book Publ., Chicago.

Slepyan, A.H., Burks, J.W. & Fox, J. (1961) Persistent denudation of the scalp in cicatricial pemphigoid. Treatment by skin grafting. *Archives of Dermatology*, **84**, 444.

Susi, F.R. & Sklar, G. (1971) Histochemistry and fine structure of oral lesions of mucous membrane pemphigoid. *Archives of Dermatology*, **104**, 244.

Erosive pustular dermatosis of the scalp
(References p. 357)

Aetiology

This clinical entity (Pye *et al.* 1979) has so far been reported only in women over 70 years of age. Its cause is unknown but there is no evidence that it is primarily infective in origin, though Gratton *et al.* (1988) suggested that local trauma and sun-damage are important in their study of twelve cases.

Pathology

Histological examination shows atrophy, some parakeratosis, and areas of epidermal erosion. A chronic inflammatory infiltration in the dermis consists predominantly of lymphocytes and plasma cells. Small foci of foreign body giant cells may be seen where hair follicles have been destroyed.

Clinical features

Initially a small area of scalp becomes red and crusted and may be irritable. On examination crusting and superficial pustulation overlie a moist eroded surface (Fig. 11.7). As the condition extends areas of activity co-exist with areas of cicatricial alopecia. There is little or no tendency to spontaneous cure. Squamous carcinoma has developed in the scars (Lovell *et al.* 1980).

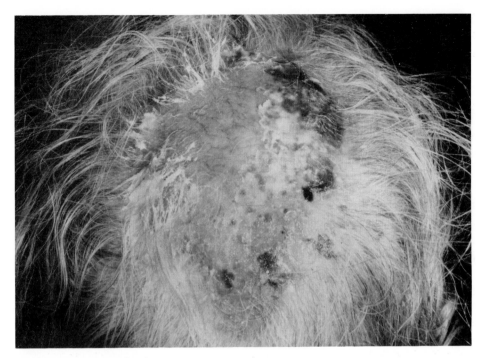

Fig. 11.7 Erosive pustular dermatosis.

Differential diagnosis
Pyogenic and yeast infection is excluded by bacteriological examination and the lack of response to antibacterial or antifungal agents. Biopsy may be necessary to exclude pustular psoriasis, cicatricial pemphigoid, 'irritated' solar keratosis or squamous carcinoma. The cases described by Jacyk (1988) in young African patients would seem to be of different aetiology, possibly pyoderma gangrenosum.

Treatment
The stronger topical corticosteroids such as 0.05% clobetasol propionate will suppress the inflammatory changes. Ikeda *et al.* (1983) suggested oral zinc sulphate can be curative in some cases.

References

Grattan, C.E.H., Peachey, R.D. & Boon, A. (1988) Evidence for a role of local trauma in the pathogenesis of erosive pustular dermatosis of the scalp. *Clinical and Experimental Dermatology*, **13**, 7.

Ikeda, M., Arata, J. & Isaka, H. (1983) Erosive pustular dermatosis of the scalp successfully treated with oral zinc sulphate. *British Journal of Dermatology*, **105**, 742.

Jacyk, W.K. (1988) Pustular erosive dermatitis of the scalp. *British Journal of Dermatology*, **118**, 441.

Lovell, C.R., Harman, R.R.M. & Bradfield, J.W.B. (1980) Cutaneous carcinoma arising in erosive pustular dermatosis of the scalp. *British Journal of Dermatology*, **102**, 325.

Pye, R.J., Peachey, R.D.G. & Burton, J.L. (1979) Erosive pustular dermatosis of the scalp. *British Journal of Dermatology*, **100**, 559.

Cicatricial alopecia resulting from physical trauma
(References p. 359)

The diagnosis and treatment of the consequences of physical injuries of the scalp will seldom confront the dermatologist, but he may be consulted as to the cause of an apparent physical injury, for example aplasia cutis may be falsely attributed to a forceps injury at childbirth.

The attachment of an electrode to the scalp for monitoring the foetal heartbeat during labour may occasionally cause some superficial damage to the scalp and, particularly if secondary infection supervenes, this may be followed by a small scar. Aplasia cutis has sometimes been mistaken for such a lesion (Brown *et al.* 1977).

An unusual case of cicatricial alopecia in a boy aged 13 was due to injury to the scalp by an intravenous infusion given in infancy for gastroenteritis (Strong 1979).

Exceptionally, self-inflicted injuries may involve the scalp and may leave scars (Fig. 11.8).

See also Chapter 9.

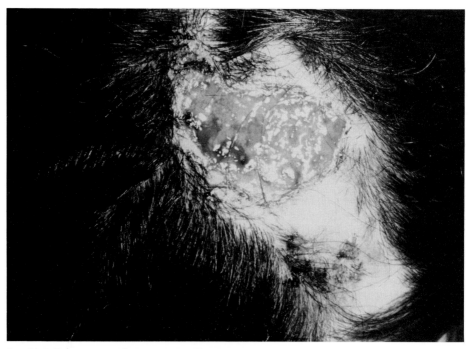

Fig. 11.8 Dermatitis artefacta—erosions becoming scars.

References

Brown, Z.A., Jung, A.L. & Stenehuver, M.A. (1977) Aplasia cutis congenita and the fetal scalp electrode. *American Journal of Obstetrics and Gynecology,* **129**, 351.

Strong, A.M.M.M. (1979) Extensive cicatricial alopecia following a scalp vein infusion. *Clinical and Experimental Dermatology,* **4**, 197.

Halo scalp ring. A type of alopecia which may be temporary or permanent, is an area of scalp hair loss due to prolonged pressure on the vertex by the uterine cervix during or prior to delivery, resulting in a haemorrhagic form of caput succedaneum.

Scalp necrosis after surgical embolization. Adler *et al.* (1986) described a case in which ischaemic necrosis of the occipital scalp occurred following embolization and surgery for a large convexity meningioma.

References

Adler, J.R., Upton, J., Wallman, J. & Winston, K.R. (1986) Management and prevention of necrosis of the scalp after embolization and surgery for meningioma. *Surgery and Neurology,* **25**, 357.

Prendiville, J.S. & Esterly, N.B. (1987) Halo scalp ring: a cause of scarring alopecia. *Archives of Dermatology,* **123**, 992.

Chronic radiodermatitis
(References p. 361)

History (Albert & Omran 1968; Getzrow 1976)

Roentgen discovered X-rays in 1895. The first carcinoma of the skin attributable to X-rays was reported 7 years later. X-ray epilation of the face for hirsutism was frequently employed during the first two decades of the 20th century, and although Schultz, an international authority, condemned this treatment as early as 1912, it continued to be used irresponsibly to such an extent that in 1947 Cipollaro & Einhorn entitled their paper on this subject 'The use of X-rays for the treatment of hypertrichosis is dangerous'.

X-ray epilation for the treatment of scalp ringworm was introduced by Sabouraud in 1904 and the technique was improved and standardized by Kienbock and by Adamson. The discovery of griseofulvin in 1958 gradually made X-ray epilation unnecessary, but it has been estimated that between 1904 and 1959 some 300,000 children throughout the world were treated with X-rays for ringworm of the scalp. The Kienbock–Adamson technique, strictly followed, did not cause clinically evident chronic cutaneous damage. However, technical errors were frequent, particularly in the early days, from inadequate and poorly calibrated apparatus. The object of the technique was to divide the scalp into five fields and give to each 300–400 rads at 75–100 kV. This produced complete epilation in about 3 weeks and regrowth after 2 months. The most frequent mistake to be made in carrying out X-ray epilation was to allow overlap of the fields so that certain areas of the scalp received double the intended dose. The follow-up of 2,043 patients treated in childhood showed a higher incidence of cancer and of mental illness in the patients than in a control group (Albert & Omran 1968).

Radiodermatitis of the scalp may occur also as an unavoidable consequence of skin damage during the treatment of internal malignant disease and also inevitably occurs when malignant disease of the skin is treated.

Pathology

The use of X-rays for epilation depends on the high susceptibility of anagen hairs to radiation. Epilating and sub-epilating doses produced dystrophic changes in human hairs as early as the 4th day after exposure (Van Scott & Reinertson 1957). Unfortunately the dose required to produce permanent epilation inevitably produces atrophy and telangiectasia. Doses of 500–800 rads produced in 20% of subjects a generalized reduction of the follicle population of the scalp and a reduction in follicle size (Albert *et al.* 1968).

Chronic radiodermatitis may follow acute radiodermatitis but may develop only slowly as degenerative changes induced by sun-exposure and ageing are superimposed on those directly due to the ionizing radiation.

In chronic radiodermatitis the epidermis is generally atrophic with loss of hair follicles and sebaceous glands but there are also irregular areas of acanthosis. Degenerative changes and nuclear abnormalities are frequent in the epidermis. Dermal collagen stains irregularly. Superficial small vessels are telangiectatic but deeper vessels are partially or completely occluded by fibrosis. The unstable anaplastic epidermis readily gives rise to keratoses and to squamous or basal cell carcinomas. The occlusive vascular changes may result in necrosis.

Clinical features (Fig. 11.9)

Chronic radiodermatitis of the scalp may present clinically in a number of different ways. The development of a basal cell carcinoma in middle-age or later in a still hairy area of the scalp should lead the dermatologist to enquire about X-ray epilation for ringworm in childhood (Anderson & Anderson 1951; Ridley 1962). Patients sometimes refer to this as 'light treatment'. Sometimes the area of the scalp around the lesion may show sparser and finer hairs than the rest of the scalp, and there may be evident atrophy and telangiectasia.

In other cases the patient complains of ordinary baldness which is apparently accentuated in certain areas and these areas are found to show both common baldness and reduction of follicle population as a result of the earlier radiation. If the initial dose of radiation was large enough to produce acute radiodermatitis this is rapidly followed by chronic radiodermatitis.

Chronic radiodermatitis produced by radiation therapy of a malignant tumour of the scalp presents a circumscribed area of cicatricial alopecia.

In chronic radiodermatitis of any region, but particularly when the dosage

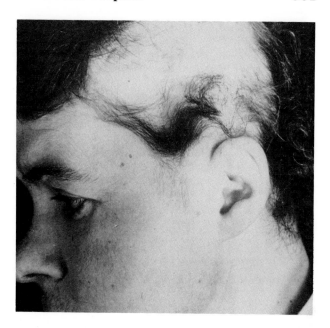

Fig. 11.9 Cicatricial alopecia as a sequel to X-ray epilation of the scalp for ringworm.

was high, as in the treatment of a malignant tumour, late radiation necrosis may occur (Traenkle & Mulay 1960). Exposure to sunlight and to cold may precipitate necrosis in an area of skin with a blood supply already precarious. Radiation necrosis is an important condition for it may simulate a recurrence of carcinoma but the edges of the necrotic ulcer are not raised. The diagnosis should be confirmed by a biopsy. Superficial X-ray of Grenz ray type, used in many countries for treating scalp psoriasis, does not penetrate deeply enough to damage scalp follicles.

Treatment

For alopecia of chronic radiodermatitis there is no treatment unless the affected area is small enough to be covered by a graft. Malignant tumours arising in radiodermatitis should be excised, preferably by a plastic surgeon (Conway & Hugo 1966).

References

Albert, R.E. & Omran, A.R. (1968) Follow-up study of patients treated X-ray epilation for tinea capitis. I. Population characteristics, posttreatment illness and mortality experience. *Archives of Environmental Health*, **17**, 899.

Albert, R.E., Omran, A.R., Brauer, E.W., Cohen, N.C., Schmidt, H., Dove, D.C., Becker, M., Baumring, R. & Baer, R.L. (1968) II. Results of clinical and laboratory examination. *Archives of Environmental Health*, **17**, 919.

Anderson, N.P. & Anderson, H.P. (1951) Development of basal cell epithelioma as a consequence of radiodermatitis. *Archives of Dermatology and Syphilology*, **63**, 586.

Cipollaro, A.C. & Einhorn, M.B. (1947) The use of X-rays for the treatment of hypertrichosis is dangerous. *Journal of the American Medical Association*, **135**, 349.

Conway, H. & Hugo, N.E. (1966) Radiation dermatitis and malignancy. *Plastic and Reconstructive Surgery*, **38**, 255.

Getzrow, P.L. (1976) Chronic radiodermatitis and skin cancer. In *Cancer of the Skin*, p. 458, eds. R. Andrade, S.L. Gumport, G.L. Popkin & T.D. Rees. Saunders, Philadelphia.

Ridley, C.M. (1962) Basal-cell carcinoma following X-ray epilation of the scalp. *British Journal of Dermatology*, **74**, 222.

Schultz, F. (1912) *The X-ray Treatment of Skin Diseases*, p. 139. Rebman, London.

Traenkle, H.L. & Mulay, D. (1960) Further observations on late radiation necrosis following therapy of skin cancer. *Archives of Dermatology*. **81**, 988.

Van Scott, E.J. & Reinertson, R.P. (1957) Detection of radiation effects on hair roots of the human scalp. *Journal of Investigative Dermatology*. **29**, 205.

Necrobiosis lipoidica
(References p. 363)

Necrobiosis occurs in 0.2–0.3% of cases of diabetes mellitus, and approximately 70% of patients with necrobiosis have diabetes. The diabetic cases begin in childhood or early adult life and the non-diabetic cases rather later and usually in women.

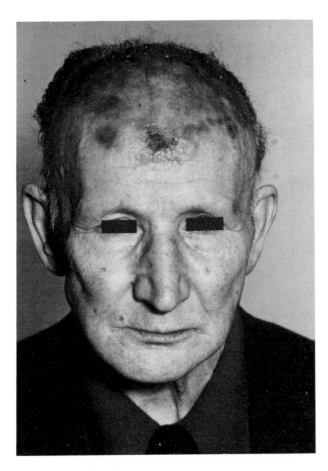

Fig. 11.10 Necrobiosis lipoidica of forehead and anterior scalp margin.

The oval atrophic plaques classically occur on the shins but may be seen in other parts of the body including the scalp. The patches are glazed and yellowish, often with conspicuous telangiectases. Scarring may be dense. The clinical features in the scalp have varied from large plaques of cicatricial alopecia (Gaethe 1964) to multiple small areas of scarring resembling the clinical entity described as 'alopecia parvimaculata' (Gartmann & Dickmans-Burmeister 1969).

An atrophic form affecting predominantly the forehead and the scalp has been described (Wilson Jones 1971; Navaratnan & Hodgson 1973). It occurs mainly in women and in middle-age. The earliest onset was at 25. Round or oval lesions appear on the forehead and the scalp margins; when they invade the scalp there may be little or no alopecia. There may be similar patches in other parts of the body. The degree of atrophy is slight. The edge is slightly raised; the centre is at first red but becomes brown or depigmented (Fig. 11.10).

In general the differential diagnosis is from sarcoidosis (Maurice & Goolamali 1988).

References

Gaethe, G. (1964) Necrobiosis lipoidica diabeticorum of the scalp. *Archiv für Dermatologie und Syphilologie*, **89**, 865.

Gertmann, H. & Dickmans-Burmeister, D. (1969) Ungewöhnliche Hautveränderungen bei einem 4 jahrigen Kinde mit Diabetes mellitus, 'Nekrobiosis diabetica acute parvimaculata'. *Hautarzt*, **20**, 265.

Navaratnan, A. & Hodgson, G.A. (1973) Necrobiosis lipoidica presenting on the face and scalp. *British Journal of Dermatology*, **89** (Suppl. 9), 100.

Wilson Jones, E. (1971) Necrobiosis lipoidica presenting on the face and scalp. *Transactions of the St John's Hospital Dermatological Society*, **57**, 202.

Maurice, D.D.L. & Goolamali, S.K. (1988) Sarcoidosis of the scalp presenting a scarring alopecia. *British Journal of Dermatology*, **119**, 116.

Circumscribed scleroderma
(Reference p. 365)

Circumscribed scleroderma is rare in the scalp, but may occur there as a single or multiple lesions. Females are affected almost three times more frequently than males with an age range from 10–30.

The early stages of morphoea are rarely seen in the scalp unless a bald area is affected. Morphoea appears as a lilac macule which slowly extends centrifugally. The centre becomes pearly or ivory white, smooth and shining and attached to deeper structures. A lilac ring persists as long as active extension is taking place. Morphoea tends to regress spontaneously after 3–5 years, but the plaque may continue to enlarge for much longer periods. The hair is shed at an early stage to leave a cicatricial alopecia (Fig. 11.11), which may show no distinctive features, but the diagnosis may be suggested by the presence of morphoea in other parts of the body (Fig. 11.12). The diagnosis must be confirmed histologically.

Linear circumscribed morphoea in the frontal region—'en coup de sabre'

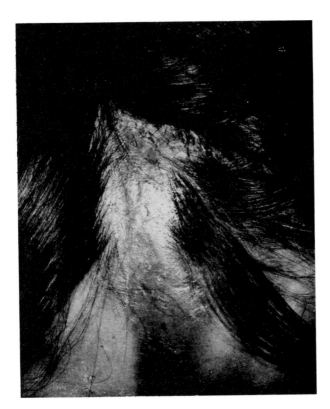

Fig. 11.11 Cicatricial alopecia at an early stage of facial hemiatrophy.

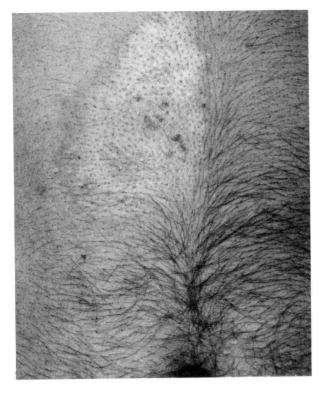

Fig. 11.12 A plaque of morphoea of the abdominal wall showing loss of hair in the affected area.

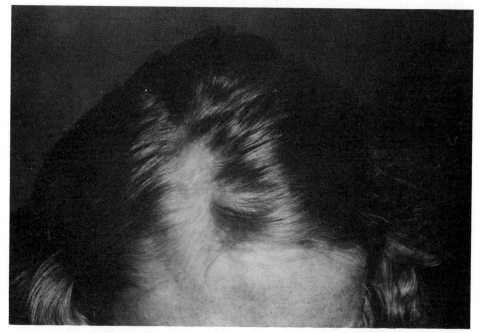

Fig. 11.13 Paramedian circumscribed scleroderma, 'en coup de sabre' morphoea.

from its fancied resemblance to the scar of a sabre cut—may be associated with facial hemiatrophy. Paramedian greying or loss of hairs may be the earliest sign; soon the lesion's scar-like structure is apparent (Fig. 11.13). If hemiatrophy supervenes facial asymmetry is usually apparent within 1 year.

Recently Hulsmans *et al.* (1986) described a case of 'en coup de sabre' morphoea associated with hereditary deficiency complement C2.

Reference

Hulsmans, R.F.H.J., Asghar, S.S., Siddiqui, A.H. & Cormane, R.H. (1986) Hereditary deficiency of C2 in association with linear scleroderma 'en coup de sabre'. *Archives of Dermatology*, **122**, 76.

Lichen sclerosus et atrophicus
(References p. 366)

The relatively uncommon disease affects females ten times more often than males. It involves the vulva only, or the vulva and perineum in a high proportion of women (Wallace 1972), but lesions may also be present on the trunk or limbs, and in some cases such sites may be affected in the absence of genital lesions.

Lichen sclerosus of the scalp appears to be rare. In one case (Foulds 1980), in an elderly woman, it caused extensive cicatricial alopecia (Fig. 11.14). The scalp lesions were pruritic. There were also lesions of the trunk and of the vulva.

The diagnosis must be established histologically.

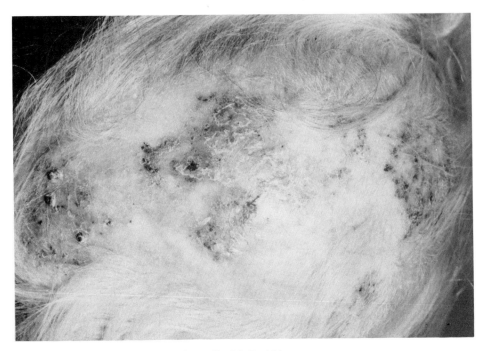

Fig. 11.14 Lichen sclerosus et atrophicus (Dr I.S. Foulds).

References

Foulds, I.S. (1980) Lichen sclerosus et atrophicus of the scalp. *British Journal of Dermatology*, **103**, 197.
Wallace, H.J. (1972) Lichen sclerosus et atrophicus. *Transactions of the St John's Hospital Dermatological Society*, **57**, 148.

Porokeratosis of Mibelli
(References p. 367)

This is a rare disorder of keratinization characterized by extending plaques of hyperkeratosis succeeded by atrophy. The rapid extension of a previously minimal lesion in a patient receiving immunosuppressive agents, suggested that in porokeratosis there is a mutant clone of cells in the epidermis, the proliferation of which is normally controlled by immune processes (Macmillan & Roberts 1974). There is also evidence of chromosomal instability of fibroblasts from affected areas of skin (Taylor *et al.* 1973). Most cases are sporadic but some pedigrees show autosomal dominant inheritance.

Histologically the lesion shows hyperkeratosis and irregular acanthosis, penetrated by a furrow filled by a dense horny plug with a column of parakeratotic cells in its centre. Serial sections may be needed to identify this diagnostic feature, the 'cornoid' lamella.

Porokeratosis of Mibelli commonly begins in childhood (Saunders 1961) but may first appear at any age. It is most frequent on limbs, particularly the hands and feet, the neck, the shoulders and the face but may occur anywhere including the scalp (Savage & Lederer 1952; Sehgal & Dube 1967). The initial lesion is a crateriform horny papule which gradually extends to form a circinate or irregular atrophic plaque with a raised horny margin which may be surmounted by a furrow from which the lamina of horn projects. In the scalp there is loss of hair in the atrophic phase. Squamous carcinoma (Court & Abdel-Aziz 1972) may occur in porokeratosis as early as the third decade and these patients should therefore be kept under regular supervision if excision and grafting are not practicable. Individual lesions of porokeratosis respond well to cryosurgery but this may itself cause alopecia on areas with coarse hair.

References

Cort, D.F. & Abdel-Aziz, A.H.M. (1972) Epithelioma arising in porokeratosis of Mibelli. *British Journal of Plastic Surgery*, **25**, 318.

Macmillan, A.L. & Roberts, S.O.B. (1974) Porokeratosis of Mibelli. *British Journal of Dermatology*, **90**, 45.

Saunders, T.S. (1961) Porokeratosis. *Archives of Dermatology*, **84**, 98.

Savage, J. & Lederer, H. (1952) Porokeratosis (Mibelli). *British Journal of Dermatology*, **63**, 187.

Sehgal, V.M. & Dube, B. (1967) Porokeratosis (Mibelli) in a family. *Dermatologica*, **134**, 269.

Taylor, A.M.R., Harnden, D.G. & Fairburn, E.A. (1973) Chromosomal instability associated with susceptibility to malignant disease in patients with porokeratosis of Mibelli. *Journal of the National Cancer Institute*, **51**, 371.

Cicatricial alopecia in hereditary syndromes

Incontinentia pigmenti (References p. 368)

This rare syndrome occurs almost exclusively in females; its inheritance is probably determined by an X-linked gene, usually lethal in the male (Carney & Carney 1970; Gordon & Gordon 1970).

Cicatricial alopecia has been present in at least 25% of reported cases; it appears in early infancy and ceases to extend after a variable period of up to 2 years, but the loss of hair is of course permanent. Other hair defects present in some cases have been hypoplasia of the eyebrows and eyelashes and woolly-hair naevus of the scalp (Wiklund & Weston 1960).

The diagnosis is based on the skin lesions which occur in three overlapping phases. The first phase, which begins soon after birth, consists of erythema and bullae; after 3–5 months these are succeeded by hypertrophic warty papules which may be present for several months, to be succeeded in turn by a bizarre pattern of pigmentation which gives the syndrome its name, and which eventually fades. Dental and ocular anomalies are frequent.

Confusion in diagnosis is largely terminological. The name incontinentia pigmenti is best reserved for the present syndrome, associated with the names of

Bloch and Sulzberger. It is sometimes applied also to the two different pigmentary syndromes associated respectively with the names of Naegele and of Ito.

References
Carney, R.G. & Carney, R.G. Jr. (1970) Incontinentia pigmenti. *Archives of Dermatology*, **102**, 157.
Gordon, H. & Gordon, W. (1970) Incontinentia pigmenti: clinical and genetical studies of two familial cases. *Dermatologica*, **140**, 150.
Wiklund, D.A. & Weston, W.L. (1960) Incontinentia pigmenti. *Archives of Dermatology*, **115**, 701.

Generalized follicular hamartoma

Cicatricial alopecia, beginning in childhood was a feature of a syndrome described by Mehregan & Hardin (1973).

Their patient was a woman aged 23. From infancy she had widespread horny plugs over the trunk and limbs and small pits on the palms and soles. She later developed cicatricial alopecia, in which, from the age of 8, appeared follicular tumours.

The tumours of the scalp were proliferating tricholemmal cysts. The lesions of palms and soles showed funnel-shaped dilatation of sweat ducts, which were plugged with parakeratotic material containing acid mucopolysaccharide.

Ridley and Smith (1981) described this entity associated with alopecia and myasthenia gravis.

References
Mehregan, A.H. & Hardin, I. (1973) Generalized follicular hamartoma. *Archives of Dermatology*, **107**, 435.
Ridley, C.M. & Smith, N.P. (1981) Generalized hair follicle hamartoma associated with alopecia and myasthenia gravis. *Clinical and Experimental Dermatology*, **6**, 283.

Epidermolysis bullosa (References p. 369)

History and nomenclature
The term epidermolysis bullosa is applied to a group of distinct genetically determined disorders characterized by the formation of bullae of skin, and often also of mucous membranes, in response to trauma or spontaneously. Only one of these diseases is accompanied by abnormalities of scalp or hair—recessive dystrophic epidermolysis bullosa; however, Gambrog-Nielsen and Sjolund (1985) described a new syndrome of localized epidermis bullosa simplex associated with hair, nail and teeth abnormalities.

Histopathology
Bullae form at the dermo-epidermal junction and fragments of dermis may adhere to the roof.

Clinical features

The inexorable blistering of skin and mucous membranes dominates the picture. The blisters are followed by atrophic scarring. This may give rise to more or less extensive cicatricial alopecia of the scalp (Wagner 1956). In addition the hair generally may be fine and sparse (Vuorinen 1970).

In many case reports the state of the hair is not mentioned. Of 30 cases studied by Videl (1974) three had cicatricial alopecia.

References

Gambrog-Nielsen, P. & Sjolund, E. (1985) Epidermolysis bullosa simplex localisation associated with anodontia, hair and nail abnormalities. *Acta Dermato-Venereologica*, **65**, 526.

Videl, J. (1974) Epidermolisis ampollares. *Actas Dermo-Sifiliograficas*, **65**, 3.

Vuorinen, E. (1970) Über ein Zwillingspaar mit Epidermolysis bullosa dystrophica polydysplastica. *Dermatologica*, **140** (Suppl. II), 3.

Wagner, W. (1956) Alopezia und Nagelveränderungen bei Epidermolysis bullosa hereditaria. *Zeitschrift für Haut und Geschlechtskrankheiten*, **20**, 278.

Cleft lip–palate, ectodermal dysplasia and syndactyly

Aetiology

This rare, or rarely recognized syndrome is probably hereditary, and determined by an autosomal recessive gene.

Clinical features

The constant features of the syndrome are mental retardation, cleft palate, genital hypoplasia, cicatricial alopecia and defective teeth. Other features include syndactyly.

Reference

Brown, P. & Armstrong, H.B. (1976) Ectodermal dysplasia, mental retardation, cleft lip/palate and other anomalies in three sibs. *Clinical Genetics*, **9**, 35.

Polyostotic fibrous dysplasia

The progressive enlargement over a period of 10 years of a bald patch present since childhood was shown histologically to be due to the replacement of the follicles by coils of fibrous tissue. The patient had polyostotic fibrous dysplasia (Shelley & Wood 1976).

Reference

Shelley, L.B. & Wood, M.G. (1976) Alopecia with fibrous dysplasia and osteoma of the skin. *Archives of Dermatology*, **112**, 715.

Chapter 12
The Colour of the Hair

Normal hair colour
(Zviak & Dawber 1986; Prunieras 1986; Bolognia & Pawelek 1988)
(References p. 380)

Melanin literally means black but scientists have long used the term to describe a range of pigments from yellow to black (Robin 1873). Animal biologists usually define melanin as pigment derived from the melanophore, the melanocyte. The superficial structures of most vertebrates contain such melanin pigments—skin, hair, scales and feathers.

If one is to understand and study the nature of the basic mechanisms that regulate pigmentation in man, one should consider the process in sequence (Prunieras 1986).

Four major classes of factors regulate mammalian melanin pigmentation:

1 those regulating the number and position of melanocytes in the hair and skin;

2 those regulating tyrosinase and melanin synthesis;

3 those governing the morphology and distribution of melanosomes in melanocytes; and

4 factors modulating the transfer of melanosomes from melanocytes to keratinocytes and the distribution of melanomes in the latter cells.

Genetic and epigenetic factors are operative in controlling all of these stages and many of the disease states to be described later in this chapter show examples of specific defects within this overall scheme of events.

In man, hair pigmentation depends entirely on the presence of melanin from melanocytes, but the actual colour perceived may sometimes also depend on physical phenomena. The range of colours produced by melanins is limited to shades of grey, yellow, brown, red and black. In contrast, many lower animals display colours due to such pigments as porphyrins and carotenoids in addition to melanins (Munro Fox & Vevers 1960).

It is important to remember that much of the research done on melanogenesis and its cellular control is in relation to cells in other epithelial surfaces, mainly the epidermis. There is no reason to believe that the biochemical events in hair bulb melanocytes are different and the work that has been carried out suggests that they are similar.

Melanin chemistry

Many problems remain to be resolved regarding the structure of natural melanins. They usually exist bound to protein and cannot be solubilized without degradation. They bind various other substances avidly thus making purification and exact chemical analysis difficult, and X-ray diffraction patterns cannot be obtained. This implies that melanins do not form crystal structures and furthermore suggests that they are mixtures of related but dissimilar molecules which are likely to result at least partly from a chemical condensation rather than from a purely enzyme-catalysed reaction (Mier and Cotton 1976).

The whole range of human hair colour is due to two types of melanin; eumelanins, which are mainly black and brown hair, and phaeomelanins, which are yellow or red and give auburn and blonde hair. Figure 12.1 shows their suggested sub-unit structure (Riley 1974). Whatever the hair colour seen by the eye, isolated melanin is brown in colour and gives a dark brown solution in aqueous alkaline hydrogen peroxide (Arnaud and Bore 1981).

Eumelanins

These appear to be polymers of irregular structure often occurring conjugated to proteins. They are insoluble in almost all solvents, resist chemical treatment and lack well-defined spectral and other physical characteristics. Eumelanins are derived from tyrosine, dopa and perhaps, dopamine (Fig. 12.2).

In the presence of the enzyme tyrosinase and molecular oxygen, via various intermediates, melanin is produced (Mason 1948; Lerner & Fitzpatrick 1950). The exact status of tyrosinase in man remains controversial (Jimbow & Kukita 1971). In the melanin biosynthetic pathway, tyrosinase plays an important regulatory role—in skin its level of activity usually correlates with the degree of pigment produced (Lerner & Fitzpatrick 1950). Several forms of tyrosinase have been described, differing primarily in their cellular localization and patterns of

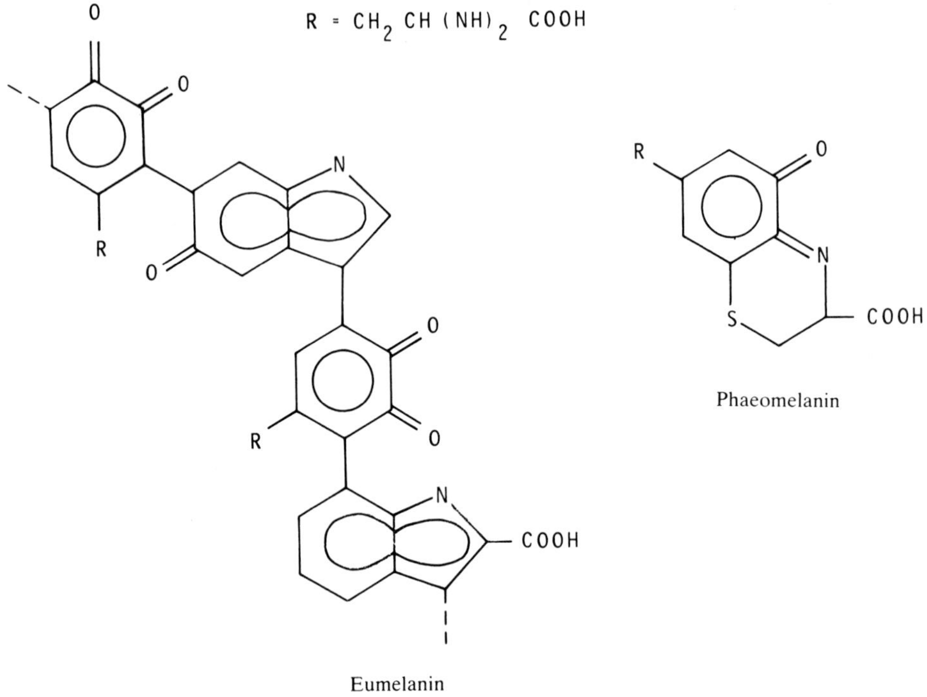

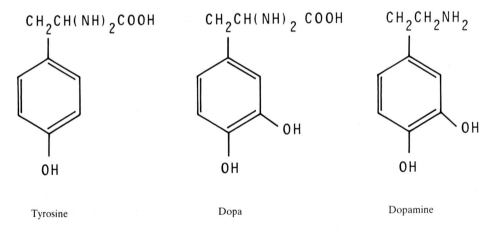

R = CH2 CH (NH)2 COOH
O
O
R
O
N
O
O
R
N
COOH
Eumelanin
R
O
N
S
COOH
Phaeomelanin

Fig. 12.1 The suggested sub-unit structure of eumelanins and phaeomelanins.

CH2CH(NH)2COOH
OH
Tyrosine
CH2CH(NH)2 COOH
OH
OH
Dopa
CH2CH2NH2
OH
OH
Dopamine

Fig. 12.2 Eumelanins.

glycosylation; these post-translational modifications are thought to occur within the cysternae of the Golgi apparatus prior to the enzymes' incorporation into the melanosomes (Hearing *et al.* 1978). Lloyd *et al.* (1987) have shown that, in general, hair bulb tyrosinase activity does not decline linearly with age but it tends to be maximal in middle-age. A probable relationship of specific tyrosinases to human hair colours is still controversial (King & Olds 1981). There seems little doubt that the hair bulb produces eumelanin similar to that found in other sites (Nicolaus *et al.* 1964).

Phaeomelanins

These are formed in nature by a modification of the eumelanin pathway (Prota 1972) which involves an interaction of dopaquinone with cysteine (Fig. 12.3).

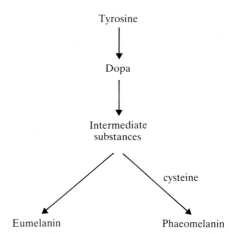

Tyrosine

Dopa

Intermediate substances

cysteine

Fig. 12.3 Pathways of melanin production (phaeomelanins).

Eumelanin

Phaeomelanin

Early workers used acid treatment for isolation of pigments from red hair or feathers. This is now known to be unsuitable since it gives only minor fragments, the so-called trichosiderins, and even these may be structurally modified. Prota *et al.* (1970) using an alkaline extraction procedure from the feathers of New Hampshire chickens produced a red-brown precipitate and a yellow-orange supernatant. Chromatographic analysis of the dialysed precipitate gave rise to four gallophaeomelanin fractions which have not yet been structurally characterized, but they are probably based on the sub-unit structure shown in Fig. 12.1; they were polymeric and contained sulphur; some also contained protein. Further treatment of the orange-yellow supernatant yielded a number of pigments; one group of these, the acid-soluble fraction, was considered to be that fraction previously regarded as trichosiderins. They did not contain iron as had previously been suggested (Fletch 1968). The structure shown in Fig. 12.4, has been proposed for three of these pigments (Prota *et al.* 1971).

In support of melanin structures obtained from work based on degradation fractions of natural melanins, both eu- and phaeomelanins have been produced *in vitro* (Cleffman 1963).

It has been traditional to believe that each individual produces only eumelanin or phaeomelanin throughout life. This is probably untrue. Juhlin and Ortonne (1986), for example, described a 57-year-old man whose red scalp hair began to

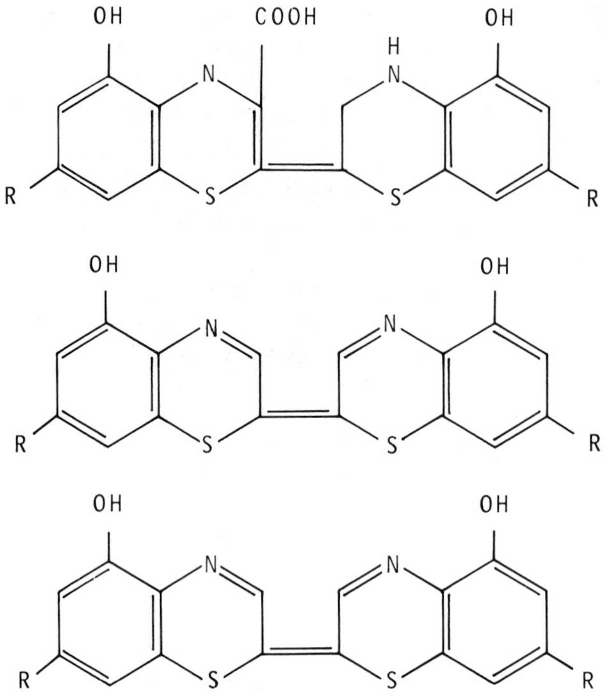

Fig. 12.4 Suggested structures of three acid-soluble pigments (formerly called trichosiderins).

turn dark brown at 50 years of age and suggested a change from phaeo- to eumelanogenesis as the basis for this. Many other natural hair colour changes may reflect similar biochemical changes.

Melanocytes

The melanocyte is the site of pigment production in the hair bulb. Functional melanocytes are situated in the bulb at the apex of the dermal papilla among the germinative cells of the hair matrix, the main body of the cell being in contact with the basement membrane (Fig. 12.5). Melanocytes are also present in the external root sheath and other parts of the follicle (Montagna & Chase 1956; Starrico 1960). Prior to the work of Rawle (1948) melanocytes were considered by many authorities to derive from the local cell population (Bloch 1927); Rawle (1948) showed them to be of neural crest origin (Weston 1970). Transmission electron microscopic studies (Birbeck *et al.* 1956) established clearly the secretory nature of the melanocyte and the structure of its product, the melanosome. The presence of developing melanosomes and the scarcity of tonofilaments in the cytoplasm, together with the absence of desmosomal attachments, easily differentiates melanocytes from adjacent matrix cells.

Biochemical, histochemical, electron microscopic and autoradiographic studies have shown that melanosome formation proceeds in an orderly fashion. The

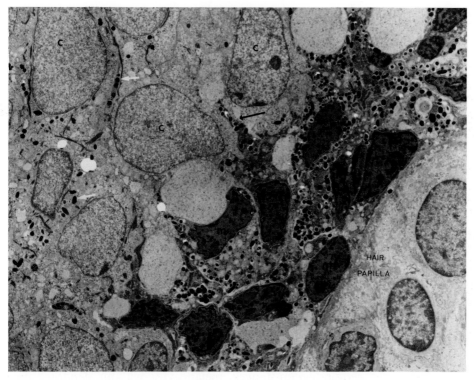

Fig. 12.5 A melanocyte (M) is present adjacent to the dermal papilloma: the dark-staining nucleus (M) is surrounded by large numbers of cytoplasmic melanosomes in the melanocyte (black arrows) and matrix cells (white arrows). Many paler staining matrix cells are present (C).

process involves the construction of four basic components that include structural proteins, tyrosinase, 'membranes' and possibly also certain auxiliary enzymes. The process has been well reviewed (Jimbow & Kukita 1971). The main constructional theory (Birbeck 1963; Seiji & Iwashita 1965) states that tyrosinase is synthesized on membrane-bound ribosomes and transported via endoplasmic reticulum to the Golgi region where it accumulates in small, round, membrane-limiting vesicles. These increase in size either by enlargement or fusion, become oval and acquire a characteristic patterned internal structure consisting of an ordered arrangement of tyrosinase molecules on a protein matrix. Alternative theories to this sequence of events have been proposed (Welling & Siegal 1963; Overbeck & Philipp 1968; Jimbow *et al.* 1971), but all lead to the stage-one melanosome (unmelanized) containing inactive tyrosinase. Subsequent stages involve the activation of tyrosinase and increasing deposition of electron-dense melanin within the melanosomes. The complete development of melanosomes has been divided into four stages (Zelickson & Mottaz 1974). Stage four is the fully mature melanosome; in the past, many studies have intimated that this electron-dense, melanin-laden structure is amorphous. However, Jimbow and Kukita (1971) have shown that completely mature melanosomes contain spherical translucent structures of unknown function called vesico-globular bodies; they are present throughout all stages of melanosome development and increase in number as the melanosomes mature (Jimbow & Fitzpatrick 1974).

Within the cytoplasm of melanocytes, early melanosomes are distributed close to the nucleus in the Golgi region. With increasing maturity, the melanosomes enlarge (Zelickson & Mottaz 1974), move away from the nuclear region and enter the dendritic processes (Jimbow & Kukita 1971).

In black hair follicles deposition of melanin within melanosomes continues until the whole unit is uniformly dense. Lighter coloured hair shows less melanin deposition and blonde hair follicles show melanosomes with a moth-eaten appearance. Red and blonde hair follicles have spherical melanosomes; those in brown and black hair are ellipsoidal (Montagna & Parakkal 1974).

Melanocytes in the hair bulb (and epidermis) differ from those found in internal structures in donating pigment to receptor cells, i.e. the hair matrix cells (keratinocytes) that ultimately differentiate to produce the hair cortex. No pigment is donated to presumptive cuticular and internal root sheath cells (Orfanos & Ruska 1968) though pigment granules have been detected in the cuticle of human nostril hair and in the coat of many animals (Swift 1977). In the epidermis each melanocyte has a relationship to a determined pool of adjacent keratinocytes to which, under suitable conditions, it donates melanosomes usually via dendritic processes; under certain circumstances, melanocytes without dendrites may transfer pigment (Fitzpatrick & Breathnach 1963; Hadley & Quevado 1966). At present, there is no evidence to show whether a similar defined pool of receptor cells exists for each melanocyte in the hair follicle but it remains a probability.

Much speculation has arisen regarding the mechanism of transfer of melano-somes. Melanocytes were thought to inject pigment into recipient cells, the so-called 'cytocrine' activity (Masson 1948). It has become evident that receptor cells actively phagocytose melanin-laden dendritic fragments (Fitzpatrick & Breathnach 1963; Mottaz & Zelickson 1967). Within the matrix cells the engulfed dendritic tips undergo partial lysosomal digestion releasing some pigment granules into the cytoplasm. As the presumptive cortical cells differentiate, they harden prior to keratinization, thus fixing the position of the melanin granules between keratin fibrils.

Melanocytes are functionally active only during the anagen phase of the hair cycle. They were formerly thought to disappear during telogen but it is now known that they remain at the surface of the papilla in a shrunken adendritic form. Jimbow *et al.* (1974) found melanocytes with mature melanosomes in resting feather follicles, whilst other workers detected aggregated pigment granules in clear cells of telogen hair follicles (Silver *et al.* 1969). It is possible that the full complement of melanocytes present during successive anagen phases is the result not only of reactivation of 'dormant' cells but also new cells due to melanocyte replication (Jimbow *et al.* 1975).

Definitive hair pigmentation

Melanin granules are distributed throughout the hair cortex (Fig. 12.6) but in greater concentration towards the periphery. Paracortex is thought to contain more granules than the less dense orthocortex (Laxer *et al.* 1954). The pigment granules of black and brunette hair have oval pigment grains with a more or less homogeneous inner structure and sharp boundaries; the surface is finely grained with a thin surrounding membrane-like layer of osmophilic material (Orfanos & Ruska 1968). Black hair granules are also relatively hard as judged from ultramicrotome sectioning, have a high refractive index (Swift 1977) and a greater absolute number of such granules are present in dark hair compared to lighter shades. Blonde hair granules are smaller, partly ellipsoid and partly rod-shaped in longitudinal section and frequently have a rough, irregular and pitted surface.

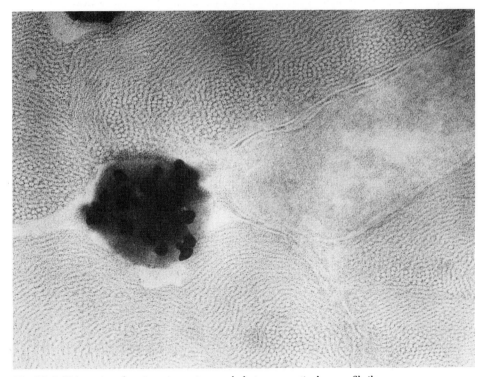

Fig. 12.6 Hair cortex showing pigment granule between cortical macrofibrils.

Hair colour due to physical phenomena

The white colour of hair seen when melanin is absent is an optical effect due to reflection and refraction of incident light from various interfaces at which zones of different refractive index are in contact (Fig. 12.7).

Thus, in general, non-pigmented hair with a broad medulla appears paler than

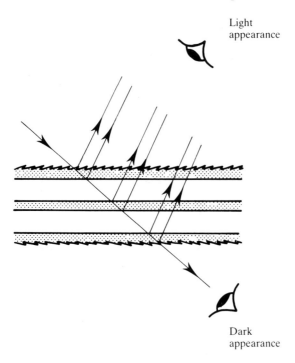

Light
appearance

Dark
appearance

Fig. 12.7 Diagrammatic view
of main hair structure
interfaces which reflect and
refract light (cuticle and
central medulla).

non-medullated hair. Many arctic animals have such broadly medullated hair
which contributes to the whiteness necessary for camouflage. Normal 'weathering'
of hair along its length may lead to the terminal part appearing lighter than the rest
due to a similar mechanism—the cortex and cuticle become disrupted and form
numerous interfaces from internal reflection and refraction of light. This also
applies in trichorrhexis nodosa (excessive 'weathering') in which patients often
note a lightening in colour of the brittle hair, and in the white bands of pili annulati
(Dawber 1972). Since these optical whitening effects are due to reflection and
refraction of incident light, when such hairs are viewed by transmitted light
microscopy they appear dark. Newly formed unpigmented hair with no medulla
appears yellowish rather than white. This is probably the intrinsic colour of dense
keratin as orientated in hair fibres. Findlay (1982) showed that the perceived
colour is affected by the physical characteristics of the hair shaft and may bear
little relationship to the true chromaticity of the shaft.

Function of hair colour

In lower animals coat colour and patterning are important as camouflage, for
sexual attraction, in releasing certain behaviour patterns and for protection
against sunlight (Cott 1956; Lorenz 1970). Hair colour in man is purely decorative
and has no essential biological function. The racial and genetic colour differences
that have evolved are probably related to the UVR protective colours seen in the

skin, i.e. dark-skinned races have dark hair. Hair pigment, however, is not important in protection against the effects of sunlight, though there is evidence to suggest that hair bleached by sunlight and hair with less natural amounts of melanin 'weather' less well, i.e. the structure degenerates more easily (Zviak & Dawber 1986). The decorative function of hair colour thus appears to be a matter of serendipity.

Colour variation

Lanugo hair present *in utero* is unpigmented. Vellus hair is also typically unpigmented but, in men, in particular, some vellus fibres may pigment slightly after puberty. Hair colour varies according to body site in most people (Wasserman 1974). Eyelashes are usually the darkest. Scalp hair is generally lighter than genital hair, which often has a reddish tint even in subjects having essentially brown hair. Grobbelaar (1952) showed that hair on the lower and lateral scrotal surfaces is lighter than on the pubes. He also noted the frequent presence of a red tint in axillary hairs even in the absence of auburn hair on other body sites; this change was not seen in Rehoboth coloureds. Apart from individuals with red scalp hair, a red tint to axillary hair is commonest in brown-haired individuals.

Hair on exposed parts may be bleached by sunlight. Very dark hair first lightens to a brownish-red colour but rarely becomes blonde even after strong sunlight exposure; brown hair, however, may be bleached white.

Slow oxidation of hair melanin occurs after death with consequent colour lightening (Brothwell and Spearman 1963).

Control of hair colour

Hair colour is primarily under close genetic supervision; however, the exact hormonal and cellular mechanisms that control melanocyte function are not clearly worked out. An intimate relationship must exist between the factors controlling melanocyte and matrix cell activity since melanocyte mitosis and melanosome production and transfer occur only during the anagen phase of the hair cycle. A negative-feedback system has been postulated. Enzyme degradation products of melanosomes within matrix cells may cross cell membranes to melanocytes and control further melanin production or transfer (Jimbow *et al.* 1975). Melanosome degradation within melanocytes may also have an inhibitory effect on melanogenesis and even destroy melanocytes. A melanocyte-specific 'chalone' acting within a negative feedback system may well exist for follicular melanocytes (Bullough 1975). Voorhees *et al.* (1973) have proposed that such control mechanisms utilize the 'second messenger' adenyl cyclase–cyclic AMP system (Sunderland 1970). Lerner (1971) suggested that cAMP controls hormonal and neural regulation of melanosome movement and stimulates tyrosinase synthesis prior to increased melanogenesis. Follicular melanocytes are known to respond like epidermal melanocytes to melanocyte stimulating hormone (MSH) which can darken light-coloured hair. A summary of the current structure and function of MSH is present in the review by Bolognia and Pawelek (1988). Three forms of MSH have been described: α, β and γ. These are small peptide hormones consisting of 12 to 18 amino acids. In vertebrates they are produced from the intermediate lobe of the pituitary gland. All three melanotrophins are cleavage products of a common precursor peptide, pro-opiomelanocortin. Corticotrophin (ACTH) and α-MSH contain homologous internal sequences and thus the hyperpigmentation that occurs in Addison's disease, Nelson's syndrome and ectopic ACTH syndrome may be the result of ACTH, α-MSH and even other peptides with common sequences. Current evidence suggests the following mechanism of action of MSH:

1 binding of MSH to specific high-affinity receptors on the cell's surface during the G_2 phase of the cell cycle;

2 formation of the hormone–receptor complex followed by stimulation of the adenyl system and a net increase in intra-cellular levels of cAMP;

3 the cAMP increase results in increased tyrosinase activity and melanin deposition, together with changes in morphology and proliferation rates;

4 these changes are partly mediated by cAMP dependent protein kinases.

α-MSH may act on tyrosinase by converting it to an active form by inactivation of an inhibitor (Wong & Pawelek 1975). cAMP may also control replication of melanocytes which show mitosis during the anagen phase (Jimbow *et al.* 1975); whether cGMP is active in controlling matrix cell division is not clear. The effect of hormones other than MSH on hair pigmentation has yet to be clearly elucidated. Oestrogens and progestogens may increase hair colour in view of their effect on the epidermis during pregnancy.

References

Arnaud, J.C. & Bore, P. (1981) Isolation of melanin pigments from human hair. *Journal of the Society of Cosmetic Chemists*, **32**, 137.

Birbeck, M.S.C. (1963) Electron microscopy of melanocytes: the fine structure of hair bulb premelanosomes. *Annals of the New York Academy of Sciences*, **100**, 540.

Birbeck, M.S.C., Mercer, E.H. & Barnicot, N.A. (1956) The structure and formation of pigment granules in human hair. *Experimental Cell Research*, **10**, 505.

Bloch, B. (1927) *Das Pigment Anatomie der Haut*, p. 434, eds. B. Bloch, F. Pinkus & W. Spalteholz, Springer Verlag, Berlin.

Bolognia, J.L. & Pawelek, J.M. (1988) Biology of hypopigmentation. *Journal of the American Academy of Dermatology*, **19**, 217.

Brothwell, D. & Spearman, R.I.C. (1963) The hair of earlier people. In *Science in Archaeology*, p. 111, eds. D. Brothwell & E. Higgs. Thames & Hudson, London.

Bullough, W.S. (1975) Chalcone control mechanisms. *Life Science*, **16**, 323.

Cleffman, G. (1963) Agouti pigment cells *in situ* and *in vitro*. *Annals of the New York Academy of Sciences*, **100**, 749.

Cott, H.B. (1956) *Adaptive Colouration in Animals*. Methuen, London.

Dawber, R.P.R. (1972) Investigations of a family with pili annulati associated with blue naevi. *Transactions of the St John's Hospital Dermatology Society*, **58**, 51.

Findlay, G. (1982) An optical study of human hair colour in normal and abnormal conditions. *British Journal of Dermatology*, **107**, 517.

Fitzpatrick, T.B. & Breathnach, A.S. (1963) Das epidermale Melanin Einheit System. *Dermatologische Wochenschrift*, **147**, 481.

Fletch, P. (1968) Inhibitory action of extracts of mammalian skin on pigment formation. *Proceedings of the Society of Experimental Biological Medicine*, **70**, 136.

Grobbelaar, C.S. (1952) The distribution of, and correlation between eye, hair and skin colour in male students at the University of Stellenbosch. *Annals of the University of Stellenbosch*, **28**, Sect A/1.

Hadley, M.E. & Quevado, W.C. (1966) Vertebrate epidermal melanin unit. *Nature*, **209**, 1334.

Hearing, V.J., Nicholson, J.M. & Montague, P.M. (1978) Mammalian tyrosinase structural and functional interrelationship of isozymes. *Biochimica Biophysica Acta*, **522**, 327.

Jimbow, K., Roth, S., Fitzpatrick, T.B. & Szabo, G. (1975) Mitotic activity in non-neoplastic melanocytes *in vivo* as determined by histochemical autoradiographic and electron microscopic studies. *Journal of Cell Biology*, **66**, 663.

Jimbow, K., Szabo, G. & Fitzpatrick, T.B. (1974) Ultrastructural investigation of autophagocytosis of melanosomes and programmed death of melanocytes in white Leghorn feathers. *Developmental Biology*, **36**, 8.

Jimbow, K. & Fitzpatrick, T.B. (1974) The characterization of a new melanosomal body—the vesiculo-globular body—by conventional transmission, high voltage and scanning electron microscopy. *Journal of Ultrastructural Research*, **48**, 269.

Jimbow, K. & Kukita, A. (1971) In *Biology of Normal and Abnormal Melanocytes*, p. 1, eds. T. Kawamura, T.B. Fitzpatrick & M. Seiji. University Park Press, Baltimore.

Jimbow, K., Takahashi, M., Sato, S. & Kukita, A. (1971) Ultrastructural and cytochemical studies on melanogenesis in melanocytes of normal human hair matrix. *Journal of Electron Microscopy*, **20**, 87.

Juhlin, L. & Ortonne, J.P. (1986) Red scalp hair turning dark-brown at 50 years of age. *Acta Dermato-Venereologica*, **66**, 71.

King, R.A. & Olds, D.P. (1981) Electrophoretic patterns of human hair bulb tyrosinase. *Journal of Investigative Dermatology*, **77**, 201.

Laxer, G., Sikorski, J., Whewell, C.S. & Woods, H.J. (1954) The electron microscopy of melanin granules isolated from pigmented mammalian fibres. *Biochimica Biophysica Acta*, **15**, 174.

Lerner, A.B. (1971) Neural control of pigment cells. In *Biology of Normal and Abnormal Melanocytes*, p. 1, eds. T. Kawamura, T.B. Fitzpatrick & M. Seiji. University Park Press, Baltimore.

Lerner, A.B. & Fitzpatrick, T.B. (1950) Biochemistry of melanin formation. *Physiology Review*, **30**, 91.

Lloyd, T., Garry, F.L., Manders, E.K. & Marks, J.G. (1987) The effect of age and hair colour on human hair bulb tyrosinase activity. *British Journal of Dermatology*, **116**, 485.

Lorenz, K. (1970) *Studies in Animal and Human Behaviour*, vol. 1. Methuen, London.

Mason, H.S. (1948) The chemistry of melanins. *Journal of Biological Chemistry*, **172**, 83.

Masson, P. (1948) Pigment cells in man. In *The Biology of Melanosomes*, p. 15, eds. R.W. Miner & M. Gordon. Special publication of New York Academy of Sciences.

Mier, P.D. & Cotton, D.W.K. (1976) *The Molecular Biology of Skin*. Blackwell Scientific Publications, Oxford.

Montagna, W. & Chase, H.B. (1956) Histology and cytochemistry of human skin. X. X-irradiation of the scalp. *American Journal of Anatomy*, **99**, 415.

Montagna, W. & Parakkal, P.K. (1974) *The Structure and Function of Skin*, p. 232. Academic Press, New York.

Mottaz, J.H. & Zelickson, A.S. (1967) Melanin transfer: a possible phagocytic process. *Journal of Investigative Dermatology*, **49**, 605.

Munro Fox, H. & Vevers, G. (1960) *The Nature of Animal Colours*. Sidgwick & Jackson, London.

Nicolaus, R.A., Piattelli, M. & Fattorusso, E. (1964) The structure of melanins and melanogenesis. IV. On some natural melanins. *Tetrahedron*, **20**, 1163.

Orfanos, C. & Ruska, H. (1968) Die Feinstruktur des menschlichen Haares. III. Das Haarpigment. *Archiv für klinische und experimentelle Dermatologie*, **231**, 279.

Overbeck, L. & Philipp, E. (1968) Zur Melanogenese in menschlichen Tumorzellen. *Naturwissenschaften*, **55**, 232.

Prota, G., Crescenzi, S., Miscuraca, G. & Nicolaus, R.A. (1970) New intermediates in phaeomelano-genesis *in vitro. Experientia*, **26**, 1058.

Prota, G., Suarato, A. & Nicolaus, R.A. (1971) The isolation and structure of trichosiderin B. *Experientia*, **27**, 1381.

Prota, G. (1972) Structure and biogenesis of phaeomelanins. In *Pigmentation, its Genesis and Biological Control*, p. 615, ed. V. Riley. Appleton-Century-Corfts, New York.

Prunieras, M. (1986) Melanocytes, melanogenesis and inflammation. *International Journal of Dermatology*, **25**, 624.

Rawle, M.E. (1948) Origin of melanophores and their role in development of color patterns in vertebrates. *Physiology*, **28**, 383.

Riley, P.A. (1974) The nature of melanins. In *Physiology and Pathophysiology of the Skin*, vol. 3, p. 1102, ed. A. Jarrett. Academic Press, London.

Robin, C.P. (1873) *Anatomie et Physiologie Cellulaire.* Baillière et Fils, Paris.

Seiji, M. & Iwashita, S. (1965) Intracellular localisation of tyrosinase and site of melanin formation in the melanocyte. *Journal of Investigative Dermatology*, **45**, 305.

Silver, A.F., Chase, H.B. & Potten, C.F. (1969) Melanocyte precursor cells in the hair follicle germ during the dormant stage (telogen). *Experientia*, **25**, 209.

Staricco, R.G. (1960) The melanocyte and the hair follicle. *Journal of Investigative Dermatology*, **35**, 185.

Sunderland, W.E. (1970) On the biological role of cyclic AMP. *Journal of the American Academy of Dermatology*, **214**, 1281.

Swift, J.A. (1977) The histology of keratin fibres. In *The Chemistry of Natural Protein Fibres*, p. 1, ed. R.S. Asquith. Wiley, London.

Voorhees, J.J., Duell, E.G., Bass, L.J. & Harrell, E.R. (1973) Role of cyclic AMP in the control of epidermal cell growths and differentiation. In *Chalones: Concept and Current Researchers*, eds. B.K. Forscher & J.C. Houck. National Cancer Institute Monograms, **38**, 47.

Wasserman, H.P. (1974) *Ethnic Pigmentation.* Excerpta Medica, Amsterdam.

Welling, S.R. & Siegal, B.V. (1963) Electron microscopic studies on the subcellular origin and ultrastructure of melanin granules in mammalian melanosomes. *Annals of the New York Academy of Sciences*, **100**, 548.

Weston, J.A. (1970) The migration and differentiation of neural crest cells. In *Advances in Morphogenesis*, p. 41, eds. M. Abercrombie, J. Brachet & T. King. Academic Press, New York.

Wong, G. & Pawelek, J. (1975) Melanocyte-stimulating hormone promotes activation of pre-existing tyrosinase molecules in Cloudeman 591 melanoma cells. *Nature*, **255**, 644.

Zelickson, A.S. & Mottaz, J.H. (1974) Ultrastructure of hair melanomes. In *The First Human Hair Symposium*, p. 277, ed. A.C. Brown. Medcom Press, New York.

Zviak, C. & Dawber, R.P.R. (1986) Hair colour. In *The Science of Hair Care*, p. 23, ed. C. Zviak. Marcel Dekker, New York.

Variation in hair colour
(References p. 392)

Genetic and racial aspects (Baker 1974)

Mammalian hair colour has long been a subject of considerable interest to geneticists and in a variety of species, including man, a number of genetic variants have been described. Most of the large studies have been in species which provide many hair colour mutations, e.g. the house mouse; in such animals the required stocks demonstrating the mutations are available and easily produced in view of the large number of inbred strains in existence (Silvers 1968). Genetic studies of hair colour do not only provide us with knowledge of gene function; they also give insight into the mechanism of hair pigmentation (Takeuchi 1975). From laboratory and animal studies a general conformity has been shown in the complement of genes affecting hair colour (Fitzpatrick *et al.* 1958; Rife 1967) and it is reasonable to assume that an essentially similar complex of genes may be involved in man. Human hair (and skin) colour is influenced by at least four gene loci which are probably allelic (Harrison & Owen 1965; Livingston 1969; Stern 1970; Harrison 1973); several of the allelic series of other mammals (Deol 1963) are probably present in man but the agouti allele is not. The chief obstacle to more detailed studies of hair colour inheritance in man is the absence of clear data on crosses between individuals with 'pure' Caucasoid, Negroid and Mongoloid skin. Much has been read into crosses between American Negroids and Caucasoids but such studies to not provide clear answers since American blacks are not a pure race. Stern (1953) estimated the Caucasoid alleles in the American Negroid at 30%; Reed (1969) suggested 20%.

Ethnic differences in hair colour are very conspicuous, as are the differences in hair morphology, though colour and hair form are inherited separately (Trotter & Duggins 1950). Many early studies on ethnic hair colour differences are difficult to relate since they did not compare like with like, using different descriptive terms of hair colour (Wassermann 1974). Verbal description has been used widely for general studies: blonde hair colour is considered with 'bamboo' and 'flax'. Other terms often used are flaxen, platinum blonde, dark blonde, golden brown and hairbrown. Grey variations of hair include ash blonde, golden grey and ash grey. Golden or reddish variations are: golden blonde, reddish blonde, red-haired, golden, golden yellow, reddish golden, titian (red) and henna (Kornerup & Wanscher 1963). Colour matching is the usual method now used to describe hair colour more specifically, e.g. the Fischer–Saller Hair Colour Scale (Sunderland 1956). When sufficient hair is available reflectance spectrophotometry may be usefully used (Reed 1952; Sunderland 1956; Barnicott 1956). Hanna (1956) used colorimetric estimation of extracted pigment.

Dark hair predominates in the world. Among Caucasoids there is wide variation in colour within geographical regions (Sunderland 1956). Blonde hair is most frequent in Northern Europe and black hair in Southern and Eastern Europe; foci of blondness are to be found even in North Africa, the Middle East and in some Australoids. Congoid, Capoid, Mongoloid and Australoid hair is mainly black. Previous description has shown that melanin pigment is synthesized in the melanocyte and deposited in melanosomes; the chemical nature of melanin and the shape, number and final position of pigment granules in the hair cortex determine the exact colour. Density of cortical pigment shows greater variation between, rather than within, races. In dark-haired populations there is variation in the quantity of pigment and as hair tends towards black, differentiations of shades become more difficult. In specific countries, variations in hair colour may be found associated with eye colour changes. Blonde hair is often linked with blue eyes.

Red hair (Rutilism)

This has attracted more attention than other colours because it is less common and because it is so distinctive. The melanin pigment is phaeomelanin, not eumelanin — the differences of melanin distribution and melanosome structures are described elsewhere. In the United Kingdom and Italy the distribution of red hair is similar to that of blood group O, excluding East Anglia (Harrison *et al.* 1964). The incidence of red hair varies from 0.3% in Northern Germany, 1.6% in Paris to 3.7% in England; it is as high as 11% in parts of Scotland. Red-hair inheritance is dominant to non-red but hypostatic to brown and black (Rife 1967). This contrasts with earlier reports that it is recessive to non-red (Singleton & Ellis 1964). Reddish hair may occur as an isolated abnormality or in association with xanthism in certain areas (Barnicott 1952). Like hair of many other colours, red hair often darkens with age from red through brown to sandy or auburn in the adult. The skin of red-heads is generally pale, burns easily in sunlight and pigments very little even after prolonged and frequent sun exposure; there is also poor resistance to skin irritants, e.g. red-haired psoriatic patients receiving topical dithranol will tolerate only relatively low strengths without burning. The evidence for the widely held view that red-haired individuals are more susceptible to tuberculosis and rheumatic fever is only anecdotal.

Heterochromia

This implies the growth of hair of two distinct colours in the same individual. A colour difference between scalp and moustache is not uncommon. In fair-haired individuals pubic and axillary hair, eyebrows and eyelashes are much darker than scalp hair. In humans, eyelashes are generally the most darkly pigmented hairs. Black- and brown-haired subjects often have red or auburn sideburns. In other than the fair-haired, genital hair is usually lighter than scalp hair and it may have a reddish tint even in those with brown pubic hair: 33% of a series of South African whites had red axillary hair whilst this was only occasionally seen in coloureds; also hair on the lower and lateral aspect of the scrotum was lighter than on the pubes (Grobbelaar 1952). In brown-haired individuals a reddish tint is more common in axillary hair than on the scalp.

In general, scalp hair darkens with age (Sunderland 1956). Many fair-haired children have brown hair by adult life; in a Polish population, blonde-haired children between 13 and 24 months of age changed to dark colouring by the age of 15 years.

Rarely, a circumscribed patch of hair occurs of different colour. This generally has a genetic basis, though the type of inheritance is not known in man. In the mouse, haphazard colour patterns may be due to somatic mutations during embryonic life; clones of altered melanocytes, or keratinocytes with changed inductive effects form a mosaic pattern in the skin (Russell 1964). Patchy differences of hair colour are of five types:

1 tufts of very dark, coarse hair growing from a melanocytic naevus;

2 hereditary, usually autosomal dominant heterochromia, e.g. tufts of red hair at the temples in a black-haired subject or a single black patch in a blonde;
3 perhaps as a result of somatic mosaicism, partial asymmetry of hair and eye colour may occur sporadically;
4 the white forelock of piebaldism;
5 the 'flag' sign in kwashiorkor.

Greying of hair (Canities)

Greying of hair is usually a manifestation of the ageing process and is due to a progressive reduction in melanocyte function. The larger medullary spaces of older people may contribute to the process. There is no gross change in the cuticle or cortex with age but it has been suggested that increased reflection of light may occur on cell interfaces and islets of interfibrillary matrix (Orfanos *et al.* 1970).

There is a gradual dilution of pigment in greying hairs, i.e. the full range of colour from normal to white can be seen both along individual hairs and from hair to hair. Loss of hair shaft colour is associated with decrease and eventual cessation of tyrosine activity in the lower bulb (Kukita & Fitzpatrick 1955). Transmission electron microscopic studies (Orfanos *et al.* 1970) have shown that many melanocytes are still present in their normal anatomical position in grey hairs; however, many contain large cytoplasmic vacuoles and others, normal looking but incompletely melanized melanosomes. In white hairs melanocytes are infrequent or absent (Herzberg & Gusck 1970) or possibly dormant (Fitzpatrick *et al.* 1966). It has been suggested that autoimmunity plays a part in the pathogenesis of greying: grey hair certainly has an association with the autoimmune disease pernicious anaemia. Dawber (1970) found that 55% of patients with pernicious anaemia were grey before 50 years of age compared with only 30% in a matched control group. Altered nerve supply may also be relevant (Lerner 1966); compared to the normal side the sympathectomized scalp shows fewer grey hairs. In this respect it is interesting that there have been reports of pilocarpine taken orally, darkening white hair (Savill 1944). True canities is probably never associated with pathological processes such as malabsorption syndrome and vitamin B deficiencies (Savill 1944; Klaus 1980).

The age of onset of canities is primarily dependent on the genotype of the individual though acquired factors may play a part. The visual impression of greyness is more obvious (seen earlier) in the fair-haired. In Caucasoid races, white hair first appears at the age of 34.2 ± 9.6 years, and by the age of 50 years, 50% of the population have at least 50% grey hairs (Keogh & Walsh 1965). The onset in Negroes is 43.9 ± 10.3 years, and in Japanese between 30 and 34 years in men and 35 and 39 years in women (Wassermann 1974). The beard and moustache areas commonly become grey before scalp or body hair. On the scalp the temples usually show greying first, followed by a wave of greyness spreading to the crown and later to the occipital area.

Rapid onset, allegedly 'overnight' greying of hair, has excited the literary, medical and anthropological worlds for centuries (Jelinek 1972). Many reports have been over-dramatized but it certainly occurs. Historical examples often quoted include Sir Thomas More and Marie Antoinette whose hair became grey over the night preceding their execution. Henry de Navarre showed white hair in his moustache within hours of hearing that the edict of Nemours had been conceded. Brown-Séquard (1869) studied the rate of hair whitening of his own beard. He pulled out all the white hair and carefully observed the remainder. Two days later, apart from many hairs which were grey near the root, five were white along their entire length. Further similar observations over several weeks confirmed this finding; unfortunately no microscopic studies were carried out and the length of affected hairs was not stated. The probable mechanism for rapid greying is the selective shedding of pigmented hairs in diffuse alopecia areata, the non-pigmented hairs being retained. Most grey-haired individuals have both grey and pigmented hair and the visual impression of greyness may not be obvious until the dark hairs are lost. The flaw in his hypothesis is the frequent absence of hair loss associated with rapid whitening, though often as much as 50% of scalp hair may not need to be lost before alopecia is noted.

Despite occasional reports to the contrary, in general greying of hair is progressive and permanent, though melanogenesis during anagen may be intermittent for a time before finally stopping. Most of the reports of the return of normal hair colour from grey are examples of a pigmented regrowth following alopecia areata, which eventually repigments in many cases. The reported repigmentation of grey hair in association with Addisonian hypoadrenalism may result from a mechanism similar to that in alopecia areata or vitiligo, in view of the known association between these diseases (Addison 1855; Dunlop 1963; Cunliffe *et al.* 1968; Main *et al.* 1975). The mechanism of repigmentation of grey hair and persistence of well-pigmented hair into old age associated with hypothyroidism remains unknown (Wright 1984; Morris & Wright 1986). Darkening of grey hair may occur following large doses of p-aminobenzoic acid; Sieve (1941) gave 100 mg three times per day by mouth to 460 grey-haired people and noted a response in 82%. Pigmentation was obvious within 2–4 months of starting treatment. The hairs became grey again 2–4 weeks after stopping therapy.

Premature greying of hair

Premature greying of hair (Fig. 12.8) has been defined as onset of greying before 20 years of age in Caucasoids and 30 years of age in Negroids. It probably has a genetic basis and occasionally occurs as an isolated autosomal dominant condition. The association between premature greying and certain organ-specific autoimmune diseases is well documented. The relationship is probably not one of common pathogenesis but on the basis of genetic linkage. It is often stated that premature greying may be an early sign of pernicious anaemia, hyperthyroidism and, less commonly, hypothyroidism, all autoimmune diseases which individually have

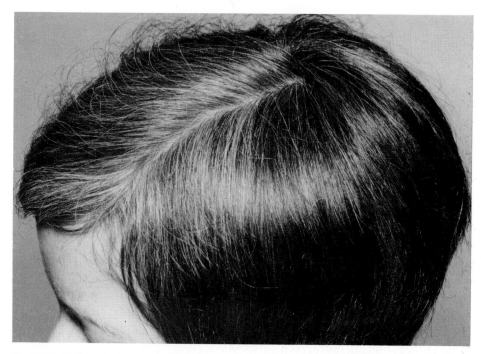

Fig. 12.8 Well-marked greying of the hair in a healthy woman aged 22 years.

a genetic predisposition. In a controlled study of the integumentary associations of pernicious anaemia, 11% had premature greying (Dawber 1970). It has been suggested that coronary artery disease, hypertension and left bundle branch block are significantly associated with premature greying, but the evidence is largely anecdotal and the relationship remains unproven.

In Böök's syndrome, an autosomal dominant trait, premature greying is associated with premolar hypodontia and palmoplantar hyperhidrosis (Böök 1950).

The premature ageing syndromes, progeria and Werner's syndrome (pangeria), may have very early greying as a prominent feature. It does not occur in metageria, acrogeria, or total lipodystrophy (Gilkes *et al.* 1974). In progeria it is associated with marked loss of scalp hair as early as 2 years of age. Werner's syndrome is inherited as an autosomal recessive condition. Temporal greying usually commences in adolescence, rarely as early as 8 years of age. Further spread of grey hair on the scalp is followed by progressive baldness by 25 years of age in association with other manifestations of premature ageing in many tissues (Fleischmajer & Nedwich 1973).

In dystrophia myotonica the onset of grey hair may precede the myotonia and muscle wasting.

Premature canities is an inconstant feature on the Rothmund–Thomson syndrome; when present, it typically commences in adolescence.

One-third of patients with chromosome 5 p-syndrome (cri du chat syndrome) have prematurely grey hair (Breg 1975).

Poliosis

Poliosis is defined as the presence of a localized patch of white hair due to the absence or deficiency of melanin in a group of neighbouring follicles. Essentially the changes in melanogenesis are the same in the hair follicle as in the affected epidermis.

Hereditary defects (Mosher & Fitzpatrick 1988)
Piebaldism (white spotting or partial albinism) is an autosomal dominant abnormality with patches of skin totally devoid of pigment, which remain unchanged throughout life (Comings & Odland 1966). Most commonly a frontal white patch occurs—the white forelock—which may be the only sign. Melanocytes are decreased in number, but are morphologically abnormal and contain normal non-melanized pre-melanosomes, and also pre-melanosomes and melanosomes of abnormal appearance (Grupper *et al.* 1970). Similar pathological changes are seen in Tietz's syndrome of generalized 'white spot' loss of skin and hair pigment, complete deaf mutism and eyebrow hypoplasia (Witkop 1971). Whether melano-cytes are present or not in the affected areas remains controversial. Stains for functioning melanocytes are usually negative but clear cells with unusual organelles may be found; Grupper *et al.* (1970) considered the clear cells to be Langerhans cells.

The debate on the histological 'variability' from study is well reviewed by Mosher & Fitzpatrick (1988) as is the discussion of whether piebaldism should be considered as three conditions (Hayashibe & Mishima 1988).

Waardenburg's syndrome (Waardenburg 1951; Bolognia & Pawlek 1988) shows skin changes so similar to piebaldism that they are presumed to have a similar pathogenesis. Symptoms and signs are present from birth and include dystopia cantharum with lateral displacement of the medial canthi, hypertrophy of the nasal root and hyperplasia of the inner third of the eyebrows with confluent brows. Total or partial iridial heterochromia may occur as may perceptive deafness. The white forelock is present in 20% of cases. Premature greying may develop with or without the white forelock (Rugel & Keats 1965; Pantke & Cohen 1971); a minority have piebaldism and congenital nerve deafness but no other overt signs of Waardenburg's syndrome, suggesting that this association may be genetically distinct.

Vitiligo is an acquired cutaneous achromia probably determined by an autosomal gene, in which the white patches of skin frequently have white hairs within them. The histological changes are consistent with an 'autoimmune injury' to the melanocytes.

The Vogt–Koyanagi–Harada syndrome (Harada 1926; Koyanagi 1929) consists of a post-febrile illness comprising bilateral uveitis, labrynthine deafness, tinnitus and vitiligo, poliosis and alopecia areata (Rosen 1945; Howsden 1973). Alezzandrini's syndrome combines unilateral facial vitiligo, retinitis and poliosis of eyebrows and eyelashes (Alezzandrini 1964); perceptive deafness is rarely associated.

In alopecia areata regrowing hair is frequently white. It may remain so, particularly in cases of late onset. Though absent hair pigment is only evident at this stage of resolution, melanocytes are lost from the hair bulb quite early and migrate to the dermal papilla. The last formed hair above the catagen root in 'exclamation-mark' hairs is poorly pigmented, indicating impaired melanization of keratinocytes before matrix cell division ceases.

Poliosis occurs in 60% of cases of tuberose sclerosis (Nickel & Read 1962); depigmented hair may be the earliest sign (McWilliam & Stephenson 1978).

The pathognomonic signs of Von Recklinghausen's multiple neurofibromatosis (Canale & Bebin 1972) relate to hyperpigmented areas — café au lait macules and axillary and perineal freckling. Scalp neurofibromas may have a patch of poliosis overlying them; this must not be mistaken for vitiliginous changes, though the latter may occur as a halo around neurofibromata since they are neuroectodermal in origin.

Acquired defects

Permanent pigmentary loss may be induced by inflammatory processes which damage melanocytes, e.g. herpes zoster. X-irradiation often causes permanent hair loss but less intense treatment leads to hypopigmented and, rarely, hyper-pigmented hair. Patchy white hair may develop on the beard area after dental treatment.

Albinism (Bolognia & Pawelek 1988)

In autosomal recessive oculocutaneous albinism (complete, perfect, or generalized albinism) similar changes are found in the hair bulb melanocytes as in the epidermis (Witkop 1971). This applies to tyrosine positive and negative types. Melanocytes are structurally normal and active in producing melanosomes of grades I and II. They are, however, enzymically inactive. The melanocyte system is never completely devoid of melanin. In Caucasoids the hair is typically yellowish-white though it may be cream, yellow, yellowish-red or vibrant red. This range of colour parallels those seen in normal blonde Caucasoids. In Negroid albinos the hair colour is white or yellowish brown (Barnicott 1952).

Chediak–Higashi syndrome

This syndrome is basically an autosomal recessive defect of the membrane-bound organelles of several cell types (White & Clawson 1980). It combines oculocutaneous hypopigmentation with a lethal defect of leucocytes (Clawson *et al.* 1979; White & Clawson 1979). Most patients die of recurrent infections by 10 years of age. Melanocytes contain very large melanosomes derived from defective pre-melanosomes. Continued growth and fusion of the latter give rise to the giant melanosomes which eventually degenerate (Zelickson & Mottaz 1974). The hair is silvery grey or light blonde and may be sparse.

Colour changes induced by drugs and other chemicals

Some topical agents temporarily change hair colour. Dithranol and chrysarobin stain light-coloured or grey hair mahogany brown. Resorcin, formerly used a great deal in a variety of skin diseases, colours black or white hair yellow or yellowish-brown.

Some systemic drugs alter hair colour by interfering with the eumelanin or phaeomelanin pathway; in others, the mechanism is not known. Chloroquine interferes with phaeomelanin synthesis, i.e. it only affects blonde- and red-haired individuals. After 3–4 months' treatment hair becomes increasingly silvery or white; it is usually patchy and first affects the temples or eyebrows (Fig. 12.9). The changes are completely reversible. Mephenesin, a glycerol ether used for diseases with muscle spasms, causes pigmentary loss in dark-haired people (Spillane *et al.* 1963). Triparanol, an anti-cholesterolaemic drug, and fluoro-butyrophenone, an anti-psychotic drug, both interfere with keratinization and

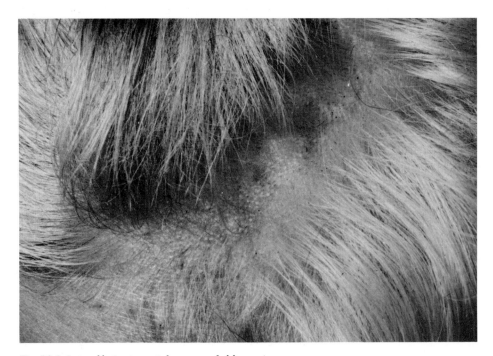

Fig. 12.9 Loss of hair pigment from use of chloroquine.

cause hypopigmented and sparse hair; the altered colour may be due to impaired phagocytosis of melanosomes by presumptive cortical cells or an optical effect due to micropathological changes in the definitive cuticle or cortex. Minoxidil and diazoxide (Burton & Marshall 1979; Ridgley & Kassassieh 1979), two potent anti-hypertensive agents, both cause hypertrichosis and darkening of hair. The colour produced by diazoxide is reddish, whilst minoxidil darkens hair mainly by converting vellus hair to terminal hair, i.e. the increased colour equates with other body hair of the affected individual. Hydroquinone and phenylthiourea interfere with tyrosine activity causing hypopigmentation of skin and hair (Dieke 1947).

Darkening of white hair occurred in a patient with Parkinson's disease following the addition of carbidopa and bromocryptine therapy (Reynolds *et al.* 1989).

Colour changes due to nutritional deficiencies

Because specific dietary deficiencies are rare in man, most clinical knowledge of their effects is derived from laboratory and animal studies. Copper deficiency in cattle causes achromotrichia since it is the prosthetic group of tyrosinase. Loss of hair colour from this mechanism occurs in humans as Menkes' kinky hair syndrome. In protein malnutrition, exemplified by kwashiorkor, hair colour changes are a prominent feature; normal black hair becomes brown or reddish, and brown hair becomes blonde (Bradfield 1974; Bradfield & Jellife 1974). Intermittent protein malnutrition leads to the 'flag' sign of kwashiorkor (signe de la bandera) — alternating white (abnormal) and dark bands occur along individual hairs (Fitzpatrick *et al.* 1979). Similar changes to kwashiorkor have been described in severe ulcerative colitis and after extensive bowel resection.

The lightening of hair colour from black to brown described in severe iron-deficiency anaemia may be an effect on keratinization rather than melanocytic function (Sato *et al.* 1989).

Noppakun and Swasdikul (1986) described a case of reversible white hair in vitamin B_{12} deficiency and commented on a variety of reversible and other hair colour changes in adult coeliac disease and drugs.

Hair colour in metabolic disorders

Phenylketonuria is an autosomal recessive disorder in which the tissues are unable to metabolize phenylalanine to tyrosine because of phenylalanine hydroxylase deficiency (Scriver & Rosenberg 1973). Mental retardation, fits and decreased pigmentation of skin, eyes and hair occurs with eczema and dermographism. Black hair may become brown whilst older institutionalized phenylketonurias may have pale blonde or grey hair. Tyrosine treatment causes darkening towards normal colour within 1–2 months (Bolognia & Pawelek 1988).

The paling of hair, seen in homocystinuria, is probably due to keratinization changes in view of the error in methionine metabolism (Fitzpatrick *et al.* 1979).

Light, almost white, hair and recurrent oedema are the surface manifestations of the hair condition, 'oast-house' disease. Methionine concentration in the blood is raised.

Accidental hair discoloration

Hair avidly binds many inorganic elements and thus hair colour changes are occasionally seen after exposure to certain substances.

Exposure to high concentrations of copper in industry or from inadvertently high concentrations in tap water (Goldschmidt 1979) or in swimming pools (Goette 1978), may cause green hair, particularly visible in blonde-haired subjects (Melnik *et al.* 1986; Blanc *et al.* 1988). Cobalt workers get bright blue hair whilst a deep blue tint may be seen in indigo handlers (Beigel 1965). A yellow hair colour is not uncommon in white- or grey-haired heavy smokers due to tar in cigarette smoke; yellow staining may also occur from picric acid and dithranol. Trinitrotoluene (TNT) workers sometimes develop yellow skin and reddish-brown hair.

References

Addison, T. (1855) *On the Constitutional and Local Effects of the Diseases of the Supra-renal Capsule.* Highly, London.
Alezzandrini, A.A. (1964) Manifestations unilatérales de dégénérescence tapetoretinienne de vitiligo, de poliose, de cheveux blancs et hypoacousie. *Ophthalmologica*, **147**, 409.
Baker, J.R. (1974) *Race.* Oxford University Press, London.
Barnicott, N.A. (1952) Albinism in South-western Nigeria. *Annals of Eugenics*, **17**, 38.
Barnicott, N.A. (1956) The relation of the pigment trichosiderin in hair colour. *Annals of Human Genetics*, **21**, 31.
Beigel, H. (1965) Blue hair in indigo handlers. *Archives of Pathology, Anatomy and Physiology*, **83**, 324.
Blanc, D., Zultak, M. & Rochefort, A. (1988) Les cheveux vert; étude clinique, chimique et épidémiologique. *Annales de Dermatologie et de Vénéréologie*, **115**, 807.
Bolognia, K. & Pawlek, S. (1988) Hair colour. In *Dermatology in General Medicine*, eds T.B. Fitzpatrick *et al.*, 3rd edn. McGraw-Hill, New York.
Böök, J.A. (1950) Clinical and genetic studies of hypodontia. I. Premolar aplasia, hyperhidrosis and canites prematura: a new hereditary syndrome in man. *American Journal of Human Genetics*, **2**, 240.
Bradfield, R.B. (1974) Hair tissue as a medium for the differential diagnosis of protein–calorie malnutrition: a commentary. *Journal of Pediatrics*, **84**, 294.
Bradfield, R.B. & Jellife, D.B. (1974) Hair colour changes in kwashiorkor. *Lancet*, i, 461.
Breg, W.R. (1975) Abnormalities of chromosomes 4 and 5. In *Endocrine and Genetic Diseases of Childhood and Adolescence*, ed. L.I. Gardner. Saunders, Philadelphia.
Brown-Séquard, C. (1869) Rapid hair whitening. *Archives de Physiologie*, **2**, 442.
Burton, J.L. & Marshall, A. (1979) Hypertrichosis due to minoxidil. *British Journal of Dermatology*, **101**, 593.
Canale, D. & Bebin, J. (1972) Von Recklinghausen's multiple neurofibromatosis. In *Handbook of Clinical Neurology*, p. 132. North-Holland, Amsterdam.
Clawson, C.C., Repine, J.E. & White, J.G. (1979) The Chediak–Higashi syndrome: quantitation of a deficiency in maximum bacterial capacity *American Journal of Pathology*, **94**, 539.

Comings, D.E. & Odland, G.F. (1966) Partial albinism. *Journal of the American Medical Association*, **195**, 519.

Cunliffe, W.J., Hall, R., Newell, D.J. & Stevenson, C.J. (1968) Vitiligo, thyroid disease and auto-immunity. *British Journal of Dermatology*, **80**, 135.

Dawber, R.P.R. (1970) Integumentary associations of pernicious anaemia. *British Journal of Dermatology*, **82**, 221.

Deol, M.S. (1963) Inheritance of coat colour in laboratory rodents. In *Animals for Research*, ed. W. Lane-Petter, Academic Press, London.

Dieke, S.H. (1947) Pigmentation and hair growth in black rats as modified by the chronic administration of thiourea, phenylthiourea and alpha-naphthylthiourea. *Endocrinology*, **40**, 123.

Dunlop, D. (1963) Eighty-six cases of Addison's disease. *British Medical Journal*, **2**, 887.

Fitzpatrick, T.B., Brunet, P. & Kukita, A. (1958) The nature of hair pigmentation. In *Biology of Hair Growth*, eds. W. Montagna & R.A. Ellis. Academic Press, New York.

Fitzpatrick, T.B., Eisen, A.Z., Wolff, K., Freedberg, I.M. & Austen, F. (1979) *Dermatology in General Medicine*, 2nd edn. McGraw-Hill, New York.

Fitzpatrick, T.B., Quevedo, W.C., Levene, A.L., McGovern, V.J., Mishima, Y. & Oettle, A.C. (1966) Terminology of vertebrate melanin-containing cells. *Science*, **152**, 88.

Fleischmajer, R. & Nedwich, A. (1973) Werner's syndrome. *American Journal of Medicine*, **54**, 111.

Gilkes, J.J.H., Shavrill, D.E. & Wells, R.S. (1974) The premature ageing syndromes. Report of eight cases and description of a new entity named metageri. *British Journal of Dermatology*, **91**, 243.

Goette, D.K. (1978) Swimmers' green hair. *Archives of Dermatology*, **114**, 127.

Goldschmidt, H. (1979) Green hair. *British Journal of Dermatology*, **115**, 1288.

Grobbelaar, C.S. (1952) The distribution of and correlation between eye, hair and skin colour in male students at the University of Stellenbosch. *Annals of University of Stellenbosch*, **28**, sect A/1.

Grupper, C., Brunieras, M., Hincky, M. & Garelly, E. (1970) Albinisme partiel familial: étude ultra-structurale. *Annales de Dermatologie et Syphilologie*, **97**, 267.

Hanna, B.L. (1956) Colorimetric estimation of the pigment concentration in hair of various color grades. *American Journal of Physical Anthropology*, **14**, 153.

Harada, Y. (1926) Fruhzeitiges Ergrauen der Cillen und Bemerkungen über den sogenannten plötzlicher Einstritt dieser Veränderung. *Klinische Monatsblatt für Augenheilkunde*, **44**, 228.

Harrison, G.A. (1973) Differences in human pigmentation; measurement, geographical variation and causes. *Journal of Investigative Dermatology*, **60**, 418.

Harrison, G.A. & Owen, J.J.T. (1965) Studies on the inheritance of human skin colour. *Annals of Human Genetics*, **28**, 27.

Harrison, G.A., Weiner, J.S., Tanner, J.M. & Barnicott, N.A. (1964) *Human Biology, An Introduction to Human Evolution, Variation and Growth*. Oxford University Press, London.

Hayashibe, K. & Mishima, Y. (1988) Tyrosine positive melanocyte distribution and induction of pigmentation in human piebald skin. *Archives of Dermatology*, **124**, 381.

Herzberg, J. & Gusck, W. (1970) Das Ergrauen des Kopfhaares. Eine histo- und fermentschemische sowie elektronen-mikroskopische Studie. *Archiv für Klinische und experimentelle Dermatologie*, **236**, 368.

Howsden, H.M. (1973) Vogt–Koyanagi–Harada syndrome and psoriasis. *Archives of Dermatology*, **108**, 395.

Jelinek, J.E. (1972) Sudden whitening of hair. *Bulletin of the New York Academy of Medicine*, **48**, 1003.

Keogh, E.V. & Walsh, R.J. (1965) Rate of greying of human hair. *Nature*, **207**, 877.

Klaus, S.N. (1980) Acquired pigment dilution of the skin and hair; a sign of pancreatic disease in the tropics. *International Journal of Dermatology*, **19**, 508.

Kligman, A.M. (1961) Pathologic dynamics of human hair loss. *Archives of Dermatology*, **83**, 175.

Kornerup, A. & Wanscher, J.H. (1963) *Methuen's Handbook of Colour*. Methuen, London.

Koyanagi, Y. (1929) Dysacusis, alopecia, und poliosis bei schwerer uveitis nicht traumatischen Ursprungen. *Klinische Monatsblatt für Augenheilkurde*, **82**, 194.

Kukita, A. & Fitzpatrick, T.B. (1955) The demonstration of tyrosinase in melanocytes of the human hair matrix by autoradiography. *Science*, **121**, 893.

Lerner, A.B. (1966) Vitiligo. *Archives of Dermatology*, **93**, 235.

Livingston, F.B. (1969) Polygenic models for the evolution of human skin colour differences. *Human Biology*, **41**, 480.

Main, R.A., Robbie, R.B., Gray, E.S., Donald, D. & Horne, C.H.W. (1975) Smooth muscle antibodies and alopeca areata. *British Journal of Dermatology*, **92**, 389.

McWilliam, T.S. & Stephenson, J.B.P. (1978) Depigmented hair: the earliest sign of tuberose sclerosis. *Archives of Disease in Childhood*, **53**, 961.

Melnik, B.C., Plewig, G. & Daldrup, T. (1986) Green hair: guidelines for diagnosis and therapy. *Journal of the American Academy of Dermatology*, **15**, 1065.

Morris, D.E. & Wright, F.K. (1986) Hair turning from grey to black in a patient with auto-immune hypothyroidism. *British Medical Journal*, **292**, 1430.

Mosher, D.B. & Fitzpatrick, T.B. (1988) Piebaldism. *Archives of Dermatology*, **124**, 346.

Nickel, W.R. & Reed, W.B. (1962) Tuberose sclerosis. Special reference to microscopic alterations in the cutaneous hamartoma. *Archives of Dermatology*, **85**, 209.

Noppakun, N. & Swasdikul, D. (1986) Hyperpigmentation of skin and nails with white hair due to vitamin B_{12} deficiency. *Archives of Dermatology*, **122**, 896.

Orfanos, C., Ruska, H. & Mahle, G. (1970) White hair of older people. *Archiv für klinische und experimentelle Dermatologie*, **236**, 395.

Pantke, O.A. & Cohen, M.M. Jr. (1971) The Waardenburg syndrome. In Part XI, *Orofacial Structures. Birth Defects. Original Article Series*, vol. VII, No. 7, ed. D. Bergsma. Williams & Wilkins, Baltimore.

Prunieras, M. (1986) Melanocytes, melanogenesis and inflammation. *International Journal of Dermatology*, **25**, 624.

Reed, T.E. (1969) Caucasian genes in American Negroes. *Science*, **165**, 762.

Reed, T.W. (1952) Red hair colour as a genetic character. *Annals of Eugenics*, **17**, 115.

Reynolds, N.J., Crossley, J., Ferguson, I & Peachey, R.D.G. (1989) Darkening of white hair in Parkinson's disease. *Clinical and Experimental Dermatology*, **14**, 317.

Ridgley, G.V. & Kassassieh, S.D. (1979) Minoxidil. *Lahey Clinic Foundation Bulletin*, **28**, 80.

Rife, D.E. (1967) The inheritance of red hair. *Acta Geneticae Medicae et Gemellologiae (Rome)* **16**, 342.

Rosen, E. (1945) Uveitis with poliosis, vitiligo, alopecia and dysacousia. *Archives of Ophthalmology*, **33**, 281.

Rugel, S.J. & Keates, E.U. (1965) Waardenburg's syndrome in six generations of one family. *American Journal of Diseases of Children*, **109**, 579.

Russell, L.B. (1964) Genetic and functional mosaicism in the mouse. In *Role of Chromosomes in Development*, ed. M. Locke. Academic Press, New York.

Sato, S., Jitsukawa, K., Sato, H., Yoshino, M., Seta, S., Ito, S., Hayashi, Y. & Anzai, T. (1989) Segmental heterochromia in black scalp hair associated with Fe-deficiency anaemia. *Archives of Dermatology*, **125**, 531.

Saunders, T.S., Fitzpatrick, L.E., Seiji, M., Brunet, P. & Rosenbaum, E.E. (1977) Decrease in human hair colour and feather pigment of fowl following chloroquine diphosphate. *Journal of Investigative Dermatology*, **33**, 87.

Savill, S. (1944) *The Hair and Scalp*, 3rd edn. Edward Arnold, London.

Scriver, C.R. & Rosenberg, L.E. (1973) Phenylketonuria. In *Amino Acid Metabolism and its Disorders. Major Problems in Clinical Pediatrics*, vol. X, p. 290. Saunders, Philadelphia.

Sieve, B.F. (1941) Darkening of grey hair following *para*-aminobenzoic acid. *Science*, **94**, 257.

Silvers, W.K. (1968) Genes and the pigment cells of mammals. *Science*, **134**, 368.

Singleton, W.R. & Ellis, B. (1964) Inheritance of red hair for six generations. *Journal of Heredity*, **55**, 261.

Spillane, J.D. (1963) Brunette to Blond. Depigmentation of hair during treatment with oral mephenesin. *British Medical Journal*, **1**, 997.

Stern, C. (1953) Model estimates of the frequency of white and near white segregants in the American Negro. *Acta Genetica (Basel)*, **4**, 281.

Stern, C. (1970) Model estimates of the number of gene pairs involved in pigment variability of the Negro American. *Human Heredity*, **20**, 165.

Sunderland, E. (1956) Hair colour variation in the United Kingdom. *Annals of Human Genetics*, **20**, 312.

Takeuchi, T. (1975) Genetic control of mammalian hair colour. In *Biology and Diseases of the Hair*, eds. T. Kobori & W. Montagna. University Park Press, Baltimore.

Trotter, M. & Duggins, O.H. (1950) Age changes in head hair from birth to maturity. *American Journal of Physical Anthropology*, **8**, 467.

Waardenburg, P.J. (1951) New syndrome combining developmental abnormalities of the eyelids, eyebrows, nose root with pigmentary defects of the iris and head hair and with congenital deafness. *American Journal of Human Genetics*, **3**, 195.

Wassermann, H.P. (1974) *Ethnic Pigmentation: Historical, Physiological and Clinical Aspects*, 1st edn. Excerpta Medica, Amsterdam.

White, J.G. & Clawson, C.C. (1979) The Chediak–Higashi syndrome: ring-shaped lysosomes in circulating monocytes. *American Journal of Pathology*, **96**, 781.

White, J.G. & Clawson, C.C. (1980) The Chediak–Higashi syndrome: the nature of the giant neutrophil granules and their interaction with cytoplasm and foreign particles. *American Journal of Pathology*, **48**, 151.

Witkop, C.J. Jr (1971) Albinism. In *Advances in Human Genetics*, eds H. Harris & K. Hirschorn. Plenum Press, New York.

Wright, C.B. (1984) Clinical curio: myxoedema and dark hair in old age. *British Medical Journal*, **288**, 1517.

Zelickson, A.S. & Mottaz, J.H. (1974) Ultrastructure of hair melanomes. In *The First Human Hair Symposium*, p. 277, ed. A.C. Brown. Medcom Press, New York.

Chapter 13
Infections and Infestations

Scalp ringworm (Tinea capitis)

History and nomenclature (References p. 398)

Scalp ringworm is an infection of the scalp by a ringworm fungus or dermatophyte (Elewski & Hazen 1989). The disease has been known for centuries, and had become a worldwide public health problem until the last two decades; it remains a problem in those parts of the world where the antibiotic griseofulvin is not freely available.

Although the disease has long been recognized, its diagnostic features were poorly defined until the causative fungi were isolated and identified, and non-infective disorders such as alopecia areata were frequently confused with it. The discovery of the ringworm fungi occupies an important, often unacknowledged, place in the development of knowledge of the microbial causes of disease.

The old nomenclature of skin diseases was devastatingly simple. All skin diseases affecting the scalp were called porrigo, which was then qualified by a descriptive adjective. Tinea was an old word used by the Arab physicians, and it too was applicable to any disease of the scalp. All skin diseases affecting any other part of the body were tetters (dartres in France). Herpes, which had had a more precise meaning in antiquity, had come to be a more scientific sounding synonym for a tetter. Ringworm was the popular term for any annular or expanding lesion. Scalled head was the usual English term for scaling of the scalp and hair loss in children. At the end of the 18th century Plenck of Vienna introduced a classification of skin diseases based on morphology, and his classification was later modified by Willan. Both authors used the old terms with new meanings. The porrigos were classified with the pustular eruptions and came to include porrigo scutulata and lupinosa, which were different stages of favus, porrigo tonsurans and porrigo decalvans. Very gradually tinea replaced porrigo to leave tinea favosa (favus), tinea tonsurans and tinea decalvans, the last including what we now call alopecia areata. This classification contained the seeds of future controversies.

The improvement in and increased availability of microscopes in the 1830s led to the discovery by Agostino Bassi in 1834 of a fungus as the cause of the disease muscardin in silkworms. J.L. Schoenlein, later Professor of Medicine in Berlin, repeated Bassi's observations which led him to discover a fungus in a patient with favus (Schoenlein 1839). Between 1841 and 1844 David Gruby, born in Austro-Hungary, but working in Paris, independently discovered a fungus in favus, and also in what is now called scalp ringworm. Gruby's discoveries were soon widely known, but it was many years before fungi were universally accepted as the cause of ringworm. Erasmus Wilson (1809–84), the most influential British dermatologist of his day, believed that the granules visible with the microscope were merely degenerative products. Jabez Hogg (1817–99), a leading microscopist, accepted that fungi were present in the lesions, but did not accept them as their cause. Opinion in other countries was equally divided (see Rook 1978). The controversy was long and often bitter. Microscopes were still regarded with suspicion, the concept of vegetable parasites causing contagious disease was too revolutionary, and clinical definitions were inadequate, so that alopecia areata was often still confused with ringworm. Gradually the microbial origin of fungus and other diseases was recognized and the conceptual barrier was surmounted.

The acceptance of fungi as the cause of ringworm brought further controversy, because of the inadequacy of mycological techniques. The contamination of cultures by *Aspergillus* and other common airborne mould fungi led many authors to suggest that the ringworm fungi and the moulds were forms of a single organism. After this problem had been resolved there was still no agreement concerning the interrelationship of the ringworm fungi themselves. Was there a single variable species, or were there numerous distinct species? The French dermatologist Raymond Sabouraud (1864–1938) played a very large part in establishing the status and characteristics of dermatophyte species. Since his time further taxonomic studies have clarified the classification of these organisms.

The greatest therapeutic advance has been the discovery of griseofulvin.

References

Rook,A.J. (1978) Early concepts of the host–parasite relationship in mycology. *International Journal of Dermatology*, 17, 371.

Schoenlein, J.L. (1839) Zur Pathogenese der Impetigines. *Archiv für Anatomie, Physiologie und wissenschaftliche Medizin*, p. 82.

The dermatophytes (References p. 402)

The dermatophytes are a group of fungi which colonize and keratinize structures in man and other animals. They may be considered in three groups — anthropophilic, zoophilic or geophilic — according to whether the natural habitat is on humans, animals or in the soil. Fungi in all three groups are able to invade hair. The pathogenic dermatophytes are classified in three genera, *Microsporum*, *Trichophyton*, and *Epidermophyton* (Table 13.1). Most of the many species in the first two genera can invade in varying degree the horny layer, the nails and the hair. The species of *Epidermophyton*, and *Trichophyton concentricum* are unable to parasitize hair and will not be further discussed. The genera *Microsporum* and *Trichophyton* both include species whose natural host is man, and others which occur naturally in one or more other animal species, and parasitize man only accidentally. The distinction between the former, anthropophilic species, and the latter, zoophilic species is important from the epidemiological and clinical points of view, as the natural history of the two groups of infections differs in important respects. In Western Europe before 1945 zoophilic fungi accounted for only a small proportion of cases of scalp ringworm, e.g. 2.4% of cases in Rome in 1910 (Caprilli *et al.* 1979, 1980). Now scalp ringworm of any kind is rare in most of Europe, and zoophilic species account for the majority, e.g. *Microsporum canis* 87.9% of cases in Rome in 1972–7.

Microsporum gypseum

At least one species, *M. gypseum*, normally occurs in the soil, from which man and other animals may acquire the infection. Table 13.1 lists all the important known causes of scalp ringworm and, in the case of the zoophilic species, the animals from which human infections are usually contracted. The geographical distribution of the various dermatophytes indicated in Table 13.1 is necessarily incomplete.

Table 13.1 Fungi causing scalp ringworm

Type	Distribution and host
Anthropophilic	
Microsporum audouini	Worldwide
M. ferrugineum	China, Japan, parts of Russia, Central and E. Africa*
Trichophyton rubrum (rarely affects the scalp)	Widespread endemic; extension from Asia
T. schoenleini	Widespread, but uncommon in most areas: common in the Middle East, N. Africa
T. tonsurans	Widespread; common in parts of Latin America
T. violaceum	Dominant in many parts of Africa*, Central and S. Europe, Middle East†
T. gourvilii	W. Africa
T. megninii	S. Europe, Africa
T. soudanense	Central Africa
T. yaoundi	Africa
Zoophilic	
Microsporum canis	Worldwide (Cats and dogs)
M. equinum	(Horses)
M. nanum	(Pigs)
M. persicolor	W. Europe (Field-vole)
Trichophyton mentagrophytes	Worldwide (Many species; reservoirs in rodents)
T. verrucosum	Widespread (Cattle)
T. equinum	Widespread (Horses)
T. erinacei	Europe, New Zealand (Hedgehogs)
T. quinckeanum	Widespread, but generally rare (Mice; may be transmitted to man by cats and dogs)
T. simii	India (Monkeys)
Geophilic	
Microsporum gypseum	Widespread (Soil; man infected by contact with soil or from infected animals)

* Verhagen (1976).
† Asgari & Satevi (1973).

Movements of population are introducing tropical species to temperate regions. A further source of error is introduced by the uneven world distribution of mycologists.

Whenever it is practicable the infecting species should be reliably identified by culture, for without an identification reliable epidemiological surveys and preventive measures are impossible.

Pathogenesis

The type of tissue response induced in a given individual by parasitization by a dermatophyte depends on a multitude of variables which determine the inherent mode of growth of the species concerned in relation to the hair shaft, and the immune response of the host. Thus, with some species in some patients scalp ringworm may be acutely inflammatory and rapidly self-limiting, whilst with other species, or in other patients, extensive scaling and broken hairs persist for months or years, but eventually resolve without scarring. In other cases, usually but not invariably induced by species different from those associated with the syndromes already mentioned, there may be a prolonged course and permanent residual scarring.

Our knowledge of the pathogenesis of scalp ringworm is derived largely from the experimental studies of A.M. Kligman with *M. audouini* (Fig. 13.1) (Kligman

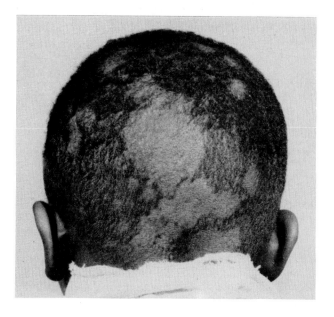

Fig. 13.1 *Microsporum audouini* ringworm of the scalp.

1955). Minor trauma favours the successful inoculation of a child's scalp. From the point of inoculation the fungal hyphae grow centrifugally in the stratum corneum. By the 6th or 7th day a narrow band of fluorescence can be detected with Wood's light 1 mm above the hair bulb; only hairs in the growing phase are attacked. The fungus grows downwards, invading keratin as it is formed, so that the zone of fluorescence extends upwards at the rate at which the hair grows, and is visible above the surface by the 12th–14th days. The infected hair is brittle, and by the 3rd week broken hairs are evident. The infection continues to spread in the stratum corneum to involve other hairs for 8–10 weeks, by which time the infected area is usually about 3.5 cm, but may be up to 7 cm in diameter. In some cases only a few scattered hairs around the inoculated site become infected. In the usual centrifugally spreading infection, the period of extension is followed by a refractory period, during which host–parasite equilibrium is maintained in the infected follicles, but mycelium is no longer present in the horn of the scalp surface. Inoculation of another area of scalp during this period usually fails, but may produce a trivial infection which rapidly resolves. The primary experimental infection tended to resolve spontaneously in under 7 months, even in the absence of inflammatory changes, but occasionally persisted for over 1 year; spontaneous infections tended to last still longer. Even in the absence of clinically apparent inflammation, histological examination shows that intense inflammatory changes are in fact present (Graham *et al.* 1964). Adult scalps showed relative immunity to experimental inoculation. The spontaneous cure of naturally occurring infection at puberty is a familiar clinical observation, but the precise mechanism is not fully understood (Kligman & Ginsberg 1950).

The experimental inoculation of *M. canis* in children showed essentially the same sequence of events, but the hairs were invaded more rapidly, and resolution, frequently accomplished by inflammatory changes, usually occurred within 3 months.

Equally detailed studies of the pathodynamics of infection with other species have not been published but it is highly probable that with most species the various stages of infection differ only in detail and in duration, according to the degree of inflammatory response evoked in the host. There are, however, differences in mode of growth in relation to the hair shaft.

Type of hair invasion
Two main forms of scalp ringworm may be differentiated on mycological grounds according to the type of hair invasion that occurs (Clayton 1986).

Ectothrix infection. The intra-pilary hyphae emerge through the hair surface and fragment into masses of spores. The spores here are predominantly outside the hair shaft and are either small (2–3 μm) and arranged in masses (small-spored ectothrix) or large (3–5/5–10 μm) when they occur usually in straight chains on the surface of the hair. Small-spored ectothrix invasion is produced by *Microsporum* species and larger ectothrix by *Trichophyton mentagrophytes* and *T. verrucosum*. The infected hair grows upwards and usually breaks off a few millimetres above the scalp surface.

Endothrix infection. The intra-pilary hyphae break up to form spores which become rounded, fill the cortex of the hair and remain confined to the hair shaft. This type of invasion is produced by *Trichophyton tonsurans*, *T. violaceum* and *T. soudanense*. Because of the greater degree of shaft damage, hairs break off close to the scalp surface.

In favus, a chronic endothrix form of tinea capitis due to *T. schoenleinii*, the hyphae grow irregularly down the hair shaft and do not fragment into masses of spores, with the result that the shaft is not weakened and long lengths of hair are carried beyond the follicle by growth of the hair. Degeneration of the hyphae in the infected hair leads to formation of elongated air spaces.

The *Microsporum* species form an irregular mosaic of small spores outside the hair shaft. This ectothrix mode of growth is shown also by *Trichophyton mentagrophytes*, but with this species the spores which ensheath the shaft are arranged in chains; polymorphic mycelia within the hair are broken up into large quadrangular elements. *Trichophyton tonsurans*, *T. rubrum* and *T. violaceum* produce longitudinal chains of large spores within the shaft (endothrix); *T. schoenleinii* does likewise, and the combination of chains of large spores, narrow flat budding mycelium and scattered air bubbles is sometimes distinctive.

The favus fungi (*T. schoenleinii* and *T. quinckeanum*) give rise to additional pathological changes. They cause spongiosis and acanthosis of the epidermis and form *scutula*, which consist of spores and cellular debris in a dense feltwork of mycelium.

References

Asgari, M. & Satevi, H. (1973) Common mycoses in Bandon Abbas, Iran. 2. Scalp ringworm. *Iran Journal of Public Health*, **2**, 65.

Caprilli, F., Marcantini, R., Farotti, E. *et al.* (1979) Etiologia delle dermatofitosi in Roma. *Bolletino del'Istituto San Gallicano*, **10**, 123.

Caprilli, F., Marcantini, R. Marsella, R. & Farotti, E. (1980) Etiology of ringworm of the scalp, beard and body in Rome, Italy. *Sabouraudia*, **18**, 129.

Clayton, Y.M. (1986) Scalp ringworm in superficial fungal infections. New clinical applications. In *Dermatology*, p. 1, ed. Verbov. MTP Press, Lancaster.

Graham, J.H., Johnson, W.C., Burgoon, C.F. & Helwig, E.B. (1964) Tinea capitis. *Archives of Dermatology*, **89**, 528.

Kligman, A.M. (1955) Tinea capitis due to *Microsporum audouini* and *Microsporum canis*. *Archives of Dermatology*, **71**, 313.

Kligman, A.M. & Ginsberg, D. (1950) Immunity of the adult scalp to infection with *Microsporum audouini*. *Journal of Investigative Dermatology*, **14**, 345.

Verhagen, B.A. (1976) Distribution of dermatophytes causing tinea capitis in Africa. *Tropical and Geographical Medicine*, **26**, 101.

Epidemiology (References p. 404)

There have been worldwide changes in the prevalence and patterns of certain dermatophytes causing scalp ringworm. Before 1950 *Microsporum audouinii* was the dominant cause of tinea capitis in Britain, although in London, infections by *M. audouinii* and *M. canis* were approximately equal in number. Since 1970 the number of *M. audouinii* infections has declined steadily so that very few cases are now recorded in Britain (Clayton 1977). *Microsporum canis* has become the commonest cause of fluorescent scalp ringworm in most of Europe (Clayton 1986). In Japan and Korea, where *M. ferrugineum* predominated prior to 1970, *M. canis* is isolated more frequently. *Microsporum canis* is also the species most commonly isolated from tinea capitis in Australia (McAleer 1980), New Zealand (Allred 1982) and South America (Philpot 1978). In Denmark, tinea capitis in equal numbers by *M. canis* and *T. verrucosum* (Foged and Jepsen 1984).

Previously, tinea capitis has always been recorded as being up to three times more common in boys than girls (Clayton 1977; Benedek & Felsher 1944; Blank *et al.* 1974). It was suggested that this was because of shorter haircuts allowing access for infecting spores. More recently, whichever fungus species causes the scalp infection, cases are more equally distributed between the sexes (McAleer 1980). In London, in 1973, 76 cases of tinea capitis occurred in boys compared to 35 in girls, whereas in 1984, 50 cases were seen in boys compared to 57 in girls (Clayton 1986). Longer hairstyles for boys, which may provide a natural barrier to infection, may have influenced these changes.

Microsporum audouini and *M. ferrugineum*, the two most important anthropophilic *Microsporum* species, are spread directly or indirectly from child to child *Microsporum audouini* infection has occurred in dogs (Kaplan & Georg 1957) but the rare animal infections are seldom of epidemiological significance. The spores remain viable in shed human hairs for a year or more (Glass 1948), and allow the transmission of the disease by brushes, combs, hats or caps, or the seats of cinemas and public vehicles. In some children there may be only a few infected hairs, undetectable without Wood's light, and it is the difficulty of identifying such cases and the ease with which spores are disseminated in the hair (Alexander *et al.* 1965; Friedman *et al.* 1960; Gip 1966) which explain the very high incidence of the infection in susceptible age groups during the epidemics which occur periodically in so many populations. In a Nigerian school about 10% of children were shown to be asymptomatic carriers of *M. audouini* (Ive 1966). When treatment facilities are poor the endemic rate may remain constantly high.

Infectivity varies; at the height of an epidemic all or almost all children in a family or an institution may be infected. Far more commonly only some 30–50% of those exposed are infected, and the disease is rare in older children or adults. In most school epidemics the peak age of incidence is 6 or 7 and boys are affected more often than girls (Curry & Daniels 1958) but in one epidemic in a mixed residential school boys and girls appeared to be equally susceptible and the greatest incidence was in younger children, aged 2 and 3 years (Walby 1952).

Microsporum canis ringworm is particularly a disease of kittens and puppies and its incidence in humans reflects the incidence in the small animal population, and the size of the latter (Stephens *et al.* 1989). The spores remain viable in infected hair for a shorter period than those of *M. audouini* (Glass 1948) and almost all human infections are acquired by direct contact with animals. Child-to-child transmission occurs only to a very limited extent. Boys and girls are equally affected and, although the age in children has varied in different epidemics, the cases are usually fairly evenly distributed throughout the various ages (Curry & Daniels 1958); infants may be affected, though rarely (Hubener 1957). In some outbreaks the infectivity has been very high, up to 93% of all children exposed developing the infection (Lawson & McLeod 1957).

Microsporum equinum rarely infects man, even where it is prevalent in horses, but it is occasionally acquired by direct contact with their associates and has been reported in children and in an adult (O'Grady *et al.* 1972). The other zoophilic *Microsporum* species also are rare causes of scalp ringworm, and are acquired by contact with their primary hosts.

Microsporum gypseum is primarily a soil saprophyte and most human infections result from direct contact with soil (e.g. Meinhof 1964). This fungus was isolated from 4% of samples of soil from children's playgrounds in Mannheim, Germany (Bojanovsky *et al.* 1979). However, infections are not rare in cats (Kaplan *et al.* 1957), dogs (Menges & Georg 1957), and other animals, and human infections may be acquired by contact with them.

The anthropophilic *Trichophyton* infections (see Table 13.1) are spread by direct or mediate contact (Babel & Baughman 1974). Adults are susceptible to infection, and although there is a tendency for some males and for many females to develop a resistance to infection, some females fail to do so (Seale & Richardson 1960). Spontaneous cures occur, but are unpredictable in the individual patient. Lesions may be insignificant and overlooked for years, and many members of a household may acquire the infection from adult carriers, usually women (Raubitschek 1959). Immigrants may introduce infections which, unsuspected, cause outbreaks in hospitals, schools and homes (Rosenthal *et al.* 1958; Putkonen & Blomqvist 1959). In parts of the United States, notably the South, *Trichophyton tonsurans* has replaced *Microsporum* as the predominant cause of scalp ringworm (Prevost 1974). As these infections show no fluorescence under Wood's light the diagnosis is readily overlooked. Similar diagnostic problems are reported from Benghazi, Libya (Malhotra *et al.* 1979) while 4.5% of school- children have tinea capitis caused by *Trichophyton schoenleinii* or *T. violaceum* and these infections tend to simulate seborrhoeic dermatitis. The mode of spread of human favus is essentially similar; reserves of infection are maintained in backward communities (Hannell & Partridge 1955). 'Witkop', relatively frequent among Bantu children in Africa, is a severe form of favus; poor nutrition is probably a factor in its wide extension (Murray *et al.* 1957).

The zoophilic *Trichophyton* species (see Table 13.1) may be contracted by direct contact with the host species, but mediate transmission is very frequent. *Trichophyton verrucosum*, for example, is acquired from stalls or fences against which infected cattle have rubbed their lesions. *Trichophyton mentagrophytes* often follows a minor abrasion in the region of farm buildings, but may also be contracted from cats or dogs. Similarly *T. quinckeanum* infection may result from direct contact with infected mice, or with a dog as intermediate host (Schneider 1954).

References

Alexander, S., Clayton, Y.M. & North, W.C. (1965) Tinea capitis in a primary school. *British Journal of Dermatology*, **77**, 373.
Allred, B.J. (1982) Dermatophyte prevalence in Wellington, New Zealand. *Sabouraudia*, **20**, 75.
Babel, D.E. & Baughman, S.A. (1989) Evaluation of the adult carrier state in juvenile tinea capitis caused by *Trichophyton tonsurans*. *Journal of the American Academy of Dermatology*, **21**, 1209.
Benedek, T. & Felsher, I.M. (1944) Epidemiology of tinea capitis. *Archives of Dermatology*, **49**, 120.
Blank, F., Mann, S.J. & Reale, R.A. (1974) Distribution of dermatophytoses according to age, ethnic group and sex. *Sabouraudia*, **12**, 352.
Bojanovsky, A., Mueller, H. & Freigang, K. (1979) Zur Vorkommen von Dermatophyten und anderen Keratophilen Pilze auf Kinderspeilplatzen. *Mykosen*, **22**, 149.

Clayton, Y.M. (1977) Epidemiological aspects of dermatophyte infections. *Current Therapeutic Research Clinical and Experimental*, **22**, 2.

Clayton, Y.M. (1986) Superficial fungal infections in new clinical applications. In *Dermatology*, p. 12, ed. Verbov. MTP Press Ltd, Lancaster.

Curry, J. & Daniels, G. (1958) Ringworm of the scalp in school children in the Manchester region. *Medical Officer*, **93**, 165.

Elewski, B.E. & Hazen, P.G. (1988) The superficial mycoses and the dermatophytes. *Journal of the American Academy of Dermatology*, **21**, 655.

Foged, E.K. & Jepson, L.V. (1984) Hair loss following kerion celsi — a follow-up examination. *Mykosen*, **27**, 411.

Friedman, L., Derbes, V.J., Hodges, E.P. & Gimshi, J.T. (1960) The isolation of dermatophytes from the air. *Journal of Investigative Dermatology*, **35**, 3.

Gip, L. (1966) Investigation of the occurrence of dermatophytes on the floor and in the air of indoor environments. *Acta Dermato-Venereologica*, **46**, (Suppl. 58).

Glass, F.A. (1948) Viability of fungus in hairs from patients with tinea capitis and *Microsporum audouini*. *Archives of Dermatology and Syphilology*, **57**, 122.

Hannell, J. & Partridge, B.M. (1955) Favus: a report of some selected cases. *British Medical Journal*, **i**, 1509.

Hubener, L.F. (1957) Tinea capitis (*M. canis*) in a thirty day old infant. *Archives of Dermatology*, **76**, 242.

Ive, F.A. (1966) The carrier stage of tinea capitis in Nigeria. *British Journal of Dermatology*, **78**, 219.

Kaplan,W. & Georg, L.K. (1957) Isolation of *M. audouini* from a dog. *Journal of Investigative Dermatology*, **28**, 313.

Kaplan, W., Georg, L.K. & Bronley, C.L. (1957) Ringworm of cats caused by *Microsporum gypseum*. *Veterinary Medicine*, **52**, 374.

Lawson, G.T.N. & McLeod, W.J. (1957) *Microsporum canis* — an intensive outbreak. *British Medical Journal*, **ii**, 1159.

McAleer, R. (1980) Fungal infection of the scalp in Western Australia. *Sabouraudia*, **18**, 185.

Malhotra, V.K., Gang, M.D. & Kanwar, A.J. (1979) A school survey of tinea capitis in Benghazi. *Journal of Tropical Medicine and Hygiene*, **82**, 59.

Meinhof, W. (1964) Endogene und exogene Faktoren der Entstellung von *Microsporum gypseum* Infektionen. *Hautarzt*, **15**, 352.

Menges, R.W. & Georg, L.K. (1957) Canine ringworm caused by *Microsporum gypseum*. *Cornell Veterinarian*, **47**, 1.

Murray, J.F., Freedman, M.L. Lurie, H.I. & Merriweather, A.M. (1957) Witkop: a synonym for favus. *South African Medical Journal*, **31**, 657.

O'Grady, K.J., English, M.P. & Warin, R.P. (1972) *Microsporum equuum* infection of the scalp in an adult. *British Journal of Dermatology*, **86**, 175.

Philpot, C.M. (1978) Geographical distribution of dermatophytes; a review. *Journal of Hygiene*, **80**, 301.

Prevost, E. (1974) Nonfluorescent tinea capitis in Charleston S.C.: a diagnostic problem. *Journal of the American Medical Association*, **242**, 1765.

Putkonen, T. & Blomqvist, K. (1959) *Trichophyton violaceum* infection in a home for mental defectives in Finland. *Acta Dermato-Venereologica*, **39**, 310.

Raubitschek, F. (1959) Infectivity and family incidence of black-dot tinea capitis. *Archives of Dermatology*, **79**, 477.

Rosenthal, S.A., Fisher, D. & Farneri, D. (1958) A localized outbreak in New York City of tinea capitis due to *Trichophyton violaceum*. *Archives of Dermatology*, **78**, 689.

Schneider, W. (1954) Favusepidemic durch Feldmause. *Hautarzt*, **5**, 348.

Seale, E.R. & Richardson, J.B (1960) *Trichophyton tonsurans*. *Archives of Dermatology*, **81**, 87.

Walby, A.L. (1952) Tinea capitis (*M. audouini*) in a residential school. *British Medical Journal*, **i**, 1114.

Stephens, C.J.M., Hay, R.J. & Black, M.M. (1989) Fungal kerion—total scalp involvement due to *M. canis*. *Clinical and Experimental Dermatology*, **14**, 442.

Wood's light in diagnosis

Wood's light, named after the American physicist R.W. Wood, is ultraviolet light passed through glass containing 9% nickel oxide. It was first used in dermatology by Margarot and Deveze in 1925. The responsible fluorescent substance is formed only when the keratin of the hair is invaded and its presence in detectable amounts under a Wood's lamp may depend on the degree to which the hairs are infected.

The fungi of the genus *Microsporum*, and also *Trichophyton schoenleinii*, when growing in hair, give a green fluorescence in Wood's light. Non-fluorescent variants of *Microsporum audouini* and *M. canis* have been reported, but are rare (Beare & Walker 1955). Non-fluorescent *M. gypseum* has also been reported (Wilson & Plunkett 1951; Funt 1959). In *Microsporum* infections the light-green fluorescence may be limited to a narrow band just above the scalp. Hairs infected by *Trichophyton schoenleinii* show a duller fluorescence, but along the whole length of the hair.

The effective use of Wood's light requires some experience. The examination must be made in a fully darkened room. The reflected light from white coats or uniforms may make occasional lesions difficult to detect. If the scalp has been smeared with ointment, this must be washed off with a detergent shampoo. The actinic fluorescence of scales and exudates soon becomes familiar and can then be ignored.

References

Beare, J.M. & Walker, J. (1955) Non-fluorescent *Microsporum audouini* and *canis* ringworm of the scalp. *British Journal of Dermatology*, **67**, 101.

Funt, T.R. (1959) Nonfluorescent *Microsporum* in tinea capitis. *Journal of the Florida Medical Association*, **45**, 1021.

Margarot, J. & Deveze, P. (1925) Aspect de quelques dermatoses en lumière ultraviolette; note préliminaire. *Bulletin de la Société des Sciences Medicales et Biologiques de Montpellier et du Languedoc Méditerranéen*, **6**, 375.

Wilson, J.W. & Plunkett, O.A. (1951) Lack of fluorescence of scalp hairs infected with *Microsporum gypseum*. *Journal of Investigative Dermatology*, **16**, 119.

Clinical features (References p. 414)

The patient's immune responses, their modification by medication, whether prescribed for the infection or for concomitant disease, the nutritional status of the patient, and the special properties of the strain of fungus concerned introduce such a multiplicity of variables that almost any species of dermatophyte can be associated with any of the ringworm syndromes. Nevertheless each group of species produces a reasonably consistent clinical picture, in the majority of cases.

Anthropophilic Microsporum species

Infections with *M. audouini* have been extensively studied. The less comprehensive literature on *M. ferugineum* infections suggests that the behaviour of the two species is similar. Most patients present with single or multiple rounded or irregular patches in which the hairs are broken off a few millimetres above the scalp; the stumps are twisted and brittle and are often greyish-white. The individual patch seldom exceeds 5 cm in diameter, but by confluence of neighbouring patches large areas may be involved. Less commonly only scattered hairs are infected and clinical diagnosis without Wood's light is impossible. During the earliest stages of infection the scalp may be reddened but the redness soon fades to leave superficial scaling. Persistent inflammatory changes with kerion formation occur in 2–3% of cases. Associated lesions of the glabrous skin occur rather uncommonly.

If inflammatory changes occur spontaneous cure takes only a few weeks. Even in the absence of clinically obvious inflammation the infection rarely extends for more than 10 weeks, but it may then persist apparently unchanged for many months, even for 3 or 4 years. Almost all infections resolve at puberty and the many non-inflammatory infections in younger children are self-limiting within a few months (Rivalier 1950; Whittle 1953); in a small proportion of cases the natural duration, without treatment, is about 3 years (Friedman *et al.* 1964).

It seems probable that cases of very long duration are unusual except in the presence of malnutrition or of other factors impairing the immune response. *Microsporum audouini* has been isolated from a young adult with cicatricial alopecia since childhood (Avram & Porojan 1962); such exceptional cases require immunological investigation.

Zoophilic and geophilic Microsporum species

Although there are probably significant differences between the reactions to species within this group, the characteristic clinical features as compared with infections with anthropophilic species are the greater incidence of grossly inflammatory lesions, with kerion formation in over 40% of cases in some outbreaks (Sonck 1965) and the frequent presence of associated lesions on glabrous skin. However, there are racial differences in the response to *M. canis*, which causes little evident inflammation in Australian aboriginals (Donald *et al.* 1965) (Fig. 13.2).

Anthropophilic Trichophyton species

(i) *Favus. Trichophyton schoenleinii* classically gives rise to distinctive, readily recognisable lesions. In fact such lesions occur in a minority of infections in individuals of good nutritional status and the less-striking changes which are commonly present are readily overlooked. The classical lesion is the scutulum; a yellowish concretion at the orifice of a hair follicle, it enlarges to form a concave disc 1 cm or more in diameter and is firmly attached at its centre to the underlying scalp. The coalescence of large scutula may give rise to crumbling asbestos-like masses. The less distinctive changes, now more often seen, vary greatly in morphology and extent (Jung 1955; Hakendorf *et al.* 1965). The concretions may be small and plug-like but otherwise typical, or they may be replaced by patchy

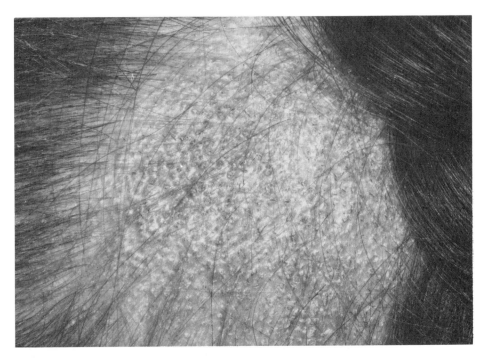

Fig. 13.2 *Microsporum canis* infection. Inflammatory changes in this case are slight.

pityriasiform scaling or crusting. Rarely there may be marked inflammatory changes and even kerion formation. The hairs in the affected regions become opaque, and later sparse, but broken hairs are not a common finding. In long-standing cases there may be widespread cicatricial alopecia. Under Wood's light affected hairs give a dull greenish fluorescence along their entire length.

Lesions of the glabrous skin are sometimes associated; they may be of tinea circinata or herpetiform type or may consist of scattered or grouped scutula. Rarely the nails are involved (Jung 1955).

Favus of the scalp, contracted as it often is in early childhood, shows some tendency to spontaneous cure between the ages of 8 and 14 (Cantanei 1950) but many infections persist long into adult life (Kalter & Wolf 1984), particularly in women (Fig. 13.3). Up to four generations have been found to be infected (Blank 1962). Lesions of the glabrous skin commonly clear without treatment.

(ii) *Trichophyton tonsurans* (formerly *T. sulphureum*), *T. violaceum, T. gourvilii, T. megninii, T. soudanense* and *T. yaoundi*. The lesions produced by these species have many features in common and it is difficult to determine whether such differences as have been noted are inherent, or result from genetic variation in the host, or environmental factors.

The classical lesion produced by these species is 'black-dot' ringworm, in which numerous small plaques of irregular shape are studded with black dots—hairs broken off at scalp level. Long healthy hairs in groups of three or four may persist

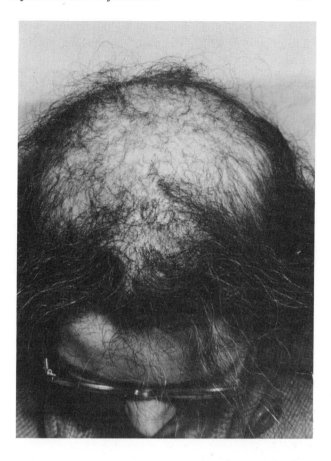

Fig. 13.3 Favus with extensive scarring. In such a scalp foci of active infection may still be present.

within the plaques. In most outbreaks, however, such cases form a minority, and the clinical manifestations are very variable. To some extent the type of lesions may be correlated with the duration of the infection (Howell *et al.* 1952). Scaling without loss of hair (Putkonen & Blomquist 1959) or with occasional broken hairs (Joseph & Halde 1955; Beare 1956; Mackenzie *et al.* 1960) provides the only clinical evidence of infection in many cases. In very long-standing infections large areas of cicatricial alopecia dominate the picture, and scaling or broken hairs are found only with difficulty. The nails are sometimes infected (Calnan *et al.* 1962).

Although an inflammatory phase is not uncommon, trichophytides are not often recorded. They tend to be follicular (Conerly & Greer 1988) but may take the form of erythema nodosum (Franks *et al.* 1952).

While active inflammatory changes lead often to spontaneous cure, this failed to occur in a generalized vegetating granulomatous infection with *T. tonsurans* (Beirana & Novales 1959). Those cases in which inflammatory changes are neither conspicuous nor prolonged tend eventually to clear spontaneously, but may take many years to do so, and may persist indefinitely in some adult women (Kamalam & Thambiah 1976). Adult carriers are apparently exclusively women (Raubitschek 1959).

(iii) *Trichophyton rubrum.* This species is considered apart from those in the above group because, unlike them, it is in many areas an extremely common cause of tinea of glabrous skin and nails, but very rarely causes scalp ringworm (Borda 1969). In the majority of cases in which infection extends far beyond the hands, feet and genitocrural region it is probable that cell-mediated immunity is impaired. It may well be so in all patients with scalp involvement. One such patient was an elderly diabetic in whom impaired cellular immunity was demonstrated (Kind *et al.* 1974). She had pustules, erythema, scaling, and loss of hair. Some patients have developed black-dot tinea (Price *et al.* 1963), others breaking of hairs at different levels, and still others kerion formation (Bazex *et al.* 1963).

Zoophilic Trichophyton species
(i) The species listed in Table 13.1 (excluding *T. quinckeanum*) usually cause severely inflammatory lesions leading to kerion formation in the scalp and spontaneous cure in a matter of months. The morphology and the course of infections with *T. verrucosum* and *T. mentagraphytes* are identical (Rook & Frain-Bell 1954; Rook 1954). Reported differences between the lesions induced by other species must be assessed in the light of possible genetic and nutritional variations in the hosts, and of the site involved (Fig. 13.4).

These infections tend to show marked inflammatory changes from the first appearance of the lesions; after an interval of 7–10 days severe pustulation develops, as a reaction to the fungus, and not as a result of secondary bacterial

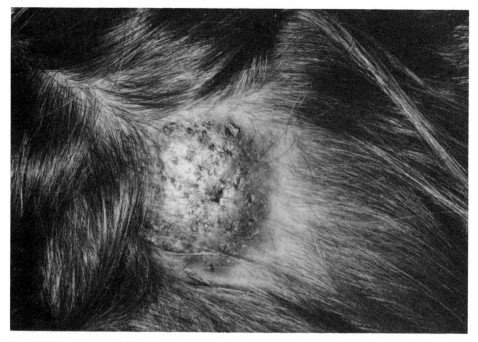

Fig. 13.4 Kerion caused by *Trichophyton mentagrophytes.*

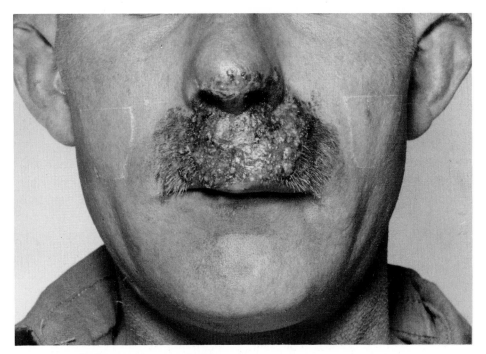

Fig. 13.5 *Trichophyton verrucosum* infection.

infection (Birt & Wilt 1954; Even-Paz & Raubitschek 1960). Immunological defects modify the course of the infection. *Trichophyton verrucosum* (Fig. 13.5) caused chronic lesions in a boy with a reticulosis (Hval 1936). Black-dot ringworm with scarring persisted for over 50 years in a patient infected with this same species (Altéras 1962).

The normal course of a scalp infection, however, is the rapid development of a plaque of erythema, which becomes increasingly oedematous and studded with large follicular pustules, the so-called agminate folliculitis, which in most cases is succeeded by a kerion, a raised boggy mass of pustules. Less often, firm inflammatory nodules are formed—Majocchi's granuloma. Scalp involvement may be very extensive, when malaise and low fever may occur. Spontaneous healing is the rule and although scarring is inevitable the degree of regrowth of hair is often greater than the severity of the reaction leads the inexperienced to expect.

(ii) *Mouse favus.* The lesions produced by *T. quinckeanum* are seldom immediately recognizable as such. Most distinctive is an inflammatory infiltrated plaque, with small sulphur-yellow scutula (Blank *et al.* 1961). More often there are erythematous patches with scaling and hair loss (Christmas & Clayton 1966), or kerion formation (Altéras 1959; Kabur & Plotz 1962). There may be only impetigo-like crusting.

The infection is self-limiting.

Diagnosis of scalp ringworm (References p. 414)

The possibility of ringworm must be considered in the presence of alopecia, scaling, broken hairs or folliculitis, singly or in any combination. Since throughout this book the need to exclude a ringworm infection is stressed in the discussion of each of the conditions which ringworm may simulate, differential diagnosis will not be considered in detail in this chapter.

In the child the commonest sources of error are traumatic alopecia, alopecia areata, pityriasis simplex and pityriasis amiantacea (Honig & Smith 1979). In the commonest form of traumatic alopecia as a habit hairs are twisted and broken, but of normal texture. In alopecia areata the scalp is not scaly. In pityriasis amiantacea the masses of sticky scale may cover a moist red area of scalp from which the hair readily falls, but the hair is not broken or abnormal in texture.

Pyogenic infections of the scalp are rare in childhood, except impetigo complicating head louse infestation. A history of trauma is often given by patients with zoophilic ringworm infections, and the diagnosis of 'infected abrasion' of the scalp is suspect.

In the older child or adult scarring alopecia without evident cause is ringworm until proved not to be so.

Where the diagnosis of ringworm is under consideration the scalp should be examined under Wood's light. If fluorescent hairs are present, some should be removed for microscopy and culture. If no fluorescent hairs are detected, but the lesions are otherwise suggestive of *Microsporum* infections, hairs which appear abnormal in texture or length when viewed in ordinary light should be extracted, to exclude the rare non-fluorescent strains. If there is no fluorescence and ringworm cannot be excluded on clinical grounds any broken or abnormal hairs, scale or crust must be examined by microscopy and culture.

Microscopy of infected hairs may provide immediate confirmation of the diagnosis of ringworm, and will also establish whether fungus is small or large spore, ectothrix or endothrix.

Culture should always be carried out, since precise identification of the species is essential for epidemiological purposes.

Treatment (Hay 1990)

The choice of treatment will be determined by the species of fungus, the degree of inflammation, and of the facilities available. In some cases the immunological and nutritional status of the patient may have to be taken into account. A severe agminate folliculitis or kerion caused by a zoophilic species may well resolve but co-existing non-inflammatory lesions in other regions of the scalp may persist. Totally non-inflammatory lesions run a long course, though the anthropophilic *Microsporum* infections tend to clear at puberty. If for economic or other reasons griseofulvin is in short supply or unobtainable, it is reasonable to leave untreated those cases which can be expected to resolve, but if it is available it is the treatment of choice in all ringworm of the scalp. Given late in inflammatory infections it may have little influence on the course of existing lesions, but it will prevent the development of new ones.

Griseofulvin (Lesher & Smith 1987)

Griseofulvin is an antibiotic derived from *Penicillium griseofulvum*. It is active against the dermatophytes, but not against yeasts or bacteria. Resistant strains of dermatophytes are unusual. After oral administration, griseofulvin is poorly absorbed from the gut, although micronization (reduced particle size) (Davies 1980) significantly enhances absorption as does taking fatty food simultaneously (Ogunbona *et al.* 1985). Once absorbed, it is primarily protein-bound to serum albumin, with free drug plasma concentrations determining tissue distribution. The drug is demethylated in the liver and then excreted by the kidneys. Griseofulvin accumulates in the keratin of the stratum corneum, hair and nails, rendering them resistant to invasion by the fungus. Treatment must be continued for long enough for the infected keratin to be replaced by resistant keratin.

The drug has a fungistatic effect, that is, it works best on actively growing dermatophytes. Its mechanism of action may include inhibition of synthesis of fungal cell walls, interference with DNA synthesis and mitosis, binding to RNA, and inhibition of cellular microtubules (Davies 1980).

Griseofulvin has proved to be remarkably non-toxic but side effects such as gastrointestinal upset, headache, fatigue and transient rashes occasionally occur. Headache due to the drug may sometimes be overcome by decreasing the dose and slowly increasing it again (Blank 1982). Griseofulvin may interact with other medications such a phenobarbitone and warfarin.

Griseofulvin microsize is usually given in a total daily dose of 500–1000 mg for adults, or 10 mg/kg body weight daily for children. The hair in and around the infected areas of scalp should be cut short and tolnaftate cream or Whitfield's ointment should be applied daily. Therapy for 6–8 weeks is usually effective but treatment should be continued until there is good regrowth of hair and mycological cure has been achieved. Progress must be monitored by regular clinical examination (and Wood's light for fluorescent species). In inflammatory lesions compresses may be necessary to remove pus and scale.

A single dose of griseofulvin has been used successfully to treat cases of tinea capitis. Friedman *et al.* (1960) treated 22 children infected by *M. audouini* with a single dose of 3 g and obtained cure in 21, while in a study carried out in the Congo (Van Breuseghem *et al.* 1970), cure was achieved in 93% of 72 children after a single dose of 1.5 g. Single-dose therapy may have a place in developing countries where daily administration may be expensive and difficult to monitor.

Griseofulvin treatment of kerion does not necessarily reduce the development of scarring alopecia, and additional anti-inflammatory treatment with corticosteroids may be reasonable and beneficial (Foged & Jepsen 1984).

Azole compounds and allylamines (Hay 1990)

The development of this group of synthetic antifungal agents has made a significant impact in the therapy of fungal infections. The imidazoles offer the first broad-spectrum coverage against a variety of yeasts and fungi. Ketoconazole is the first oral agent to be generally available but its use is limited by expense and hepatotoxicity. Fluconazole has less hepatotoxicity and may prove a useful alternative although it is only recommended for *Candida* infections at present. Itraconazole is a triazole drug developed for oral use, which has a wide spectrum of activity against yeast and fungi, and appears to be safe and non-toxic, but hair loss during therapy may occur. Azoles and allylamines are fungicidal at normal therapeutic concentrations cf. griseofulvin which is fungistatic.

Public health measures

The diagnosis of ringworm of the scalp imposes the obligation to determine the source of infection so that action may be taken to prevent its further dissemination. The infecting species must therefore be identified.

If the species is anthropophilic, family and school contacts must be examined, using Wood's light where this is appropriate. In the control of an outbreak caused by *Microsporum audouini* the use of a plastic scalp massager proved more reliable than Wood's light in identifying carriers with minimal sub-clinical infection (Dixon 1968). Three of eight cases thus detected had shown no abnormality under Wood's light. All infected individuals must be isolated until they have been successfully treated.

The source of infection with some zoophilic species is often difficult to trace. Outbreaks of *M. canis* infection can be large. Patients' cats and dogs must be inspected under Wood's light, and referred for treatment. In some cases the help of the police may be required in rounding up stray animals. *Trichophyton mentagrophytes* may follow known contact with rodents, but often no source can be traced.

References

Altéras, M.I. (1959) Kérion de celse du cuir chevelu dû à l'*Achorion quinckeanum*. *Annales de Dermatologie et de Syphiligraphie*, **86**, 518.

Altéras, M.I. (1962) A propos d'un cas de trichophytie chronique du cuir chevelu, à type de pseudopelade, dû au *Trichophyton violaceum*. *Dermatologica*, **125**, 382.

Avram, A. & Porojan, I. (1962) Un cas isolite de microsporose chronique de l'adulte simulant le favus. *Dermatologica*, **125**, 259.

Bazex, A., Salvador, B. & Dupre, A. (1963) Sur le polymorphism clinique réalisé par le *Trichophyton rubrum*. *Annales de Dermatologie et de Syphiligraphie*, **90**, 361.

Beare, J.M. (1956) Tinea capitis due to *Trichophyton sulphureum*. *British Journal of Dermatology*, **68**, 193.

Beirana, L. & Novales, J. (1959) Tiña universal y granulomatose por *Trichophyton tonsuras*. *Dermatologia Revista Mexicana*, **3**, 4.

Birt, A.R. & Wilt, J.C. (1954) Mycology, bacteriology and histopathology of suppurative ringworm. *Archives of Dermatology and Syphilology*, **69**, 441.

Blank, F. (1962) Human favus in Quebec. *Dermatologica*, **125**, 369.

Blank, F., Tech, S., Leclerc, G. & Telner, P. (1961) Clinical manifestations of mouse favus in man. *Archives of Dermatology*, **83**, 587.

Blank, H. (1982) Commentary: treatment of dermatomycoses with griseofulvin. *Archives of Dermatology*, **118**, 835.

Borda, J.M. (1969) El *Trichophyton rubrum* en dermatologia. *Archivos Argentinos de Dermatologia*, **19**, 1.

Calnan, C.D., Djavahiszwili, N. & Hodgson, C.J. (1962) *Trichophyton soudanense* in Britain. *British Journal of Dermatology*, **74**, 144.

Catanei, A. (1950) Les teignes en Afrique du Nord. *Maroc Medical*, **29**, 955.

Christmas, R.J. & Clayton, Y.M. (1966) Studies in mycology. I. *T. quinckeanum*. *Transactions of the St. John's Hospital Dermatological Society*, **52**, 241.

Conerly, S.L. & Greer, D.L. (1988) Tinea capitis in adults over fifty years of age. *Cutis*, **41**, 251.

Davies, R.R. (1980) Griseofulvin. In *Antifungal Chemotherapy*, p. 149, ed. D.C.E. Speller. John Wiley, Chichester.

Dixon, P.N. (1968) The mycological control of an epidemic of tinea capitis due to *Microsporum audouini*. *Medical Officer*, **120**, 59.

Donald, G.F., Brown, G.W. & Sheppard, A.A.W. (1965) The dermatophytic flora of South Australia. A survey of 1819 cases of tinea studied between 1954 and 1964. *Australian Journal of Dermatology*, **8**, 78.

Even-Paz, Z. & Raubitschek, F. (1960) Epidemics of tinea capitis due to *Trichophyton verrucosum* contracted from cattle or sheep. *Dermatologica*, **120**, 74.

Foged, E.K. & Jepsen, L.V. (1984) Hair loss following kerion celsi—a follow up examination. *Mykosen*, **27**, 411.

Franks, A.G., Rosenbaum, E.M. & Mandel, E.H. (1952) *Trichophyton sulphureum* causing erythema nodosum and multiple kerion formation. *AMA Archives of Dermatology and Syphilology*, **65**, 95.

Friedman, L., Derbes, V.J. & Tromovitxh, T.A. (1960) Simple dose therapy of tinea capitis. *Archives of Dermatology*, **82**, 415.

Friedman, L., Derbes, V.J. & Hodges, E.P. (1964) The course of untreated tinea capitis in Negro children. *Journal of Investigative Dermatology*, **42**, 237.

Hakendorf, A.J., Donald, G.F. & Linn, H.W. (1965) Favus. *Australian Journal of Dermatology*, **8**, 22.

Hay, R.J. (1990) Antifungal drugs—an introduction. *Journal of Dermatological Treatment*, **1** (Supplement), 1.

Honig, P.J. & Smith, L.R. (1979) Tinea capitis masquerading as atopic or seborrhoeic dermatitis. *Journal of Pediatrics*, **94**, 604.

Howell, J.B., Wilson, J.W. & Caro, M.R. (1952) Tinea capitis caused by *Trichophyton tonsurans* (sulfureum or crateriforme). *AMA Archives of Dermatology and Syphilology*, **65**, 194.

Hval, E. (1936) A case of reticulosis of the regional lymph glands in association with a chronic skin infection. *Acta Dermato-Venereologica*, **17**, 402.

Joseph, H.L. & Halde, C. (1955) Tinea capitis due to *Trichophyton tonsurans*. *California Medicine*, **83**, 371.

Jung, H.-D. (1955) Zur Diagnose und Therapie des Favus. *Hautarzt*, **6**, 12.

Kabur, U. & Plotz, W.-D. (1962) Mausefavus im Bereich des behaarten Kopfes. *Dermatologische Wochenschrift*, **146**, 270.

Kalter, D.C. & Wolf, (1984) Tropical and unusual superficial fungal infections. *Dermatology Clinics*, **2**, 45.

Kamalam, A. & Thambiah, A.S. (1976) *Trichophyton violaceum* infection in an Indian school. *International Journal of Dermatology*, **15**, 136.

Kind, R., Hornstein, O.P., Meinhof, W. & Weidner, F. (1974) Tinea capitis durch *Trichophyton rubrum* und multimorbidität im Senium, mit partiellem Defekt der zellularem Immunität. *Hautarzt*, **25**, 606.

Lesher, J.L. & Smith, J.G. (1987) Antifungal agents in dermatology. *Journal of American Academy of Dermatology*, **17**, 383.

Mackenzie, D.W.R., Burrows, D. & Walby, A.L. (1960) *Trichophyton sulphureum* in a residential school. *British Medical Journal*, **ii**, 1055.

Ogunbona, F.A., Smith, I.F. & Olawoye, O.S. (1985) Fat contents of meals and bioavailability of griseofulvin in man. *Journal of Pharmacy and Pharmacology*, **37**, 283.

Price, V.H., Rosenthal, S.A. & Villafane, J. (1963) Black dot tinea capitis caused by *Trichophyton rubrum. Archives of Dermatology*, **87**, 487.

Putkonen, T. & Blomquist, K. (1959) *Trichophyton violaceum* infection in a home for mental defectives in Helsinki. *Acta Dermato-Venereologica*, **39**, 310.

Raubitschek, F. (1959) Infectivity and family incidence of black-dot tinea capitis. *Archives of Dermatology*, **79**, 477.

Rivalier, E. (1950) Les microspories spontanément curables. *Annales de Dermatologie et de Syphiligraphie*, **10**, 518.

Rook, A.J. (1954) Cattle ringworm in man. *Medical Illustration*, **8**, 12.

Rook, A.J. & Frain-Bell, W. (1954) Cattle ringworm. *British Medical Journal*, ii, 1198.

Sonck, C.E. (1965) Mikrospori i Finland. *Nordisk Medicin*, **60**, 1100.

Van Breuseghem, R., Gatti, F. & Ceballos, J.A. (1970) Mass treatment of scalp ringworm by a single dose of griseofulvin. *International Journal of Dermatology*, **9**, 59.

Whittle, C.H. (1953) Is scalp ringworm a self-limiting disease? *Lancet*, ii, 10.

Mycetoma of the scalp

Aetiology and epidemiology

An uncommon manifestation of dermatophytosis of the scalp is the formation of a mycetoma. A mycetoma is an indolent infection of soft tissue, characterized by tumefaction, draining sinus tracts to the skin with dark or pale granules. Eumycetomas are produced by true fungi, but actinomycetomas result from branching, filamentous bacteria. Dermatophytes have caused scalp mycetomas almost exclusively in Africans (Van Breuseghem and Vandeputte 1959; Camain *et al.* 1971). *Trichophyton rubrum*, *T. verrucosum*, *T. mentagrophytes*, *T. violaceum*, *Microsporum ferrugineum*, *M. canis* and *M. audouini* have been isolated from such cases (Strobel *et al.* 1980). Traumatic inoculation of the aetiological agent from the soil or a plant occurs in the tropics or hot, temperate climates.

Clinical features

The mycetoma presents a relatively painless, smooth, firm mobile nodule with or without discharging sinuses. Pus and granules may drain through the skin via multiple intercommunicating fistulae. The disease can proceed very slowly for years, with underlying scalp involvement producing periostitis, sclerosis, loss of trabecular pattern and small areas of osteolysis. Hideous deformities may result after many years of infection (Hickey 1956).

References

Camain, R., Baylet, R., Nonhouayi, Y. *et al.* (1971) Note sur les mycétomes de la nuque et du cuir chevelu de l'Africain. *Bulletin de la Société de Pathologie Exotique et de ses Filiales*, **64**, 447.

Hickey, B.B. (1956) Cranial maduromycosis. *Transactions of the Royal Society of Tropical Medicine and Hygiene*, **50**, 393.

Strobel, M., Ndiaye, B., Machaund, J.-P., Ravisse, P. & Baisset, M. (1980) Mycétome à dermatophyte du cuir chevelu. *Annales de Dermatologie et de Vénéréologie*, **107**, 1181.

Van Breuseghem, R. & Vandeputte, M. (1959) Mycétome de la nuque chez un noir du Congo Belge. *Annales de la Société Belge de Médecine Tropicale*, **39**, 227.

Ringworm of the beard

Aetiology
Ringworm of the beard is necessarily confined to adult males. Most cases are caused by zoophilic species, especially *Trichophyton mentagrophytes*, *T. verrucosum* and *Microsporum canis* (Loewenthal 1965), but some are caused by anthropophilic fungi such as *Trichophyton rubrum* (Avram 1963). In Western Australia *T. rubrum* was the most frequent species in urban cases, followed by *T. mentagrophytes* and *Microsporum canis*, whilst in rural areas all the cases were caused by *Trichophyton mentagrophytes* (McAleer 1980). Such cases are occasionally inappropriately treated with corticosteroids, which profoundly modify the course of the infection.

Clinical features
Plaques of large follicular pustules or fully developed kerions are usually seen. However, in some cases there is a diffuse area of erythema and scaling with irregularly distributed pustules. Cases treated with corticosteroids are particularly liable to show this appearance. Such lesions may slowly extend over months. Untreated agminate folliculitis too may persist for long periods, but tends eventually to resolve (Fig. 13.5).

Diagnosis
Hairs from the follicular pustules should be extracted for microscopy and culture.

Treatment
See p. 412.

References
Avram, A. (1963) Sur les pilomycoses déterminées par le *Trichophyton rubrum*. *Dermatologica*, **126**, 354.
Loewenthal, K. (1965) Tinea barbae due to *Microsporum canis*. *Archives of Dermatology*, **91**, 60.
McAleer, R. (1980) Fungal infections as a cause of skin diseases in Western Australia. III. Tinea barbae. *Australian Journal of Dermatology*, **21**, 40.

Pediculosis capitis
(References p. 422)

History
Lice have been man's frequent companions for millenia (Essig 1931) and no race is known to be spared their attentions. Two species of louse infest man, *Pediculus humanus* and *Phthirus pubis*. *Pediculus humanus* occurs in two distinct populations; *P. humanus capitis* the head louse, and *P. humanus corporis*, the body louse. It seems probable that the body louse evolved from the head louse when man began to wear

clothes. The two races, which can interbreed, show marked physiological, and some inconstant anatomical differences. The head louse is occasionally found on the body, but the body louse is rarely seen in the scalp (Buxton 1947).

Pediculosis humanus capitis
(Orkin *et al.* 1977; Parish *et al.* 1989)
The female head louse is 3–4 mm long; the male is slightly smaller and banded across the back. Its colour ranges from greyish-white to brown according to the skin colour of the human population it habitually parasitizes (Ferris 1935). The eggs, which are oval-lidded white capsules (Fig. 13.6) are each firmly cemented to

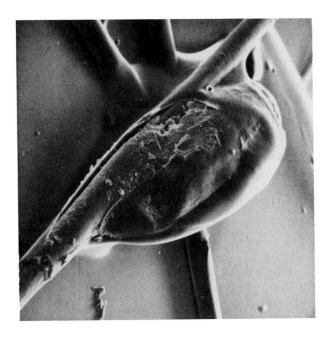

Fig. 13.6 Egg capsule (nit) of the head louse under the scanning electron microscope.

a hair shaft adjacent to the scalp. After about a week the eggs hatch to produce larvae (nymphs) which resemble small adults. Feeding begins soon after hatching, each nymph filling with blood until they look like 'rubies on legs' (Maunder 1983). They undergo three moults during their first 10 days of life to reach maturity, darken in colour and commence mating.

The factors which regulate the larvae population in the individual scalp are not fully understood. The temperature and humidity of the scalp provide a favourable environment for incubation; hatching is slowed, or will not occur, at temperatures below 22°C. In most established infestations there are fewer than 10 adult lice (Mellanby 1942), but Buxton (1947) found 1286 adults and nymphs in one head in West Africa and 774 adults on one head in Colombo; in general, counts of over

100 are uncommon, and those of over 1000 are rare. The population tends to be related to the total weight of hair, and seasonal climatic changes appear not to be relevant, nor is there reliable evidence that the nutritional status of the host influences the population (Buxton 1947). However, 67 refugees from Burma, who had suffered severe deprivations, showed average counts of 130 adults and 418 nymphs (Roy & Ghosh 1944). When the population is large the ratio of males to females is high and the mortality of young females is increased (Buxton 1937).

Lice and their eggs are most numerous in the occipital and post-auricular regions of the scalp (Fig. 13.7).

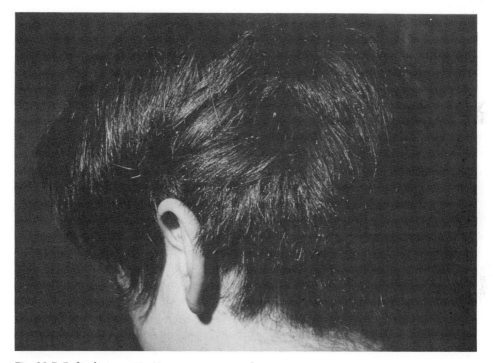

Fig. 13.7 Pediculosis capitis. Numerous egg capsules are present.

Epidemiology and incidence
The head louse occurs throughout the world. It is transmitted by direct contact, or by shared hats, caps, brushes or combs. The louse can travel directly from one head to another on a pillow or a chair or may be transferred as eggs on shed hairs. Long fine hair and poor hygiene favour the establishment of infestation. Girls of low intelligence showed a higher incidence than others living under the same conditions (Rollin 1943). Members of large families have greater opportunities of exposure (Mellanby 1942) as do members of schools or other communities.

Mellanby's (1941) detailed studies in a large industrial city showed up to 50%

of girls infested at all ages between 2 and 13, over 20% between 14 and 18 and some 40% aged 1. The incidence of boys was lower in all age groups, and reached a peak of about 45% in those aged 2–4 years. During the school years the percentage of boys infested fell rapidly. Other statistics show similar age and sex differences, but no age is immune. The usually low incidence in adults, and particularly in adult males, has been said to be related to their lower total weight of hair, but this cannot be the sole explanation (Askew 1971). In some communities where living conditions are crowded and hygiene standards are low the prevalence in adults of both sexes may remain high (Davis *et al.* 1944).

The importance of social conditions in determining the prevalence of head lice was emphasized by a study of school children in Kassel in Germany (Letz 1980). Infestation was most frequent among children of foreign workers and in children who were physically or mentally handicapped.

The prevalence of head lice in Britain was high in 1940 and the years that followed, but by 1960 was relatively uncommon, especially in rural areas. In recent years the infestation has again become more common. In Glasgow in 1969 nearly 10% of girls and 4% of boys had lice (Wilson 1969). The relatively greater increase in the infestation rate of boys, which has been noted also in some surveys has been attributed to changes in hairdressing styles but in one survey the prevalence was highest in children with short hair (Juranek 1977). On Teeside (Coates 1971) about 12% of children returning to school after the summer holidays were infested. The incidence continued to rise (Department of Education and Science 1974), partly no doubt because some lice were becoming resistant to DDT and gammexane (Maunder 1971a). Davidson (1975) estimated the national prevalence at 2.4%, since when it has fallen. The prevalence in some other parts of the world is discussed by Gretz (1977). An interesting observation, which is not fully explained, is that the prevalence of head lice is more than 30 times greater in American whites than in blacks attending the same school classes (Juranek 1977). This observation was confirmed in Kenya where Negroid children had lower infestation rates than non-Negroid children (Churge 1986), and the prevalence of infestation was higher in private schools because non-Negroid children predominated (of 1270 school children, 17.1% were infested). In the Niger Delta 5.7% of inhabitants harboured head lice, but the prevalence rose to 13.5% in the 6–13 year group (overall, more females were affected than males) (Arene & Ukaular 1985). The incidence is high in some villages in India, reaching about 18% (Hati *et al.* 1980).

Pathology

Nymphs and adults of both sexes suck blood, and in doing so inject their saliva. The pruritus which leads to scratching and hence to the secondary bacterial infection which may dominate the clinical picture is a manifestation of hypersensitivity to antigenic constituents of the saliva. There have been few investigations in man of the immunological response to lice. Peck *et al.* (1943) used human volunteers. Experimental feeding at first produced pinpoint areas of erythema without pruritus. After about a week pruritus was first experienced. Thereafter bites provoked an immediate irritable weal followed by a persistent papule. There was wide individual variation in response and some subjects showed little or no reaction after months of daily exposure. In the investigation of home contacts of our patients we have seen very heavily infested subjects with no symptoms.

Clinical features

The clinical features of pediculosis are surprisingly variable. Pruritus, which may be intense, depends on the immune response to the salivary antigens of the louse and on the host's threshold of perception. It is seldom completely absent. Characteristically it is most severe in the occipital region where the infestation is usually most heavy. Scratching introduces secondary bacterial infection, leading to impetiginous crusts and cervical adenitis. In severe cases a child may be pale, listless and febrile. A generalized erythematous dermatitis has been reported (Ronchese 1946).

If the infestation is of long duration and secondary infection is severe and persistent the hair may become densely matted by malodorous pus and exudate to give rise to the state formerly known as 'plica polonica'.

In those individuals in whom pruritus is slight or absent, the infestation may not be recognized until it is deliberately sought.

Except in those few cases in which the population of lice as nymphs or adults is high, there is no 'mechanized dandruff' to be seen. The diagnostic feature is the presence of oval egg-capsules, popularly known as nits, firmly cemented to the hair shafts. They are most easily confused with hair casts but the latter slide freely along the shaft and are annular. Other foreign bodies (Kutz 1969; Gemrich 1974) have been responsible for misdiagnoses, which may have embarrassing consequences for public health administrators. With a hand-lens the distinctive shape of the egg is easy to identify. It is particularly easy to see under Wood's light, which is useful if a large school population has to be screened.

Impetigo of the scalp is never an acceptable diagnosis until pediculosis has been reliably excluded.

Treatment

If secondary infection is severe, and particularly in the presence of adenitis or toxaemia, an antibiotic should be administered systemically. If the hair is densely matted it may be necessary to cut it.

In most cases, however, treatment with a parasiticide is sufficient provided it is carried out thoroughly. Preparations of gammexane or 5% emulsion of DDT have been widely used with success for some years. The chosen application is rubbed into the scalp once daily for 5 days, and thoroughly washed off a week later. The hair is then carefully examined and any remaining eggs are removed with a fine-toothed comb.

Where lice are resistent to gammexane and the DDT (Maunder 1971a), malathion 0.5% in spirit has been successfully used (Ares Mazaz *et al.* 1988; Maunder 1971b). The lotion is applied liberally and allowed to dry. After 12–24 hours the hair is washed and combed. *In vitro* testing has shown that 0.5% malathion lotion killed lice within 5 minutes and was highly ovicidal, with only 5% of eggs hatching (Meinking *et al.* 1986).

Other preparations which may be successful are 1% lindane shampoo (Rasmussen 1984), pynethine (Lange *et al.* 1980) and 10% crotamiton (Kovacic & Yawalker 1982).

In one investigation of school children (Maguire & McNally 1972) 20% of treated children were reinfected within 2 months. This experience emphasizes the need to examine and treat all school and home contacts, including of course those who are allegedly symptom-free.

References

Arene, F.O.I. & Ukaular, A.L. (1985) Prevalence of head louse infestation among inhabitants of the Niger Delta. *Tropical Medicine and Parasitology,* **36**, 140.

Ares Mazaz, M.E., Fandino Salerio, M.L., Silva Viller, M.J. *et al.* (1988) Efficacy of a malathion lotion for the treatment of *Pediculosis capitis. International Journal of Dermatology,* **27**, 267.

Askew, R.R. (1971) *Parasitic Insects.* Heinemann, London.

Buxton, P.A. (1937) The numbers of males and females in natural populations of head lice. *Proceedings of the Royal Entomological Society (London),* A, **12**, 12.

Buxton, P.A. (1947) *The Louse,* 2nd edn. Arnold, London.

Churge, R.N. (1986) A study of head lice among primary schoolchildren in Kenya. *Transactions of the Royal Society of Tropical Medicine and Hygiene,* **80**, 42.

Coates, K.G. (1971) Control of head infestation in schoolchildren. *Community Medicine,* **126**, 148.

Davis, W.A., Juvera, F.M. & Lira, P.H. (1944) Studies on louse control in a civilian population. *American Journal of Hygiene,* **39**, 177.

Department of Education and Science (1974) *The Health of the School Child 1971–2.* HMSO, London.

Davidson, R.J. (1975) *The Head Louse in England.* Health Education Council, U.K.

Essig, E.O. (1931) *A History of Entomology — Report 1965,* p. 18. Hafner, New York.

Ferris, G.F. (1935) *Contributions toward a Monograph of the Sucking Lice,* Part VIII. *Publications in the Biological Sciences,* **2**, No. 5. Stanford University.

Gemrich, E.G., Brady, J.G., Lee, B.L. & Parham, P.H. (1974) Outbreak of head lice in Michigan misdiagnosed. *American Journal of Public Health,* **64**, 805.

Gretz, N.G. (1977) Epidemiology of louse infestations. In *Scabies and Pediculosis,* p. 157, eds. M. Orkin, H.C. Maibach, L.C. Parish & R.M. Schwartzman. Lippincott, Philadelphia.

Hati, A.K., Bhetkolapyya, L., Chakerobody, A.K., Choudhuri, A.K. & Chowdhury, B.J.R. (1980) The incidence and extent of head louse infestation in a West Bengal village. *Indian Journal of Dermatology,* **24/25**, 4.

Juranek, B.D. (1977) Epidemiologic investigation of *Pediculosis capitis* in school children. In *Scabies and Pediculosis,* p. 168, eds. M. Orkin, H.C. Maibach, L.C. Parish & R.M. Schwartzman. Lippincott, Philadelphia.

Kovacic, I. & Yawalker, S.J. (1982) A single application of crotamiton lotion in the treatment of patients with *Pediculosis capitis. International Journal of Dermatology,* **21**, 611.

Kutz, F.W. (1969) Problem with diagnosis of head lice. *Entomological News,* **80**, 27.

Lange, K., Nielsen, A.O., Jensen, O. *et al.* (1980) Pyriderm shampoo in the treatment of *Pediculosis capitis. Acta Dermato-Venereologica,* **61**, 91.

Letz, A. (1980) Verbreitung von Kopflausbefall in kasseler Schulen. *Öffentliche Gesundheitswesen*, **42**, 228.

Maguire, J. & McNally, A.J. (1972) Head infestation in school-children: extent of the problem and treatment. *Community Medicine*, **128**, 374.

Maunder, J.W. (1971a) Resistance to organochlorine insecticides in head lice and trials using alternative compounds. *Community Medicine*, **125**, 27.

Maunder, J.W. (1971b) Using malathion in the treatment of louse infestation. *Community Medicine*, **126**, 145.

Maunder, J.W. (1983) The appreciation of lice. *Proceedings of the Royal Institute of Great Britain*, **55**, 1.

Meinking, Th., Taplin, D., Kalter, D.C., & Eberle, M.W. (1986) Comparative efficacy of treatments for *Pediculosis capitis* infestations. *Archives of Dermatology*, **122**, 267.

Mellanby, K. (1941) The incidence of head lice in England. *Medical Officer*, **65**, 39.

Mellanby, K. (1942) Relation between family size and incidence of head lice. *Public Health*, **56**, 31.

Ministry of Education (1951) *Report of the Chief Medical Officer for the Years 1950–51*, p. 36. HMSO, London.

Orkin, M., Maibach, H.C., Parish, L.C. & Schwartzman, R.M. (1977) *Scabies and Pediculosis*. Lippincott, Philadelphia.

Parish, L.C., Witkowski, J.A. & Millikan, L.E. (1989) Pediculosis capitis and the stubborn nit. *International Journal of Dermatology*, **28** (7), 436.

Peck, S.M., Wright, W.H. & Gant, J.U. (1943) Cutaneous reactions due to the body louse (*Pediculus jumanus*). *Journal of the American Medical Association*, **123**, 821.

Rasmussen, J.E. (1984) Controversies in paediatric dermatology. *Australian Journal of Dermatology*, **25**, 37.

Rollin, H.R. (1943) *Pediculosis capitis* and intelligence in WAAF recruits. *British Medical Journal*, **1**, 475.

Ronchese, F. (1946) Generalized dermatitis from *Pediculosis capitis*. *New England Journal of Medicine*, **234**, 605.

Roy, D.N. & Ghosh, S.M. (1944) Studies on the population of head lice—*Pediculus humanus* var. *capitis*. *Parasitology*, **36**, 69.

Wilson, T.S. (1969) Scabies and pediculosis: a study of the incidence in Glasgow from the early nineteen twenties. *Medical Officer*, **122**, 125.

Phthiriasis pubis
(References p. 425)

History and nomenclature
The pubic louse belongs to a different genus from body and head lice, and is correctly termed *Phthirus pubis*. Infestation with this louse is often loosely referred to as pubic pediculosis, but the somewhat pedantic phthiriasis is preferable as this louse differs structurally and ecologically from the body louse, and as its activities are by no means confined to the pubic region.

Phthirus pubis
The descriptive term crab-louse effectively draws attention to the distinctive shape of this parasite, which is 1.5–2 mm long, and about as broad (Herms & James 1961). The middle and hind pairs of legs are armed with very short claws. The female attaches her eggs to coarse hairs; they hatch in 6–8 days, and maturity is reached in 15–17 days after hatching. The lice tend to be stationary in their habits and may remain attached to the skin at one point for days. When the infestation is heavy the lice may roam over all the hair regions of the body, including the axillae, eyebrows and eyelashes and the scalp. However, the width of the louse prevents it

from colonizing more than the scalp margins. The colonization of all areas of the body in a hirsute patient was a consequence of prolonged application of topical corticosteroids (Nielsen & Secker 1980).

Epidemiology
The louse is usually transmitted by sexual contact, or by shed hairs in borrowed clothing, towels or sleeping bags. Eyelash infestation of infants has been derived from the breast hairs of their mothers (Ronchese 1953).

Among the promiscuous the incidence may be high. Sylvest (1951) found 30% of Copenhagen prostitutes to be infested in winter but only 15% in summer, and suggested that the seasonal difference might be explained by less frequent bathing in the cold northern winter. In Britain the incidence tends to parallel that of gonorrhoea in that it occurs predominantly in the same age groups and often in the same individuals (Fisher & Morton 1970).

Pathology
The immunological reactions to the salivary antigens of the pubic louse appear not to have been investigated. On clinical evidence the variation in host response would seem to be comparable to that to the head louse, in that in some subjects intense irritation can be present with a small lice population, whilst in others there are few or no nymphs although lice are very numerous.

Clinical features
The classical symptom is intense irritation of the pubic region, but it may extend, as may the lice, to the entire anogenital region, the abdominal wall and the axillae. On examination the lice are easily detected, unless self-treatment has produced eczematization, or scratching has introduced gross secondary infection.

In may cases blue-grey macules, known as maculae caeruleae, are present on the abdominal wall and thighs. They are probably due to altered blood pigments at the sites of bites. In massive infestations (Safdi & Farrington 1947) there may also be lymphadenopathy, fever and malaise. Phthiriasis of the scalp is rare and is perhaps commoner in children than in adults (Heilesen & Lindgren 1946; Gartmann & Dickmans-Bermeister 1970). The eyebrows and lashes may also be infested. In such cases maculae caeruleae may be found on the shoulders, upper arms or trunk.

Infestation confined to the eyelashes (Korting 1967) usually occurs in infants, but is occasionally reported in older children (Bose 1955). It may occasionally be a manifestation of child abuse (Scott & Esterly 1983).

Exceptionally a bullous reaction to the bites has occurred (Kern 1952).

Diagnosis
Difficulties in diagnosis arise mainly where overtreatment has caused eczematous dermatitis.

Lice in the anterior scalp margin in a child, particularly if no eggs can be discovered, should raise the suspicion that pubic rather than head lice are present. The distinction is readily made under the lower power of the microscope.

Parasitophobia is common and a diagnosis of pubic louse infestation should not be accepted unless lice or their eggs have been positively identified.

Treatment

A 5% emulsion of DDT applied once and washed off after 24 hours is usually effective. If resistant strains emerge it may be necessary to use 0.1% malathion in spirit. The possible co-existence of other sexually transmitted diseases should be remembered.

Lice may be removed manually from eyelashes or eyebrows, although in children this may be difficult. Many topical applications may be tried including petrolatum, 0.25% physostigmine eye ointment, yellow mercuric oxide eye ointment and 20% fluorescein drops; an excellent review is provided by Burns (1987). Cryotherapy and argon laser treatment have also been used (Awan 1986) although this would rarely be necessary.

References

Awan, K.J. (1986) Argon laser phototherapy of *Phthiasis palpebrarum. Ophthalmic Surgery*, **17**, 813.
Bose, J. (1955) Phthiriasis palpebrarum. *American Journal of Ophthalmology*, **39**, 211.
Burns, D.A. (1987) The treatment of *Phthirus pubis* infestation of the eyelashes. *British Journal of Dermatology*, **117**, 741.
Fisher, I. & Morton, R.S. (1970) *Phthirus pubis* infestation. *British Journal of Venereal Diseases*, **46**, 326.
Gartmann, H. & Dickmans-Bermeister, D. (1970) Phthiri im Bereia der Kopfhaare, Augenbrauen und Wimpern bei 2½ jährigen Mädchen. *Hautarzt*, **21**, 279.
Heilesen, B. & Lindgren, I. (1946) *Phthirus pubis* in capillitum, cilia et supercilia. *Acta Dermato-Venereologica*, **26**, 533.
Herms, W.B. & James, M.T. (1961) *Medical Entomology*, 5th edn., p. 106. Churchill Livingstone, Edinburgh.
Kern, A.B. (1952) Bullous eruption due to pediculosis pubis. *AMA Archives of Dermatology and Syphilology*, **65**, 334.
Korting, G.W. (1967) Phthiriasis palpebrum und ihre ersten historischem Erwährungen. *Hautarzt*, **18**, 73.
Nielsen, A.O. & Secker, L.S. (1980) Pediculosis pubis in a patient treated with topical corticosteroids. *Cutis*, **25**, 655.
Ronchese, F. (1953) Treatment of pediculosis ciliorum in an infant. *New England Journal of Medicine*, **249**, 897.
Safdi, S.A. & Farrington, J. (1947) Constitutional reactions and maculae caeruleae attending phthiriasis pubis. *American Journal of Medical Science*, **214**, 308.
Scott, M.J. & Esterly, N.B. (1983) Eyelash infestation by *Phthirus pubis* as a manifestation of child abuse. *Paediatric Dermatology*, **1**, 179.
Sylvest, B. (1951) Seasonal variation in the incidence of crab lice among loose women in Copenhagen. *Acta Dermato-Venereologica*, **31**, 676.

Insect bites

The cutaneous reactions to the bites of most insects depend on an acquired allergic sensitivity to antigens in the insect's saliva. This allergic reaction may be of Type

I manifest as an immediate weal of rapid onset, or of Type IV manifest as a firm and more persistent papule developing in 24–48 hours. The intensity of the reaction shows wide variation and in the most severe cases there may be bulla formation or necrosis.

Many biting insects occasionally bite in the scalp and the resulting inflammatory reaction may lead to some temporary shedding of hair from the site of the bites and from a narrow zone surrounding each of them. The minute gnats and midges of the family Ceratopogonidae particularly favour the scalp. On summer evenings they may be present in such vast swarms that they cause quite intolerable irritation. The reaction to the bites and secondary infection following the scratching may lead to patchy loss of hair but this normally regrows rapidly (Fig. 13.8).

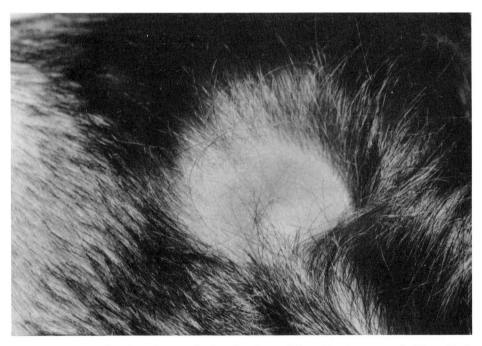

Fig. 13.8 An insect bite, heavily secondarily infected, was followed by temporary shedding of hair in the oedematous skin around the lesion. The hair regrew leaving a barely detectable central scar without hair.

Tick bites
(References p. 427)

Ticks can carry a variety of infections by their bites and they can induce a wide range of allergic reactions (Marshall 1967), and also nodular reactions which can last for months or indefinitely.

The saliva of the tick contains numerous antigens and other substances, including anticoagulant. It seems possible that the anticoagulant is responsible for the alopecia which is associated with tick bites and which may be far more extensive than the narrow zone of temporary hair loss which may be associated with the inflammatory changes induced by other arthropods.

After 7–10 days following a tick bite in a child's scalp the hair may be shed in an area up to 4 cm in diameter. The bald patch resembles alopecia areata, except for the central area of crusting at the site of the bite (Saughar 1921; Marshall 1966). Complete regrowth of hair is usual except in a small central area of scarring. In two cases in which there were multiple tick bites (Ross & Friede 1955) multiple small areas of cicatricial alopecia up to 1.3 cm in diameter persisted.

References
Marshall, J. (1966) Alopecia after tick bite. *South Africa Medical Journal*, **40**, 555.
Marshall, J. (1967) Ticks and the human skin. *Dermatologica*, **135**, 60.
Ross, M.S. & Friede, H. (1955) Alopecia due to tick bite. *Archives of Dermatology*, **71**, 524.
Saughar, L. (1921) Alopécie peladoide consecutive à une piqûre de tique. *Bulletin de la Société Française de Dermatologie et Syphiligraphie*, **28**, 442.

Cutaneous myiasis
(References p. 428)

Myiasis is the infestation of the body by the larvae of certain species of Diptera—two-winged flies. Some species lay their eggs in existing wounds or ulcers but others deposit them on normal skin, and others such as *Dermatobia hominis*, important in Latin America, lay them on mosquitoes or house flies, which transfer them to the human body (Hubler *et al.* 1974).

The lesions of obligate and specific cutaneous myiasis in man are usually on exposed skin and sleeping babies are particularly at risk. The lesions present as furuncular nodules, single or multiple. There may be mild constitutional symptoms and eosinophilia. In one outbreak (Macias *et al.* 1973) the affected children were already suffering from pediculosis and pyoderma of the scalp. Around each nodule there may be temporary shedding of hair in a zone up to 3 cm in width. When the infection is controlled, only the small central area at the site of the actual lesion remains bald. In a distinctive but uncommon clinical variant the larva migrates under the skin to produce one form of creeping eruption.

The lesions in myiasis in which the eggs are laid in a wound has complicated an infected ulcer of the scalp (Calero 1949).

Myiasis is more common in tropical than in temperate climates, but the species of fly (bot-fly or warble-fly) causing myiasis are widely distributed in temperate regions as well, and cases can occasionally occur there (Morgan *et al.* 1964).

In treating cutaneous myiasis the larvae should be evacuated from the nodules—they can sometimes be removed with fine forceps—and an antibiotic should be given systemically to control secondary infection.

References

Calero, C. (1949) Cutaneous myiasis due to *Chryosostomomyia bergi*. *Journal of Parasitology*, **35**, 545.

Hubler, W.R., Rudolph, A.H. & Dougherty, E.F. (1974) Dermal myiasis. *Archives of Dermatology*, **110**, 109.

Macias, E.G., Graham, A.J., Green, M. & Pierce, A.W. (1973) Cutaneous myiasis in South Texas. *New England Journal of Medicine*, **289**, 1239.

Morgan, R.J., Moss, H.B. & Hansker, W.L. (1964) Myiasis. *Archives of Dermatology*, **90**, 180.

Demodex folliculorum

Demodex folliculorum is the most common ectoparasite of man (Rufli & Muncuoglu 1981). The hair follicle mites (*D. folliculosum* and *D. brevis*) are common inhabitants of the human pilosebaceous unit. In a recent review Aylesworth and Vance (1982) found that 10% of 1124 skin biopsies and 12% of 1692 follicles studied contained follicular mites. Roth (1979) examined 100 biopsies of eyelid skin and found follicular mites in 84% of all cases and in 100% of cases in which the patients were over 70 years of age. Because of its prevalence on human skin its role as a pathogen remains controversial. Although demodex in animals is known to produce alopecia and a cutaneous eruption (demodectic mange), the mite has not clearly been shown to cause disease in man.

Demodex has been circumstantially implicated in the aetiology of several clinical entities: Pityriasis folliculorum (Demodex) is described as diffuse flushing of the face associated with follicular plugging and a fine, white scale resulting in a 'dry-nutmeg grater' appearance (Ayres & Ayres 1960). Acne rosacea (Demodex) is described as a dry type of rosacea characterized by superficial vesicopustules and small papules or papulopustules. In both conditions numerous mites were identified by KOH examination of follicular scale or secretions and scabicidal preparations produced a rapid improvement.

Similar findings have been implicated in papulopustular dermatosis of the scalp (Miskjian 1951), blepharitis (Ayres & Nihan 1967), granulomatous rosacea (Ecker & Winkelmann 1979) and pustular folliculitis (Purcell, *et al.* 1986; Watzig & Zollman 1987).

It is thought that demodex induces the formation of a perifollicular lympho-histiocytic infiltrate in sensitized individuals, via the follicular epithelium (Rulfi & Buchner 1984). This infiltrate tends to attack the follicle; when the mites multiply the infiltrate is more often present but not necessarily more aggressive (Forton 1986).

References

Aylesworth, R. & Vance, J.C. (1982) *Demodex folliculorum* and *Demodex brevis* in cutaneous biopsies. *Journal of American Academy of Dermatology*, **7**, 583.

Ayres, S. & Ayres, S. (1960) Demodectic eruptions (Demodicidosis) in the human. *Archives of Dermatology*, **83**, 154.

Ayres, S. & Nihan, R. (1967) Rosacea-like demodicidosis involving the eyelids. *Archives of Dermatology*, **95**, 63.

Ecker, R.I. & Winkelmann, R.K. (1979) Demodex granuloma. *Archives of Dermatology*, **115**, 343.

Forton, F. (1986) Demodex et inflammation perifolliculaire chez l'homme. *Annales de Dermatologie et de Vénéréologie*, **113**, 1047.

Miskjian, H.G. (1951) Demodicidosis (Demodex) infestation of the scalp. *AMA Archives of Dermatology and Syphilology*, **63**, 282.

Purcell, S.M., Hayes, T.J. & Dixon, S.L. (1986) Pustular folliculitis associated with Demodex folliculorum. *Journal of the American Academy of Dermatology*, **15**, 1159.

Roth, A.M. (1979) Demodex folliculorum in hair follicles of eyelid skin. *Annals of Ophthalmology*, **11**, 37.

Rufli, T. & Buchner, S.A. (1984) T-cell subsets in acne rosacea lesions and the possible role of *Demodex folliculorum*. *Dermatologica*, **169**, 1.

Rufli, T. & Muncuoglu, Y. (1981) The hair follicle mites *Demodex folliculorum* and *Demodex brevis*: biology and medical importance. *Dermatologica*, **162**, 1.

Watzig, von V. & Zollman, C. (1987) Demodicose — eine rosazeaartige Dermatose. *Dermatologische Monatsschrift*, **173**, 158.

Piedra
(References p. 431)

Black piedra

Epidemiology and aetiology

The term piedra is applied to two distinct infections of the hair. Black piedra is caused by the ascomycete *Piedraia hortai*, which is unique among pathogenic fungi in that it reproduces sexually while in its parasitic state. Black piedra is endemic to tropical regions of South and Central America, Malaysia and South East Asia, but rare cases have been reported in the United States and South Africa. Prevalence surveys show that in some areas, e.g. the Matto Grosso in Brazil, it is common at all ages, but particularly in young adults (Fischman 1973). The infection is endemic in a number of wild mammals which may serve as reservoirs of infection (Kaplan 1959). Transmission may occur from person to person, through close contact, or through shared combs. Epidemics have occurred among school children in Thailand (Kneedler 1939) and Puerto Rico (Carion 1965). In South America, black piedra is more common after puberty and in those with long hair whether male or female (Fischman 1965). In Malaysia the hair nodules are considered beautiful and fungal growth is encouraged by sleeping with their heads in the soil (Rippon 1982).

Pathology

Piedraia hortai penetrates the hair cuticle, proliferates in the shaft and then breaks out to surround the shaft forming hard, brown to black nodular concretions consisting of branched hyphae and containing asci and ascospores. The concretions may achieve 1.5 mm in length, attaching via hyphae to the superficial cortex.

Clinical features

Black piedra is characterized by discrete, hard, black nodules that cling firmly to the scalp hairs. Piedra ('stone' in Spanish) describes these gritty, adherent concretions, which are difficult to scrape off. Combing of the affected hairs with a metal comb is said to produce a characteristic rattling sound. Nodules may be present along the length of the hair. Hair is normal between the nodules and is not weakened. Other hairy regions, including the backs of the hands (Adams *et al.* 1977), may be affected.

Wood's lamp examination is negative, but light microscopy reveals compact, dark, thick-walled, septate hyphae in an organized geometric mass. Within the mature nodule paler loculi or asci appear like honeycombs, containing two to eight fusiform ascospores.

Fungal culture produces a slow-growing black colony, initially glabrous but later developing short, greenish-brown, aerial mycelia.

White piedra may exist concurrently with black piedra.

Treatment
Affected hairs may be cut short and the hair washed daily.

White piedra

Epidemiology and aetiology
White piedra is a rare mycotic infection of the hair caused by the imperfect yeast-like fungus *Trichosporum cutaneum* (formerly known as *T. beigelii*). It is usually encountered in tropical and temperate climates although it is known to be cosmopolitan and has been seldom reported from very cold climates like Scandinavia. *Trichosporum* may be recovered in abundance from the environment, as well as from mammals and from human sputum, stools, and skin in the absence of clinical disease.

Young, active, black males and male homosexuals are more susceptible than others to genital infection with *T. cutaneum*. A recent study (Kalter *et al.* 1986) confirmed this and found a 40% incidence in men and only 14% in women. There was no relationship between infection and foreign travel. Transmission may rarely occur from person to person after prolonged intimate contact. Many patients have recurring and remitting disease which is more symptomatic in warm, humid environments.

Systemic infection has been reported in immunocompromised and predisposed hosts.

Pathology
Trichosporum cutaneum invades the hair shaft cortex, damaging it so that breaking and splitting and trichorrhexis nodosa readily occur. The soft whitish nodules consist of hyphae which fragment into arthrospores.

Clinical features
Initially thought to affect the hairs of the scalp, beard, and moustache, white piedra

has been discovered on eyelashes, eyebrows and axillary and perigenital hairs. Infection of genital hairs is now thought to be the most common manifestation, although concurrent infection of multiple sites can occur.

The infection, which may be either asymptomatic or irritating, is manifest by whitish, soft, spongy, nodular concretions that cling to the hair shafts either as discrete nodules or a coalesced sheath. The fusiform swellings can be scraped off — unlike the hard, dark ovoids in black piedra. In the genital area intertrigo may also be present; in the scalp, pruritus may be the presenting complaint.

Clinically, white piedra may be difficult to distinguish from trichomycosis axillaris or pubis.

Light microscopic examination of hairs in KOH confirms the diagnosis. The nodules are composed of closely packed septate hyphae and blastoconidia in a dense geometric array. Wood's light examination is negative.

Treatment

Affected hairs should be cut short and the hair washed daily. Eradication is difficult; however, spontaneous remissions may occur (Kalter *et al.* 1986). Topical 1% econazole nitrate may improve symptoms and signs.

References

Adams, B.A., Soottoo, T.S. & Chung, K.C. (1977) Black piedra in West Malaysia. *Australasian Journal of Dermatology*, **18**, 45.

Carion, A. (1965) Dermatomycoses in Puerto Rico. *Archives of Dermatology*, **91**, 431.

Fischman, O. (1965) Black piedra in Brazil. *Mycopathologia*, **25**, 201.

Fischman, O. (1973) Black piedra among Brazilian Indians. *Revista do Instituto de Medicina Tropical de São Paolo*, **15**, 103.

Kalter, D.C., Tschen, J.A., Cernoch, P.L. *et al.* (1986) Genital white piedra: epidemiology, microbiology and therapy. *Journal of the American Academy of Dermatology*, **14**, 982.

Kaplan, W. (1959) Piedra in lower animals. *Journal of the American Veterinary Association*, **134**, 113.

Kneedler, W.H. (1939) Tinea nodosa of the scalp hair in school children of South Siam. *Archives of Dermatology and Syphilology*, **39**, 121.

Rippon, J.W. (1982) *Medical Mycology*, p. 148. W.B. Saunders Co., Philadelphia.

Stenderup, A., Schonheyder, H., Ebberson, P. *et al.* (1986) White piedra and *Trichosporon beigelii* carriage in homosexual men. *Journal of Medical and Veterinary Mycology*, **24**, 401.

Trichomycosis axillaris and pubis

(References p. 433)

Aetiology and pathology (Wilson & Dawber 1989)

In trichomycosis axillaris nodules consisting of masses of bacteria develop in the axillae and sometimes the pubic hairs. Paxton described the disorder in 1869 and attributed the infection to fungi and named the disease. Later investigators saw cocci and bacilli in histologic sections of trichomycosis hairs but were unable to culture any bacteria. In 1911 Catellani incriminated a streptothrix which he named *Nocardia tenuis*, but he could not culture the organism from the concretions.

Nocardia was considered to be the cause until 1952 when Crissey *et al.* cultured a *Corynebacterium* from each of 28 patients and named the organism *Corynebacterium tenuis*. Savin *et al.* (1970) in a large series found on average three distinct isolates of corynebacteria in each individual. It has been suggested that the different types give rise to different colours (Freeman *et al.* 1969); there are three colour varieties, yellow, black and red, but the black and red are unusual outside the Tropics (Crissey & Murray 1954).

The condition is common in many populations. It was found in 23 of 100 consecutive patients examined in the United States (Crissey *et al.* 1952) and in an institution for the mentally retarded in England (Savin *et al.* 1970) trichomycosis was found in the axillae of 26 and 2% had involvement of scrotal hair. Men are affected more frequently than women; the prevalence of the infection among patients in a mental institution was 35% in males and 5% in females (Noble & Savin 1985). Axillary sweating and low hygiene standards are said to favour the infection.

Electron microscopic studies (Fig. 13.9) have shown that the bacteria elaborate a virtually insoluble cement substance enabling adherence to the hair shaft (Shelley & Miller 1984). Occasionally colonies of bacteria may be seen invading and destroying cuticular and cortical keratin (Montes *et al.* 1963; Orfanos *et al.* 1971; Wilson & Dawber 1989).

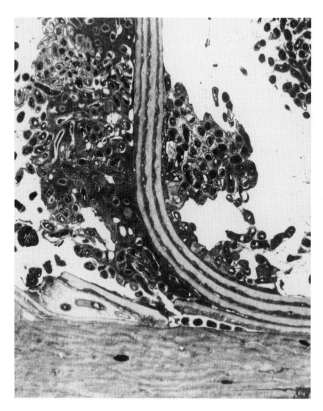

Fig. 13.9 Corynebacteria within the hair cuticle of an axillary hair. The cortex, seen at the bottom of the picture, is not affected.

Clinical features

Usually the patient is not aware of the presence of the infection but sometimes yellow, red or black staining of clothing brings it to his notice. The hair shaft is not weakened, so there is no alopecia or brittleness.

Wood's lamp examination yields a dull yellow fluorescence of the affected hairs, and irregularly nodular granules adherent to the hairs can be seen with a hand-lens.

Trichomycosis may sometimes be associated with other *Corynebacterium* infections such as erythrasma and pitted keratolysis. Trichomycosis pubis may accompany white piedra of the scrotum, from which it can be distinguished microbiologically. Artefacts from deodorants, creams or soaps should be excluded.

Treatment

Regular washing usually suffices to clear the condition. Clindamycin 1% lotion in alcohol has been found to be effective (White & Smith 1979).

References

Castellani, A. (1928) Fungi and fungous diseases. *Archives of Dermatology and Syphilology,* **17**, 194.

Crissey, J.T. & Murray, P.F. (1954) Trichomycosis axillaris. *New York State Journal of Medicine,* **54**, 2841.

Crissey, J.T., Rebell, G.C. & Laskas, J.J. (1952) Studies on the causative organism of trichomycosis axillaris. *Journal of Investigative Dermatology,* **19**, 187.

Freeman, R.G., McBride, M.E. & Knox, J.M. (1969) Pathogenesis of trichomycosis axillaris. *Archives of Dermatology,* **100**, 96.

Montes, L.F., Vasquez, C. & Cataldi, M.S. (1963) Electron microscopic study of infected hairs in trichomycosis. *Journal of Investigative Dermatology,* **40**, 273.

Noble, W.C. & Savin, J.A. (1985) Trichomycosis of scrotal hair. *Archives of Dermatology,* **121**, 25.

Orfanos, C.E., Schloesser, E. & Mahrle, G. (1971) Hair-destroying growth of *Corynebacterium tenuis* in the so-called trichomycosis axillaris. *Archives of Dermatology,* **103**, 632.

Paxton, F.V. (1869) On a diseased condition of the hairs of the axilla, probably of parasitic origin. *Journal of Cutaneous Medicine,* **3**, 133.

Savin, J.A., Somerville, D.A. & Noble, W.C. (1970) The bacterial flora of trichomycosis axillaris. *Journal of Medical Microbiology,* **3**, 352.

Shelley, W.B. & Miller, M.A. (1984) Electron microscopy, histochemistry, and microbiology of bacterial adhesion in trichomycosis axillaris. *Journal of the American Academy of Dermatology,* **10**, 1005.

White, S.W. & Smith, J. (1979) Trichomycosis pubis. *Archives of Dermatology,* **115**, 444.

Wilson, C. & Dawber, R.P.R. (1989) Trichomycosis axillaris—a different view. *Journal of the American Academy of Dermatology,* **21**, 325.

Impetigo

(References p. 435)

Definition

Impetigo is a contagious superficial infection of the skin due to streptococci, staphylococci or both (Dillon 1972).

Normal skin is relatively resistant to invasion by bacteria; impetigo is very difficult to produce in laboratory animals (Johnson 1961).

Primary impetigo occurs as two types, impetigo contagiosum of Tilbury Fox, typically due to Group A streptococci, and bullous impetigo due to pyogenic staphylococci.

Secondary impetigo implies colonization and infection of already abnormal skin by streptococci or staphylococci.

Epidemiology and bacteriology (Marples 1965)

The relative importance of streptococci or staphylococci as the cause of impetigo varies from epidemic to epidemic and from country to country. Pure staphylococci impetigo is common in temperate climates, typically due to Group II type 71 or 80/81. The streptococcal strains involved are usually of Group A though rare cases may be due to Groups B (impetigo neonatorum), C or G.

Primary impetigo is highly communicable and mainly affects pre-school children in late summer and early autumn. Staphylococci may infect the skin following initial nasal colonization whilst streptococci may directly infect the skin. Crowding, poor hygiene, and neglected minor trauma may contribute to the spread in epidemics. Localized outbreaks may occur in athletes taking part in contact sports.

Pathology

The inflammatory changes are superficial and commonly found near hair follicles. Vesiculation occurs in the epidermis at the level of the stratum granulosum. Epithelial cell debri, leucocytes and organisms are present in the vesicle. Smears for cytodiagnosis may show acantholytic cells. The skin heals without scarring.

Clinical findings

Primary impetigo. Streptococcal impetigo begins as a transient thin-roofed vesicle with a surrounding inflammatory halo; in this type pustulation and crusting occur early. Removal of established crusts leads to rapid drying of serous exudate and further crust formation. The face, particularly around the nose and mouth, is the site of predilection; lesions may be multiple and become generalized. Staphylococcal impetigo is characterized by intact blisters often without any surrounding inflammatory reaction. Impetigo neonatorum is usually staphylococcal.

Secondary impetigo 'impetiginization' may occur in skin altered by minor trauma, insect bites, pediculosis capitis and eczema. Scalp infection with increasing serous matting of hair is usually associated with pediculosis capitis, atopic eczema, lichen simplex or insect bites.

Regional lymphadenitis and fever may both occur.

Laboratory findings include neutrophil leucocytosis and Gram smears showing positive staining cocci. Swab cultures readily yield colonies of staphylococci or streptococci.

Complications

The most severe complication of streptococcal impetigo is acute glomerulonephritis, less commonly acute guttate psoriasis and erythema multiforme may be precipitated. Toxic epidermal necrolysis ('scalded skin syndrome') may develop from staphylococcal impetigo (Lyell 1967).

Treatment

Very mild cases may respond simply to removal of crusts and bathing with saline or hydrogen peroxide. The use of topical antibiotics for treating impetigo is limited by the tendency of many to cause allergic sensitization. Sodium fucidate is active against most staphylococci.

Impetigo remits most quickly when oral antibiotics are used. A single dose of intra-muscular soluble penicillin G sodium followed by oral phenoxymethyl penicillin for 1 week is satisfactory for streptococcal infection; in childhood the dose will depend on the age of the patient. Most staphylococci respond to the same regime though penicillinase-producing strains may require flucloxacillin. Erythromycin is the treatment of choice for patients who are allergic to penicillins.

In impetigo secondary to pediculosis capitis, eczema or lichen simplex, treatment of the infection is the first priority. Once bacterial inflammation has subsided, treatment appropriate to the primary disease must be started; if such treatment is inadequate, impetigo may recur. Since the normal bacterial flora may protect against virulent pathogens in diseases such as eczema, only organisms causing inflammatory signs should be treated (Savin & Noble 1977).

References

Dillon, H.C. (1972) Streptococcal infections of the skin and their complications: impetigo and nephritis. In *Streptococci and Streptococcal Diseases*, p. 571, eds. L.W. Wannamaker & J.M. Matson. Academic Press, New York.

Johnson, L.E. (1961) Studies on the pathogenesis of staphylococcal infection. I. The effect of repeated skin infections. *Journal of Experimental Medicine*, 113, 235.

Lyell, A. (1967) A review of toxic epidermal necrolysis. *British Journal of Dermatology*, 79, 662.

Marples, M.J. (1965) *The Ecology of the Human Skin*, 1st edn. Thomas, Springfield.

Savin, J.A. & Noble, W.C. (1977) Opportunism and skin infections. In *Recent Advances in Dermatology*, vol 4, ed. A. Rook. Churchill Livingstone, Edinburgh.

Furuncles and carbuncles
(References p. 437)

Aetiology

The furuncle is an acute, usually necrotic, infection of the hair follicle with *Staphylococcus aureus*, causing a perifollicular abscess. Furuncles occur most commonly in later childhood and in adolescence and reach a peak incidence in young adult life. They are more frequent in males than in females. Episodes of furunculosis may be short and acute but they may consist of crops at irregular intervals over a long period. Fatigue and stress are among many predisposing factors incriminated but without any statistical evidence that they are relevant. Malnutrition is however certainly a predisposing factor but otherwise most cases occur in apparently healthy young males.

A carbuncle is a deep infection with *Staphylococcus aureus* of a group of neighbouring hair follicles; the inflammatory changes involve the surrounding connecting tissues and subcutaneous fat. Carbuncles occur in the middle-aged and elderly, particularly in men, and systemic diseases, notably diabetes and cardiac failure, and corticosteroid therapy are among the important predisposing factors.

In both furuncles and carbuncles the patient may himself have been a chronic carrier of *Staphylococcus aureus* in the nose, axillae, perineum, toe-clefts or on the hair (Noble 1981). In other cases there is repeated reinfection from an asymptomatic carrier in the household or among nursing and medical attendants. The patient who has clinically recovered from these infections may remain a carrier.

Clinical features
Furuncles affect predominantly vellus hair follicles and are unusual in the scalp although they may frequently occur in the face and neck; they are also common around the axillae and in the anogenital region and on the hands and arms. They present single or multiple tender red follicular nodules which become pustules from which a necrotic core is discharged. They heal to leave small scars.

Carbuncles, on the other hand, are most often seen on the nape of the neck within the scalp margin; they may also occur on the shoulder, hips or thighs. An acutely tender smooth red nodule may reach a diameter of 8–10 cm within a few days. Focal necrosis is followed by the discharge of pus from multiple follicular orifices. This is followed by more extensive necrosis and the separation of the whole central core, or such necrosis may occur rapidly without the preliminary follicular discharge. In either case a large ulcer results and heals to leave a permanent scar. Fever and other constitutional symptoms occur during the acute stage

Chronic follicular infection with *Staphylococcus aureus* may result in multiple tufted hairs arising from single follicular openings at the epidermal surface. It is postulated that infection may be confined to the dermis where the follicular wall and sebaceous glands are destroyed. The hair shafts continue to grow from healthy roots situated below the inflammation. Bundles of hairs appear on the surface as they clump together during healing. *Staphylococcus aureus* is cultured from the scalp and biopsies show a granulomatous infiltrate with plasma cells, polymorphs and histiocytes in the dermis superficial to single hair roots (Smith 1978; Oakley & Scollay 1985).

Diagnosis
Furunculosis in the scalp is sufficiently unusual for this diagnosis to be suspect. Superficial pustules complicating pediculosis must be excluded as must ringworm infection and myiasis.

A carbuncle is simulated by anthrax but the haemorrhagic crust and vesicular margin of the latter infection are distinctive.

In all cases of furunculosis or carbuncle a swab should be taken for bacteriological confirmation of the diagnosis and it is an advantage if phage typing can be carried out and antibiotic sensitivities established although treatment should not be postponed until this information is available.

The urine should be tested and underlying disease should be sought.

Treatment

Treatment of furunculosis and the careful search for the source of infection in the patient or his environment are described in general textbooks of dermatology. In chronic cases prolonged courses of antibiotics are not the ideal solution.

For carbuncles penicillin G, the full dosage, should be given at the earliest opportunity.

References

Noble, W.C. (1981) *Microbiology of the Human Skin*, 2nd edn., p. 159. Lloyd Luke, London.
Oakley, A. & Scollay, D. (1985) Hair bundles: a presentation of folliculitis. *Australian Journal of Dermatology*, **26**, 139.
Smith, N. (1978) Tufted folliculitis of the scalp. *Proceedings of the Royal Society of Medicine*, **71**, 606.

Neonatal scalp infections

Since the head is commonly the presenting part of the baby the scalp is prone to trauma and infection. Bacterial infection is usually caused by slight injury inflicted by instrumentation, especially the use of scalp electrodes for monitoring foetal heart rate occurring in 0.3–5% of cases (Siddiqi & Taylor 1982; Feder *et al.* 1976). Gonococcal scalp abscesses have also occurred via such a portal of entry (Reveri & Krishnamurthy 1979)

Trauma from forceps and aplasia cutis may also be responsible. Other predisposing factors include prolonged duration of monitoring, prolonged rupture of membranes, vaginal contamination by faeces, puerperal infection and trauma to the neonate's head.

The clinical infection varies from a solitary pustule at the site of the electrode attachment to abscess, cellulitis, necrotizing fasciitis and osteomyelitis. Bacterial infections are usually evident within a few days after birth, whereas anaerobic infections may take several days or weeks to present (Siddiqi & Taylor 1982). A variety of organisms may be responsible for infections and include *Staphylococcus aureus, S. epidermidis, β* haemolytic streptococci, *Haemophilus influenzae* type B, *Neisseria gonorrhoeae, Pseudomonas* and *Klebsiella* and many anaerobes.

References

Feder, H.M.V., MacLean, W.C. & Moxon, R. (1976) Scalp abscess secondary to fetal scalp electrode. *Journal of Pediatrics*, **89**, 808.
Reveri, M. & Krishnamurthy, C. (1979) Gonococcal scalp abscess. *Journal of Pediatrics*, **94**, 819.

Siddiqi, S.F. & Taylor, P.M. (1982) Necrotizing fasciitis of the scalp. A complication of fetal
    monitoring, *American Journal of Diseases of Children*, **136**, 226.

Erysipelas

Aetiology
Erysipelas is an acute superficial cellulitis, caused by streptococci, usually of Group
A. It occurs most frequently in infants and in the elderly, but can occur at any age.
A wound or a non-infective skin lesion may provide an obvious point of entry for
the infection but in many cases no portal of entry is evident. Defective lymphatic
drainage favours the development of erysipelas and the infection tends to recur in
such areas. Erysipelas most commonly affects the legs but the face is the next most
frequent site (Schneider 1973). The scalp may be spared in erysipelas which may
stop short at the scalp margin. However, the scalp may be involved by extension
from the face or pinna or primarily in the presence of a scalp wound.

Clinical features
Fever and malaise often precede the development of visible cutaneous lesions and
the patient may be severely ill; without effective treatment high fever may continue
for several days and, particularly in the malnourished, the disease can be fatal.
    Soon after the onset of the fever a sharply marginated plaque of erythema and
oedema appears, sometimes with vesicles or bullae. The hair in affected areas of the
scalp may be shed within a week to 10 days. Before antibacterial agents were
available, the early localized hair loss was followed after about 3 months by diffuse
alopecia of the whole of the scalp as a result of the prolonged high fever.

Diagnosis
Streptococci are not easily isolated from the skin lesions and are by no means
always present in the patient's throat. The clinical diagnosis is not difficult.

Treatment
A course of systemic penicillin or other appropriate antibiotic should be given at the
earliest possible stage.

Reference
Schneider, I. (1973) Klinik und Pathogenese des rezidivierenden Erysipels. *Hautarzt*, **24**, 145.

Viral warts
(References p. 440)

Warts are benign tumours of the skin or adjacent mucous surfaces and are due to
a DNA virus, the human papilloma virus (HPV); most clinical types regress
spontaneously (Rees 1979).

Viral spread is by direct inoculation into damaged skin. The incubation period varies from 1 to 20 months with a mean value of approximately 4 months. Warts appear to have increased in incidence during the last 20 years.

Pathology

Individual lesions show irregular acanthosis and hyperkeratosis; the stratum granulosum contains foci of virus-infected vacuolated cells whilst the horny layer may be parakeratotic with basophilic nuclear inclusions. Lesions present for more than 1 year may show little or no evidence of active viral presence.

Local immunity against the wart virus is cell-mediated, as with most viral infections; during the phase of resolution complement-fixing (IgG) antibodies are detectable. Until recently all the clinical manifestations of HPV infection were considered to be due to a single strain of HPV. It is now evident that several distinct sub-types exist (Gissmann *et al.* 1977; Coggin & Zur Hausen 1979). The suggested types and their relationship to the clinical groups are as follows (Rees 1981):

Virus type	Clinical type
HPV 1 a,b,c,	Plantar or common
HPV 2	Common
HPV 3	Plane, or epidermodysplasia verruciformis (EV)
HPV 4	Plantar, common or EV
HPV 5	EV (scaly lesions)
HPV 6	Genital (?); laryngeal (?)

Warts may occur at any age but their peak incidence is in childhood.

Recent work by Viac *et al.* (1977) suggests that once HPV virus can be harvested in culture it will be possible to produce an effective anti-HPV vaccine.

Warts tend to involute spontaneously within months (Massing & Epstein 1963), but there is wide individual variation in their course. There is a suggestion that T-lymphocytes may be reduced in patients with persistent warts (Chretien *et al.* 1978). The cell-mediated response and humoral complement-fixing IgG antibodies are both involved (Ivanyi & Morrison 1976; Pyrhonen & Johansson 1975). Very numerous warts may be present in patients with immune deficiencies, especially Hodgkin's disease (Morrison 1975) and warts are particularly prevalent in elderly patients with systemic lupus erythematosus (Johansson *et al.* 1977).

Clinical types

Common warts (verruca vulgaris) are firm papules with a horny surface; sites of predilection are the hands and knees though any part of the body may be affected including the scalp.

Generalized verrucosis, which may be associated with impaired cell-mediated immunity, consists of common and sometimes plane warts disseminated widely over the body surface; individual lesions may coalesce to produce large verrucous plaques.

Plane warts are small (1–5 mm) smooth, flat or slightly elevated lesions. The colour varies from skin colour, to grey or brown. The face, shins and hands are commonly affected. Multiple plane or filiform warts of the beard area are due to seeding of the wart virus into sites of minor damage from shaving. Individual lesions may affect follicular opening. Plane warts often last for several years. The differential diagnosis depends on the site and number of lesions present but flat epidermal naevi and lichen planus may give a similar appearance.

Filiform or digitate warts occur more frequently in men than women; most lesions are found on the head or neck but hundreds of small filiform warts may develop in the beard area. Grouped filiform lesions on the scalp may mimic epidermal naevi.

Treatment

In carrying out treatment for warts one must constantly temper enthusiasm with the knowledge that most lesions will remit spontaneously within a few months of onset leaving no permanent scar (Rees 1981); warts that are causing little in the way of symptoms may therefore be left untreated or a placebo may be appropriate.

Plane warts may be treated with salicylic acid preparations. Therapy of common warts depends on their size and site; single large lesions can be removed by curettage or cryosurgery, preferably using liquid nitrogen spray. Filiform or digitate warts can be treated by electrocautery or cryosurgery; isolated large lesions on the scalp are best treated by curettage under local anaesthetic.

References

Chretien, J.H., Esswin, J.G. & Garagus, P.F. (1978) Decreased T-cell levels in patients with warts. *Archives of Dermatology*, **114**, 313.

Coggin, J.R. & Zur Hausen, H. (1979) Workshop on papilloma viruses and cancer. *Cancer Research*, **39**, 545.

Gissmann, L., Pfister, H. & Zur Hausen, H. (1977) Human papilloma viruses (HPV): characterization of four different isolates. *Virology*, **76**, 569.

Ivanyi, L. & Morrison, W.C. (1976) *In vitro* lymphocyte stimulation by wart antigen in man. *British Journal of Dermatology*, **94**, 523.

Johansson, E., Pyrohonen, S. & Rostili, T. (1977) Warts and wart virus antibodies in patients with systemic lupus erythematosus. *British Medical Journal*, **i**, 74.

Massing, A.M. & Epstein, W.C. (1963) Natural history of warts. *Archives of Dermatology*, **87**, 306.

Morrison, W.C. (1975) Viral warts, herpes simplex and herpes zoster in patients with secondary immune deficiencies or neoplasms. *British Journal of Dermatology*, **92**, 625.

Pyrhonen, S. & Johansson, E. (1975) Regression of warts: an immunological study. *Lancet*, **i**, 592.

Rees, R.B. (1979) Warts. *Cutis*, **23**, 588.

Rees, R.B. (1981) The characterization, immunopathology and treatment of viral warts. *International Journal of Dermatology*, **20**, 110.

Viac, J., Thivolet, J. & Chardonnet, Y. (1977) Specific immunity in patients suffering from recurring wart before and after repetitive intra-dermal tests with human papilloma virus. *British Journal of Dermatology*, **91**, 365.

Molluscum contagiosum
(References p. 442)

Molluscum contagiosum is a common infection of skin and rarely of mucous membranes due to a large (200–300 nm) DNA poxvirus which usually affects children (Postlethwaite 1970). It is mainly a human infection but has been described in chimpanzees in captivity and in a kangaroo (Bagnall & Wilson 1974).

It occurs in all races and has a worldwide distribution. In Britain, school-age children up to 15 years of age are commonly affected; the increased incidence in the age group 20–30 years is mainly due to venereal spread. Transmission of the virus is by direct contact or via infected fomites. Communal living is associated with a high incidence of infection; however, multiple family cases are rare. In children under 14 years of age, boys are more frequently affected than girls.

The incubation period is from 14 to 50 days.

The earliest stage pathologically shows minute intra-cellular granules which coalesce into large eosinophilic hyaline bodies (molluscum, or Henderson–Paterson bodies); these infected cells associated with increased cell proliferation give characteristic light microscopic appearance of scrapings or curettings.

Clinical features
Individual lesions are shiny, pearly white, umbilicated papules varying in size from 1–10 mm (Fig. 13.10). Cheesy white material can be expressed from the centre of

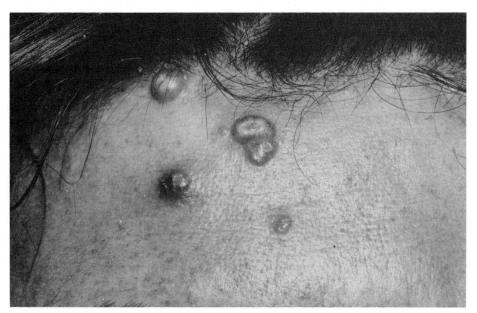

Fig. 13.10 Molluscum contagiosum of the forehead: smooth, pearly umbilicated lesions.

any papule. In hairy areas, follicular lesions may mimic furunculosis though careful observation will always reveal associated pearly-white lesions.

The sites affected vary with factors such as climate, the mode of contact and the presence of an eczematous diathesis. Atopic subjects may develop hundreds of papules (Solomon & Telner 1966). In non-atopic subjects the infection is usually localized to one area, often on the trunk or axilla—apart from in-patients who are immunosuppressed or taking cytotoxic or steroid therapy (Rosenberg & Yusk 1970; Schorfinius 1972).

In temperate regions the neck and trunk are sites of predilection whilst in the tropics the limbs are more aften involved; less commonly the face, scalp and mucous membranes are affected. Not infrequently, molluscum contangiosum causes conjunctivitis and an eczematous reaction in the affected area; these clear on resolution of the viral lesions.

In normal subjects most cases clear within 3–4 months; a minority may persist for up to 3–4 years. However, occasionally a solitary lesion or more rarely a cluster of contiguous lesions may reach a diameter of 2 cm or more and persist for years. Such giant mollusca have been reported in the scalp (Fox 1902; Foelsche 1965).

True follicular involvement rarely occurs in molluscum contagiosum producing deeper waxy papules without central umbilication with an occasional coarse hair growing through the centre. Squeezing fails to produce any discharge. Atopic adults tend to be affected. Skin biopsy shows dermal aggregation of molluscum bodies in a contiguous follicular arrangement (Ive 1985).

Clinical diagnosis of the typical lesions presents no difficulty. The diagnosis of a giant molluscum is rarely suspected and is made histologically after the lesion has been curetted or excised.

Treatment is not necessary in most cases due to the good prognosis and absence of symptoms. Large, visible or irritating and sore lesions may require treatment. All the recommended therapeutic modalities involve irritating the papules, i.e. using trichloroacetic acid or phenol applied on a pointed orange-stick, or cryosurgery. Localized large lesions may be removed by curettage. Topical retinoic acid has been suggested by some authorities. Associated eczema may require treatment with topical anti-pruritic agents, or weak local corticosteroid creams; oral antihistamines are helpful particularly if eczematous itching leads to sleeplessness.

References

Bagnall, B.G. & Wilson, G.R. (1974) Molluscum contagiosum in red kangaroo. *Australasian Journal of Dermatology*, **15**, 115.

Foelsche, W. (1965) Mollusca contagiosa seitener Extensität und Lokalisation. *Zeitschrift füt Haut und Geschlechtskrankheiten*, **37**, 268.

Fox, T.C. (1902) Case presentation. Dermatological Society of London. *British Journal of Dermatology*, **14**, 216.

Ive, A. (1985) Follicular molluscum contagiosum. *British Journal of Dermatology*, **113**, 493.

Poselthwaite, R. (1970) Molluscum contagiosum: a review. *Archives of Environmental Health*, **21**, 432.

Poselthwaite, R., Watt, J.A., Horley, T.G., Simpson, I. & Adam, H. (1967) Features of molluscum contagiosum in the north east of Scotland and in Fijian settlements. *Journal of Hygiene (Cambridge)*, **65**, 281.

Rosenberg, E.W. & Yusk, J.W. (1970) Molluscum contagiosum: eruption following treatment with prednisolone and methotrexate. *Archives of Dermatology*, **101**, 439.

Schorfinius, H.H. (1972) Molluscum Contagiosum als Symptom. *Hautarzt*, **23**, 34.

Solomon, L.M. & Telner, P. (1966) Eruptive molluscum contagiosum in atopic dermatitis. *Canadian Medical Association Journal*, **95**, 978.

Orf

Orf, a poxvirus, has a world-wide distribution and is common in young lambs. In man, it characteristically produces lesions on the hands from direct inoculation of infected material. Rarely trauma to the scalp may be the means of viral inoculation via infected material producing a scalp nodule. Lesions subside spontaneously.

Reference
Rees, J. & Marks, J.M. (1988) Two unusual cases of Orf following trauma to the scalp. *British Journal of Dermatology*, **118**, 445.

Acquired Immune Deficiency Syndrome (AIDS)
(References p. 445)

AIDS is caused by the human T-cell leukaemia virus type III (HTLV III/LAV). This virus has recently been renamed human immunodeficiency virus (HIV). The clinical picture of HIV infections varies from an asymptomatic state to a state with nonspecific symptoms, the so-called AIDS-related complex (ARC), and finally to manifest AIDS disease (the two latter being based on strict diagnostic criteria (Ebbesen *et al.* 1984).

The conditions occur in male homosexual and intravenous drug abusers, but also at risk are recipients of blood products, and the heterosexual partners and children of AIDS patients.

Non-specific manifestations include an acute exanthematic flu-like illness, fatigue, malaise, night sweats, diarrhoea, weight loss and generalized persistent lymphadenopathy. Dermatological manifestations have featured prominently in descriptions of AIDS and include malignant processes such as Kaposi's sarcoma and cutaneous infections such as chronic genital herpes simplex (Siegel *et al.* 1981), herpes zoster, mucocutaneous candidiasis (Gottlieb *et al.* 1981), fungal infections, chronic pyoderma, molluscum contagiosum and sporotrichosis. Several other skin disorders seen in HIV infections involve hair, hair follicles and hair bearing sites.

The development or aggravation of seborrhoeic dermatitis has been noted frequently varying from mild to explosive with extensive reddening and scaling of the face (Eisenstat & Wormser 1984). The severe form has distinctive histological features which include necrotic keratinocytes and a dermal infiltrate containing plasma cells and neutrophils showing leukocytoclasis (Soeprono & Schinella 1986). Farthing *et al.* (1985) suggested that *Pityrosporum* yeasts may be aetiologically related to seborrhoeic dermatitis as first proposed by McGinley in 1975. *Demodex folliculorum* may also be present in greater number than normal (Sindrup *et al.* 1987).

Follicular eruptions may also be useful clinical indicators of the infection. These may present as a recurrence of teenage acne or a relapsing folliculitis concentrated around the axillae (Farthing *et al.* 1985). A chronic, widespread, pustular acneiform folliculitis diffusely affecting the face, chest, buttocks and back has been described as an early warning skin sign in AIDS and persistent generalized lymphadenopathy (Muhlemann *et al.* 1986). Biopsies showed a mixed perifollicular infiltrate with polymorphs, lymphocytes and plasma cells. Folliculitides have also been observed in asymptomatic seropositive homosexuals (Farthing *et al.* 1985) and in individuals at risk from HIV infection (Muhlemann *et al.* 1986). Treatment with flucloxacillin, dilute topical steroids and emollients is initially successful but relapse is frequent.

Staphylococcus aureus has been isolated from half of the patients in whom cultures have been performed. The remainder yielded normal skin flora or were negative (Farthing *et al.* 1985; Muhlemann *et al.* 1986).

Another pattern, a florid impetigo, localized to the beard area and anterior neck was seen in 22% of patients with recently diagnosed AIDS and 50% of patients in the high-risk group (Muhlemann *et al.* 1986). In association extensive fungal infections of the feet and groins were also often seen.

The rare dermatosis eosinophilic pustular folliculitis has also been described in AIDS and ARC patients. Aetiologically, hypersensitivity of the skin to *Demodex folliculorum* and dermatophytes associated with immunologic aberrations of AIDS was suggested (Soeprono & Schinella 1986; Jenkins *et al.* 1988). UVB therapy may be of benefit for this condition in AIDS patients (Buchness *et al.* 1988).

A severe necrotizing folliculitis with an underlying vasculitis has also been described. Erythematous follicular papules symmetrically affect the forearms, back and thighs, leaving scaly hyperpigmented macules and papules, 3–6 mm in diameter. A vascular pathogenesis for the papulonecrotic eruption was presumed (Barlow & Schulz 1987).

Alterations in the scalp hair of black patients with AIDS may be seen producing longer, lighter, softer and occasionally discoloured hair (Leonides 1987). This 'AIDS trichopathy' has since been estimated to occur in at least 50% of black patients with AIDS (Kinchelow *et al.* 1988). The naturally 'curly' hair gradually becomes straighter with time and is independent of the patient's nutritional status. Hair changes were also noticed among white patients with AIDS, although not as frequently or consistently.

Hypertrichosis of the eyelashes has rarely been reported in patients suffering from AIDS and appears not to be iatrogenically induced (Casanova *et al.* 1987).

Alopecia areata in association with AIDS has been described in a single patient (Schonwetter & Nelson 1986). The authors suggested that the immunological effects in AIDS could lead to the syndrome of alopecia areata.

References

Barlow, R.J. & Schulz, E.J. (1987) Necrotizing folliculitis in AIDS-related complex. *British Journal of Dermatology*, **116**, 581.

Buchness, M.R., Lim, H.W., Hatcher, V.A., Sanchez, M. & Soter, N.A. (1988) Eosinophilic pustular folliculitis in AIDS. *New England Journal of Medicine*, **318**, 1183.

Casanova, J.M., Puig, T. & Rubio, M. (1987) Hypertrichosis of the eyelashes in Acquired Immunodeficiency Syndrome. *Archives of Dermatology*, **123**, 1599.

Ebbesen, T., Biggar, R.J. & Melbye, M., (eds.) (1984) *AIDS: A Basic Guide for Clinicians*. W.B. Saunders, Philadelphia.

Eisenstat, B.A. & Wormser, G.P. (1984) Seborrhoeic dermatitis and butterfly rash in AIDS. *New England Journal of Medicine*, **311**, 189.

Farthing, C.F., Staughton, R.C.D. & Rowland Payne, C.M.E. (1985) Skin disease in homosexual patients with AIDS and lesser forms of human T-cell leukaemia virus (HTLV–III) disease. *Clinical and Experimental Dermatology*, **10**, 3.

Gottlieb, M.S., Schroff, R., Schanker, H.M. *et al.* (1981) *Pneumocystis carinii* pneumonia and mucosal candidiasis in previously healthy homosexual men: evidence of a new acquired immunodeficiency. *New England Journal of Medicine*, **305**, 1425.

Jenkins, D., Fisher, B.K., Chalvardjian, A. & Adam, P. (1988) Eosinophilic pustular folliculitis in a patient with AIDS. *International Journal of Dermatology*, **27**, 34.

Kinchelow, T., Schmidt, U. & Ingato, S. (1988) Changes in the hair of black patients with AIDS. *Journal of Infectious Diseases*, **157**, 394.

Leonidas, J.R. (1987) Hair alteration in black patients with AIDS. *Cutis*, **39**, 537.

McGinley, K.J., Leyden, J.J., Marples, R.R. *et al.* (1975) Quantitative microbiology of the scalp in non-dandruff, dandruff and seborrhoeic dermatitis. *Journal of Investigative Dermatology*, **64**, 401.

Muhlemann, M.F., Anderson, M.G., Paradinas, F.J. *et al.* (1986) Early warning signs in AIDS and persistent generalized lymphadenopathy. *British Journal of Dermatology*, **114**, 419.

Schonwetter, R.S. & Nelson, E.B. (1986) Alopecia areata and the acquired-immunodeficiency-syndrome-related complex. *Annals of Internal Medicine*, **104**, 287.

Siegal, F.P., Lopez, C., Hammer, G.S. *et al.* (1981) Severe acquired immunodeficiency in male homosexuals manifested by chronic perianal ulcerative herpes simplex lesions. *New England Journal of Medicine*, **305**, 1439.

Sindrup, J.H., Lisby, G., Weismann, K. *et al.* (1987) Skin manifestations in AIDS, HIV infection and AIDS-related complex. *International Journal of Dermatology*, **26**, 267.

Soeprono, F.F. & Schinella, R.A. (1986) Eosinophilic pustular folliculitis in patients with acquired immunodeficiency syndrome. *Journal of the American Academy of Dermatology*, **14**, 1020.

Candida

Candida septicaemia with folliculitis in heroin addicts (References p. 447)

A distinctive syndrome of systemic candidiasis in intravenous heroin addicts has presented in small epidemics in France, Australia, United Kingdom, Italy and Spain. It occurred wherever brown 'Iranian' heroin was introduced to a susceptible population. *Candida albicans* spores are probably injected into the blood stream along with the heroin, as indicated by the short latency period between the injection and the first symptom (Davies *et al.* 1986). Healthy guinea pigs injected intravenously with *Candida albicans* developed cutaneous candidiasis with pseudo-hyphae in the hairshafts and in the cornified layers of the epidermis (Franden *et al.* 1984; Van Cutsen *et al.* 1985). Similarities between this experimental disease and heroin addict cutaneous infection suggest that the source of dissemination is the same. This type of heroin is relatively insoluble in water and requires acidification with lemon juice or vinegar, and heating. Contaminated lemon has been suggested as the source of infection (Hay 1986) since it has been demonstrated that *Candida albicans* can survive for several days at room temperature inside a lemon (Newton-John *et al.* 1984; Davies 1986). Cultures of the heroin have always been negative for *Candida*. The habit of licking the needle and the use of lavatory water have also been incriminated as the possible source of fungus.

The syndrome due to septicaemia appears suddenly within a few hours (but occasionally after a few days) after the intravenous injection of heroin, with an initial pyrexial phase with severe headache, myalgia, vomiting and chills. Normally within 4 days a second phase follows, characterized by cutaneous lesions.

Multiple painful nodules appear on the scalp and either suppurate or resolve spontaneously leaving areas of alopecia. Painful follicular papules and pustules appear over the beard, neck, scalp and other hairy areas including thorax, axillae and pubis. Occipital lymphadenopathy may occur.

Ocular involvement may appear a few days later, characterized by unilateral or bilateral eye pain, redness, photophobia and reduced visual acuity. Fundoscopy may show a typical fluffy exudate with hyalitis at the posterior pole. This is the most serious manifestation of the syndrome, necessitating early treatment to prevent blindness; in one-third of cases there may be total loss of vision or reduced visual acuity to less than 30% of normal (Davies *et al.* 1986).

Jaundice accompanied by abnormal liver function tests often occurs during this phase. Bone and osteoarticular involvement may appear some weeks or months later, costochondritis, spondylodiskitis and abscesses of the chest being the most common manifestations. Pulmonary lesions are rare.

Blood cultures are usually negative but smears from pustules yield *Candida albicans* and microscopic examination of a 10% KOH preparation (or chlorazole black E stain) of a hair plucked from a follicular lesion may show characteristic pseudohyphae of *Candida* within the hair and occasional budding around it (Puig *et al.* 1987). The diagnosis is confirmed by cultures on Sabouraud medium. Urine and sputum may also yield *Candida albicans* on culture. High titres of anticandidal antibody are present and *Candida* skin test is positive.

Histopathology reveals dense, nodular, mixed cell infiltrate of lymphocytes, macrophages and neutrophils especially around the base of the hair bulb and periadnexally. Pustules form by accumulation of neutrophils between hair shafts and follicular epithelium. PAS reaction demonstrates multiple pseudohyphae in the pustules and invading the hair shafts.

Although spontaneous resolution may occur, ketoconazole (400–600 mg/day for 15 days) is the treatment of choice for cutaneous candidiasis in this syndrome. When ocular or osteoarticular involvement is present, a course of combined therapy with intravenous amphotericin B and flucytosine is advisable.

Follicular lesions together with fever in heroin addicts are highly suggestive of this condition, which is completely different from the usual features of septicaemia that occur in immunocompromised patients. Also, in contrast, the immunological status of heroin addicts with *Candida* septicaemia appears normal.

References

Darcis, J.M., Etienne, M., Christophe, J. & Pierard, G.E. (1986) *Candida albicans* septicemia with folliculitis in heroin addict. *American Journal of Dermatology*, **8**, 507.

Fransen, J., Van Cutsen, J., Vandersteene, R. *et al.* (1984) Histopathology of experimental systemic candidosis in guinea pigs, Sabouraudia. *Journal of Medical and Veterinary Mycology*, **22**, 465.

Hay, R.J. (1986) Systemic candidiasis in heroin addicts. *British Medical Journal*, **292**, 1096.

Newton-John, H.F., Wise, K. & Looke, D.F.M. (1984) The role of lemon juice in disseminated candidiasis of heroin abusers. *Medical Journal of Australia*, **140**, 780.

Puig, L., Garcia, P. & de Moragas, J.M. (1987) KOH preparation for early diagnosis of systemic candidiasis in heroin addicts. *International Journal of Dermatology*, **26**, 257.

Van Cutsen, J., Fransen, J. & Janssen, P.A.J. (1985) Animal models for systemic dermatophyte and candida infection with dissemination to the skin. *Models in Dermatology*, **1**, 196.

'Candida folliculitis'

Candida albicans does not normally produce folliculitis (Chauvin *et al.* 1988), although there are examples of folliculitis developing after prolonged intravenous hyperalimentation (Schleppner *et al.* 1972), after administration of topical or systemic antibiotics (Meinhof *et al.* 1970).

Dekio *et al.* (1987) described facial follicular erythematous papules and pustules due to *Candida albicans* in association with hypothyroidism. There were no signs of oral, genital or other candidiasis.

References

Chauvin, M.F., Cosnes, A., Benkhraba, F. & Touraine, R. (1988) Folliculite du cuir chevelu et de la barbe a *Candida albicans*. *Annales de Dermatologie et de Venereologie*, **115**, 1164.

Dekio, S., Imeoka, C. & Jidoi, J. (1987) Candida folliculitis associated with hypothyroidism. *British Journal of Dermatology*, **117**, 663.

Meinhof, W., Balda, B.R., Vogel, H. & Braun-Falco, O. (1970) Zum Krankheitsbild der Folliculitis barbae Candida Mycetica. *Hautarzt*, **21**, 312.

Schleppner, O.L.A., Shelley, W.B., Ruberg, R.L. & Dudrick, S.J. (1972) Acute papulopustular acne associated with prolonged intravenous hyperalimentation. *Journal of the American Medical Association*, **219**, 877.

Chronic mucocutaneous candidiasis

This is a chronic cutaneous disease without systemic candidiasis. There are several variants in existence, most beginning early in childhood.

Clinical manifestations include chronic oral thrush, paronychia, nail dystrphy, vulvovaginits, balanitis and cutaneous granuloma formation. Scalp and face are often involved when granulomatous, hypertrophic plaques occur. Verrucous growth is progressive and responds poorly to treatment. Gross disfigurement may ensue.

Candida infection in immunocompromised patients

Immunosuppressed hosts such as patients with lymphoma, leukaemia, diabetes, neutropenia and receiving immunosuppressive therapy are at risk of developing *Candida* infection.

Disseminated candidiasis in such patients produces a maculopapular rash, nodular lesions, erythematous papules, purpura and skin necrosis. The lesions usually affect the trunk, proximal extremities and legs and may be associated with severe myalgia. The *Candida* organism most often isolated is *Candida tropicalis* (Grossman *et al.* 1980).

Candida granuloma may also be seen as a crusted hypertrophic non-inflammatory lesion frequently involving the scalp. They can be simple or multiple and may be associated with septicaemia (Kaidbey & Kurban 1971).

Erosive candidiasis of the scalp is also recognized in diabetes as recurrent, deep scalp abscesses (Verbov 1981; Goldstein *et al.* 1986).

References

Kaidbey, K.H. & Kurban, A.K. (1971) Unusual granulomas of the skin seen in Lebanon. *Acta Dermato-Venereologica*, 51, 225.

Goldstein, N., Tuazon, C.U. & Lessin, L. (1986) Carbuncles caused by *Candida albicans*. *Journal of the American Academy of Dermatology*, **14**, 511.

Grossman, M.E., Silvers, D.N. & Walther, R.R. (1980) Cutaneous manifestation of disseminated candidiasis. *Journal of the American Academy of Dermatology*, **2**, 111.

Verbov, J. (1981) Erosive candidiasis of the scalp, followed by the reappearance of black hair after 40 years. *British Journal of Dermatology*, **105**, 595.

Syphilis
(References p. 450)

Precise figures for the prevalence of syphilis are seldom obtained because only a proportion of identified primary infections are notified and because unidentified primary infections are frequent, particularly in women and male homosexuals. The widespread use of antibiotics in common diseases of adolescents and young adults, such as acne vulgaris, also distorts the natural history of syphilitic infections. In 1935, Hazen reported a 5% incidence in his study of skin lesions in a population of 2844 patients with secondary syphilis. Secondary syphilis and its classic manifestations are becoming less common in dermatological practice today.

Hair loss does not occur in primary syphilis, except in the case of the primary lesion on the scalp (Druella 1923). Syphilis may involve the scalp in the secondary stage of the infection. In its classic form (Fig. 13.11) the irregular, 'moth-eaten' appearance is highly suggestive of the diagnosis, but a somewhat similar appearance may occasionally be seen in acute disseminated lupus erythematosus.

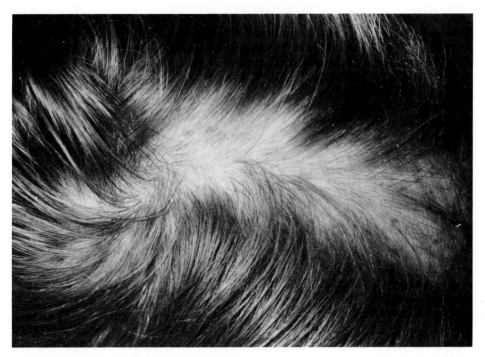

Fig. 13.11 Irregular, patchy alopecia in secondary syphilis.

The eyebrows may be shed, particularly in their lateral third, and there may be patchy alopecia of the beard. The pattern of hair loss is indeed very variable; in one patient loss of eyebrows was accompanied by only moderate alopecia of pubic hair (Pirozzi *et al.* 1972).

Three to five months after infection, however, a diffuse shedding of telogen hairs (telogen effluvium) may occur, differing in no way from the alopecia which may follow certain other infections. Not only the scalp but other hairy areas may be affected. Hair growth resumes spontaneously after a few months. A very rarely reported phenomenon is the acceleration of hair loss in secondary syphilis as a feature of a febrile Jarisch–Herzheimer reaction, a few hours after initiating treatment with penicillin (Pareek 1977). Serological tests for syphilis are advisable in unexplained acute diffuse alopecia.

Trichogram studies have shown a decrease in anagen hairs and an increase in catagen hairs in both the primary and secondary stages of syphilis (Van der Willigen *et al.* 1987).

A less common presentation of secondary syphilis is the folliculopapular variant which is seen more in blacks than whites. Small, closely set, non-coalescing but well-disseminated groups of papules occur without scaling or follicular plugging on the beard or trunk (Winchell *et al.* 1985). Studies have shown a correlation between secondary syphilis of the follicular papulopustular type and neurosyphilis (Stokes 1945; Mikhail & Chapel 1969).

The two principal forms of cutaneous syphilis in the tertiary stage may also involve the scalp. The serpiginous nodulo-squamous syphilide can occur anywhere but it favours the face, back and extensor aspects of the limbs. The grouped reddish-brown indolent scaly papules may spread into the scalp from the forehead or from the nape of the neck. This eruption can be mistaken for psoriasis or for sarcoidosis. Later the nodules break down to form crusted ulcers. The syphilitic gumma may begin in the skin or in bone. It gradually forms a painless mass of rubbery consistency, breaking down to form a punched-out ulcer. Subsequent alopecia is scarring and atrophic.

The confirmation of a suspected diagnosis depends on positive serological tests for syphilis. Full clinical evaluation and proper planned course of treatment and careful follow-up are essential. Inadequate treatment which merely heals the cutaneous lesions expose the patient to the serious risk of later cardiovascular or neurological involvement.

References

Druella, M. (1923) *Le Chancre du Cuir Chevelu.* Thèse, Lyon.

Hazen, H.H. (1935) Syphilis and skin disease in the American Negro. *Archives of Dermatology and Syphilology,* **31**, 316.

Mikhail, G.R. & Chapel, T.A. (1969) Follicular papulopustular syphilid. *Archives of Dermatology,* **100**, 471.

Pareek, S.S. (1977) Syphilitic alopecia in Jarisch–Herzheimer reaction. *British Journal of Venereal Disease,* **53**, 389.

Pirozzi, D.J., Lockshia, N.A. & Rosenberg, P.E. (1972) An unusual manifestation of cutaneous syphilis. *Cutis,* **20**, 451.

Stokes, J.H., Beerman, H. & Ingram, N.R. (1945) *Modern Clinical Syphilology,* p. 250. W.B. Saunders, Philadelphia.

Van der Willigen, A.H., Peereboom-Wynia, J.D.R., Van der Hoek, J.C.S. *et al.* (1987) Hair root studies in patients suffering from primary and secondary syphilis. *Acta Dermato-Venereologica (Stockholm),* **67**, 250.

Winchell, S.A., Tschen, J.A. & McGavran, M.H. (1985) Follicular secondary syphilis. *Cutis,* **35**, 259.

Tuberculosis
(Reference p. 451)

Apart from lupus vulgaris, which is itself uncommonly found in the scalp, tuberculosis in the scalp is excessively rare. At the end of his career Sabouraud (Boutelier 1953) had great difficulty in recalling a single case.

Where tuberculosis is prevalent lupus vulgaris is usually the most frequent cutaneous form. It occurs as a post-primary infection in patients with some degree of immunity to tuberculosis. The distribution of the lesions depends on the extent to which the body is covered by clothing. In temperate climates 80% of lesions are on the head and neck; in the Tropics lesions on the trunk are relatively more frequent. The scalp is protected to some extent from inoculation of the infection, but lupus may extend into the scalp from contiguous non-hairy skin and it may at times begin in the scalp itself.

Soft reddish-brown nodules extend slowly but irregularly, leaving scarring in their wake. Without treatment the lesion tends to persist indefinitely and, particularly in the malnourished, may be very destructive. The diagnosis should be considered in the presence of soft granulomatous nodules and should be confirmed histologically. After full investigation to establish whether tuberculosis is present in other organs, treatment with antituberculous drugs may be initiated.

Reference

Boutelier, A. (1953) Tuberculose du cuir chevelu. In *Affections de la Chevelure et du Cuir Chevelu*, p. 606, ed. A. Desaux. Masson, Paris.

Leprosy
(References p. 452)

Loss of scalp hair caused by leprosy is very unusual. In lepromatous leprosy the lateral third of the eyebrows may be shed, body hair may be lost, but scalp lesions are exceptional (Fig. 13.12) (Parikh *et al.* 1974, 1985; Malaviya *et al.* 1987).

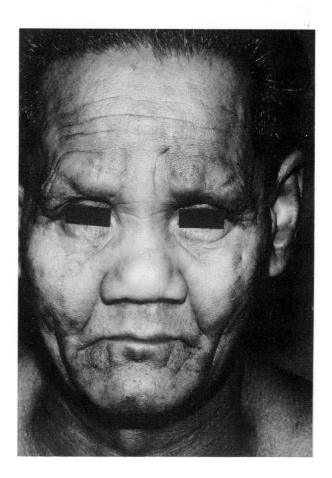

Fig. 13.12 Leprosy. Loss of eyebrows.

However Lepra bacilli were found in 100% of apparently normal scalps of patients with lepromatous leprosy and 75 % of those with borderline leprosy (Kaur & Kumar 1978). It has been suggested that the sparing of the scalp in clinical leprosy may be due to the higher surface temperature in the skin in this site, resulting from the abundant blood supply and further increased by a normal covering of hair (Dutta *et al.* 1983). *Mycobacterium leprae* is known to favour the cooler parts of the body (Binford & Meyers 1978).

Jopling (1978) suggested that the testicular atrophy which occurs in lepromatous leprosy reduces testosterone levels and thus may retard the development of androgenetic alopecia.

References

Binford, C.H. & Meyers, W.M. (1978) Leprosy. In *A Window on Leprosy*, p. 153, ed. B.R. Chatterjee. Statesman Commercial Press, Calcutta.

Dutta, A.K., Mandal, S.B. & Jopling, W.H. (1983) Surface temperature of bald and hairy scalp in reference to leprosy affection. *Indian Journal of Dermatology*, **28**, 1.

Jopling, W.H. (1978) *Handbook of Leprosy*, 2nd edn., p. 20. Heinemann, London.

Kaur, S. & Kumar, B. (1978) Study of apparently uninvolved skin in leprosy as regards bacillary population at various sites. *Leprosy in India*, **50**, 38.

Malaviya, G.N., Girdhar, B.K., Husain, S., Ramu, G., Lavania, R.K. & Desikan, K.V. (1987) Scalp lesion in a lepromatous patient—case report. *Indian Journal of Leprosy*, **59**, 103.

Parikh, A.C., D'Souza, N.G., Chaulawala, R. & Ganapati, R. (1974) Leprosy lesions in the scalp. *Leprosy in India*, **46**, 39.

Parikh, D.A., Oberai, C. & Ganapati, R. (1985) Involvement of scalp in leprosy—case report. *Indian Journal of Leprosy*, **57**, 883.

Atypical mycobacterium

The 'atypical' mycobacteria are a heterogeneous group of non-motile, aerobic, acid-fast rods, differing from 'typical' mycobacteria (*M. tuberculosis* and *M. leprae*) in their clinical and cultural characteristics, and *in vivo*/*in vitro* resistance to antimycobacterial drugs. They are classified into four groups based on colonial pigmentation morphology and other bacteriologic data (Runyon 1959). Cutaneous infections caused by *M. kansasii* are rarely seen. Large crusted, exudative and verrucous plaques affecting the forehead and scalp producing patchy alopecia and cervical lymphadenopathy in a black woman have been described (Hanke *et al.* 1987). Treatment with rifampicin and ethambutol produced complete resolution with normal regrowth of hair.

References

Hanke, C.W., Temofeew, R.K. & Slama, S.L. (1987) *Mycobacterium kansasii* infection with multiple cutaneous lesions. *Journal of the American Academy of Dermatology*, **16**, 1122.

Runyon, E.H. (1959) Anonymous mycobacteria in pulmonary disease. *Medical Clinics of North America*, **43**, 272.

Leishmaniasis
(References p. 454)

The protozoan parasite *Leishmania* occurs in three forms: *L. tropica*, associated with dermal leishmaniasis, *L. donovani*, associated with kala-azar, and *L. braziliensis*, associated with South American (mucocutaneous) leishmaniasis. The three 'species' are morphologically identical by normal criteria, but show antigenic differences (Zuckerman 1975). The natural reservoirs of infection are wild rodents, dogs and foxes, from which the parasites are conveyed to man by the bites of the sandfly *Phlebotomus*, and possibly sometimes by mosquitoes.

Dermal leishmaniasis (Haghighi *et al.* 1971)
This disease is widely distributed throughout the Tropics and subtropics. In Europe it is endemic, in the Mediterranean littoral, including some areas of the South of France (Rioux *et al.* 1968). The lesions are commonly on exposed skin, particularly the face and arms. Most infections occur in childhood and in the indigenous population of an endemic area, but may develop at any age in previously unexposed tourists and other visitors. We have seen lesions in the scalp margin and they can occur in bald areas of the scalp. Clinically the lesion, single or multiple, forms a granulomatous nodule, dry or ulcerated, which heals after months or years to leave an ugly or depressed scar.

Kala-azar
Skin lesions do not occur except in the 10% who, one or more years after apparent cure, develop post-kala-azar dermal leishmaniasis with an extensive maculo-papular eruption on the face, which later spreads to other parts of the body.

Mucocutaneous leishmaniasis (Azulay 1968)
The initial lesions are granulomatous ulcers which occur on exposed skin including that of the scalp. Progressive involvement of the mucous membranes occurs some 3 years later.

Diagnosis of leishmaniasis
The diagnosis is suggested when granulomatous skin lesions develop in an individual at an appropriate interval of weeks or months after the patient has visited an area in which either dermal or mucocutaneous leishmaniasis is endemic. The diagnosis is confirmed by the demonstration of *Leishmania* in a biopsy or in a smear taken from the edge of the lesion.

Treatment
Treatment is not entirely satisfactory and when this diagnosis has been reliably established advice should be sought from a physician with experience in the management of these diseases.

References

Azulay, R.D. (1968) Leishmaniasis americana. *Dermatologia Ibero Latino Americano*, **3**, 235.

Haghighi, I., Kavoussi, A. & Hayat-Davendi, G.H. (1971) Some practical aspects of cutaneous leishmaniasis. *International Journal of Dermatology*, **10**, 129.

Rioux, J.A., Golvan, Y., Lauret, H., Haim, R. & Tour, S. (1968) Enquête écologique sur les leishmanioses dans le sud de la France. *Bulletin de l'I.N.S.E.R.M.*, **23**, 1125.

Zuckerman, A. (1975) Parasitological review: current status of the immunology of blood and tissue parasites. I. *Leishmania. Experimental Parasitology*, **38**, 374.

Onchocerciasis (Convit 1975)

Onchocerciasis is caused by the filarial parasite *Onchocerca volvulus*, which is transmitted by the bites of small flies of the genus *Simulium*. The disease is endemic in much of equatorial Africa, and in the Yemen, and there are smaller foci in several Central American countries and in Venezuela and Colombia. The biting habits of the vector influence the clinical picture of the disease, notably the distribution of the nodules which are on the lower part of the body in Africa but tend to be on the upper trunk and in the scalp in Latin America.

About a year after infection a pruritic eruption develops with weals and oedema and sometimes with fever and joint pains. Gradually over the years the skin becomes thickened and lichenified from scratching and there are often patchy areas of decreased pigmentation.

Firm painless nodules develop over the bony prominences and in Latin America these nodules are often in the scalp, particularly in the occipital region. The serious manifestation of the late stage of the disease is eye involvement leading to blindness.

During the earlier stages the diagnosis is made by taking a skin 'snip' and examining a smear in saline for microfilariae. If nodules are present they may be excised to confirm the diagnosis and when this has been done the remainder should be excised as a stage in the therapeutic attack on the disease, which should include the administration of diethyl carbamazine.

The diagnosis should be suspected in a patient with scalp nodules who has the associated lichenified pruritic lesions on the trunk and who has visited, however briefly, an endemic area.

Reference

Convit, J. (1975) In *Clinical Tropical Dermatology*, p. 220 ed. O. Canizares. Blackwell, Oxford.

Varicella–herpes zoster
(References p. 456)

Varicella is the usual response of the previously unexposed subject to infection with the varicella–zoster virus, and zoster is commonly due to reactivation of the latent virus, but it is probable that zoster can also follow exogenous infection (Nally & Ross 1971; Luby 1973).

The eruption of varicella occurs in successive crops of small clear vesicles on the trunk, face and scalp. Scalp involvement may be extensive but there is little or no permanent scarring unless secondary infection has been severe or the normal immune response is depressed by disease or by drugs. There is temporary hair loss from the affected areas of scalp.

Herpes zoster is often preceded by localized pain and tenderness. The eruption consists of closely grouped vesicles in segmental distribution (Fig. 13.13). In the elderly or malnourished the lesions may be haemorrhagic, necrotic or even gangrenous (Fig. 13.14). The scalp is involved in zoster of the ophthalmic division of the trigeminal nerve or of cervical segments 1–3. Zoster of C23–herpes occipito–collaris (Payten & Dawes 1972)—is associated with an eruption of the pre-auricular region of the cheek, the pinna, the side of the neck and the occipital scalp.

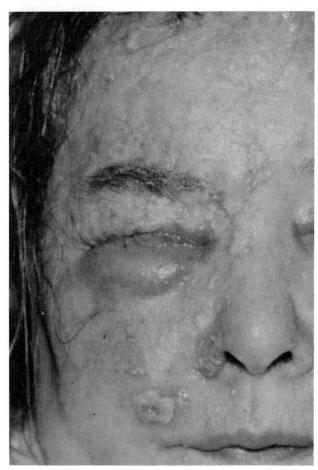

Fig. 13.13 Herpes zoster of the ophthalmic division of the trigeminal nerve.

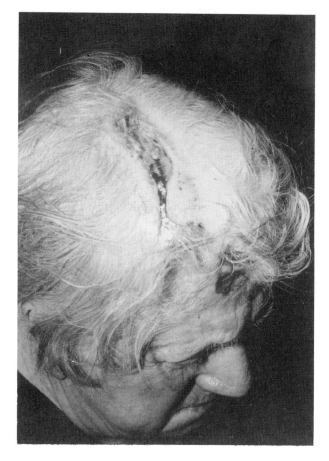

Fig. 13.14 Ulceration following herpes zoster.

Severe herpes zoster is treated by intravenous or oral acyclovir which, when given early in the disease, significantly reduces pain and accelerates skin healing (Bean *et al.* 1983; Cobo *et al.* 1986). Systemic corticosteroids have been recommended for the treatment of herpes zoster since 1951 to reduce inflammation and resultant scarring; however, their prescription conferred no further benefit over acyclovir and their use remains controversial (Esmann *et al.* 1987). Topical antiseptics are usually prescribed and probably reduce some of the scarring and hair loss.

References

Bean, B., Aeppli, D. & Balfour, H.H. Jr. (1983) Acyclovir in shingles. *Journal of Antimicrobial Chemotherapy*, **12** (suppl. B), 123.

Cobo, L.M., Foulkes, G.N., Liesegang, T., Lass, J., Sutphin, J.E., Wilhelmus, K., Jones, D.B., Chapman, S., Segreti, A.C. & King, D.H. (1986) Oral acyclovir in the treatment of acute herpes zoster ophthalmicus. *Ophthalmology*, **93**, 763.

Esmann, V., Geil, J.P., Kroon, S., Fogh, H., Peterslund, N.A., Petersen, C.S., Rønne-Rasmussen, J.O. & Danielsen, L. (1987). Prednisolone does not prevent post-herpetic neuralgia. *Lancet*, **ii**, 126.

Luby, J.P. (1973) Varicella-zoster virus. *Journal of Investigative Dermatology*, **61**, 212.

Nally, F.F. & Ross, I.H. (1971) Herpes zoster of the oral and facial structures. *Oral Surgery, Oral Medicine, Oral Pathology*, **32**, 221.

Payten, R.J. & Dawes, J.D.K. (1972) Herpes zoster of the head and neck. *Journal of Laryngology and Otology*, **86**, 1031.

Chapter 14
Psychological Factors and Disorders
of the Hair

Introduction

The effective diagnosis, assessment and management of many disorders of the hair is impossible without some appreciation of the special psychological significance of the hair. Diseases which produce patterns of hair growth which deviate even slightly from that which the patient regards as normal may in extreme cases cause emotional stress of such a degree as may perpetuate the abnormality, whether or not stress played a role in initiating it.

The unconscious significance of hair
(References p. 460)

In a monograph with this title Charles Berg (1950) reviewed the anthropological and psychiatric literature. He emphasized the importance of the hair in many rituals in a variety of primitive peoples. He pointed out that hair has, in modern man, practically no other significance except as a sexual symbol and he claimed that there is no normal person without some degree of hair fetishism. He referred to a young women with total alopecia who stated that she would rather have lost an arm or a leg, and he discussed the general overvaluation of hair. He mentioned that even minimal facial hair in a woman may cause great distress—'these affects are not based upon reality values, but like all the affects connected with hair have their source in those unconscious constellations which we are endeavouring to plumb'.

Charles Berg was a psychoanalyst of the Freudian school and he believed that the normal concern about the hair becoming thin, falling out or greyish was a displacement of castration anxiety and that shaving the head was symbolic castration.

This explanation may seem extreme, but in many societies and religions shaving the head is associated with celibacy or chastity, as is to a lesser extent covering the hair in Muslim and orthodox Jewish society. The Christian wedding veil similarly represents modesty and chastity.

The association of hair with sexual attractiveness as perceived both objectively and subjectively is obvious from even the most superficial survey of the visual arts, literature, and the output of the advertising industry. The cliché 'a woman's crowning glory' exemplifies this attitude, and the anguish at the loss of head hair and thus of sexual attractiveness is well-described and illustrated in the self-help book *Coping with Sudden Hair Loss* (Steel 1988).

This heavy freight of symbolism pertaining to head hair is outweighed by that of body hair, the presence and depiction of which is hedged with taboos. Classical painting from the 15th–19th centuries does not show any body hair on female nudes. This omission led the art critic and historian John Ruskin to consider his wife abnormal because of her body hair which prevented the consummation of their marriage and resulted in its annulment. Pubic hair is often considered forbidden, and may be an object of fetishism (Cooper 1971). Axillary hair is considered normal and attractive in continental Europe, but is regarded as abhorrent in women or as a sign of rampant feminism in the UK and USA. Hairiness of the head, face and body of men is often equated with barbarism, violence and rape (Cooper 1971).

There can be no doubt that some disorders of hair give rise to anxieties more profound than their objective severity would appear to justify, and this may reflect the symbolic significance of hair.

Disturbance of the body image

In 1965 Meador introduced the concept of non-disease and pointed out that the absence of diagnostic signs and symptoms need not imply an absence of significant symptomatology. Of 28 such patients studied by Cotterill (1981) the symptoms were confined to the scalp in 9, the face in 8 and to the perineum in 8; there were 16 females and 12 males. The age ranged from 16 to 76 years with a mean age of 46. The scalp symptoms were more common in women and were chiefly of excess hair loss (7 of 8) but 2 also had irritation and burning. None of these patients had objective signs of hair loss. Many of these patients had a depressive illness. Three female patients were preoccupied with excess facial hair, which was not clinically apparent, 2 were suicidal so this symptom must be taken seriously. We have seen similar patients whose principal scalp complaint apart from hair loss was extreme tenderness of the scalp. In all these patients the objective changes, if indeed there are any, are so slight as to seem trivial even to the most sympathetic observer, yet the patients insist that the symptoms are ruining their life.

From the psychiatric point of view these patients are not a uniform group. Most have a disturbed body image and the majority are depressed. They require most careful management and the more severely affected, who are potential suicide risks, should be referred to a psychiatrist.

Common causation of emotional and hair disorders

Depressive illness in young women may be accompanied by androgenetic cutaneous changes. Although the patient may herself tend to blame her alopecia, hirsutism or acne for her depression, a detailed history often establishes that the emotional and cutaneous changes developed in parallel. There is controversy and doubt as to the relationship between depression, stress and androgenetic syndromes.

References

Berg, C. (1950) *The Unconscious Significance of Hair.* Allen & Unwin, London.
Cooper, W. (1971) *Hair: Sex, Society and Symbolism.* Alden Books, London.
Cotterill, J.A. (1981) Dermatological non-disease: a common and potentially fatal disturbance of cutaneous body image. *British Journal of Dermatology,* **104**, 661.
Meador, C.K. (1965) The art and science of non-disease. *New England Journal of Medicine,* **272**, 92.
Steel, E. (1988) *Coping with Sudden Hair Loss.* Thorsons Publishing Group, Wellingborough.

Stress as a precipitating factor in diseases of the hair
(References p. 461)

Diffuse shedding of hair can occur in patients under very severe stress but diffuse alopecia should not be glibly attributed to the minor stresses which, with perseverance, can be elicited in the history of most individuals. Diffuse shedding of hair beginning some 3 or 4 months after a well-defined major stressful episode may, however, be accepted as provoked by that episode and to be potentially reversible in the same way as post-partum or post-febrile alopecia. This may be due to the stress itself or to the profound anorexia and consequent weight loss that often occur with a major life crisis or stress.

However, stress, acute and severe or chronic and prolonged, may occasionally induce the androgenetic syndrome and unless early investigation and treatment are undertaken, skin changes which are not easily reversed or are irreversible may be produced. The first symptom of androgenetic alopecia is profuse but predominantly frontovertical shedding of telogen hairs. It can be seen that this symptom is very easily confused with true diffuse telogen shedding as mentioned above.

The role of stress in precipitating alopecia areata is well discussed by Whitlock (1976). The literature is conflicting. The time interval between the alleged precipitating stress and loss of hair has varied from a few days to 4 months. It follows that if stress can indeed precipitate an attack of alopecia areata, it must do so by more than one mechanism. Some writers suggest that alopecia may be an auto-immune disorder. Should this prove to be the case it does not preclude the possible precipitation of an attack by stress as the science of psychoimmunology is still in its infancy, but can already suggest possible mechanisms (Maddox 1984).

The evidence incriminating stress remains controversial, but it is probable that no dermatologist of experience would exclude its possible role in certain cases.

Stress as a perpetuating factor

In the cutaneous androgenetic syndromes the distress caused by the skin changes can contribute to their perpetuation. Acne and/or hirsutism can seriously impair the sensitive adolescent's capacity to establish normal social relationships with his contemporaries and if severe may retard his or her psychosocial development. The evidence that a self-perpetuating vicious circle can become established has not yet been proven biochemically, but clinical experience suggests that it may occur and that it may indeed be of common occurrence.

Alopecia areata can be extremely disfiguring. Whether or not stress plays a part in provoking it, it is certain that the alopecia is often itself a source of severe stress. This relationship is certainly perceived by sufferers (Steel 1988). It is not proven that this stress perpetuates the condition but the possibility should be borne in mind in the management of these patients.

Artefacts (Lyell 1972)

Artefacts are self-inflicted lesions, but the term as usually employed excludes such lesions produced accidentally through the abuse of mechanical or chemical cosmetic procedures. The most frequent form of deliberate artefact of the scalp consists of plucking the hair, so-called trichotillomania. In children the partially bald patches so produced are seldom of serious psychiatric significance, but the plucking systematically of all the head hair in an adult usually indicates a very serious personality disorder as does extensive self-mutilation of the skin in any region of the body (Sneddon & Sneddon 1975).

Deliberate physical or chemical production of other injuries of the scalp is very unusual but it is possible that some such cases are undiagnosed.

References

Lyell, A. (1972) Dermatitis artefacta and self-inflicted disease. *Scottish Medical Journal*, **17**, 187.
Maddox, J. (1984) Psychoimmunology before its time. *Nature*, **309**, 400.
Sneddon, I. & Sneddon, J. (1975) Self-inflicted injury: a follow-up of 43 patients. *British Medical Journal*, **iii**, 527.
Whitlock, F.A. (1976) *Psychophysiological Aspects of Skin Disease*, p. 181. Saunders, London.

Hair in the social sciences*
(References p. 464)

The religious significance of hair

Hair has two perceived symbolic meanings in a religious context. Shaven or shorn hair is a symbol of celibacy and chastity. Monks and nuns both Buddhist and Christian have shaven heads, as do Hindu priests and widows. Hair sacrifice and offering to the gods was widespread in many ancient religions. The hair was offered for fertility, victory, in fulfilment of vow, and in place of human sacrifice. The practice continues today. The temple of Tirupati in South India is a renowned pilgrimage site for such offerings, which it is said also contribute to the temple revenues. In contrast matted, uncut hair is seen as withdrawal from worldly concerns and vanities in the Hindu Sadhu. Sometimes long hair is a religious requirement as in the Sikh religion and for the Rastafarians, although in both groups it now also has become a symbol of identity as well as a religious tenet.

Hair cutting as punishment

Cutting off or shaving the hair as a punishment has been practised by many peoples. The Ainu of the island of Hokkaido, north of Japan, have a long-established reputation for hirsutism; they are in fact a proto-Caucasoid stock who are no more hirsute than many other Caucasoids, although very hairy by contrast with their Japanese neighbours (Harvey & Brothwell 1969). Among the Ainu great emphasis is placed on the possession of a very full beard and abundant head hair and the enforced cutting of hair was regarded as a severe punishment associated with loss of honour. Women's hair was cut as punishment for adultery. The same punishment was used in Europe after the Second World War on women who had associated with soldiers of occupying armies.

The importance placed on short hair by the armed forces of many countries reinforces the popular association between short hair and authority and discipline.

Hair style

The importance of hair as a component of the body image has been mentioned. The length, the colour and the style in which it is worn must conform to an accepted stereotype. Some knowledge of recent research on such stereotypes is helpful in increasing the dermatologist's understanding of some of his patients who appear to be perversely endeavouring to demand from their hair qualities with which nature failed to endow it.

---

*The remainder of this chapter is designed to introduce the clinician to the rapidly growing literature on the hair published in the journals of the social sciences. It is not cited in textbooks of dermatology and is largely unknown to dermatologists, but its relevance to clinical situations is evident.

Opler (1971) in discussing long hair in males in the United States feels that hair style is a reflection of group attitudes culturally defined rather than of personal feelings of sexual identity. The finding of some investigators on male students classified as 'deviant' in hair length were not unexpected (Larsen & White 1974). The deviants, with hair reaching below their shoulders, assigned more value to independence and less value to recognition and conformity than the non-deviant students. The stereotypes accepted among students have been found to vary from one university to another even during the same period, being influenced by the conservatism or liberalism of the community in which the university is situated. Long hair has been seen as a protest but, 'the increasing number of hair stylists for young men seem to indicate that many of them need an artificial aid to win or to retain a desired self-esteem' (Rom 1973).

In the 1980s short hair was again the norm, and long hair was often a badge of defiance, e.g. the Rastafarians. Short hair can also be a symbol of defiance as in the skin-heads and punks. The 1920s passion for the bob was seen as such by parents and authority figures.

Hair colour

As with other stereotypes those concerning hair colour apply only to the communities studied and to the period of the study. Nevertheless, they throw considerable light on deeply rooted concepts and prejudices.

Yellow hair or a yellow wig was the trademark of a prostitute in ancient Rome. Blonde hair is associated with both innocence, as in so many fairytales, and conversely with sexual allure as exemplified by Marilyn Monroe and other screen goddesses. Dark hair has connotations of night and mystery and is essential for the vamp. Lawson (1971) found that 79 male psychology students, rating the females by hair colour, put brunettes first in 37 of 63 possible comparisons, blondes in 17, redheads in 5 and artificial blondes in 2, suggesting that attitudes may not have changed greatly from Roman times. The 161 female students voted dark males superior to blond males in the proportion of 34 to 4 out of 42 possible comparisons.

Beards

Numerous psychological studies carried out during the 1970s on the subject of beards show a generally positive correlation between the amount of hair on the subject's face and high ratings for masculinity, maturity, good looks, dominance, self confidence and other desirable traits (Pellegreni 1973). Similar findings have been reported from the University of Chicago (Freedman 1969). However, at the rural and more conservative University of Wyoming only 12.8% of females preferred men with a very full beard whereas 40% preferred no facial hair and 42% preferred a moustache but no beard (Feinman & Gill 1977).

Moustaches

Few investigations have been made of the correlation of moustaches with personality traits or of observer reactions to them. Peberdy (1961) studied candidates for commission in the British Army. He classified moustaches into four types:

1 Trimmed, flatly covering most of the lip;
2 Clipped—'toothbrush';
3 Line;
4 Bushy.

Those with trimmed moustaches did not differ in their assessments from clean-shaven candidates. All those with clipped moustaches failed to pass the selection board (but not of course on account of their moustaches). They were limited in imagination with little appreciation of the opinions of others and they tended to create rather than to decrease interpersonal tensions. Men with line moustaches passed the board at only half the normal rate; those that failed showed obsessive health consciousness. Men with bushy moustaches passed at the normal rate; those that failed tended to self-indulgence and self-display.

Parker's (1970) study carried out in Australia is subtitled 'semi-scientific'. He presents interesting facts and figures, tending to show an association between moustaches and sexual pathology, but not allowing any firm conclusions to be drawn.

References

Feinman, S. & Gill, G.W. (1977) Females' response to males' beardedness. *Perceptual and Motor Skills*, **44**, 533.
Freedman, D. (1969) The survival value of the beard. *Psychology Today*, **3**, 36.
Harvey, R.G. & Brothwell, D.R. (1969) Biosocial aspects of Ainu hirsuteness. *Journal of Biosocial Science*, **1**, 109.
Larsen, J.P. & White, B.A. (1974) Comparison of selected perceptual and personality variables among college men deviant and non-deviant in hair length. *Perceptual and Motor Skills*, **38**, 1315.
Lawson, E.D. (1971) Hair color, personality and the observer. *Psychological Reports*, **28**, 311.
Opler, M. (1971) Long hair in contemporary males. *Medical Aspects of Human Sexuality*, **144**.
Parker, N. (1970) The moustache: a semi-scientific study. *Australia and New Zealand Journal of Psychology*, **4**, 49.
Peberdy, G.R. (1961) Moustaches. *Journal of Mental Science*, **107**, 40.
Pellegreni, R.J. (1973) Impressions of the male personality as a function of beardedness. *Psychology*, **10**, 29.
Rom, P. (1973) Hair style and life style. *Individual Psychology*, **10**, 22.

Chapter 15
Hair Cosmetics

Introduction

Women and men have always been concerned about their hair and sought to modify it by grooming, colouring, cutting and wigs. There are references in Egyptian papyruses to the importance of arranging the hair prior to seduction (Pomey-Rey, 1986). The Dowager Empress of China was so upset when her hairdresser pulled out some hairs that she was only mollified by the suggestion that he be put to death. Though perhaps extreme, many women do have an attenuated form of this relationship with their hairdresser.

Twentieth-century woman has continued this concern at modifying her appearance by cosmetic preparations and nowhere is this concern more strongly manifest than in connection with the hair, no doubt a measure of its psychological and sexual importance. The production of shampoos, dyes, waving and other hair applications has become big business in every 'Western' country. Science has benefited enormously from this industry since many of the advances in our knowledge of the structure of the hair follicle and hair have come from cosmetic science laboratories (Harry 1973; Schoen 1978; Zviak & Dawber 1986).

References

Harry, R.G. (1973) *Harry's Cosmeticology*, 6th edn., revised J.B. Wilkinson. Leonard Hill Books, London.

Pomey-Rey, D. (1986) Hair and psychology. In *The Science of Hair Care*, ed. C. Zviak. Marcel Dekker Inc., New York.

Schoen, L.A. (1978) *Skin and Hair Care*, 1st English edn. Penguin Books, Harmondsworth.

Zviak, C. & Dawber, R.P.R. (1986) Hair structure, function, and physicochemical properties. In *The Science of Hair Care*, ed. C. Zviak. Marcel Dekker Inc., New York.

Shampoos

(Corbett 1976; Robbins 1979; Zviak & Vanlerberghe 1986; Zviak & Bouillon 1986)
(References p. 468)

In modern terms a shampoo may be defined as a suitable detergent for washing hair that leaves the hair in good condition. Originally shampoos were used solely for cleansing hair but their range of function has extended in recent years to include conditioning, and the treatment of some hair and scalp diseases.

In principle, to wash hair a shampoo must remove grease since it is the latter which attracts dirt and other particulate matter. The polar group of a detergent achieves this by displacing oil from the hair surface. The evaluation of shampoo detergency is difficult and complicated. The consumer tends to equate detergency with foaming and this is scientifically incorrect; however, in Western society few shampoos sell unless they possess good foaming power. In the evaluation of detergents as shampoos no single criterion can be used though instrumental methods have been devised (Prall 1970). Efficacy can be based only on the subjective impression of the consumer. The factors taken into consideration include (i) ease of distribution of shampoo over the hair, (ii) lathering power, (iii) ease of rinsing and combing of wet hair, (iv) lustre of hair, (v) speed of drying, and (vi) ease of combing and setting of dried hair. Safety is of paramount importance.

Shampoo formulations vary enormously but the basic ingredients can be resolved into a few groups—water, detergent and some fatty material. Soap shampoos are made from vegetable or animal fats and remove dirt and grease as efficiently as detergents; however, a scum forms with hard water and the trend has therefore been increasingly towards detergents as the principal washing ingredient. Detergents are synthetic petroleum products and form no hard water scum.

Shampoos contain (i) principal surfactants for detergency and foaming power, (ii) secondary surfactants to improve and 'condition' hair, and (iii) additives which both complete the formulation and add 'special' effects; whatever the claims of some manufacturers most special additives end up down the sink! (Spoor 1973).

Principal surfactants
The main ones are anionic substances, e.g. alkyl sulphates made from alcohols obtained from fatty acids of coconut and palm kernel oil, the so-called lauryl sulphates. Other surfactants which may be the principal constituent are cationics—functionally good but in general too irritant, non-ionics—rather deficient in foaming power, and amphoterics—a low irritancy potential but rather expensive. Specific types include fatty acid soaps which are alkaline and cause 'rough' hair, alkyl benzene sulphonates which are powerful degreasers used in shampoos for greasy hair, alpha olefin sulphonates used in acid conditioning shampoos, alkyl ether sulphates which are widely used, some particularly in mild and baby shampoos, and non-ionic surfactants which are also used in baby shampoos (Zviak & Vanlerberghe 1986). All have properties that can be utilized in combination with principal anionic substances.

Secondary (auxiliary) surfactants

These are added to improve the foaming and 'conditioning' characteristics of shampoos. In practice, most are amphoteric or anionic. Examples include secondary alkyl sulphates (teepols), monoglyceride sulphates (like lauryl sulphate), turkey red oil, alkyl phosphates, methyl taurides, fatty acid alkanolamides—often combined with lauryl sulphate for richness of lather and 'after condition', acyl amino acids, sarcosines and peptides. Cationic surfactants have useful conditioning properties and are added to conditioning shampoos.

Additives

These include biocides, conditioners, pearlescents, sequestrants, colours, perfumes and preservatives.

Conditioners may be detergent in action, as already described under secondary surfactants, or non-detergent, for example natural polymers such as polyvinyl pyrrolidone (PVP), fatty materials (lanolin) or natural products such as herbs, peptides and egg fractions. Protein additives made from hydrolysed collagen have become popular. As applied to shampoo formulations, the term conditioner can only be defined qualitatively. It must act to add body to 'thin' hair and improve the appearance and manageability, particularly of damaged hair, e.g. add gloss, lustre and minimize tangling and 'flyaway'. They should perhaps be called 're-conditioners', but any changes they induce are only temporary.

Shampoo formulations

In general cosmetic shampoos can be dry (powder and liquid types), liquid, solid cream, aerosol or oily. Anti-dandruff, 'medicated' and scalp treatment shampoos contain antiseptics and active agents such as coal- and wood-tar fractions. Clear liquid shampoos are the most popular, including 'cleansing' types, sold for treating greasy hair, and 'cosmetic' types having good conditioning action and popular among women with dry or 'normal' hair. For details of other specific formulations the reader is recommended to read larger texts (Harry 1973; Zviak & Vanlerberghe 1986; Zviak & Bouillon 1986).

Shampoo safety

Shampoos evidently must be non-toxic, and at concentrations used by the consumer irritate neither skin nor eyes. New shampoo formulations are tested exhaustively prior to marketing, particularly to assess their propensity to cause eye irritation, scarring and corneal opacities. Skin irritation is not usually encountered from shampoos that have low eye irritancy potential. Eye safety is assessed by the technique known as the Draize test; standard solutions of shampoo are instilled into the conjunctival sac of an albino rabbit. In general the eye irritancy of detergents is greatest with cationics, followed by anionics, and least with non-anionics. There are exceptions to this, suggesting that shampoo irritancy may be due to properties other than detergency including surface activity, pH, wetting power, foaming power (Ross–Miles Test), and wetting and foaming power together. Most shampoos are, in fact, irritant but not dangerously so. Allergic contact dermatitis due to biocides does occur (Chapter 17).

Conditioners

Dry hair lacks gloss and lustre and is difficult to style. This results from natural weathering and is worsened by chemical and physical processes applied to the hair. Conditioners comprise fatty acids and alcohols; natural triglycerides, e.g. almond, avocado, corn and olive oil; waxes, e.g. beeswax, jojoba oil, mink oil; lanolin; phospholipids, e.g. egg yolk and soya bean; vitamins A, B and E; protein hydrolysates of silk, collagen, keratin (horn and hoof), gelatin and others; and cationic polymers. Conditioners are available in a variety of forms and are widely used. They provide lubrication and gloss and render the hair easier to comb and style. The most commonly used are creams and emulsions applied for a few minutes after washing and then rinsed off. Deep conditioners are left on for up to 30 minutes, often with damp heat. Fluids, gels and aerosol foams have become popular recently and aid styling. Hair oils are traditional conditioners. Men use brilliantines, greases or oils to leave the hair glossy and sleek (Zviak & Bouillon 1986).

References

Corbett, J.P. (1976) The chemistry of hair-care products. *Journal of the Society of Dyers and Colorists,* **92**, 285.
Harry, R.G. (1973) *Harry's Cosmeticology,* 6th edn., revised J.B. Wilkinson. Leonard Hill Books, London.
Prall, J.K. (1970) *Proceedings of the Sixth Congress of the International Federation of Societies of Cosmetic Chemists.* Unpublished.
Robbins, C.R. (1979) *Chemical and Physical Behaviour of Human Hair,* 1st edn. Van Nostrand Reinhold, New York.
Spoor, H.J. (1973) Shampoos. *Cutis,* **12**, 671.
Zviak, C. & Bouillon, C. (1986) Hair treatment and hair care products. In *The Science of Hair Care,* ed. C. Zviak. Marcel Dekker Inc., New York.
Zviak, C. & Vanlerberghe, G. (1986) Scalp and hair hygiene: shampoos. In *The Science of Hair Care,* ed. C. Zviak. Marcel Dekker Inc., New York.

Cosmetic hair colouring
(Corbett & Menkart 1973; Burnett & Corbett 1977; Zviak 1986a;
Zviak 1986b; Kalopissis 1986)
(References p. 472)

Since the days of the pharaohs, women in particular have used hair dyes both to hide grey hair and for reasons of fashion. The latter use has increased enormously during the past 50 years and now men are using them.

The penetration of dyes into hair depends on molecular size and the aqueous swelling of the hair at the time of application of the dye (Zviak 1966); basicity of the dye is also important. The most successful dyes are relatively small molecules.

Excluding bleaches, hair colouring materials can be divided into three groups: vegetable, metallic and synthetic organic dyes. In advanced countries vegetable and metallic hair colourants are almost obsolete because of the more 'natural' colours obtained with synthetic organic chemicals.

Vegetable dyes

Henna may be used to give reddish-auburn shades. It is obtained from shrubs found in North Africa and the Middle-East—*Lawsonia alba, L. spinosa* and *L. inermis*. The dye is produced from dried leaves which are removed before the plant flowers. The active principle is an acidic naphthoquinone (lawsone); it is still to be found in some hair rinses. Traditionally it is applied as a paste 'pack' which is left *in situ* for from 5 to 60 minutes. The effects last for up to 10 weeks. This process is non-toxic but messy, and finger nails may become stained. Henna rengs are mixtures of henna and powdered indigo leaves that produce blue-black shades. A wide range of colours can be obtained from henna combined with metallic salts or pyrogallol—compound henna (Natow 1986b). Ground flower heads of Roman or German chamomile yield a yellow dye, 1,3,4-trihydroxyflavone (apigenin). It stains only the cuticle and can be used to lighten or brighten hair. Other vegetable dyes include extracts from logwood and walnut shell and these can be used by patients who are paraphenylenediamine sensitive. These products are obtainable at herbalists and beauty shops.

Metallic dyes

Traditionally hair dyes for men have been of this type since the colour changes occur less rapidly and are not as immediately obvious as with the oxidative dyes. Inorganic salts are used which are altered by the hair and coat the surface as either oxides from reduction of the metal salts by keratin, or sulphides from the action of the sulphur in keratin on the metal. They all give a rather dull (metallic) appearance and may cause brittle or damaged hair if used too often.

Lead acetate, with precipitated sulphur or sodium thiosulphate, gives brown to black shades; grey hair may be changed through yellow to brown or black. Silver nitrate used alone produces a greenish-black colour; pyrogallol is used as developer. Colours from ash blond to black are possible by mixing silver nitrate variously with copper, cobalt or nickel; brownish-black skin staining is the great disadvantage. Bismuth salts give shades of brown.

Newer metallic dyes, containing a metal plus an organic ligand, are used on textile fibres and in some hair dye patents.

Metallic dyes cannot be removed without hair damage and should be left to grow out.

Synthetic organic dyes

This group have now been in use for more than 40 years. They are the most important type because of the comprehensive range of 'natural' colours that can be obtained. Most penetrate the hair cuticle, i.e. they are potentially permanent, but in recent years less-permanent types have been introduced.

Synthetic organic colourants are of three types:

1 *Temporary.* These wash out with one shampoo and last no longer than 1 week. Many temporary rinses belong to this group, including fashionable unnatural colours used by avant-garde sects and groups! They are available in aerosol sprays by incorporation into transparent polymeric plastics such as PVP; the disadvantages of such vehicles is their tendency to flake off onto clothing.

2 *Semi-permanent.* In Great Britain these have the widest appeal. They are used frequently at home and also in salons to brighten or subdue a natural colour, modify a permanent or bleached colour, or modify white or grey. They are of sufficiently small molecular size to penetrate into the cortex. They are intrinsically coloured, i.e. no developing is required, cf. the oxidative permanent group. They are relatively easy to wash out with shampoos containing ammonia; other shampoos must be used 6–10 times to remove them. The nitro group, for example the nitrophenylenediamine and nitroaminophenols, when mixed, give colours from red or yellow to blond to chestnut; satisfactory brown colours can be obtained by including anthroquinones which are intrinsically blue. Some semi-permanent dyes have an affinity for thioglycollate—waved hair. Many are now used in colour shampoos.

3 *Permanent* (developed or oxidation dyes). These do not rely on the natural colour of a single chemical dye stuff, cf. semi-permanents, but require an oxidative developer—H_2O_2—to produce the final colour:

Paraphenylenediamine (PPD)

and/or

Paratoluenediamine (PTD)

$\downarrow + H_2O_2$

Applied to hair

$\downarrow$

Quinone diimine (small molecule)

$\downarrow$

Penetrates hair—to cortex

$\downarrow$

Large molecules   (by diamine 'self' condensation and
produced   modifiers e.g. pyrogallol)

Other substances may be included in specific formulations to give greater intensity to the dye, for example resorcinol and polyhidric phenols. For the range of formulations see Zviak 1966 and Zviak 1986b.

Oxidative dyes are potentially hazardous. The need for hydrogen peroxide enables lighter shades to be obtained and is chiefly responsible for the structural damage to hair that may occur if care is not exercised. Additives such as pyrogallol and resorcinol are potential irritants. The greatest problem is the potential of PPD (less so with PTD) to cause allergic dermatitis. Up to 10% of users may develop type IV allergy (Blohm & Rajka 1970; Lubowe 1973). All dyes in this group are therefore sold with instructions to carry out preliminary patch testing 24–48 hours before the proposed dye is used, i.e. the dye system is applied to skin either behind one ear or on the forearm—any redness, swelling or blistering implies allergy and the dying should not therefore proceed. A negative patch test does not mean that subsequent allergy cannot develop, it simply shows the subject not to be allergic at the time the test was carried out. If allergy is shown, it is not sufficient merely to stop all future use of oxidative dyes—unfortunately cross sensitization occurs with other aromatic benzenes, e.g. sulphonamides and some local anaesthetics, which must also be avoided for life. Modern formulations seem to cause less problems with allergy (Calnan 1986). Hair dyes of this group have been incriminated as possible carcinogens (Burnett 1980). Chromosome breaks have occurred under experimental conditions (Kirkland *et al.* 1978) and an increased incidence of tumours has been found in regular users (Burnett & Menkart 1978). It has also been intimated that aplastic anaemia could be produced by hair dyes (Burnett *et al.* 1978). None of these reports is sufficiently conclusive to warrant the withdrawal of such dyes. The toxicology has recently been reviewed in detail (Kalopissis 1986).

Permanent dyes last for several months; they must not be applied more frequently than every 3–4 weeks since hair damage will occur. Permanent waving or straightening too soon after dyeing may also induce hair damage. Permanent dyes must therefore be allowed to grow out. However, if a light shade has been produced and the subject wishes for a darker shade, then temporary rinses may safely be used since these only coat the hair surface and have no propensity to cause structural damage.

For less commonly used permanent dye formulations the reader is referred to larger texts (Harry 1973; Zviak 1986b).

Bleaches (Wolfram *et al.* 1970; Wall 1972; Zviak 1986b).
Women have bleached their hair since Roman times. Hydrogen peroxide was first used to bleach hair in the 1860s. Bleaching is used both to lighten hair and to prepare it to take up hair dyes. Bleaching is an oxidative alkaline treatment that oxidizes and bleaches melanin. The hair lightens to reddish or yellow tones depending on the underlying hair colour, and ultimately to platinum. It is very damaging to the hair rendering it dry, porous and more prone to tangle. Overuse may cause disruption and fracture of the hair (Selzle & Wolff 1976). Thus it is advisable to perform permanent waving before bleaching. Home bleaching is usually performed with 6% H_2O_2 (20 volumes) with ammonia to speed the reaction which otherwise takes 12 hours. Salons use more powerful bleaching creams, powders, and pastes which are much faster. They are often applied to individual strands of hair, others being left untreated to give highlights, which lessens the problem of the dark new roots. Bleaching is terminated by shampooing or an acid rinse. The human eye perceives a more aesthetically acceptable blonde ('platinum' blonde) when the bleached hair is treated with a blue or lilac colourant. The pigment destruction in bleached hair is chiefly localized in the surface portion of the cortex (Orfanos & Mahrle 1971).

References

Blohm, S.G. & Rajka, G. (1970) The allergenicity of paraphenylene diamine. *Acta Dermato-Venereologica*, **50**, 49.

Burnett, C.M. & Menkart, T. (1978) Hair dyes and breast cancer. *New England Journal of Medicine*, 299, 1253.

Burnett C.M. & Corbett J.F. (1977) Chemistry and toxicology of hair dyes. In *Cutaneous Toxicity. Proceedings of the Third Conference on Cutaneous Toxicity, Washington, 1976*, eds. V.A. Drill and P. Lazar. New York, Academic Press.

Burnett, C.M., Corbett, J.F. & Lanman, B.M. (1978) Hair dyes and aplastic anaemia. *Drug and Chemical Toxicology*, **1**, 45.

Burnett, C.M. (1980) Evaluation of toxicity and carcinogenicity of hair dyes. *Journal of Toxicology and Environmental Health*, **6**, 247.

Calnan, C. (1986) Adverse reactions to hair products. In *The Science of Hair Care*, ed. C. Zviak. Marcel Dekker Inc., New York.

Corbett, J.F. & Menkart, T. (1973) Hair colouring. *Cutis*, **12**, 190.

Kalopissis, G. (1986) Toxicology and hair dyes. In *The Science of Hair Care*, ed. C. Zviak. Marcel Dekker Inc., New York.

Kirkland, D.J., Lawler, S.D. & Venitt, S. (1978) Chromosome damage and hair dyes. *Lancet*, **ii**, 124.

Lubow, I. (1973) Allergic dermatitis and cosmetics, *Cutis*, **11**, 431.

Natow, A.J. (1986a) Henna. *Cutis*, **38**, 21.

Natow, A.J. (1986b) Hair bleach. *Cutis*, **37**, 28.

Orfanos, C.E. & Mahrle, G. (1971) Human hair and its changes with cosmetic treatments *in vivo*. *Parfume Kosmet*, **52**, 203.

Selzle, D. & Wolff, H.H. (1976) Exogener Haarschaden durch Bleichen und Kaltwelle. *Hautarzt*, **27**, 453.

Wall, C. (1972) In *Cosmetics Science and Technology*, eds. B. Balsam & E. Sagarin. Wiley Interscience, New York.

Wolfram, L.J., Hall, K. & Hui, I. (1970) The mechanism of hair bleaching. *Journal of the Society of Cosmetic Chemists*, **21**, 875.

Zviak, C. (1966) *Problèmes Capillaires*, eds. E. Sidi & C. Zviak. Gauthier Villars, Paris.

Zviak, C. (1986a) Hair coloring: nonoxidation coloring. In *The Science of Hair Care*, ed. C. Zviak. Marcel Dekker Inc., New York.

Zviak, C. (1986b) Oxidation coloring. In *The Science of Hair Care*, ed. C. Zviak. Marcel Dekker Inc., New York.

Zviak, C. (1986c) Hair bleaching . In *The Science of Hair Care*, ed. C. Zviak. Marcel Dekker Inc., New York.

Permanent waving (Corbett 1976; Zviak 1986; Wickett 1987)
(References p. 475)

Permanent waving has been defined as the process of changing the shape of the hair so that the new shape persists through several shampoos. Ancient Egyptian women used wet mud for this purpose and even as recently as 1910 the only methods available were heat, using a hot curling iron, or boiling water. During the last 70 years increasing knowledge of keratin chemistry has enabled semi-permanent chemical methods to be developed. Whatever the process used, three stages are involved in hair waving: (i) physical or chemical softening of the hair, (ii) reshaping, and (iii) hardening of fibres to retain the reshaped position.

Softening
Water can extend the hydrogen bonds between adjacent polypeptides in the keratin

molecule, allowing temporary reshaping to be carried out—exposure to high humidity or rewetting immediately reverses the process. To obtain a more durable effect from water, steam may be used which in a limited way disrupts disulphide bonds. Heat and steam alone are rarely acceptable to modern women because their effects are temporary and the treatment is uncomfortable. Heat can be more effectively utilized in conjunction with ammonium hydroxide and potassium bisulphite or triethanolamine as agents to reduce −S=S− bonds; great skill is involved in this process since failure to judge the time of application of chemicals and heat may cause severe damage. Chemical heat pads are still rarely used, for example utilizing heat produced from exothermic reaction, e.g. quicklime.

Since 1945, cold wave processes utilizing substituted thiosulphates, i.e. thioglycollates, have largely superseded hot waving. Thioglycollates are potent reducers of disulphide bonds in the keratin molecule:

$$-S=S- \longrightarrow 2-SH$$

A typical cold waving lotion contains thioglycollic acid plus ammonia or monoethanolamine.

Acid permanent waves have recently become popular for salon use. They contain glyceryl monothioglycollate, and produce a softer curl and can be used on damaged and bleached hair. Their disadvantage is the high frequency of sensitization in the hairdressers using the product and occasionally sensitization of the client (Morrison & Storrs 1988).

Reshaping
The type of rollers or curlers used to reshape the softened hair depends on the training of the hairdresser and the fashion desired. The degree of curl or tightness of the permanent wave depends both on the diameter of the roller and the size of the strand wound round the roller. Increasing the time of the exposure to the perming solution up to 20 minutes increases the curl, but longer times do not give a further increase. The strength of the solution used depends on the hair type, texture and previous bleaching. Home permanent waves are weaker and cannot achieve the same degree of curl. 'Tepid' shampooing involves using a weaker thioglycollate solution plus warm air. Neutralization is carried out initially with the curlers in place and again they have been carefully removed. The reshaping stage is thus a great test of hairdressing skill and experience.

Hardening (neutralizing or setting)
In general this process involves a reversal of the softening (reduction) stages:

$$2\ SH \xrightarrow{\text{oxidation}} -S=S-$$

It is important to note that complete reversal to pre-softened 'strength' cannot occur since many free −SH groups may not be in a position for oxidation to be effective.

$$2-SH \longrightarrow -S-C-S-$$

or

$$2SH \longrightarrow -S-Ba-S-$$

Atmospheric oxidation may effectively neutralize the waving process. This method is slow and rollers must be left in position for several hours overnight. Chemical oxidation is now the rule. Hairdressers generally use hydrogen peroxide whilst most solutions for home use contain sodium perborate or percarbonate (UK) or sodium or potassium bromate (USA). This is why hair is lighter after permanent waving. Some neutralizers contain shellac which may react with alcohol groups to cause hair discoloration.

Practical procedures
Hot waving is almost never used. The procedure is:
1 shampooing,
2 the hair is divided and rollers or curlers are applied under slight tension,
3 waving solution is applied,
4 heating. This varies according to the solution used or the type of wave required. Electric rollers or exothermic reactive chemicals may be used. The latter allow free head movement during the waving. The skill of this procedure lies in good hair sectioning, judging the right amount of solution, correct winding tension and appropriate steaming time.

Cold waving also involves initial shampooing, hair division into locks, moistening with waving lotion and application of croquignole curlers. Further solution may then be applied. The softening time is from 10 to 20 minutes. Occasionally mild heat is used either using exothermic chemicals or the natural heat from the head by enclosing the scalp in a plastic bag. These may add to the comfort of the process. Rinsing then takes place, followed by neutralization with the oxidizing solution for up to 10 minutes. After removing the curlers further 'hardening' solution is usually applied. 'Loose' curl waves last for no more than a few weeks but 'tight' curl styles may persist for 4–12 months.

Evaluation of permanent waving

Fibre extension studies. These are used to assess changes in mechanical properties of hair due to waving. Hair fibres show a hysteresis curve of extension and relaxation after the application of a load (stress). It has been shown that after application of thioglycollates the total work of extending to 30% was lowered to 65% of its original value after reduction; oxidation reversed this.

Scanning electron microscopy. This is used to study anatomical changes due to permanent waving. Along with bleaching, waving is potentially very damaging (Swift & Brown 1972) which is hardly surprising in view of the molecular disruption intrinsic to the procedure.

Human trials. These are evidently important to test efficacy and potential toxicity. Factors to be assessed include (i) ambient temperature giving best results and (ii) optimum duration of the mechanical process, for example curlers, the perming and hardening solutions.

Toxicity. This depends on the process used. In view of the pH at which they are used waving solutions must be kept away from the eyes and prolonged skin contact is to be avoided. Because of the unavoidable smell of thiols, some manufacturers put perfumes into the solution and these may cause dermatitis. Other toxicity is the result of poor technique, for example over-use of heat or overlong contact with softening agents. In general, the scalp resists irritants better than most sites on the body; any reactions from skin contact are therefore more liable to occur on the face or neck or elsewhere.

References

Corbett, J.F. (1976) The chemistry of hair-care products. *Journal of the Society of Dyers and Colorists,* **92**, 285.

Morrison, L.H. and Storrs, F.J. (1988) Persistence of an allergen in hair after glyceryl monothiogly-colate-containing permanent wave solutions. *Journal of the American Academy of Dermatology,* **19**, 52.

Swift, J.A. & Brown, A.C. (1972) The critical determination of fine changes in the surface architecture of human hair due to cosmetic treatment. *Journal of the Society of Cosmetic Chemists,* **23**, 695.

Wickett, R.R. (1987) Permanent waving and straightening of hair. *Cutis,* **39**, 496.

Zviak, C. (1986) Permanent waving and hair straightening. In *The Science of Hair Care,* ed. C. Zviak. Marcel Dekker Inc., New York.

Hair straighteners (Gershen *et al.* 1972, Zviak 1986; Wickett 1987)
(References p. 476)

In principle the methods used to straighten hair are similar to those used in permanent waving. The practice is almost exclusively used to straighten Negroid hair.

Pomades. These are mostly used by men with relatively short hair. They are greasy and act by 'plastering' hair into position.

Hot comb methods. Shampooing is carried out and the hair is towelled dry; oil is then applied, e.g. petroleum jelly or liquid paraffin, which act as heat-transferring agents. Heat pressing with hot combing is then used (148–260°F) causing breakage and reforming of —S=S— bonds allowing the hair to be moulded straight. Structural damage (and breakage) of hair is common with this process and scarring alopecia may occur as a result of hot waxes entering the follicles. Sweating and rain reverse this procedure.

Cold methods. The chemical methods employed utilize alkaline reducing agents (caustics), thioglycollates, ammonium carbonate or sodium bisulphite. Caustic soda preparations are usually creams and require the application of protective scalp oil or wax. They are combed through the hair and left for 15–20 minutes, the hair is combed and straightened again, then rinsed and neutralized. These preparations are limited to salon use because of their potential to cause irritant dermatitis and damage the hair. Thioglycollate creams are the commonest agents used; the cream is applied liberally to the hair, which is then combed until it is straight. The cream is then washed off and a neutralizer (oxidizing agent) applied (Corbett 1976). Other straighteners ('relaxers') do not contain thioglycollates, e.g. sodium bisulphite and ammonium carbonate, acidic ethylene glycol or 1,3-propylene glycol. Bisulphite straighteners are suitable for home use in combination with alkaline stabilizers.

References

Corbett, J.F. (1976) The chemistry of hair-care products. *Journal of the Society of Dyers and Colorists*, **92**, 285.
Gershen, J., Goldberg, B. & Reiger, A. (1972) Hair straighteners. In *Cosmetics, Science and Technology*, 2nd edn., eds. B. Balsam & E. Sagarin. Wiley Interscience, New York.
Wickett, R.R. (1987) Permanent waving and straightening of hair. *Cutis*, **39**, 496.
Zviak, C. (1986) Permanent waving and hair straightening. In *The Science of Hair Care*, ed. C. Zviak. Marcel Dekker Inc., New York.

Hair setting lotions and sprays (Zviak 1986)

Setting lotions have changed considerably in recent years. The traditional semi-liquid gels based on water-soluble gums, for example tragacanth, karaya and acasia, have been replaced by various synthetic polymers in a bewildering array of forms—aerosol foams and sprays, liquids and gels. Most are bases on PVP in a gelled aqueous solution and give an attractive glossy, non-greasy appearance (Friefeld *et al.* 1962). Some preparations incorporate other ingredients to condition or to add antistatic action, lustre or sheen.

Setting lotion and spray formulations are considered safe, after early reports of foreign body granulomatous inflammation (Bergmann *et al.* 1958; Edelston 1959) had been questioned and not supported by further cases. Hair sprays were incriminated as a possible cause of peripilar keratin casts (Scott 1959) but this was not confirmed by later work (Dawber 1979). There is now grave concern about the damage to the ozone layer from the chlorofluorocarbon propellants.

References

Bergmann, M., Flance, I.J. & Blumenthal, A.T. (1958) Thesaurosis following inhalation of hair spray; a clinical and experimental study. *New England Journal of Medicine*, **258**, 471.
Dawber, R.P.R. (1979) Hair casts. *British Journal of Dermatology*, **100**, 417.
Edelston, B.G. (1959) Thesaurosis following inhalation of hair spray (Letter). *Lancet*, **ii**, 465.
Friefeld, M., Lyons, J. & Martinelli, A.T. (1962) Polyvinylpyrrolidone in cosmetics. *American Perfumery*, **77**, 25.
Scott, M.J. (1959) Peripilar keratin casts. *Archives of Dermatology*, **79**, 654.
Zviak, C. (1986) Hair setting. In *The Science of Hair Care*, ed. C. Zviak. Marcel Dekker Inc., New York.

Hair strengtheners

Many cosmetic preparations, by their action on the keratin molecule, irreversibly weaken the hair. The cosmetic scientist has produced chemicals that attempt to combat this problem. The formulations contain methylolated compounds of varying strength depending on the type of hair under treatment and the solubility of the compound. Early preparations were not satisfactory and released more than the legally permitted level of formaldehyde whilst in contact with the hair. Later preparations containing alkylated methylol compounds have greater stability and release very little formaldehyde.

Reference

Zviak, C. & Bouillon, C. (1986) Hair treatment and hair care products. In *The Science of Hair Care*, ed. C. Zviak. Marcel Dekker Inc., New York.

Hair removers
(References p. 479)

The terms 'epilation' and 'depilation' have varied in their exact definition over the years. It is more convenient to define the exact process used, or the principle behind it, under the general term 'hair removers'. Superfluous hair may be masked by bleaching or removed by a variety of methods such as plucking, waxing, shaving, chemical processes and electrolysis—only the latter is permanent. No method is entirely satisfactory and the one adopted will depend on personal preference and the character, area and amount of hair growth.

Bleaching is widely used for hair, particularly on the upper lip and the arms. It is painless, and when repeated often inflicts sufficient damage to cause hair breakage. However, bleached hair can look very obvious against dark skin. A simple method may be used such as 6% hydrogen peroxide (20 vol. peroxide) with 20 drops ammonia (household ammonia or common ammonia water) per 25 ml of peroxide. The bleach is added immediately on mixing and left for approximately 30 minutes. Some individuals develop an irritant reaction to bleach; it is therefore advisable to carry out a preliminary test—if irritation occurs within 30–60 minutes the peroxide strength and the duration of application should be reduced.

Shaving is unacceptable to some women as being too 'masculine': however, the majority are happy to shave axillary and leg hair. Modern bathing costumes are very brief and require the wearer to shave the inner thighs and even part of the pubic region. In these sites it is common to experience folliculitis during regrowth, sometimes also due to infection with *Staphylococcus aureus*. There is no scientific basis for the belief that shaving stiffens hair or increases its pigmentation.

Waxing is one of the oldest methods known to man. Typically the wax is preheated, applied to the area to be treated, allowed to cool, then stripped off taking the embedded hair with it. Some 'cold' waxes are available that act in the same way. Glucose and zinc oxide waxing has the advantage of lasting up to several weeks before a repeat is required. Only relatively long hair can be treated in this way. Some women find it painful and irritating. It is more often used by beauticians than in the home (Rentoul & Aitken 1980).

Plucking is really satisfactory only for individual or small groups or scattered coarse hairs. It is useful for sparse nipple or abdominal hairs. It is usually done with tweezers. As with waxing, it requires to be repeated only every few weeks.

Chemical hair removers are now widely used for superfluous hair removal from most sites including the face. Their use on the face is limited by their irritancy potential. Sulphides and stannites, widely used in the past, have now been largely superseded by substituted mercaptans. Sulphides were unsatisfactory both because of skin irritancy and because of their odour—hydrogen sulphide—generated particularly when the preparation was washed off; strontium sulphide preparations are still available. Stannites, popularized some 30–40 years ago, had good hair-removing properties but were rather unstable. Substituted mercaptans form the basis of virtually all modern chemical depilatory preparations. They are slower in action than the sulphides but are safe enough for facial use if necessary. Thioglycollates are used in a concentration of 2–4% and typically act wthin 5–15 minutes (Turley & Windus 1937). Of the thioglycollates, the calcium salt is most favoured as it is the least irritant—the pH is maintained by an excess of calcium hydroxide which also acts to prevent the excess alkalinity known to irritate skin. Attempts to formulate products which accelerate the rather slow thioglycollate action have not been particularly successful. Modern preparations are available in foam, cream, liquid and aerosol forms, the one chosen depending on personal preference. Since thioglycollates attack keratin, not specifically hair, they may have adverse effects on the epidermis if manufacturers' recommendations are not adhered to; it is generally suggested that a small test site should first be treated in order to prevent more extensive irritant reactions in susceptible individuals. The ideal hair-removing chemical has still to be found—new substances are tested constantly for hair removal properties using *in vitro* methods such as the hair swelling test.

Electrolysis (Savill & Warren 1962; Richards & McKenzie 1986)
All the above methods are temporary, the only practical permanent procedure being electrolysis. This involves passing a fine wire needle into the hair follicle and destroying the bulb with an electric current passed along it—the hair is loosened and plucked from each treated follicle. Disposable needles should be used to prevent transmission of infection. Either a galvanic or modified high frequency electric current is used. Galvanic electrolysis is slower but destroys more follicles in one treatment. High-frequency current (electrocoagulation) is quicker but more regrowth is seen with this method. Relatively cheap, battery-operated machines have recently been developed for home use. These have all the disadvantages and potential hazards of those used by electrolysists with the added problem of an amateur operator.

The limitations of electrolysis in skilled hands are those of cost and time; even the best operators can only deal with 25–100 hairs per sitting and hair regrows in up to 40% of the follicles treated. Shaving, a few days prior to electrolysis, increases the number of hairs in anagen and these are more easily destroyed (Richards & McKenzie 1986). In general, electrolysis is mostly used for localized coarse facial hair and alternative methods employed for excess hair on other body sites. Apart from regrowth of hair the problems that can occur with this mode of hair removal include discomfort during treatment, perifollicular inflammation and scarring, punctate hyperpigmentation and rarely, bacterial infection.

A controlled investigation was carried out comparing the results of electrolysis with those of diathermy depilation. Permanent destruction of the hairs could be achieved by either method and the time required for the total destruction of all hair roots in a given area was the same, but the diameter of hairs regrowing after diathermy was greater than that of hairs regrowing after electrolysis (Peereboom-Wynia 1975). The results of depilation depend on the skill and dexterity of the operator (Blackwell 1973). In countries such as Britain, in which a Diploma in Medical Electrolysis exists, patients should wherever possible be referred to technicians who have obtained this certification of their proficiency. In the United States the American Electrolysis Association regulates professional standards.

References

Blackwell, G. (1973) Permanence in electrolysis epilation. *Cutis*, **11**, 753.
Peereboom-Wynia, J.D.R. (1975) The effect of electrical epilation on the beard hair of women with idiopathic hirsutism. *Archives of Dermatological Research*, **254**, 15.
Rentoul, J.R. & Aitken, A.A. (1980) The cosmetic treatment of hirsutism. *Practitioner*, **24**, 1171.
Richards, R.N. and McKenzie, M.A. (1986) Electroepilation (electrolysis) on hirsutism. *Journal of the American Academy of Dermatology*, **15**, 693.
Savill, A. & Warren, C. (1962) *The Hair and Scalp*, 5th edn, p. 304. Arnold. London.
Turley, H.G. & Windus, W. (1937) In *Stiasny Festschrift*, 1st edn. Edward Roether, Darmstadt.

Complications of hair cosmetics

Matting of scalp hair is most commonly a sudden, usually irreversible, tangling of scalp hair due to shampooing (Wilson *et al.* 1990).

Excessive bleaching, permanent waving and straightening procedures may induce excessive weathering and fragility of hair.

Reference

Wilson, C.L., Ferguson, D.J.P. & Dawber, R.P.R. (1990) Matting of scalp hair during shampooing—a new look. *Clinical and Experimental Dermatology*, **15**, 139.

Chapter 16
Hair and Scalp in Systemic Diseases

Introduction

Throughout this book emphasis has been placed on the frequency with which abnormalities of hair growth are caused by, are related to, or are associated with systemic processes. The most important examples are the disturbances in the cyclical activity of hair follicles described in Chapter 5 and the disorders of hair patterns described in Chapter 4. The present chapter contains a number of conditions in which the hair or scalp may be affected, and which are not readily classified in other chapters.

Sarcoidosis

Sarcoidosis rarely involves the scalp. Most cases have occurred in Negroid women (Goltiz *et al.* 1968; Rudolph *et al.* 1975; Smith *et al.* 1986), but elderly Europeans, male and female, have also been affected (Anderson 1977; Fazio *et al.* 1979).

The lesions may be initially nodular or papular, coalescing to form plaques, which flatten to leave an area of cicatricial alopecia, which is not pathognomonic. The typical cutaneous or systemic lesions of sarcoidosis must be sought elsewhere.

The diagnosis is made on the histological appearances and by a positive Kveim test.

References

Anderson, K.E. (1977) Systemic sarcoidosis with necrobiosis lipoidica-like scalp lesions. *Acta Dermato-Venereologica*, **57**, 367.

Fazio, M., Bassetti, F., Santucci, B., Argentieri, R. & Gentili, G. (1979) Sarcoidosi anulare cicatriziale e necrobiosi lipoidica atipica del cuoio capelluto. *Bollettino dell'Istituto Dermatologico San Gallicano*, **10**, 85.

Golitz, L.E., Shapiro, L., Hurwitz, E. & Stritzler, R. (1968) Cicatricial alopecia of sarcoidosis. *Archives of Dermatology*, **107**, 758.

Rudolph, R.I., Holzwanger, J.M. & Heaton, C.L. (1975) Diffuse cicatricial alopecia of the scalp caused by sarcoidosis. *Cutis*, **15**, 524.

Smith, S.R., Kendall, M.J. & Kondratowicz, G.M. (1986) Sarcoidosis—a cause of steroid responsive total alopecia. *Postgraduate Medical Journal*, **62**, 205.

Histiocytic reticuloendotheliosis

This term groups together the conditions known as Letterer–Siwe disease, eosinophilic granuloma of bone, Hand–Schüller–Christian disease, and xanthoma disseminatum. Each condition is usually encountered as a distinctive clinico-pathological entity, but intermediate cases also occur.

Letterer–Siwe disease

Skin lesions are a characteristic and almost constant feature of this rare disease of infancy and very early childhood. Discrete yellow-brown scaly papules appear in crops on the scalp, neck and face, trunk and buttocks. They may become haemorrhagic, particularly on the trunk. Larger nodules are occasionally seen, mainly in the flexures, and both scalp and flexures may develop crusting and secondary infection (Nyholm *et al.* 1967).

Apparent seborrhoeic dermatitis in an obviously ill child, especially if the spleen is enlarged, is an indication for urgent biopsy, as early diagnosis is important. In some cases the disease is apparently confined to the skin (Esterly & Sevick 1969) but the skin lesions may precede other evidence of the disease by weeks or months (Jones *et al.* 1967). Scalp involvement of 'seborrhoeic' type is much rarer in other forms of histiocytic reticuloendotheliosis, but has been recorded in children (de Graciansky *et al.* 1953) and in adults (Bender & Holtzman 1958).

References

Bender, B. & Holtzman, I.N. (1958) Histiocytosis X (granulomatous reticuloendotheliosis). *Archives of Dermatology*, **78**, 692.

Esterly, N.B. & Sevick, H.M. (1969) Cutaneous Letterer–Siwe disease. *American Journal of Diseases of Children*, **117**, 236.

de Graciansky, P., Leclerq, R. & Janet (1953) A propos d'un cas de reticulose histiomonocytaire subaiguë chez un nourrisson. *Semaine des Hôpitaux*, **29**, 1643.

Jones, B., Welton, W.A. & Gilbert, E.F. (1967) Congenital Letterer–Siwe disease, *Cutis*, **3**, 750.

Nyholm, K., Reed, G. & Sjalin, K.E. (1967) Letterer–Siwe disease. *Acta pathologica et microbiologica Scandinavica*, **70**, 481.

Amyloidosis
(References p. 482)

In primary systemic amyloidosis the most characteristic skin lesions are yellowish, waxy papules, which may be haemorrhagic and occur most commonly on the face, particularly affecting the eyelids, and the scalp. Papules also occur on the neck and in the anogenital region. There may also be nodules and plaques but these are not commonly found in the scalp.

Alopecia may be conspicuous (Brownstein & Helwig 1970). There may be diffuse or patchy loss of scalp hair, and body hair may be completely or partially lost (Wheeler & Barrows 1981). There is destruction of the pilosebaceous units. The diagnosis must be confirmed histologically.

The tumefactive form of cutaneous amyloidosis is very rare. Waxy nodules have been reported in the scalp (Ratz & Bailin 1981). Vascular amyloid with amyloid deposits along the course of scalp blood vessels was reported by Henry *et al.* (1986).

References

Brownstein, M.H. & Helwig, E.B. (1970) The cutaneous amyloidoses. II. Systemic form. *Archives of Dermatology*, **102**, 20.
Henry, R.B., Fisher, G.B. Jr. & Cooper, P.H. (1986) Vascular amyloid in a patient with multiple myeloma. *Journal of the American Academy of Dermatology*, **15**, 379.
Ratz, J.L. & Bailin, P.L. (1981) Cutaneous amyloidosis. *Journal of the American Academy of Dermatology*, **4**, 21.
Wheeler, G.E. & Barrows, G.H (1981) Alopecia universalis. A manifestation of occult amyloidosis and multiple myeloma. *Archives of Dermatology*, **117**, 815.

Lupus erythematosus

Scalp changes are not uncommon in both the systemic and the chronic discoid forms of lupus erythematosus. Alopecia is present in at least 50% of cases of acute systemic lupus erythematosus (Armas-Cruz *et al.* 1958) and is more common before the age of 50 years (Ward & Polisson 1989). There is diffuse shedding of hair and there may be some erythema of the scalp. The hair is dry, fragile and broken, and short hairs are often seen, particularly at the frontal margin—so-called 'lupus hair' (Alarcón-Segovia & Cetina 1974). Cicatricial alopecia is seen much less frequently in systemic lupus erythematosus, usually in cases in which the systemic phase has been preceded by chronic discoid lupus erythematosus. Alopecia closely simulating alopecia areata, but with the histological features of lupus erythematosus, has been reported.

Discoid lupus erythematosus (DLE) of the scalp affects women more than men. The disease usually begins on the face, but scalp lesions ultimately develop in 20% of men and 50% of women. When DLE involves the scalp it is often accompanied by pruritus. Typical DLE presents as an area of erythema and scaling which extends irregularly, leaving scarring. At this stage a tentative clinical diagnosis is possible; follicular plugging and basal liquefaction on histological examination and a positive lupus band test are confirmatory. Later, only the scarring remains and a confident diagnosis may not be possible.

Squamous carcinoma has been reported in chronic cicatricial lupus erythematosus of the scalp (Vidal-Lliteras & Cabré 1971; Sulica & Kao 1988).

References

Alarcón-Segovia, D. & Cetina, J.A. (1974) Lupus hair. *American Journal of Medical Science*, **267**, 241.

Armas-Cruz, R., Harmaker, J., Ducaun, G., Jebil, J. & Gonzales, F. (1958) Clinical diagnosis of systemic lupus erythematosus. *American Journal of Medicine*, **25**, 409.

Sulica, V.I. & Kao, G.F. (1988) Squamous cell carcinoma of the scalp arising in lesions of discoid lupus erythematosus. *American Journal of Dermatophathology*, **10**, 137.

Vidal-Lliteras, J. & Cabré, J. (1971) Carcinoma espinocelular sobre alopecia cicatricial eritematodica. *Acta Dermosifilograficas*, **62**, 63.

Ward, M.M. & Polisson, R.P. (1989) A meta-analysis of the clinical manifestations of older-onset systemic lupus erythematosus. *Arthritis and Rheumatology*, **32**, 1226.

Dermatomyositis

Dermatomyositis is a rare disorder which affects the skin and the muscles. Its cause is unknown but immunological mechanisms are probably involved. Over 50% of patients who present when over the age of 40 have malignant disease, which may be covert at the time of presentation.

Diffuse alopecia is present in 15–20% of cases (O'Leary & Waisman 1940; Roberts & Brunsting 1954). Complete or almost complete regrowth is possible. Also during the acute stage hypertrichosis may be conspicuous, especially on the face and limbs (Reich & Reinhardt 1948) (see Chapter 8).

In the chronic stage poikilodermatous changes with marked atrophy may replace the acute inflammatory lesions, and when such lesions involve the scalp or other hairy regions cicatricial alopecia results. In some unusual cases reported in Hong Kong (Wong 1969) cicatricial alopecia was associated with horny follicular papules.

References

O'Leary, P.R. & Waisman, M. (1940) Dermatomyositis. *Archives of Dermatology and Syphilology*, **41**, 1001.

Reich, M.E. & Reinhardt, J.B. (1948) Dermatomyositis associated with hypertrichosis. *Archives of Dermatology and Syphilology*, **57**, 725.

Roberts, H.M. & Brunsting, L.A. (1954) Dermatomyositis in childhood. *Postgraduate Medicine*, **16**, 393.

Wong, K.O. (1969) Dermatomyositis: a clinical investigation of twenty-three cases in Hong Kong. *British Journal of Dermatology*, **81**, 544.

Giant-cell arteritis (temporal arteritis, Horton's disease)
(References p. 484)

This granulomatous arteritis affects the larger and medium-sized arteries in the elderly. It forms part of the polymyalgia rheumatica complex (Fritsch *et al.* 1980). The acute phase of temporal arteritis may be precipitated by over-exposure to sunlight (Kinmont & McCallum 1965). Giant-cell arteritis is probably an auto-immune disorder.

The skin over the scalp arteries may be red, tender and pigmented; there may be localized loss of hair. Bullae, ulceration and necrosis may occur (Kinmont & McCallum 1964). Necrosis of the scalp may be unilateral or bilateral and can be very extensive (Tirschek 1957; Schucke & Kaul 1967; Baum *et al.* 1982; Berth-Jones & Holt 1988). Of those patients with scalp necrosis, 67% will develop irreversible visual loss and the mortality rate is higher than among patients who have giant-cell arteritis without scalp necrosis (Soderstrom & Seehafer 1976).

The diagnosis is made on the clinical features and a high erythrocyte sedimentation rate (ESR), and may be confirmed by biopsy. Although occasional cases with a normal ESR have been reported (Wong & Korn 1986; Berth-Jones & Holt 1988). Treatment with systemic corticosteroids is necessary; a maintenance dose may be required for many months.

References

Baum, E.W., Sams, W.M. Jr. & Payne, R.R. (1982) Giant cell arteritis: a systemic disease with rare cutaneous manifestations. *Journal of the American Academy of Dermatology*, **6**, 1081.

Berth-Jones, J. & Holt, P.J.A. (1988) Temporal arteritis presenting with scalp necrosis and a normal erythrocyte sedimentation rate. *Clinical and Experimental Dermatology*, **13**, 200.

Fritsch, P., Gschnait, F. & Wolff, K. (1980) Temporal arteritis. In *Vasculitis*, p. 285, eds. K. Wolff & R.K. Winkelmann. Lloyd-Luke, London.

Kinmont, P.D.C. & McCallum, D.I. (1964) Skin manifestations of giant-cell arteritis. *British Journal of Dermatology*, **76**, 299.

Kinmont, P.D.C. & McCallum, D.I. (1965) Aetiology, pathology and course of giant-cell arteritis. *British Journal of Dermatology*, **77**, 193.

Schucke, G. & Kaul, A. (1965) Doppelseitige Kopfschwentennekrosis an Parietalberion bei Riesen-zellarteritis. *Dermatologische Wochenschrift*, **153**, 825.

Soderstrom, C.W. & Seehafer, J.R. (1976) Bilateral scalp necrosis in temporal arteritis: a rare complication of Horton's disease. *American Journal of Medicine*, **61**, 541.

Tirschek, H. (1957) Gangraena regionis temporo-parietalis durch Arteriitis temporalis. *Wiener klinische Wochenschrift*, **69**, 610.

Wong, R.L. & Korn, J.H. (1986) Temporal arteritis without an elevated erythrocyte sedimentation rate. *American Journal of Medicine*, **80**, 959.

Sjögren's syndrome
(References p. 485)

In this syndrome, which occurs mainly in women between the ages of 30 and 70, but occasionally in younger women and in men, the hair may be dry, sparse and brittle, and diffuse alopecia may involve the pubic and axillary hair as well as the scalp.

The syndrome is divided into primary and secondary types. Both include keratoconjunctivitis sicca with or without xerostomia but secondary Sjögren's adds a connective tissue disease such as rheumatoid arthritis, Hashimoto's thyroiditis, lupus erythematosus or alopecia areata (Moutsopoulos *et al.* 1980).

The clinical picture is very variable. In the patient presenting with fine, dry sparse hair the diagnosis will be suggested by the general dryness of the skin, by the presence of red, sore dry eyes, a dry mouth or dry and sore anogenital mucous membranes.

The opinions of an ophthalmologist and an oral physician will be helpful to confirm the diagnosis. No single investigation is diagnostic (see review by Daniels

& Talal 1987). Screening for autoantibodies may be informative. Salivary gland radiographs may show the characteristic signs of duct ectasia. Biopsy of the labial salivary glands is advisable if the diagnosis is in doubt (Greenspan *et al.* 1974).

There is lymphocytic and plasma cell information of the exocrine glands, which may include the salivary glands, sweat glands, the lacrymal glands and the submucous glands of the respiratory tract, the upper alimentary tract and the vagina. The glands become atrophic and ectatic. Degenerative changes have been reported also in the external root sheath of hair follicles (Ferreira-Marques 1960).

Only symptomatic treatment is possible.

References

Bunim, J.J. (1961) A broader spectrum of Sjögren's syndrome and its pathogenic implications. *Annals of Rheumatic Diseases*, **20**, 1.

Daniels, T.E. & Talal, N. (1987) Diagnosis and differential diagnosis of Sjögren's syndrome. In *Sjögren's Syndrome*, p. 193, eds. N. Talal, H.M. Moutsopoulos & S.S. Kassan, Springer-Verlag, Berlin.

Ferreira-Marques, J. (1960) A contribution to the study of Sjögren's syndrome. *Acta Dermato-Venereologica*, **40**, 485.

Greenspan, J.S., Daniels, T.E., Talal, N. & Sylvester, R.A. (1974) The histopathology of Sjögren's syndrome in labial salivary gland biopsies. *Oral Surgery*, **37**, 217.

Moutsopoulos, H.M., Chused, T.M., Mann, D.L., Klippel, J.H., Fauci, A.S., Frank, M.M., Lawley, T.J. & Hamburger, M.J. (1980) Sjögren's syndrome (sicca syndrome): current issues. *Annals of Internal Medicine*, **92**, 212.

Benign and malignant lymphoproliferative disorders
(References p. 491)

Classification of both benign and malignant lymphoreticular proliferative disorders is difficult because cells of this type have a degree of biological versatility that is first expressed in their change from the stem cell to lymphoblasts and histiocytes or to reticulum cells and histiocytic cells. This position is further complicated by the fact that many factors in health and in diseases such as neoplasia may modify this versatility and give rise to changes in the morphological stability of the cell.

At present, the benign lymphoreticular proliferative disorders are classified according to clinical, pathological and cytological characteristics. The malignant lymphomas are typed by their degree of differentiation and also according to the relative presence of lymphocytes and histiocytic cells together with the identification of lymphoid cells as either thymus-dependent (T-cell) or bone-marrow-dependent (B-cell) in type. Monoclonal antibody techniques have advanced greatly our understanding of these diseases and their responses to treatment.

Benign lymphoplasias

Benign lymphoreticular proliferation may be caused by external influences such as insect bites (Gross 1971; Horen 1972) or mechanical trauma, and inflammatory diseases such as lupus erythematosus. Excluding these specific factors, there remains a number of cryptogenic conditions which have been described under many titles and have distinct clinical and morphological characteristics (Clark 1974; Stiegleder 1976). They are classified according to clinical differences and the type of cellular infiltrate (from 1979).

Lymphocytic infiltrate of skin (Jessner & Kanof 1953)
This is a superficial benign skin disease characterized by erythematous plaques which become annular. It waxes and wanes for several years before spontaneous resolution occurs with no residual scarring; it mainly affects men under 50 years old (Calnan 1957).

Histology
There is a dense lymphocytic infiltrate in the dermis without germinal centre formation; the cells are often predominantly around hair follicles, sweat pores and blood vessels. Elastic tissue shows basophilic degeneration, and hyaluronic acid can be demonstrated using toluidine blue or colloidal iron stains. The histological changes may be difficult to differentiate from lupus erythematosus (LE) and polymorphic light eruption. IgG and C_3 are usually found at the dermo-epidermal junction in LE by direct immunofluorescence, which is universally negative in lymphocytic infiltration. Monoclonal antibody studies have shown the lymphocytes to be T-cell in origin (Willemze *et al.* 1984).

Clinical features
Individual lesions consist of infiltrated erythematous papules which spread peripherally with central clearing. There is no follicular hyperkeratosis. Any part of the body may be affected, but typical cases affect the face, temples, ears and the interscapular region of the upper back. The bald scalp may be affected. Sunlight may be a provoking factor in some cases.

Treatment
No curative therapy is known but oral antimalarials give the best results. Other treatments that have been suggested include sunscreens, topical steroids, gold and X-irradiation.

Lymphocytoma cutis (Spiegler–Fendt pseudo-lymphoma or sarcoid; miliary lymphocytoma; benign lymphocytomatoid granuloma)
Many authors have attempted to define specific sub-types of lymphocytoma cutis but clinical overlap is so frequent that they are considered here as a single condition.
　　Lymphocytoma cutis is a benign lymphoproliferative condition in which single or multiple papules or plaques develop around the face and ears (Gross 1971). No cause has been found but infection, rudimentary lymphoid hyperplasia and other factors have been suggested as possibly important.

The dense dermal lymphocytic infiltrate usually spares a small band below the epidermis but is most dense in the upper and mid dermis (Caro & Helwig 1969). Hair follicles are not often affected. In some cases lymphocytes are organized into lymphoid germinal follicles. Monoclonal antibody studies have shown the mixed cellular infiltrate to be composed of T-lymphocytes, with Langerhan's cells and clusters of polyclonal B-cells (Ralfkiaer *et al.* 1984).

Women are more frequently affected than men; onset may be from childhood to old age. Unlike lymphocytic infiltration of Jessner–Kanof, the lesions do not become annular. Differential diagnosis includes granuloma faciale, angiolymphoid hyperplasia and insect bite reactions; the latter two conditions show a greater predominance of eosinophils in the dermal infiltrate and may affect the scalp and other sites. Diffuse and disseminated forms may resemble polymorphic light eruption and adenoma sebaceum.

No uniformly successful treatment is known. Localized lesions with a mainly lymphoid follicular infiltrate may respond to X-irradiation. Some cases improve with sunscreens. Unlike the lymphocytic infiltration of Jessner–Kanof, antimalarials are not useful.

Prognosis is poor, particularly in the diffuse and disseminate types; most cases last many years or even decades. The condition requires careful observation since malignant features have been demonstrated histologically in typical cases.

Malignant lymphomas

Mycosis fungoides

Mycosis fungoides is an uncommon, slowly growing neoplastic disease of the reticuloendothelial system in which skin manifistations are the first, and often the only, expression of the disease. It is now considered to be a tumour of the thymus-dependent lymphocyte (T-cells). The early ill-defined pre-mycotic phase may show no clear evidence of neoplasia in the pathological sense but the later stages of infiltration and tumour formation have all the hallmarks of a malignant lymphoma. This three-phase description of mycosis fungoides is attributable to Bazin (1876), though the earliest description of mycosis fungoides was by Alibert (1835), who first used the name mycosis fungoides because of the mushroom-like tumours. Although the condition was originally considered to be a lymphoma which was exclusively localized to skin, extra-cutaneous changes are well recognized (Long & Mihm 1974; Rappaport & Thomas 1974). Erythrodermic mycosis fungoides (Hallopeau & Besnier 1892) and the Sézary syndrome (Sézary 1949) can now be classified pathologically with the commoner Alibert type, but the exact status of the 'tumeur d'emblée' variety (Vidal & Brocq 1885) remains unclear.

Pathogenesis. Electron microscopic techniques have shown that the T-lymphocyte is the cell undergoing malignant transformation in mycosis fungoides but the cause of this is still not known; in particular, no infective agent has ever been found. In both the classical and leukaemic (Sézary) forms, T-cells have been noted to have 'helper' cell function in that such cells will promote B-cell transformation into immunoglobulin-producing cells (Broder 1976). There are two schools of thought which remain unreconciled. The first regards mycosis fungoides as a monoclonal T-cell malignancy *ab initio* (Edelson *et al.* 1979). The second, and more widely favoured, suggests that early mycosis fungoides represents a reactive process to chronic antigen stimulation, only a proportion of which develops true malignancy (MacKie 1981).

Histology (Rappaport & Thomas 1974). Even in the earliest stage some histological change consistent with mycosis fungoides will be evident, particularly if several biopsies are taken. Characteristic changes include: (i) a band-like infiltrate in the upper dermis 'hugging' the epidermis; the main cell type is an atypical lymphoid cell with an irregular infolded nucleus. (Other cells in the infiltrate include normal lymphocytes, plasma cells, histiocytes and eosinophils.) Some spread of the infiltrate may occur into the mid and lower dermis along adnexal structures and blood vessels; (ii) epidermal Pautrier micro-abscesses consisting of local clusters of atypical lymphoid cells; (iii) mycosis, or Lutzner cells which are larger than atypical lymphocytes and possess hyperchromatic, irregular indented nuclei, the so-called cerebriform nuclei.

Follicular mucinosis (see Chapter 17) may be seen at any stage of the disease but most typically when the disease is well advanced.

Autopsy sections of tissue from many internal organs may reveal mycosis cells and occult changes consistent with mycosis fungoides.

Clinical features. The course of the disease may be divided into the pre-tumour and tumour stages; transformation into the latter may occur within months, or even several decades after the onset of the pre-tumour stage. The eruption of the pre-tumour phase may be highly characteristic; several well-defined types are known.

1 The poikilodermatous pre-mycotic eruption (poikiloderma atrophicans vasculare; parapsoriasis lichenoides; atrophic parapsoriasis).

2 Parakeratosis variegata (Stevenson 1974) is a very rare red scaly striped eruption (zebra-like) which is considered pre-reticulotic.

3 Lymphomatoid papulosis (Macaulay 1968) is divided into two types which are determined clinically by lesion size. The small variety is a papular variant of pityriasis lichenoides.

4 A follicular form of the disease has been described and appears to be a separate entity (Pierard *et al.* 1980).

Tumour phase. This phase may supervene within months or as late as 20–30 years after the onset of the pre-tumour phase. During transformation asympto-

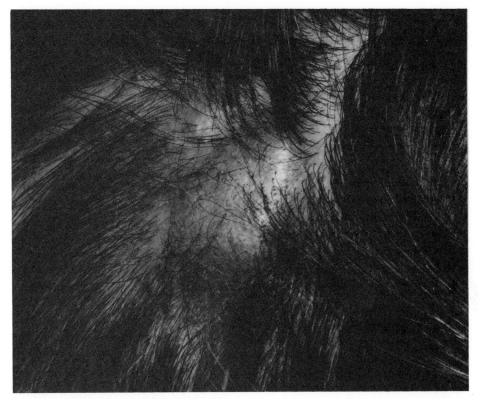

Fig. 16.1 Lymphomatous nodules of the scalp.

matic plaques may begin to itch and ecome palpable, scaly and often inflamed (Fig. 16.1). Rarely, typical infiltrated tumours may develop without a preceding pre-tumour phase, the so-called 'tumeur d'emblée' variety. Infiltrated lesions increase in number, become larger and more indurated and many eventually ulcerate. With the advent of modern suppressive treatment this phase is now rare. Any part of the body may be affected.

Variants from the above may occur. Follicular mucinosis may be manifest as widespread follicular accentuation of the eruption with hair loss (see Chapter 17). Erythroderma is usually a late stage which may be associated with diffuse hair loss. The Sézary syndrome (Sézary 1949; Winkelmann 1974) is an acute 'leukaemia' form of mycosis fungoides (T-cell erythroderma); generalized erythroderma is associated with skin histology consistent with mycosis fungoides and mycosis (or Lutzner cells) in the blood and bone marrow. Monoclonal antibody studies have shown these cells to be T-helper cells (Hamminga *et al.* 1979). Considerable generalized hair loss occurs in this type without follicular mucinosis. The nails are usually dystrophic and resemble the nails of severe psoriasis. This variant has a high mortality. Death often occurs suddenly after several years of activity of the eruption and minimal systemic findings.

B-cell lymphomas
These were formerly classified as sarcomata of lymphocytic or histiocytic types but it is now evident that the majority are tumours of the B-lymphocyte. They were thought to be seen much less by dermatologists than T-cell lymphomas (Braylan 1975), but Braun-Falco and colleagues (1981) found equal incidence. Those derived from lymphocytes in various stages of blast transformation (large cell, immunoblastic type) carry a poor prognosis; in practice, the majority of B-cell lymphomas are small cell types and are derived from plasma cell precursors which have a good prognosis for life.

Histology. Skin lesions show a dense monocytic infiltrate composed almost entirely of lymphocytes; differential diagnosis is from lymphocytoma cutis and Jessner's lymphocytic infiltration of skin.

Clinical features. Specific skin lesions are rare. They are usually firm, pink or skin-coloured papules or plaques up to several centimetres in diameter. Grouped lesions usually develop on the trunk or limbs; they may expand or coalesce to produce bizarre gyrate shapes (Graham-Brown & Calnan 1981). Cases have been described with nodules affecting only the scalp (Samman 1979).

Hodgkin's disease
Hodgkin's disease is a malignant lymphoma of the reticuloendothelial system characterized histologically by the presence of abnormal reticulum (Sternberg–Reed) cells in the cellular infiltrate of affected organs (Berard 1975). It has still not been clearly shown whether it is the Sternberg–Reed cell or the abundant T-lymphocytes that are truly malignant. Many authorities believe that Hodgkin's disease can be divided into several distinct diseases based on clinical and pathological differences.

Histologically four sub-types are recognized: lymphocytic predominance, nodular sclerosing, mixed cellularity and lymphocytic depletion—the Rye classification—(Berard 1975). The first two have a relatively good prognosis.

Hodgkin's disease is a multi-system disease; based on accurate staging using clinical, lymphangiographic and laparotomy findings (including splenectomy) four stages (each subdivided into A and B sub-types—presence or absence of systemic symptoms) can be defined.

Stage 1 Limited to one or two adjacent anatomical sites on one side of the diaphragm.

Stage 2 As for 1 but more than two regions affected.

Stage 3 Disease on both sides of the diaphragm; only lymph nodes, spleen and Waldeyer's rings are involved.

Stage 4 Involvement of many organs throughout the reticuloendothelial system, including the skin.

This classification suggests that specific skin lesions imply a bad prognosis which is generally, but not universally, true.

Clinical features. Specific infiltration of the skin with Hodgkin's disease tissue is rare. There are usually firm erythematous nodules which may ulcerate; the scalp may be the first site of involvement.

Non-specific skin symptoms and signs occur in up to 50% of cases (Bluefarb 1959). These may predate evidence of active Hodgkin's disease by months or years. Included are pruritus or prurigo, pigmentation mimicking Addison's diseae, acquired ichthyosis, generalized exfoliative dermatitis, herpes zoster and erythema nodosum. Hair loss may occur because of rubbing and scratching due to irritable dry skin, or because of pituitary or adrenal destruction by the disease process. Less commonly alopecia may be due to diffuse infiltration of the skin.

Treatment. Specific skin infiltrates are usually treated together with other sites of involvement using X-irradiation or chemotherapy or both. Pruritus and dry skin are best treated by regular oiling of the skin and by oral antihistamines.

Histiocytic medullary reticulosis (malignant histiocytosis)
This rare malignant proliferation of histiocytes (and their precursors) is a rapidly fatal tumour in all the cases so far described (Scott & Robb-Smith 1939; Berard 1975).

Men are more frequently affected than women in this condition which presents with asthenia, weight loss and pyrexia; the lymph nodes, spleen and liver are enlarged and pancytopaenia may develop. Rarely leucocytosis occurs. Jaundice and purpura are common.

The skin may be specifically infiltrated. Lesions are tender bluish/purple nodules which may coalesce to form plaques on the scalp, forehead, extremities and back.

The condition is progressive and death occurs within 1 year; no successful treatment is known.

References

Alibert, J.L.M. (1835) *Monographie des Dermatoses.* Bellière, Paris.

Bazin, P.A.E. (1876) *Maladies de la Peau Observeés à l'Hôpital.* St Louis, Paris.

Berard, C.W. (1975) Reticuloendothelial system. An overview of neoplasia. In *The Reticuloendothelial System. International Academy of Pathology Monographs,* **16,** ed. J.W. Rebuck. Williams & Wilkins, Baltimore.

Bluefarb, S.M. (1959) *Cutaneous Manifestations of the Malignant Lymphomas.* Thomas, Springfield.

Braun-Falco, O., Burg, G. & Schmoeker, C.H. (1981) Recent advances in the understanding of cutaneous lymphoma. *Clinical and Experimental Dermatology,* **6,** 89.

Braylan, R.C. (1975) Malignant lymphomas: current classification and new observations. In *Pathology Annual,* ed. S.C. Summers. Appleton–Century–Croft, New York.

Broder, S. (1976) The Sézary syndrome. A malignant proliferation of helper T-cells. *Journal of Clinical Investigations,* **58,** 1297.

Calnan, C.D. (1957) Lymphocytic infiltrate of skin. *British Journal of Dermatology*, **69**, 169.

Caro, W.A. & Helwig, E.B. (1969) Lymphocytoma cutis. *Cancer*, **24**, 487.

Clark, W.H. (1974) The lymphocytic infiltrates of the skin. *Human Pathology*, **5**, 25.

Edelson, R.L., Berger, C.L., Raffat, J. & Warburton, D. (1979) Karyotype studies of cutaneous T-cell lymphoma: evidence for clonal origin. *Journal of Investigative Dermatology*, **73**, 548.

Graham-Brown, R.A. & Calnan, C.D. (1981) Cutaneous presentation of a B-cell lymphoma. *Clinical and Experimental Dermatology*, **6**, 439.

Gross, P.R. (1971) Benign lymphoid hyperplasia. *Archives of Dermatology*, **103**, 347.

Hallopeau, H. & Besnier, F. (1892) On the erythroderma of mycosis fungoides. *Journal of Cutaneous Genetic Diseases*, **10**, 453.

Hamminga, L., Hartgrink-Groeneveld, C.A. & Van Vloten, W.A. (1979) Sézary's syndrome: a clinical evaluation of eight patients. *British Journal of Dermatology*, **100**, 291.

Horen, W.P. (1972) Insect and scorpion sting. *Journal of the American Medical Association*, **221**, 894.

Jessner, M. & Kanof, N.B. (1953) Lymphocytic infiltration of skin. *Archives of Dermatology*, **68**, 447.

Long, J.C. & Mihm, M.C. (1974) Mycosis fungoides with extracutaneous entity. *Cancer*, **34**, 1745.

Macaulay, W.L. (1968) Lymphomatoid papulosis. A continuing self-healing eruption, clinically benign—histologically malignant. *Archives of Dermatology*, **97**, 23.

MacKie, R.M. (1981) Initial event in mycosis fungoides of the skin is viral infection of epidermal Langerhans cells. *Lancet*, **ii**, 283.

Nordqvist, B.C. & Kinney, J.P. (1976) T and B cell-mediated immunity in mycosis fungoides. *Cancer*, **37**, 714.

Pierard, G.E., Ackerman, A.B. & Lapiere, C.M. (1980) Follicular lymphomatoid papulosis. *American Journal of Dermatopathology*, **2**, 173.

Ralfkiaer, E., Lange-Wantzin, G., Mason, D.Y., Stein, H. & Thomsen, K. (1984) Characterisation of benign cutaneous lymphocytic infiltrates by monoclonal antibodies. *British Journal of Dermatology*, **111**, 635.

Rappaport, H. & Thomas, L.B. (1974) Mycosis fungoides: the pathology of extracutaneous involvement. *Cancer*, **34**, 1198.

Samman, P.D. (1979) Lymphomata of B cells. In *Textbook of Dermatology*, 3rd edn., eds A.J. Rook, D.S. Wilkinson & F.J.G. Ebling, p. 1555. Blackwell Scientific Publications, Oxford.

Scott, R.B. & Robb-Smith, A.H.T. (1939) Histiocytic medullary reticulosis. *Lancet*, **ii**, 194.

Sézary, A. (1949) Une nouvelle réticulose cutanée, la réticulose maligne leucémique à histio-monocytes monstrueuses et à forme d'érythrodermie oedemateuse et pigmentée. *Annales de Dermatologie et de Syphilologie* (Paris), **9**, 5.

Stevenson, C.J. (1974) Parakeratosis variegata. *Proceedings of the Royal Society of Medicine*, **57**, 316.

Stiegleder, G.K. (1976) Benign and malignant proliferative response. *Acta Dermato-Venereologica*, **56**, 33.

Vidal, E. & Brocq, L. (1885) Étude sur le mycosis fungoides. *France Médicale*, **2**, 946.

Willemze, R., Dijkstra, A. & Meijer, C.J.L.M. (1984) Lymphocytic infiltration of the skin (Jessner): a T-cell lymphoproliferative disease. *British Journal of Dermatology*, **110**, 523.

Winkelmann, R.K. (1974) Symposium on the Sézary cell. *Mayo Clinic Proceedings*, **49**, 513.

Chapter 17
Diseases of the Scalp and Skin Diseases Involving the Scalp*

Common non-infective diseases of the scalp
    Pityriasis capitis
    Pityriasis amiantacea
    Seborrhoea
    Seborrhoeic dermatitis
    Psoriasis of the scalp
    Lichenification and lichen simplex
    Contact dermatitis
    Acne necrotica
    Folliculitis keloidalis nuchae
    Pseudofolliculitis
    Pruritus of the scalp
    Hair casts
    Rosacea
Rare diseases which characteristically affect the scalp
    Dissecting cellulitis
    Cutis verticis gyrata
    Lipedematous alopecia
Skin diseases in which lesions may occur in the scalp
    Ichthyosis
    Darier's disease
    Dermatitis herpetiformis
    Cicatricial pemphigoid
    Follicular mucinosis
    Granuloma annulare
    Elastosis perforans serpiginosa
    Eosinophilic cellulitis

Common non-infective diseases of the scalp

Pityriasis capitis (References p. 497)

History and nomenclature

In 1842 John Erichsen, later to become an eminent surgeon, published a monograph on *Diseases of the Scalp*. Of pityriasis he wrote 'The diagnosis of pityriasis from the other scaling affections is sufficiently simple, indeed it is impossible to confound the small, thin white or greyish loose scales.... It never causes the permanent loss of hair.' He regarded pityriasis as a simple cosmetic defect and not a precursor of baldness. The microbiological discoveries of the next hundred years

---

*Skin diseases causing cicatricial alopecia are considered in Chapter 11.

493

provided fuel for imaginative speculation on the relationship of pityriasis to seborrhoea, and of both to baldness. It now seems reasonable to accept pityriasis as near-physiological scaling of the scalp or other hairy regions, which may or may not be fortuitously associated with 'seborrhoea' or with baldness. Pityriasis simplex or furfuracea is popularly known as dandruff.

Aetiology
Pityriasis is a cosmetic affliction of adolescence and adult life and is relatively rare and mild in children. Its peak incidence and severity are reached at the age of about 20 and it becomes less frequent after 50. At 20 some 50% of Caucasoids are affected in some degree. Figures for other races appear not to have been published.

The age incidence suggests that an androgenic influence is important and the level of sebaceous activity may be a factor. However, gross seborrhoea may occur without pityriasis and commonly severe pityriasis may be present without clinically apparent excessive sebaceous activity. Quantitative studies have not been reported.

The microbial origin of pityriasis was accepted by Sabouraud but a number of later authors (e.g. Whitlock 1953) could establish no correlation between the degree of pityriasis and the population of *Pityrosporum ovale*. However, the role of *P. ovale* is still disputed. This yeast increases in number at puberty, and it elaborates substances which inhibit the growth of dermatophytes (Weary 1968). The large numbers of *P. ovale* in scalps with pityriasis has been regarded as secondary to the increased scaling (Ackermann & Kligman 1969). In another investigation of yeasts in subjects with and without pityriasis (Roia & Vanderwyk 1969) it was concluded that although no specific organism was significantly related to pityriasis, an increase in the total microbial flora was a factor in the increase of pityriasis. It had previously been demonstrated that the application of yeast inhibitors to one half of the scalp produced a greater reduction in pityriasis than did the application of a bacterial inhibitor to the other half of the same scalp (Vanderwyk & Hechemey 1967). When the scalp flora of 11 subjects was almost completely eliminated by the application of nystatin and neomycin, the production of pityriasis was reduced by over 60%; and when a nystatin-resistant strain of *P. ovale* was then introduced the severity of the pityriasis increased by over 80% (Gosse & Vanderwyk 1969). However, some antimicrobial agents will decrease the flora without affecting the severity of pityriasis (Ackermann & Kligman 1969). Further quantitative studies of the microflora have not finally resolved the problem of their precise role in the production of pityriasis; *P. ovale* is more abundant in pityriasis than in the normal scalp, and still more so in seborrhoeic dermatitis, while *Corynebacterium acnes* is less abundant in pityriasis than in normal scalps, and almost disappears in seborrhoeic dermatitis (McGinley *et al.* 1975); these changes could be influenced by increased blood flow since *C. acnes* is strictly anaerobic.

Some of the investigations mentioned above, tending to attribute a pathogenic role to micro-organisms, were not well controlled (Priestly & Savin 1976). The balance of evidence presented by Kligman's team (Leyden *et al.* 1976) suggests that scalp organisms play no role in causing pityriasis capitis but are present in abundance because of the increased availability of scalp nutrients; Shuster (1984), on historical and scientific grounds, presented the contrary view, particularly stressing the importance of the good effects of antipityrosporum agents as supporting the infection aetiology.

The antigenicity of *Pityrosporum* has been much investigated, but the clinical significance of allergic sensitivity to components of pityriasis scale has not been firmly established. It has been suggested that it may be of importance in some patients with atopic dermatitis. Over 75% of defatted human dandruff is non-allergenic mucopolysaccharide; the allergen is probably a glycoprotein (Berrens & Young 1964).

Similarly the significance of sensitivity to *P. ovale* is difficult to evaluate. Antibody to *P. ovale* is often present in high titre in patients with or without hair loss. However, Alexander (1967) found that patients with common baldness had more pityriasis than control subjects and that they had higher titres of antibody to *P. ovale* than had patients with alopecia areata.

Investigation on pityriasis requires a technique for the quantitative assessment of scaling, such as was described by Van Abbé (1964).

Pathology

Although their cause may be disputed, the nature of the epidermal changes resulting in pityriasis is not. In the normal scalp the horny layer consists of 25–35 fully keratinized and closely coherent cells; in pityriasis there are usually fewer than 10 layers of cells, and these are often parakeratotic and irregularly arranged, with deep crevices resulting in the formation of the flakes visible clinically (Ackermann & Kligman 1969). The permeability of such a horny layer is of course greater than normal. Autoradiographic studies (Plewig & Kligman 1969, 1970) showed a high labelling index and stratum corneum transit time of 3–4 days. Application of selenium sulphide reduced the labelling index and slowed down the transit time.

Clinical features

Small white or grey scales accumulate on the surface of the scalp in localized, more or less segmental, patches or more diffusely. After removal with an effective shampoo the scales form again within 4–7 days. The condition first becomes a cosmetic problem during the second and third decades, but there are long- and short-term variations in its severity, without obvious cause (Van Abbé 1964). There are also variations in the ease with which the scales become detached and drift unaesthetically among the hair shafts or fall on the collar and shoulders.

Although pityriasis usually clears spontaneously during the fifth or sixth decade, it may persist in old age.

In those subjects whose scalps become greasy at or after puberty, the seborrhoea binds the scale in a greasy 'paste' and it is no longer shed, but accumulates in small adherent mounds—as so-called pityriasis steatoides. The development of clinically evident inflammatory changes in such individuals leads to seborrhoeic dermatitis. Pruritus is not a feature of simple pityriasis. It is very much more common when inflammatory changes develop in seborrhoeic scalps, and such recurrent episodes may be clearly related to periods of stress. Acne necrotica, which may be intensely irritable, also can complicate pityriasis.

Diagnosis

The presence of more than very mild pityriasis in a young child throws doubt on the diagnosis. Extreme and persistent scaling, even though it lacks the characteristic features of psoriasis, is always suspect, particularly if there is a family history of this disease. Widespread scaling, sometimes with scarring, may occur in some forms of ichthyosis. At any age, if pruritus is troublesome, pediculosis must be carefully excluded.

Small areas of scaling with dull broken hair shafts are typical of *Microsporon* ringworms. Localized scaling in children is therefore an indication for examination of the scalp under Wood's light, and of the broken hairs under the microscope. A nervous hair-pulling tic may result in twisted and broken hairs of normal texture in a patch of post-inflammatory scaling.

Profuse sticky silvery scale should suggest pityriasis amiantacea.

Treatment

Pityriasis in its milder forms is a physiological process. The object of treatment is to control it at the lowest possible cost and inconvenience to the patient, appreciating that any procedure found to be effective will need to be repeated at regular intervals.

In some cases, particularly if seborrhoea is associated, a tar preparation such as Oil of Cade ointment or a proprietary preparation such as Pragmatar, may be rubbed into the scalp and washed out after a few hours with a detergent shampoo. This treatment may need to be repeated at intervals, but after two or three applications it can often be replaced by a tar shampoo, which has been shown to be more effective than the vehicle alone (Alexander 1967a,b).

In the average case one of the many proprietary shampoos may be found effective. Selenium sulphide, which has been shown to reduce epidermal turnover (Plewig & Kligman 1970) is very useful for many patients but fails inexplicably in others. The same may be said of preparations containing zinc pyrithione or zinc omadine, which are said to reduce the yeast populations (Brauer *et al.* 1966).

The evidence presented by Shuster (1984) and Shuster and Blatchford (1988) has converted many clinicians away from the above to specific antipityrosporum therapy with imidazole compounds, e.g. Nizoral shampoo (ketoconazole).

References

Ackermann, A.B. & Kligman, A.M. (1969) Some observations on dandruff. *Journal of the Society of Cosmetic Chemists*, **20**, 81.

Alexander, S. (1967a) Do shampoos affect dandruff? *British Journal of Dermatology*, **79**, 92.

Alexander, S. (1967b) Loss of hair and dandruff. *British Journal of Dermatology*, **79**, 549.

Berrens, L. & Young, E. (1964) Studies on the human dandruff allergen. *Dermatologica*, **128**, 3.

Brauer, E.W., Opdyke, D.L. & Burnett, C.M. (1966) The anti-seborrhoeic qualities of zinc pyrithione in a cream vehicle. *Journal of Investigative Dermatology*, **47**, 174.

Erichsen, J.E. (1842) *A Practical Treatise on the Diseases of the Scalp*, p. 180. Churchill, London.

Gosse, R.M. & Vanderwyk, R.W. (1969) The relationship of a nystatin-resistant strain of *Pityrosporon ovale* to dandruff. *Journal of the Society of Cosmetic Chemists*, **20**, 603.

Leyden, J.J., McGinlay, K.J. & Kligman, A.M. (1976) Role of microorganisms in dandruff. *Archives of Dermatology*, **112**, 333.

McGinley, K.J., Leyden, J.J., Marples, R.R. & Kligman, A.M. (1975) Quantitative microbiology of the scalp in non-dandruff, dandruff and seborrhoeic dermatitis. *Journal of Investigative Dermatology*, **64**, 401.

Plewig, G. & Kligman, A.M. (1969) The effect of selenium sulphide on epidermal tumours of normal and dandruff scalps. *Journal of the Society of Cosmetic Chemists*, **20**, 767.

Plewig, G. & Kligman, A.M. (1970) Zellkinetische Untersuchungen bei Kopfschuppenerkrankung. *Archiv für klinische und experimentelle Dermatologie*, **236**, 406.

Priestly, G.L. & Savin, J.A. (1976) The microbiology of dandruff. *British Journal of Dermatology*, **94**, 469.

Roia, F.C. & Vanderwyk, R.W. (1969) Residual microbial flora of the human scalp and its relationship to dandruff. *Journal of the Society of Cosmetic Chemists*, **20**, 113.

Shuster, S. (1984) The aetiology of dandruff and the mode of action of therapeutic agents. *British Journal of Dermatology*, **111**, 235.

Shuster, S. & Blatchford, N. (1988) Seborrhoeic dermatitis and dandruff—a fungal disease. *Royal Society of Medicine Publications*, London, p. 1.

Van Abbé, N.J. (1964) The investigation of dandruff. *Journal of the Society of Cosmetic Chemists*, **15**, 609.

Vanderwyk, R.W. & Hechemey, K.E. (1967) A comparison of the bacterial and yeast flora of the human scalp and their effect upon dandruff production. *Journal of the Society of Cosmetic Chemists*, **18**, 629.

Weary, P.E. (1968) *Pityrosporum ovale*. *Archives of Dermatology*, **98**, 408.

Whitlock, F.A. (1953) *Pityrosporum ovale* and some scaly conditions of the scalp. *British Medical Journal*, **i**, 484.

Pityriasis amiantacea (References p. 499)

History and nomenclature

The clinical features of this poorly documented but not uncommon syndrome were known before Alibert (1832) named it 'fausse teigne amiantacée', which may be translated as asbestos-like pseudo-ringworm. Since then it has often been referred to as tinea amiantacea, but as the term 'tinea' ordinarily implies a ringworm infection many others have preferred the non-committal 'pityriasis amiantacea'. Gschwandtner (1974) gave his etymological reasons for using the old term 'porrigo', but this term proved such a source of confusion throughout the 19th century that it seems better to let it die.

Aetiology (Becker & Muir 1929; Brown 1948)
Pityriasis amiantacea is a pattern of 'eczematous' reaction of the scalp to trauma or to infection, or without evident cause. It may complicate seborrhoeic dermatitis, psoriasis or lichen simplex. Its association with these and other conditions is difficult to evaluate. It depends on the initial clinical diagnosis. Cases which some dermatologists would accept as early psoriasis are labelled pityriasis amiantacea by others. If such cases are excluded then there is no definite association between pityriasis amiantacea and psoriasis (Hersle *et al.* 1979). In Knight's (1977) study of 71 patients, two had associated psoriasis and nine had eczema; he pointed out that it may occur at any age but the average age was 25 (range 5–40 years).

Pathology
Biopsies from 18 patients were examined by Knight (1977). The most consistent findings were spongiosis, parakeratosis, migration of lymphocytes into the epidermis, and a variable degree of acanthosis. The essential features responsible for the asbestos-like scaling are diffuse hyperkeratosis and parakeratosis together with follicular keratosis, which surrounds each hair by a sheath of horn (Kiess 1925; Jossel 1932; Gschwandtner 1974).

Clinical features (Dubreuilh 1930; Jordan & Nolting 1971; Gschwandtner 1974)
Masses of sticky silvery scales, overlapping like the tiles of a roof, adhere to the scalp and are attached in layers to the shafts of the hairs which they surround. The underlying scalp may be red and moist or may show simple erythema and scaling, or the features of psoriasis of seborrhoeic dermatitis or of lichen simplex (Fig. 17.1).

   A relatively common form seen mainly in young girls complicates recurrent or chronic fissuring behind one or both ears. The scales extend some distance into the neighbouring scalp. Another form extends upwards from patches of lichen simplex and is seen mainly in middle-aged women. The disease is usually confined to small areas of the scalp, but may be very extensive, either involving a large area diffusely, or affecting a number of small patches. The latter form in children often proves by its subsequent course to be psoriasis. The majority of patients notice some hair loss in areas of severe scaling (Knight 1977). The hair regrows when the scaling is effectively treated. If scarring alopecia occurs it may well be related to secondary infection, i.e. mixed bacterial and pityrosporum.

Diagnosis
The distinctive clinical appearance makes-the diagnosis usually easy but the identification of the underlying disease may not be easy: indeed none may be found.

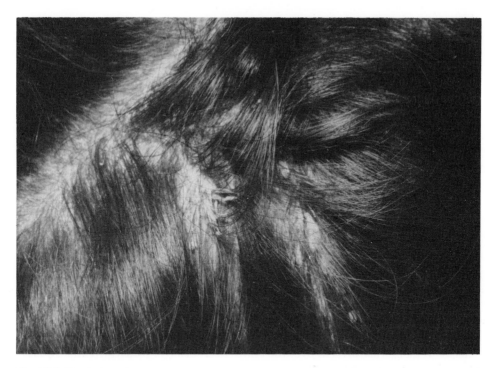

Fig. 17.1 Pityriasis amiantacea.

Treatment

Where the pityriasis complicates lichen simplex or psoriasis the underlying condition must be treated, but it may be useful initially to eliminate the abundant scale by the use of Oil of Cade ointment or a topical tar/salicylic acid ointment which is effective also in many cases in which no preceding disease of the scalp is discovered. Either preparation should be washed out of the scalp after 4–5 hours with a suitable shampoo, e.g. tar or imidazole shampoo. Even then the condition tends sometimes to recur.

If psoriasis is associated then the same local or systemic treatment principles used in general may be effective in treating the scalp (Dawber 1989).

References

Alibert, J.L. (1832) *La Porrigine Amiantacée. Monographie des Dermatoses*, vol. 1, p. 293. Imprimerie de Ridgnoux, Paris.

Becker, S.W. & Muir, K.B. (1929) Tinea amiantacea. *Archives of Dermatology and Syphilology*, **20**, 45.

Brown, W.H. (1948) Some observations on neurodermatitis of the scalp with particular reference to tinea amiantacea. *British Journal of Dermatology*, **60**, 81.

Dawber, R.P.R. (1989) Aspects of treatment of scalp psoriasis. *Journal of Dermatological Treatment*, **1** (2), 103.

Dubreuilh, W. (1930) De la forme teigne amiantacée d'Alibert. *Annales de Dermatologie et de Syphiligraphie*, **1**, 61.

Gschwandtner, W.R. (1974) Porrigo amiantacea (pityriasis amiantacea). *Hautarzt.* **25**, 134.

Hersle, K., Lindholm, A., Mobaeken, H. & Sandberg, L. (1979) Relationship of pityriasis amiantacea to psoriasis. *Dermatologica*, **159**, 245.

Jordan, P. & Nolting, S. (1971) Tinea amiantacea. *Schriften der Alfred-Marchionini-Stiftung*. **2**, 55.

Jossel, B, (1932) Zur Kenntnis der sogenannten Alibertischen tinea amiantacea. *Dermatologische Wochenschrift*. **94**, 677.

Kiess, O. (1925) Die Porrigo amiantacea. *Dermatologische Wochenschrift*. **81**, 1355.

Knight, A.G. (1977) Pityriasis amiantacea: a clinical and histopathologic investigation. *Clinical and Experimental Dermatology*, **2**, 137.

Seborrhoea (References p. 502)

Definition

Seborrhoea has been defined as the production of a quantity of sebum which is excessive for the age and sex of the individual, but this definition is inadequate in clinical practice, since many patients in whom the level of sebum excretion is not abnormal nevertheless seek advice because they find the greasiness of their hair cosmetically unacceptable. Seborrhoea in practice is that level of sebum production which the patient considers to be excessive!

Aetiology

Sebaceous glands are present over the entire skin surface except the palms and the soles and the dorsa of the feet. The largest glands are on the face and scalp and on the scrotum. The glands in the central area of the chest and back are larger than those elsewhere in the trunk. Sebaceous glands in the skin all open into hair follicles, but the pilary component of the pilosebaceous unit may be only a very small vellus hair.

The sebaceous glands are functional at birth, and in early infancy under the influence of maternal androgens, but throughout childhood they remain tiny and inactive. With the approach of puberty, at which androgen levels begin to rise, usually at about the age of 9 or 10, the sebaceous glands enlarge and the production of sebum begins. Between 13 and 16 the production of sebum is equal between males and females but the level increases in males to reach a peak at the age of about 20. From about 16 onwards the production of sebum is significantly greater in males than females. In males it remains high to extreme old age; in females there is a marked decrease after the menopause (Strauss & Pochi 1968). Sebaceous gland activity in males is dependent mainly on testicular androgen. In females it depends on adrenal and ovarian androgen.

Oestrogen decreases the size of sebaceous glands and thus the production of sebum (Pochi & Strauss 1973), but in pregnancy there is no reduction in sebum production and there is a decrease post-partum (Burton *et al.* 1970).

There is considerable variation in the normal level of sebum production in sexually normal males and those with abundant sebum may complain about it. In those genetically predisposed to acne this may accompany the seborrhoea. Men with common baldness may complain of the conspicuous greasiness of the scalp, but in such patients greasiness is merely more evident and the level of sebum production is no greater than in non-bald control subjects (Maibach *et al.* 1968). During the course of development of baldness the total number of sebaceous glands does in fact decrease significantly (Rampini *et al.*, 1968).

In women seborrhoea may have far greater significance. Seborrhoea (and acne in those so predisposed), together with hirsutism and baldness, is one of the triad of cutaneous parameters of androgenic activity.

Increased sebaceous activity, quite apart from the levels of androgenic stimulation, may occur in Parkinson's disease and in epilepsy (Grasset & Brun 1959).

There are satisfactory quantitative techniques available for the measurement of the rate of sebum excretion (Ebling 1974) and the rate of replacement sebum on the hair (Eberhardt & Kuhn-Bussiers 1975). Sebum replacement curves show wide variation and four types of curve are identified.

Clinical features

The patient complains that the scalp and hair are excessively greasy and therefore unmanageable and may insist that the frequent removal of the grease by shampooing tends to increase the rate of its production (Goldschmidt & Kligman 1968).

Management

Symptomatic treatment without any attempt to evaluate the significance of the symptom is hard to justify. Admittedly the seborrhoea may be a physiological variant and the patient be otherwise entirely normal. However, in a significant proportion of women the seborrhoea is a manifestation of increased androgenic activity which has consequences other than purely cosmetic.

The association of hirsutism or of androgenetic alopecia should be noted. The menstrual history should be recorded. If the association of hirsutism, or of alopecia of androgenetic pattern, or of menstrual irregularity, suggests the possibility of an abnormality in systemic androgen metabolism this should be investigated and treated (see Chapter 4). If the seborrhoea is an isolated symptom topical means to control it are recommended. Gloor (1979) outlined the aims of topical treatment as (i) inhibition of depletion of sebaceous glands, (ii) inhibition of lipid synthesis in the glands and (iii) inhibition of microbial lipolysis of triglycerides. He states that the use of isopropyl alcohol as a vehicle reduces sebum depletion, tar or oestrogens reduce lipid synthesis, and lipolysis is reduced by isopropyl alcohol, colloidal sulphur or selenium disulphide. The use of lotions containing oestrogens is often advocated in some European countries and its thorough investigation and evaluation is clearly desirable. It is usual in cases in which there is no indication for systemic treatment to suggest the use of proprietary, cosmetically acceptable shampoos marketed for the condition, leaving the patient to establish empirically the choice of preparation and the frequency of application to provide the greatest symptomatic relief.

References

Burton, J.L., Cunliffe, W.J., Millar, D.G. & Shuster, S. (1970) Effect of pregnancy on sebum excretion. *British Medical Journal*, **ii**, 769.

Eberhardt, H. & Kuhn-Bussius, H. (1975) Bestimmung der Ruckfettungskinetik der Haare. *Archiv für dermatologische Forschung*, **252**, 139.

Ebling, F.J. (1974) Hormonal control and methods of measuring sebaceous gland activity. *Journal of Investigative Dermatology*, **62**, 161.

Gloor, M. (1979) Aspekte zur Therapie der Seborrhoea Oleosa und des Pityriasis simplex capillitii. *Hautarzt*, **30**, 236.

Goldschmidt, H. & Kligman, A.M. (1968) Increased sebum secretion following selenium sulphide shampoo. *Acta Dermatologica et Venerealogica*, **48**, 489.

Grasset, N. & Brun, R. (1959) Étude de fonction sebacée de sujets sains et de patients atteints d'épilepsie ou de maladie de Parkinson. *Dermatologica*, **119**, 132.

Maibach, H.I., Feldmann, R., Payne, B. & Hutshell, T. (1968) Scalp and forehead sebum production in male pattern alopecia. In *Biopathology of Pattern Alopecia*, eds. A. Baccareda-Boy, G. Moretti & J.R. Frey, p. 171. Karger, Basel.

Pochi, P.E. & Strauss, J.S. (1973) Sebaceous gland suppression with ethinyl oestradiol and diethinylstilbestrol. *Archives of Dermatology*, **108**, 210.

Rampini, E., Bertamino, R. & Moretti, G. (1968) Size and shape of sebaceous gland in male pattern alopecia. In *Biopathology of Pattern Alopecia*, eds. A. Baccareda-Boy, G. Moretti & J.R., Frey, p.155. Karger, Basel.

Strauss, J.S. & Pochi, P.E. (1968) The change in human sebaceous gland activity with age. In *Biopathology of Pattern Alopecia*, eds. A. Baccareda-Boy, G. Moretti & J.R. Frey, p. 166. Karger, Basel.

Seborrhoeic dermatitis (References p. 505)

History and omenclature (Colcott Fox 1911; Shuster & Blatchford 1988)

Willan introduced the concept of pityriasis, consisting of irregular patches of small thin scales. He included both pityriasis capitis and pityriasis versicolor in this group. Hebra in 1870 introduced the term and the concept of seborrhoea oleosa, with increased sebaceous gland activity as its essential feature, and he included Willan's pityriasis capitis as seborrhoea sicca which he claimed was due to sebaceous gland dysfunction. In 1887 Unna used the term seborrhoeic eczema and emphasized the inflammatory component. Subsequent work of Sabouraud and others incriminating various micro-organisms has been discussed elsewhere.

The prevalence of seborrhoeic dermatitis shows wide geographical variation, but the extent to which this is climatic or racial is still uncertain. In Britain seborrhoeic dermatitis appears to be significantly more frequent among the Celts than in other ethnic groups. International comparisons are still more difficult to make as differences in diagnostic criteria and in nomenclature are so frequent.

Aetiology

The cause of seborrhoeic dermatitis is unknown but a genetic factor is almost certainly implicated. Clinically different syndromes with some features in common occur in the infant with sebaceous activity induced by maternal androgens and in the adolescent and adult in which sebaceous activity has been re-established by endogenous androgen production. The sebum excretion rate, however, is not increased in seborrhoeic dermatitis but the sebum contains less than the normal proportion of free fatty acids, squalene and wax esters and relatively increased quantities of triglycerides and cholesterol (Gloor *et al.* 1972). The incidence of seborrhoeic dermatitis is increased in Parkinsonism and the dermatitis in such patients is improved by L-dopa which reduces the abnormally high sebum excretion rate (Parish 1970).

Attempts to relate seborrhoeic dermatitis to the activities of pityrosporum yeasts have recently been more successful than in the previous century (Shuster & Blatchford, 1988); secondary bacterial infection is common. Claims that autoimmune mechanisms are involved (Hashimoto 1946) are also unproven. Stress seems at times to be a precipitating factor.

Pathology

The histological changes combine features of chronic eczema with features of psoriasis. The histological differential diagnosis of seborrhoeic dermatitis from psoriasis is discussed elsewhere. The ultra-microscopic appearance (Metz & Metz 1975) is not specific and resembles that seen in nummular eczema.

Clinical features (Rook 1954)

Pityriasis simplex capitis is widely regarded as the precursor or the mildest form of seborrhoeic dermatitis of the scalp but until much more knowledge of the conditions becomes available the nature of this possible relationship must remain unproven.

Pityriasis steatoides is regarded as a slightly more severe form of seborrhoeic dermatitis of the scalp. Large greasy scales often of yellow colour combine with exudate to form crusts, beneath which the scalp is red and moist (Fig. 17.2). The eyebrows and the nasolabial folds are often also involved. As the condition deteriorates perifollicular erythema and scaling gradually extends to form sharply marginated patches, dull red in colour and covered by greasy scales. There may be only a few discrete patches or the scalp may be diffusely affected with extension of the dermatitis beyond the frontal margin. Scratching and secondary infection may produce eczematization with much exudation and crusting, and secondary infection may cause an increase of these inflammatory changes or the development of pustulation.

Often associated with seborrhoeic dermatitis of the scalp is blepharitis. Small crusts form along the eyelid margins and separate to leave scars. Some eyelashes may be destroyed.

The retro-auricular region is commonly affected by seborrhoeic dermatitis either alone or in association with scalp lesions. There may be a crusted retro-auricular fissure from which dull red scaling extends into the scalp and to the back of the pinna. The concha and the external auditory canal may be similarly affected.

The renewed popularity of beards in some countries has led to an increase of

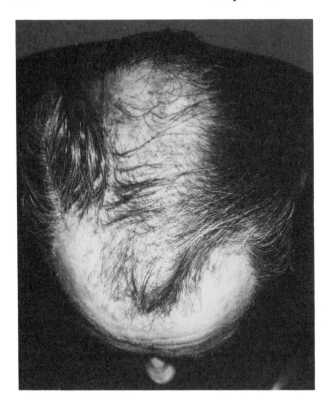

Fig. 17.2 Seborrhoeic dermatitis.

seborrhoeic dermatitis at this site (Parish & Arndt 1972). Erythema and greasy scaling are most severe on the cheeks. On the shaven chin a superficial folliculitis of the beard (barbers' rash) is common. Less often a deep follicular infection gives rise to sycosis which may leave scars.

Seborrhoeic dermatitis of other hairy regions of the body may accompany dermatitis of the scalp.

Seborrhoeic dermatitis of infancy

The relationship of this distinctive syndrome to seborrhoeic dermatitis of adults is problematical. During the early days or weeks of life grey greasy crusts form on the scalp, particularly on the frontal and parietal regions. A pink scaly erythema may develop in the neck folds and in other skin flexures (Fig. 3.4). Many authorities now state that seborrhoeic dermatitis of infancy is a manifestation of the atopic state.

Diagnosis

There is a tendency to diagnose seborrhoeic dermatitis too freely. Many other skin conditions may occur in grossly seborrhoeic subjects and the diagnostic criteria should therefore be strict.

The heavy palpable scales of psoriasis are usually easy to differentiate, particularly if psoriatic lesions can be found in the skin and on the nails. Occasionally the existence of a hybrid condition may be suspected, particularly on the face. In cases of doubt a biopsy may be helpful.

Tinea capitis may readily be confused with eborrhoeic dermatitis, particularly those forms of tinea caused by anthropophilic *Trichophyton* species; always undertake Wood's light examination and fungal culture in doubtful cases.

Lichen simplex of the nape, a relatively common condition particularly in women, can be confused with seborrhoeic dermatitis but the characteristic site and the severity and persistence of the itching suggests the correct diagnosis. Less commonly lichen simplex may occur at the side of the scalp above the ear.

Treatment

The treatment of pityriasis capitis is considered elsewhere. Seborrhoeic dermatitis of the scalp may respond to the same measures but if it is extensive or severe daily application of a corticosteroid lotion is helpful. The scalp should be shampooed twice or more each week until the dermatitis is under control. A preparation containing tar and sulphur or Oil of Cade ointment should be rubbed gently into the scalp at least 2 hours before the hair is shampooed. Imidazole shampoos (Nizoral, Janssen) are now the most commonly used agents.

If secondary infection is present a topical antibiotic/corticosteroid combination should be prescribed; if the secondary infection is severe and extensive systemic antibiotics are to be preferred.

Seborrhoeic dermatitis of the beard may be kept under control by regular washing (Parish & Arndt 1972).

Severe and extensive seborrhoeic dermatitis may tend to relapse. Some patients therefore prefer to use imidazole shampoo to prevent relapse if possible.

Gould *et al.* (1988) have suggested that topical lithium succinate is safe and effective in seborrhoeic dermatitis.

References

Colcott, Fox, T. (1911) Pityriasis. In *A System of Medicine*, vol. 4, p. 202, eds. C. Allbutt & H.D. Rolleston. Macmillan, London.

Gloor, M. (1972) Über Menge und Zusammensetzung der Hautoberflächenlipide beim sogennanten Seborrhoischer Ekzem. *Dermatologische Monatsschrift*. **158**, 759.

Gould, D.J., Davies, M.G. & Kersey, P.J.W. (1988) Topical lithium succinate—a safe and effective treatment for seborrhoeic dermatitis. *British Journal of Dermatology*, **119**, 27.

Hashimoto, I. (1946) Autoimmune phenomena in eczema seborrhoeicum. *Tohoku Journal of Experimental Medicine*, **89**, 45.

Metz, J. & Metz, G. (1975) Zur Ultrastruktur der Epidermis bei Seborrhoeischer Ekzem. *Archiv für dermatologische Forschung*, **252**, 285.

Parish, J.A. & Arndt, K.A. (1972) Seborrhoeic dermatitis of the beard. *British Journal of Dermatology*, **87**, 201.

Parish, L. (1970) L-dopa for seborrhoeic dermatitis. *New England Journal of Medicine*, **283**, 879.

Rook, A. (1954) Seborrhoeic dermatitis. *Practitioner*, **172**, 522.

Shuster, S. & Blatchford, N. (1988) Seborrhoeic dermatitis and dandruff—a fungal disease. *Royal Society of Medicine Publications*, London, p. 1.

Psoriasis of the scalp (References p. 509)

Aetiology

Psoriasis is a genetically determined disorder of the skin. There is some racial variation in its prevalence but few large-scale and reliable surveys have been reported. The prevalence in adults in north-west Europe is about 1.5–2%. The mode of inheritance of psoriasis is not known and there may indeed be more than one genotype.

In the genetically predisposed individual the first attack may develop at any age, but the mean age of onset is in the third decade and psoriasis is uncommon in the first 2 or 3 years of life. The initial attack and subsequent recurrences may be provoked by streptococcal infection, and perhaps by stress but may also occur for no discoverable reason.

The pathogenesis of psoriasis is being extensively studied and good reviews are available (Baker & Wilkinson 1979; Farber & Cox 1977). A long account of this work would be out of place in this book and a brief summary could be misleading.

Pathology

The distinctive histological features of psoriasis are acanthosis with elongation of the reti ridges and absence or reduction of the granular layer. The horny layer is parakeratotic and there are collections of polymorphonuclear lymphocytes (Monro abscesses) in the upper epidermis. The dermal papillae are oedematous. Braun-Falco *et al.* (1979) defined the criteria for the histological differential diagnosis of psoriasis from seborrhoeic dermatitis of the scalp. Features favouring psoriasis were condensed hyperkeratosis with focal parakeratosis, PAS-positive serum inclusions, Monro abscesses within the horny layer, and spongiform pustules and polymorphonuclear leucocytes within the epidermis. The criteria for seborrhoeic dermatitis were irregular acanthosis with relatively thin ortho- or para-keratotic horny layer, spongiosis and spongiotic vesicles, and exocytosis of lymphocytes.

The rate of hair growth is not increased in psoriasis (Comaish 1969). The calibre of the shafts of hairs growing in plaques of psoriasis is significantly reduced (Wyatt & Riggott 1981). Electron microscopic studies (Braun-Falco & Rassner 1966; Orfanos *et al.* 1970; Wyatt *et al.* 1972) showed changes in the hair shafts in psoriasis; the cuticular cells were irregular and dystrophic.

Using a labelling technique Shahrad & Marks (1976) found an increased index only in the upper part of the external root sheath.

Headington *et al.* (1989) noted that sebaceous gland atrophy was a frequent concomitant in the psoriatic lesion, with probable 'down-sizing' of the hair follicle and thinner hair shafts.

Clinical features

The scalp is frequently involved in psoriasis. In children and young adults it is sometimes the first site to be affected and in some patients it remains the only one. In the majority of cases, however, other sites are sooner or later involved. Sometimes the scalp remains constantly affected to some degree over many years, whilst lesions elsewhere may come and go.

The classical feature of psoriasis is a palpable bright pink plaque covered in silvery scale, and such lesions occur in the scalp (Fig. 17.3). However, the earliest changes, particularly in children, may be less distinctive. There may be patchy or a diffuse scaling without any special features, or there may be asbestos-like scale in layers (pityriasis amiantacea). The correct diagnosis may be suspected if there is a family history of psoriasis or if the patient has lesions elsewhere.

Although extensive loss of hair occurs only in the erythrodermic forms of psoriasis, some increased shedding of telogen hairs and some reduction in hair density is common in plaques of psoriasis.

In severe psoriasis of the scalp masses of heaped-up scale form a solid cap which may extend just beyond the hair margin.

Psoriasis is usually non-pruritic but irritation is sometimes severe in the scalp as elsewhere.

Seborrhoeic dermatitis is a common condition in some populations and it frequently involves the scalp, extending further beyond the scalp margins than does psoriasis, spreading behind the ears, to the forehead and into any bald areas of the scalp. In the patient predisposed to psoriasis the lesions of seborrhoeic dermatitis may become increasingly psoriasiform, showing clinical and histological features of both conditions.

Lichen simplex of the nape may be confused with psoriasis, but as with seborrhoeic dermatitis hybrid lesions occur, showing features of both conditions.

Diagnosis

The diagnosis of typical psoriasis is rarely difficult. Atypical lesions suggestive of psoriasis should lead to a thorough examination of the commonly affected sites, including the nails, for traces of psoriasis, even if the patient denies their presence. Small patches on knees or elbows are easily overlooked by the patient.

A very persistent scaly plaque on the bald scalp should be histologically examined to exclude Bowen's disease. Small psoriasiform plaques (even in the hairy scalp) remaining unchanged over many years except perhaps for some slow increase in size, should also suggest Bowen's disease.

Treatment (Dawber 1989)

A detailed explanation of the problems of psoriasis should always be given, and the patient should be reassured that although the tendency to psoriasis cannot be eradicated, the attacks can be controlled and very long complete remissions may occur.

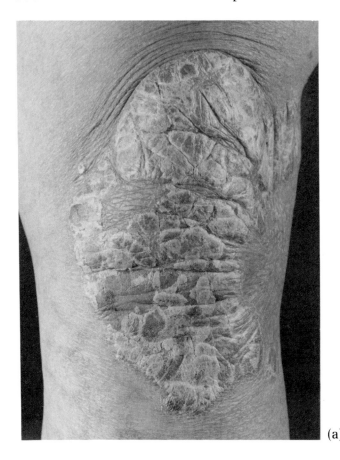

(a)

(b)

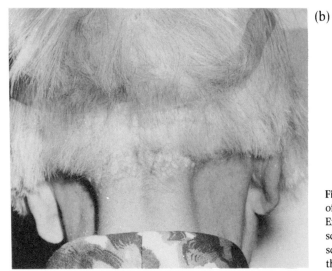

Fig. 17.3 (a) A typical plaque of chronic psoriasis. (b) Extensive psoriasis of the scalp extending below the scalp margin on the nape of the neck.

The commonest cause of treatment failure, particularly in scalp lesions, is the patient's inability to carry out the treatment thoroughly, and the lack of nursing or auxiliary help. In mild cases a tar shampoo may suffice.

In more severe cases Oil of Cade ointment is helpful:

Oil of Cade	6
Precipitated sulphur	2
Salicylic acid	2
Emulsifying ointment to	100.

Other preparations which may be effective when chronic lesions are present are the proprietary tar or dithranol preparations. These should be rubbed into the patches and washed out after a few hours.

Corticosteroid preparations are often useful, easy to comply with and are less likely to cause symptomatic atrophy within the scalp.

Patients with psoriasis require careful supervision. The disease itself can be a cause of severe stress and full discussion of the problems arising as a result forms an important part of treatment.

Where routine topical treatments prove inadequate then many of the general antipsoriatic measures should be considered, even X-irradiation (Dawber 1989).

References

Baker, H. & Wilkinson, D.S. (1979) Psoriasis. In *Textbook of Dermatology*, 3rd edn., p. 1315, eds. A. Rook, D.S. Wilkinson & F.J. Ebling. Blackwell Scientific Publications, Oxford.

Braun-Falco, O., Heilgemeir, G.P. & Lincke-Plewig, H. (1979) Histologische Differentialdiagnose von Psoriasis vulgaris und seborrhoischem Ekzem des Kapillitium. *Hautarzt*, **30**, 478.

Braun-Falco, O. & Rassner, B. (1966) Haarwurzelmuster bei Psoriasis vulgaris der Kopfhaut. *Archiv für klinische und experimentelle Dermatologie*, **225**, 42.

Comaish, S. (1969) Autoradiographic studies of hair growth in various dermatoses: investigation of a possible circadian rhythm in normal hair growth. *British Journal of Dermatology*, **81**, 283.

Dawber, R.P.R. (1989) Aspects of treatment of scalp psoriasis. *Journal of Dermatological Treatment*, **1** (2), 1.

Farber, E.M. & Cox, A.J. (1977) *Psoriasis. Proceedings of the Second International Symposium*. Yorke Medical Books, New York.

Headington, J.T., Gupta, A.K., Goldfarb, M.T. *et al.* (1989) A morphometric and histological study of the scalp in psoriasis. *Archives of Dermatology*, **125**, 639.

Orfanos, C., Mahler, G. & Christenhurz, R. (1970) Verhornungstörungen am Haar bei Psoriasis: Eine Studie im Raster-Elektronmikroscop. *Archiv für klinische und experimentelle Dermatologie*, **236**, 107.

Shahrad, P. & Marks, R. (1976) Hair follicle kinetics in psoriasis. *British Journal of Dermatology*, **94**, 7.

Wyatt, E., Bottoms, E. & Comaish, S. (1972) Abnormal hair shafts in psoriasis in scanning electron microscopy. *British Journal of Dermatology*, **87**, 368.

Wyatt, E. & Riggott, J.M. (1981) The influence of psoriasis on hair diameter. *British Journal of Dermatology*, **115**, 96.

Lichenification and lichen simplex (References p. 512)

Lichenification is a 'leathery' thickening of skin resulting from repeated rubbing and scratching. The surface skin lines and creases are exaggerated within the abnormal area. Lichenification may occur secondary to many pruritic dermatoses or develop as a localized abnormality without any predisposing diseases, the so-called lichen simplex or primary lichenification.

The pathological changes vary from site to site. Typical findings include hyperkeratosis and acanthosis; localized areas of spongiosis and parakeratosis may be present. All components of the epidermis are hyperplastic; though labelling indices are usually 25–30% greater than normal, the transit time of the thickened epidermis is longer than that of psoriasis (Marks & Wells 1973a,b). The dermal changes vary according to the primary cause and the duration of the lesion. A mixed chronic inflammatory cell infiltrate is usually present in the upper dermis sometimes associated with fibrosis and Schwann cell proliferation.

Emotional tensions play an important part in favouring the development and persistence of lichenification which may indeed persist long after the primary disease has remitted. This fact is the basis of the often-used synonym neurodermatitis. Not all individuals produce lichenified skin on rubbing and scratching; atopic subjects are particularly prone, as are the Mongoloid race. In many subjects the same disease and chronic rubbing and scratching produce nodules—nodular prurigo or nodular lichenification. Negroid subjects frequently produce papular and follicular lichenification.

The main symptom is pruritus which may be very severe despite minimal signs. The most common diseases predisposing to secondary lichenification are atopic dermatitis, nummular eczema, pruritus ani and vulvae, lichen planus, seborrhoeic dermatitis, stasis dermatitis, asteototic eczema and, rarely, psoriasis. In the condition termed actinic reticuloid (Ive *et al.* 1969) chronic photodermatoses and psoriasis may cause a lichenified appearance in areas where little scratching and rubbing occur. Lichenified patches may occur on any pruritic area that is amenable to rubbing and scratching.

Lichen simplex is defined as localized lichenification due to rubbing and scratching of skin previously apparently normal, i.e. primary lichenification (Schaffer & Beerman 1951; Cleveland 1936). In general, the local physical signs and histopathological changes are the same as in secondary lichenification.

Lichen simplex is rare before puberty, the peak incidence being between 30 and 50; women are more frequently affected than men. In lichen simplex only a few lesions are present, in 50% of cases only one lesion occurs. The commonest area affected are the nape of the neck, the shin and the calves, the upper thigh, the extensor surface of the forearms and various sites on the external genitalia (Figs 17.4, 17.5).

Lichen nuchae occurs as a single plaque on the nape of the neck; it may be very scaly and mimic psoriasis and attacks of secondary bacterial infection are common. On other parts of the scalp the presenting sign may be localized breaking of hair associated with underlying pruritus and scaling. This pattern is particularly likely to affect the temporal and parietal areas of the scalp. Allergic or irritant reactions to hair cosmetics must be carefully excluded.

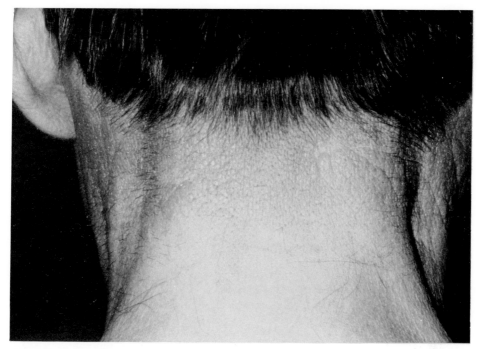

Fig. 17.4 Lichen simplex of the nape: confluent lichenoid papules.

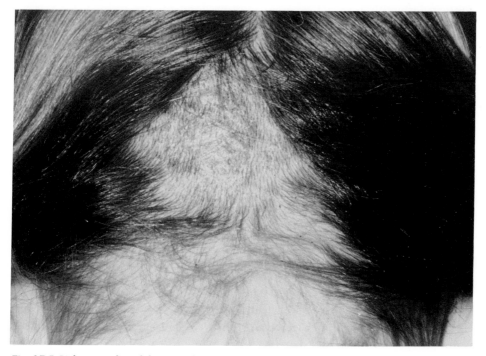

Fig. 17.5 Lichen simplex of the nape: hair loss from rubbing.

Treatment
Primary lichenification requires careful psychological assessment and treatment; the patient should be given insight into the underlying stresses and an understanding of the need to break the scratching habit. Topical treatment needs to be anti-inflammatory, occlusive in sites where this is possible such as the limbs, and antibacterial if secondary infection is present; topical steroid creams are most commonly used whilst intra-lesional triamcinolone may be effective in recalcitrant cases. Superficial X-irradiation may be helpful in the most recalcitrant cases.

References
Cleveland, D.E.H. (1936) Lichen simplex chronicus. *Archives of Dermatology and Syphilology*, **33**. 316.
Ive, F.A. Magnus, I.A., Warin, R.P. & Wilson-Jones, E. (1969) 'Actinic reticuloid', a chronic dermatosis associated with severe photosensitivity and the histological resemblance to lymphoma. *British Journal of Dermatology*, **81**, 469.
Marks, R. & Wells, G.C. (1973a) Lichen simplex; morphodynamic correlates. *British Journal of Dermatology*, **88**, 249.
Marks, R. & Wells, G.C. (1973b) A histochemical profile of lichen simplex. *British Journal of Dermatology*, **88**, 557.
Shaffer, B. & Beerman, H. (1951) Lichen simplex chronicus and its variants. *Archives of Dermatology and Syphilology*, **64**, 340.

Contact dermatitis (References p. 517)

Contact dermatitis (contact eczema) may be conveniently defined, for present purposes, as an inflammatory condition of the skin caused by an external agent. If photodermatitis is excluded, two broad divisions are recognized, irritant and allergic dermatitis.

Irritant dermatitis
A skin irritant is defined as a substance that is capable of causing cell damage in most people if it is applied for a sufficient length of time, frequently enough and in great enough concentration. The scalp is generally considered to be resistant to irritant damage, possibly because of a relatively thick epidermis and horny layer; also, the scalp has a rapid epidermal 'turn-over time', i.e. it replaces its natural barrier layer relatively quickly after any cell damage. It should be noted, however, that substances which are recognized as highly irritant on other sites are rarely applied to the scalp frequently enough, for long enough or in high-enough concentrations. For example, hairdressers frequently develop irritant contact dermatitis of the hands from contact with shampoos, but the dilute shampoo solution applied to the scalp does not cause dermatitis. Shampoos may rarely irritate the skin of the forehead and scalp margins in susceptible individuals, such as atopic eczema subjects, and inflame the conjunctival surface of the eye.

In practice, the misuse of thioglycollates, bleaching preparations and heat are the commonest causes of irritant dermatitis of the scalp. It is important to remember that irritant dermatitis affects only skin that has been in direct contact with the offending agent.

Allergic dermatitis
Allergic dermatitis implies dermatitis due to the development of allergy to a substance previously applied to the skin. Most substances causing dermatitis of this type are of small molecular weight, less than 10,000, and act only as partial antigens or haptens. To form complete antigens they must combine with epidermal protein. The immunological response requires the presence of epidermal Langerhans cells to recognize the allergen and normal regional lymph glands for the cell-mediated antibody response to occur in the epidermis. The dermatitis developing in this way may spread away from the site of contact, particularly if the allergen is applied repeatedly. The scalp is relatively resistant to allergens; as with irritants, this resistance may be due to the thick horny layer but this cannot be the only factor since eczematous contact allergy is not entirely dose related.

Less well-defined is the occurrence of immediate-type hypersensitivity with or without concurrent eczematous allergy (Calnan & Shuster 1963; Cronin 1979).

Clinical appearance
Irritant dermatitis affecting the scalp may commence with burning, or soreness and tightness of the scalp, within a short time of contact with the irritant. Liquid irritants most typically cause these symptoms at the scalp margins. The signs vary from slight erythema to marked oedema and exudation. Complete resolution usually takes no more than a few days. Hair breakage may occur from certain substances, e.g. thioglycollates; if the scalp inflammation is severe enough diffuse hair loss may occur days to weeks after the insult, due to local inflammatory telogen effluvium.

Allergic dermatitis; the clinical picture varies considerably. Irritation of the scalp or scalp margins with little visible change, and occipital lichenification due to chronic scratching may be the only signs. More severe cases present with acute, sub-acute or chronic eczema either localized to the scalp and adjacent areas or spreading to affect other parts of the head and neck. Acute signs may mimic angio-oedema, bilateral erysipelas or dermatomyositis if peri-orbital oedema occurs. Many weeks, rarely months, may elapse between the onset and the spontaneous cure of allergic dermatitis.

Agents causing contact dermatitis
In a report of 70 cases of cosmetic allergy, Schorr (1974) found that six were due to hair dyes and rinses and that two were caused by shampoos.

Hair dyes. Approximately 40% of women in the USA use some form of hair dye (Corbett & Menkart 1973).

Vegetable dyes are still used though less commonly than in the past. Henna does not cause eczematous allergy but may precipitate allergic rhinitis and asthma (Cronin 1979). Chamomile is still present in some shampoos and rinses; the dye-stuff is apigenin (trihydroxyflavone). It is a potent sensitizer in those handling the plant but not when used cosmetically.

Metallic dyes are now only rarely used. Some contain nickel and chromium which are, however, securely chelated into complex molecules.

Temporary dyes (colour rinses) and semi-permanent dyes are generally safe products though the latter are often marketed as shampoos and may give an irritant reaction in susceptible individuals, or allergic dermatitis due to *o*-nitropara-phenylenediamine (ONPPD).

Permanent dyes are more prone to cause allergic sensitization than any other hair cosmetic preparation (Fig. 17.6). Paraphenylenediamine (PPD) may cause very acute eczematous dermatitis of the head and neck though hand dermatitis in those handling PPD is the commonest pattern. PPD is a potent sensitizer; Kligman (1966) using the maximization test and 10% PPD was able to sensitize all 24 subjects tested. Such is the notoriety of PPD that it has been banned as a hair dye in many countries; this stringent abolition may soon be relaxed since the European

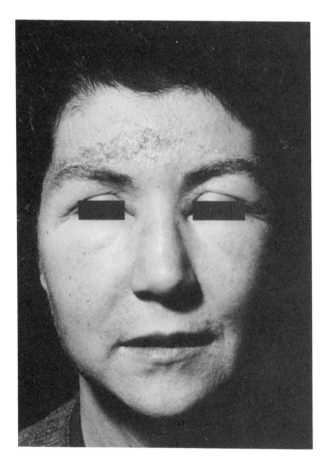

Fig. 17.6 Allergic contact dermatitis from hair dye.

Economic Community has decreed that hair dyes may contain up to 6% PPD. Cases of PPD allergy are now less common, partly from better education of hairdressers and users, and also because the chemical reaction during the dyeing process is more accurately controlled and completed, leaving little or no free PPD. Fully polymerized PPD is harmless and inert; reactions to dyed wig hair do not therefore occur. In practice, hair dyed by individuals at home is more likely to produce allergy in the user or in those afterwards in contact with the hair, due to residual free dye remaining on the hair if adequate care is not exercised during the dying process. Paratoluenediamine (PTD) is 50% less likely to cause allergy than PPD.

If allergy to a hair dye is suspected, patch testing should be carried out to 1% ONPPD, 1% PPD and 1% PTD (Fisher 1989). Cross-reactivity may be a problem; thus para-dye dermatitis may be potentiated by certain antihistamines (MacKie & MacKie 1964) and rubber antioxidants (Schønning & Hjorth, 1969).

Hair bleaches. These are commonly sold as twin packs containing hydrogen peroxide and ammonium persulphate. The latter is potentially both an irritant and a sensitizer; Calnan and Shuster (1963) showed it to be a histamine releaser causing facial swelling and scalp itching—this is more likely in dermographic subjects. The propensity of persulphate to liberate histamine was confirmed by Mahzoon *et al.* (1977). If too-high concentrations are applied for too long, an acute irritant reaction may occur with hair breakage. For patch testing, 1% aqueous ammonium persulphate should be used.

Permanent wave solutions. Sensitivity reactions to thioglycollates are extremely rare though mild transient irritant dermatitis is not uncommon (Fisher 1989). Necrosis of the scalp has been described from incorrect use of a thioglycollate solution, compounded by attempted reversal of the reaction with a borate neutralizer (Ippen & Seubert 1975); necrosis may have been due to the heat generated.

Hair straighteners and depilatories. These often contain thioglycollates but are less likely to cause significant reactions than permanent wave solutions (Foussereau & Benezra 1970).

Setting lotions. The main ingredient is usually polyvinylpyrrolidone which seems to have no allergic potential. If a reaction to such lotions occurs it is more likely to be due to added dyes.

Hair tonics, stimulants and restorers. Such preparations are generally innocuous. Kerner *et al.* (1973) described burning and exudation of the scalp due to a stimulant containing century plant extract which was used on the scalp in common baldness.

Shampoos. Since they are applied in dilute solution for a short time irritant reactions are rare though shampoos are the commonest cause of hand dermatitis in hairdressers.

Men's hair creams. Allergy to perfume, lanolin or preservations may occur.

Shaving preparations. The recorded cases of irritant and allergic reactions have been to perfumes found mostly in after-shave lotions.

Hair nets. These are no longer popular but may still be worn by some older women. Calnan *et al.* (1958) described 27 cases of nylon hair net dermatitis; 23 of the patients were over 40 years of age. The eruption affected the neck, ears and frontal hairline, simulating seborrhoeic dermatitis and lichen simplex. All the cases showed positive patch tests either to the net or to its marginal elastic. Azo- and anthroquinone dyes, PPD and certain disperse dyes are the commonest specific allergens: several of the cases had noted skin reactions to nylon stockings, clothing or gloves. Six other cases of hairnet dermatitis were documented, by Cronin (1980).

Hat-band dermatitis. The site affected by the dermatitis varies, though most cases involve the forehead (Fig. 17.7). Leather used to be the most frequent allergen (Bett

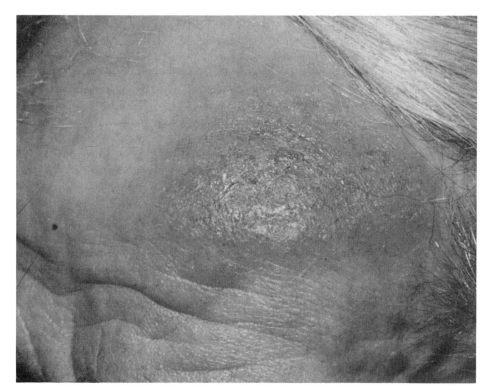

Fig. 17.7 Hat-band dermatitis.

1958) but fabric or plastic are now the more likely offenders. Dermatitis has been described from laurel oil used to add lustre to felt hats (Foussereau *et al.* 1967). Some hat bands have a varnish finish containing colophony.

Wig reactions. Ill-fitting wigs frequently cause friction and irritant damage to localized parts of the scalp, typically under the adhesion band. Allergic dermatitis may occur to adhesive substances; allergy cannot develop against completely polymerized hair dye in wigs.

References

Bett, D.C.G. (1958) The potassium dichromate patch test. *Transactions of St. John's Hospital Dermatological Society.* **40**, 41.

Calnan, C.D., Marten, R.H. & Wilson, H.T.H. (1958) Nylon hairnet dermatitis. *British Medical Journal*, **ii**, 544.

Calnan, C.D. & Shuster, S. (1963) Reactions to ammonium persulphate. *Archives of Dermatology*, **88**, 812.

Corbett, J.F. & Menkart, J. (1973) Hair colouring. *Cutis*, **12**, 190.

Cronin, E. (1979) Immediate type hypersensitivity to henna. *Contact Dermatitis*, **5**, 198.

Cronin, E. (1980) *Contact Dermatitis*, 1st edn. Churchill Livingstone, Edinburgh.

Fisher, A.A. (1989) Management of hairdressers sensitized to hair dyes or permanent wave solutions. *Cutis*, **43**, 316.

Foussereau, J., Benezra, C.I. & Durisson, G. (1967) Contact dermatitis from laurel. I. Clinical aspects. *Transactions of St. John's Hospital Dermatological Society*, **53**, 141.

Foussereau, J. & Benezra, C.I. (1970) *Les Eczemas Allergiques Professionals*, p. 385. Masson, Paris.

Ippen, H. & Scubert, A. (1975) Kopfhautnekrosen durch Haarbehandlung—eine Erklärungsmöglichkeit, *Hautarzt*, **26**, 598.

Kerner, J., Mitchell, J. & Mailbach, H.I. (1973) Irritant contact dermatitis from *Agave americana* L. *Archives of Dermatology*, **108**, 102.

Kligman, A. (1966) The identification of contact allergens by human assay. *Journal of Investigative Dermatology*, **47**, 393.

MacKie, B.S. & MacKie, L.S. (1964) Cross-sensitivity in dermatitis due to hair dyes. *Australian Journal of Dermatology*, **7**, 189.

Mahzoon, S., Yamamoto, S. & Greaves, M.W. (1977) Response of the skin to ammonium persulphate, *Acta Dermato-Venereologica*, **57**, 125.

Schønning, L., & Hjorth, N. (1969) Cross-sensitivity between hair dyes and rubber chemicals. *Berufsdermatosen*, **17**, 100.

Schorr, W.F. (1974) Cosmetic allergy: diagnosis, incidence and management. *Cutis*, **14**, 844.

Acne necrotica (References p. 519)

History and nomenclature

The variability of this clinical syndrome no doubt accounts for the multiplicity of terms applied to it. In current use for two clinical variants are acne frontalis, suggested by Hebra, and acne necrotica, suggested by Boeck. The acne pilaris of Bazin and the acne varioliformis of Hebra are commonly regarded as redundant synonyms (Pignot 1953).

Acne miliaris necrotica of Sabouraud is a third clinical variant, with some distinctive features.

Aetiology
These syndromes have been regarded as a folliculitis, probably of staphylococcal origin, occurring in seborrhoeic subjects with a possible allergic hypersensitivity to this organism (Pignot 1953). There appears to be no recent work substantiating this hypothesis and it is perhaps wisest to consider these syndromes as being of unknown origin, with stress often incriminated in precipitating recurrences (Calnan & O'Neill 1952). Men are affected more often than women; most patients are aged 30–50 but cases occur at any age past puberty.

Pathology
The histological changes are not pathognomonic. There is a folliculitis, complicated in the more severe lesions by necrosis destroying the follicle and the neighbouring dermis. Some lesions submitted to biopsy show only infected excoriations.

Clinical features (Müller 1964)
Acne necrotica and its variant acne frontalis present as indolent papulopustules with central necrosis, healing slowly to leave varioliform scars. They may be slightly painful and are sometimes pruritic. They occur most characteristically along the frontal hairs, but also involve the scalp where they may leave small patches of cicatricial alopecia; less often they occur on the cheeks and neck or on the chest and back (Stritzler *et al.* 1951). Untreated the condition runs a long course, although there may be only a small number of active lesions present at any one time.

Acne necrotica miliaris (Montgomery 1937) may co-exist with the forms just described, but much more commonly occurs alone. Pruritus, which may be distressingly severe, takes the patient to his doctor. The primary lesions are minute follicular vesicles but these are rapidly excoriated. There may be a few or many. New lesions continue to develop at irregular intervals, but the pruritus seems often to be disproportionately severe in relation to the objective change.

Diagnosis
In acne necrotica the distribution of the lesions and their orphology serve to differentiate such diseases, now uncommon in temperate regions, as papulo-necrotic tuberculides and tertiary syphilis.

The pruritic miliary form should never be diagnosed unless pediculosis and dermatitis herpetiformis have been excluded, the former by searching for the lice, and the latter by the presence of lesions elsewhere.

Treatment
All forms show a temporary response to a broad spectrum antibiotic and such treatment is useful in severe cases. Many patients find it necessary to take a small maintenance dose, e.g. oxytetracycline 250 mg twice daily, as in acne vulgaris. Topical corticosteroid/antibiotic preparations are of limited value.

References

Calnan, C.D. & O'Neill, D. (1952) Some observations on acne necrotica. *Transactions of the St. John's Hospital Dermatological Society*, **31**, 12.

Müller, H. (1964) Beitrag zur Therapie der Akne nekroticans. *Dermatologische Wochenschrift*, **149**, 495.

Montgomery, H. (1937) Acne necrotica miliaris of the scalp. *Acta Dermo-Sifiliograficas*, **36**, 10.

Pignot, M. (1953) L'Acné nécrotique du cuir chevelu. In *Affections de la Chevelure et du Cuir Chevelu*, p. 132, ed. A. Desex, Masson, Paris.

Stritzler, C., Friedman, R. & Loveman, A.B. (1951) Acne necrotica. Relation to acne necrotica miliaris and response to penicillin and other antibiotics. *AMA Archives of Dermatology and Syphilology*, **64**, 464.

Folliculitis keloidalis nuchae (acne cheloidalis)

This chronic inflammatory folliculitis of the nape of the neck occurs exclusively in males and is certainly more severe and probably also more frequent in Negroids than in Caucasoids. It may begin at any time after puberty, usually between 14 and 25. Many of those affected suffer or have suffered from acne vulgaris, many more have no other skin lesions. The cause of the condition is unknown; a genetic factor is probably implicated. Histologically chronic folliculitis and foreign body granulomata surrounding fragments of hair are the main features.

Follicular papules and pustules develop in irregularly linear clusters on the nape just below the hair line and extend in further crops at long or short intervals towards the occiput. Firm cheloid papules follow the folliculitis and become confluent to form horizontal bands or plaques. These may co-exist with new follicular papules and discharging sinuses.

Treatment with topical antibacterial agents and with systemic antibiotics may possibly restrain the progress of the inflammatory changes but not reliably or completely. The cheloids may be successfully excised by plastic surgery (Cosman & Wolff 1972).

Reference

Cosman, B. & Wolff, M. (1972) Acne keloidasis. *Plastic and Reconstructive Surgery*, **50**, 25.

Pseudofolliculitis (References p. 521)

Pseudofolliculitis is a common inflammatory disorder of the follicles, most commonly occurring when tightly coiled or very curly hair is closely shaved, and the tips of shaved hairs either penetrate the follicular wall or grow back to re-enter the skin near the follicle. Pseudofolliculitis may occur also if the hairs are plucked (Dilaimy 1976) and in such cases is caused by the abnormal regrowth of the hairs in injured follicles. Cocci can sometimes be grown from the lesions, but the condition is primarily mechanical in origin (Straus & Kligman 1956).

Pseudofolliculitis of the beard is extremely common in Negroid men, amongst whom it is almost universal in some degree (Brauner & Flandermeyer 1977) but it

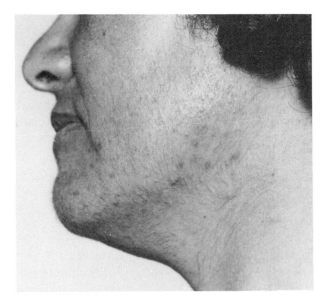

Fig. 17.8 Pseudofolliculitis in a hirsute woman aged 35 years.

occurs in other races and may be seen also in hirsute women (Fig. 17.8). The importance of genetic predisposition has been emphasized (Alexander 1974). It was present extensively in the scalps of four Negroid boys whose heads had been shaved, and regressed spontaneously as the hair regrew (Smith & Odom 1977).

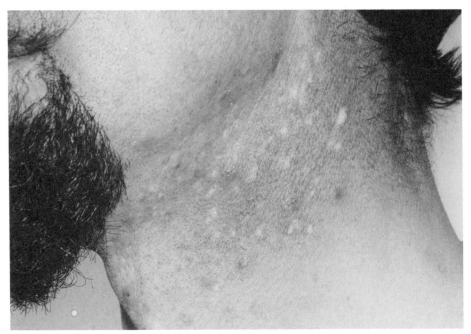

Fig. 17.9 Pseudofolliculitis leaving unsightly scars.

Pseudofolliculitis presents clinically as an eruption of follicular papules or pustules on the sides of the neck and over the angles of the jaw. In some cases unsightly nodules may form and may leave conspicuous scars (Fig. 17.9).

The logical and effective treatment is to stop shaving and there are cases in which this provides the only solution. If wearing a beard is not acceptable to the patient a corticosteroid/antibiotic cream may be helpful in mild cases. In severe cases the use of a chemical depilatory every 3 days may be recommended (Straus & Kligman 1956).

References

Alexander, A.M. (1974) Pseudofolliculitis diathesis. *Archives of Dermatology*, **109**, 729.

Brauner, C.J. & Flandermeyer, L.K. (1977) Pseudofolliculitis barbae. *International Journal of Dermatology*, **16**, 520.

Dilaimy, M. (1976) Pseudofolliculitis of the legs. *Archives of Dermatology*, **112**, 507.

Smith, J.D. & Odom, R.B. (1977) Pseudofolliculitis capitis, *Archives of Dermatology*, **113**, 328.

Straus, J.S. & Kligman, A.M. (1956) Pseudofolliculitis of the beard. *Archives of Dermatology*, **74**, 533.

Pruritus of the scalp

Many inflammatory diseases of the scalp may be associated with itching. It may both precede and accompany the development of allergic reactions to hair dyes and other chemicals and it may accompany urticaria.

Itching of the scalp may be troublesome in psoriasis especially in patients who are under stress or who are depressed. Pityriasis capitis may cause some irritation but in this condition too the irritation is rarely severe except under stress. The scalp may be involved, but seldom sufficiently severely to be a specific cause of complaint in generalized pruritus, the causes of which will not be discussed here. More frequently, in generalized pruritus without visible skin changes, the scalp is spared.

Irritation of the scalp may occur in dermatitis herpetiformis in which the lesions in other parts of the body may suggest the diagnosis.

Persistent irritation of the scalp, particularly in children but also at any age and at all levels of social respectability, may be caused by pediculosis, and in all circumstances lice and their eggs should be carefully sought.

Intense pruritus, temporarily localized to small focal sites is characteristic of acne necrotica which is seen mainly in men working under continuous tension. More diffuse irritation of the scalp, without visible lesions, may occur in either sex.

Itching or tenderness or sometimes other uncomfortable sensations may occur as a prominent symptom of mild androgenetic alopecia in a depressed patient.

The treatment of pruritus of the scalp is the treatment of its cause.

Scalp pain rarely occurs as a symptom with no overt disease—most typically in adult women.

Hair casts (References, p. 523)

Definition

Hair casts (peripilar keratin casts) are firm, yellowish-white accretions ensheathing, but not attached to, scalp hairs and freely movable up and down the affected shafts (Kligman 1957).

Such lesions found in scaly and seborrhoeic disorders of the scalp had previously been termed 'hair eaters' (Crocker 1932).

Pathology

In cross-section casts are composed of a central layer of retained internal root sheath and an outer thick keratinous layer. Scalp histology shows the follicular openings to be packed with parakeratotic squames which break off at intervals to form hair casts.

Casts are found quite commonly in scaly, mainly parakeratotic conditions of the scalp such as psoriasis, pityriasis capitas, seborrhoeic dermatitis and pityriasis amiantacea (Dawber 1979). Cases have been described in association with traction hair styles (Rollins 1961; Crovato *et al.* 1980) and hair sprays (Scott 1959).

Clinical findings

Hair casts may occur as an isolated abnormality unrelated to any overt scalp disease (Figs 17.10, 17.11); such cases may mimic pediculosis capitis (Brunner & Facq 1957) and have been termed pseudonits (Keipert 1974; Kohn 1977). Girls and young women are most commonly affected; hundreds of casts may develop within a few days. No cause is known but sex-linked inheritance has been suggested (Kligman 1957). It is possible that this type may represent an unusual manifestation of psoriasis.

If patients with scaly parakeratotic diseases of the scalp complain of persistent dandruff which resists apparently adequate treatment this is likely to be due to multiple hair casts.

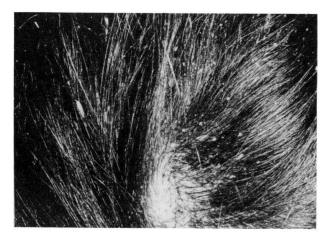

Fig. 17.10 Hair casts.

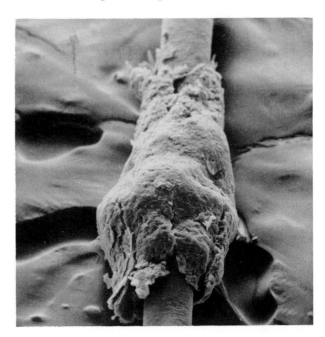

Fig. 17.11 Hair cast in the scanning electron microscope.

Diagnosis

In the absence of associated scalp disease, casts may be mistaken for pediculosis capitis, trichorrhexis nodosa or hair knots (Dawber 1974). Of these nodal shaft abnormalities, only hair casts are freely movable along the hair.

Treatment

Any causative scalp disease must be treated. Keratolytic preparations and shampoos that readily improve scalp scaling frequently fail to remove casts; prolonged brushing and combing is necessary to slide casts off the affected hairs (Bowyer 1974; Dawber 1977).

References

Bowyer, A. (1974) Peripilar keratin casts. *British Journal of Dermatology*, **90**, 231.

Brunner, M.J. & Facq, J.M. (1957) A pseudoparasite of scalp hair. *Archives of Dermatology*, **75**, 583.

Crocker, R. (1932) In *Jadassohn's Handbuch der Haut und Geschlechtskrankheiten*, vol. 13. Springer-Verlag, Berlin.

Crovato, F., Rebora, A. & Crosti, C. (1980) Hair casts. *Dermatologica*, **160**, 281.

Dawber, R.P.R. (1974) Knotting of scalp hair. *British Journal of Dermatology*, **91**, 169.

Dawber, R.P.R. (1979) The scalp and hair care in psoriasis. *Journal of the Psoriasis Association*, **16**, 5.

Keipert, J.A. (1974) Peripilar keratin casts (pseudonits) and psoriasis. *Medical Journal of Australia*, **i**, 218.

Kligman, A.M. (1957) Hair casts. *Archives of Dermatology*, **75**, 509.

Kohn, S.R. (1977) Hair casts or pseudonits. *Journal of the American Medical Association*, **2–8**, 2058.

Rollins, T.G. (1961) Traction folliculitis with hair casts and alopecia. *American Journal of Diseases of Children*, **101**, 131.

Scott, M.J. (1959) Peripilar keratin casts. *Archives of Dermatology*, **79**, 654.

Rosacea (References p. 525)

Aetiology
Rosacea is a common disorder affecting principally the facial skin. Episodes of flushing are followed by persistent telangiectasia, and development of papules and pustules. The cause of the condition is unknown. The traditionally accepted association between rosacea and gastrointestinal disease has not been confirmed (Søbye 1950; Marks *et al.* 1967). Psychological factors are widely believed to play some part in rosacea but there is not reliable evidence that they cause it (Marks 1968) although some secondary anxiety and depression are common.

Females are affected more frequently than males and usually between the ages of 30 and 50 but earlier and later onset are not unusual.

Exposure to light appears to play some part in the pathogenesis of rosacea as suggested by the predominant involvement of light-exposed skin, by the peak hospital attendance during the spring and early summer and by the histological changes. On the other hand rosacea is not confined to exposed skin.

Pathology
The papules consist of a pleomorphic lymphohistiocytic infiltrate. Granulomatous changes may be present. The dermis shows a higher degree of elastotic change than is seen in the facial skin of control subjects (Marks & Harcourt-Webster 1969).

Clinical features
Telangiectasia, papules and pustules occur in very variable proportions. There may be extensive and conspicuous telangiectasia as the only change, or this may be associated with dull red papules or the papules may predominate and the telangiectasia be relatively mild. The cheeks and the forehead are most commonly affected. Papules in areas other than the face (the limbs, sholders and the chest) are more frequent when the facial rosacea is severe, but can also occur in the presence of only mild facial changes (Marks & Wilson-Jones 1969; Röckl *et al.* 1969).

Involvement of the bald scalp (Gajewska 1975) by papules, pustules or telangiectasia is not uncommon, and may accompany severe or mild facial rosacea (Fig. 17.12)

Untreated rosacea may run a very long course and be a source of intense embarrassment to the patient. Moreover in a proportion of cases, and not necessarily in the more severe cases, ocular involvement may lead to keratitis.

Diagnosis (Steigleder 1971)
Diagnostic difficulties are likely only when rosacea of the scalp accompanies minimal facial lesions.

Treatment
The use of potent topical steroids should be avoided for they intend to increase the telangiectasia and to give rise to a troublesome folliculitis. Oral tetracycline is the

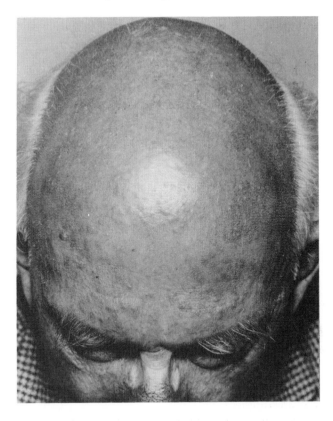

Fig. 17.12 Rosacea of the
bald scalp in an elderly man.

treatment of choice, unless contra-indicated by pregnancy or the possibility of
pregnancy. Most cases will respond to oxytetracycline 250 mg twice daily for 3–6
months. About 20% relapse rapidly when the antibiotic is discontinued, and some
others do so within a few months, but some remain symptom-free for long periods
(Knight & Vickers 1975). Oral erythromycin or clotrimazole are alternative
remedies where required.

Topical metronidasol has recently shown promising results.

References

Gajewska, M. (1975) Rosacea of common male baldness. *British Journal of Dermatology*, **93**, 65.
Knight, A.G. & Vickers, C.F.H. (1975) A follow-up of tetracycline treated rosacea. *British Journal of Dermatology*, **93**, 577.
Marks, R. (1968) Concepts in the pathogenesis of rosacea. *British Journal of Dermatology*, **80**, 170.
Marks, R., Beard, R.J., Clark, M.L., Kwok, M. & Robertson, W.B. (1967) Gastrointestinal observations in rosacea. *Lancet*, **i**, 739.
Marks, R. & Harcourt-Webster J.N. (1969) Histopathology of rosacea. *Archives of Dermatology*, **160**, 683.
Marks, R. & Wilson-Jones, E. (1969) Disseminated rosacea. *British Journal of Dermatology*, **81**, 16.
Röckl, H., Scheren, M. (1969) Rosacea mit extrafacialer Lokalisation. *Hautarzt*, **20**, 349.
Søbye, P. (1950) Aetiology and pathogenesis of rosacea. *Acta Dermato-Venereologica (Stockholm)*, **30**, 117.
Steigleder, G.K. (1971) Differentiale diagnose der Rosacea. *Hautarzt*, **22**, 91.

Rare diseases which characteristically affect the scalp

Dissecting cellulitis (References p. 527)

History and nomenclature
This rare disease was first described by Nobl of Vienna in 1905. Three years later Hoffmann (1908) gave it the name perifolliculitis capitis abscedens et suffodiens, by which it is still sometimes known. In English-speaking countries the term 'dissecting cellulitis of the scalp' (Barney 1931) is usually preferred.

Aetiology
Dissecting cellulitis occurs predominantly in males between 18 and 40 and more often in Negroids than in Caucasoids. Its cause is unknown. No specific organism has been isolated from the lesions, and although the process has much in common with acne conglobata, with which it may co-exist, the latter too is of unknown origin. The description of the pathological process as a 'keratinous granuloma' (Moyer & Williams 1962) throws no light on the source of the follicular disruption.

Some authorities have suggested that this entity may be a scalp form of hidradenitis suppurativa—apocrine gland disease (Ebling 1986).

Pathology
The follicles are destroyed by an intense folliculitis, which is succeeded by a chronic granulomatous infiltrate containing foreign-body giant cells.

Clinical features (Hoffmann 1908; Carmine 1962)
Firm skin-coloured nodules develop near the vertex, and later become softer and fluctuant. By confluence the nodules form tubular ridges in an irregularly cerebriform pattern, on a red and oedematous background. Thin blood-stained pus exudes from crusted sinuses, and pressure on one region of the scalp may cause the discharge of pus from a sinus in a neighbouring intercommunicating ridge. There is patchy loss of hair. In some cases cervical adenitis may develop, but it is usually absent even when the disease is acute (Moyer & Williams 1962).

The extent of the disease is variable but its course is prolonged with partial remission and acute exacerbations. Depressed scars at the sites of healed nodules may be seen in areas still active. Spontaneous recovery can occur, when the scarring determines the cosmetic prognosis; hair shed from temporarily oedematous skin regrows. Squamous carcinoma is a rare late complication of dissecting cellulitis (Curry *et al.* 1981).

Diagnosis
The follicular pustules of a ringworm infection should not cause confusion. In cutis verticis gyrata inflammatory changes are usually absent, and if present are follicular and only a minor and inconsistent feature of the disease.

Treatment

This is most unsatisfactory. Some authors have found no response to antibiotics (Moyer & Williams 1962) and this is certainly to be expected in the later stages of the disease. At an early stage oxytetracycline or clindamycin reduces the inflammatory reaction, and may in severe cases be combined with systemic corticosteroids. 'Scalping' and grafting have been recommended in intractable chronic cases (Moschella *et al.* 1967).

References

Barney, R.E. (1931) Dissecting cellulitis of the scalp. *Archives of Dermatology and Syphilology*, **23**, 503.

Carmine, R.L. (1962) Perifolliculitis capitis abscedens et suffodiens. *Scottish Medical Journal*, 7, 488.

Curry, S.S., Gaither, D.H. & King, L.E. (1981) Squamous carcinoma arising in dissecting perifolliculitis of the scalp. *Journal of the American Academy of Dermatology*, **4**, 673.

Ebling, F.J.G. (1986) Hair follicles and associated glands as androgen targets. *Clinics in Endocrinology and Metabolism*, **15** (2), 319.

Hoffmann, E. (1908) Sitzungsberichte. *Dermatologische Zeitschrift*, **15**, 122.

Moschella, C.L., Klein, M.H. & Miller, R.J. (1967) Perifolliculitis capitis abscedens et suffodiens. *Archives of Dermatology*, **96**, 195.

Moyer, D.G. & Williams, R.M. (1962) Perifolliculitis capitis abscedens et suffodiens. *Archives of Dermatology*, **85**, 378.

Nobl, G. (1905) Verhandlungen der wiener dermatologischen Gesellschaft, *Archiv für Dermatologie und Syphilologie*, **74**, 80.

Cutis verticis gyrata (References p. 529)

History and nomenclature

The term 'cutis verticis gyrata' describes the hypertrophy and folding of the skin of the scalp, to present a gyrate or cerebriform appearance. The term was proposed by Unna in 1907, but many cases had previously been reported under other diagnostic labels (see Polan & Butterworth (1953) for historical review). Cutis verticis gyrata (CVG) is now used by authorities on mental deficiency to describe the distinctive disorder of which the scalp changes are one feature, and which in dermatological texts has been often referred to as 'Primary' or 'Idiopathic' CVG. Dermatologists on the other hand use the term to describe a morphological syndrome with many causes. The French term pachydermie plicaturée invites further confusion with pachydermoperiostosis, of which CVG is a feature (Touraine & Golé 1938; Touraine 1955; Venencie *et al.* 1988).

Pathology

The essential abnormality appears to be overgrowth of the scalp in relation to the underlying skull. Some predisposing factor must be postulated since it occurs in only a small proportion of cases of each of the conditions with which it is associated. The histological findings depend on the essential disease. The naevoid forms usually prove to be melanocytic. Biopsies in the primary form of CVG (Paulson & Dudley 1966) showed possible sebaceous hyperplasia, but no obvious excess of collagen.

Aetiology and clinical features

Primary CVG. This syndrome, which occurs almost exclusively in males, is probably genetically determined, but its mode of inheritance is uncertain (Åkesson 1965a). In one pedigree sex-linked recessive inheritance seemed possible (Åkesson 1965b) but most cases appear to be sporadic. It has been reported in association with Darier's disease and with tuberose sclerosis. It accounts for 0.5% of the retarded population in Sweden (Åkesson 1964), Scotland (MacGillivray 1967) and the United States (Paulson 1974), and for 1–2% of institutionalized severely retarded males. The prevalence of the condition may be still higher since there is evidence that at least some patients with the Lennox–Gastart syndrome, retardation with an electroencephalograph showing slow and irregular space and wave complexes, later develop CVG (Paulson 1974).

The longitudinal and irregularly parallel folds of the scalp may appear in late childhood or at puberty and slowly become more accentuated. The IQ is rarely over 35 and cerebral palsy (spastic diplegia) and epilepsy are present (Kratter 1958; Berg & Windrath-Scott 1962; Åkesson 1964).

Pachydermoperiostosis. This genetically determined syndrome also occurs mainly in men and has often been confused with CVG. It differs from it in several particulars. The scalp is folded but the skin of the face is affected, as is that of the hands and feet. The cutaneous changes, which are accompanied by thickening of the phalanges and of the long bones of the limbs, progress for 10–15 years, then become static.

Acromegaly. Mild degrees of CVG are not uncommon in acromegaly, but more severe forms have been reported (Zeisler & Wieder 1940; Hung-Chiung 1955; Serfling & Foelsche 1959).

Other endocrine disorders. Rarely, CVG has been associated with cretinism or myxoedema, but the significance of these case reports is uncertain (Polan & Butterworth 1953).

Naevi. Naevi may assume a folded or cerebriform structure and thus simulate CVG. The naevus is present at birth and usually covers only a relatively small area (Hammond & Ransome 1937) but may slowly increase in size to cover most of the scalp (e.g. Lenormant 1920). Most of the reported cases have been naevi of melanocytic type, but neurofibromas and fibromas can assume this form (McConnell & Davies 1943).

Treatment

In the majority of cases only symptomatic measures are practicable. Plastic surgery was helpful in CVG in acromegaly (Abu-Jamra & Dinsich 1966) and may of course be indicated in cerebriform naevi.

References

Abu-Jamra, F. & Dinsich, D.F. (1966) Cutis verticis gyrata. *American Journal of Surgery,* **111,** 274.

Åkesson, H.O. (1964) Cutis verticis gyrata and mental deficiency in Sweden. *Acta medica Scandinavica,* **175,** 115.

Åkesson, H.O. (1965a) Cutis verticis gyrata and mental deficiency in Sweden. II. Genetic aspects. *Acta medica Scandinavica,* **177,** 459.

Åkesson, H.O. (1965b) Cutis verticis gyrata, thyroid aplasia and mental deficiency, *Acta Geneticae Medicae et Gemellologiae,* **14,** 200.

Berg, J.M. & Windrath-Scott, A. (1962). Cutis verticis gyrata with particular reference to its association with mental subnormality. *Journal of Mental Deficiency Research,* **6,** 75.

Hammond, G. & Ransome, H.K. (1937) Cerebriform nevus resembling cutis verticis gyrata. *Archives of Surgery,* **35,** 309.

Hung-Chiung, L. (1955) Cutis verticis gyrata associated with acromegaly. *Chinese Medical Journal.* **73,** 320.

Kratten, F.I. (1958) The incidence of cutis verticis gyrata in three low-grade mental defectives. *Journal of Medical Science,* **104,** 850.

Lenormant, C.H. (1920) La pachydermie vorticellée du cuir chevelu. *Annales de Dermatologie et de Syphiligraphie,* **1,** 225.

MacGillivray, R.C. (1967) Cutis verticis gyrata and mental retardation. *Scottish Medical Journal,* **12,** 450.

McConnell, L.H. & Davies, A.J.M. (1943) Massive fibroma of the scalp. *Annals of Surgery,* **118,** 154.

Paulson, G.W. (1974) Cutis verticis gyrata and the Lennox syndrome. *Developmental Medicine and Child Neurology,* **16,** 196.

Paulson, G. & Dudley, A.W. (1966) Cutis verticis gyrata. *Confinia Neurologica,* **28,** 432.

Polan, S. & Butterworth, T. (1953) Cutis verticis gyrata. *American Journal of Mental Deficiency,* **57,** 613.

Serfling, H.J. & Foelsche, W. (1959) Extensive Form einer *Cutis verticis gyrata* bei Hypophysenadenome, *Zentralblatt für Chirurgie,* **84,** 473.

Touraine, A. & Golé, L. (1938) La pachydermie plicaturée avec pachypériostose des extrémités. (État actuel de la question). *Progrès Médical,* **65,** 263.

Touraine, A. (1955) *L'Hérédité en Médecine,* p. 486. Masson, Paris.

Venencie, P.Y., Boffa, G.A., Delmas, P.D. *et al.* (1988) Pachydermoperiostosis with gastric hypertrophy, anaemia and increased serum bone Gla-protein levels. *Archives of Dermatology,* **124,** 1831.

Zeisler, E.P. & Wieder, L.J. (1940) Cutis verticis gyrata and acromegaly. *Archives of Dermatology and Syphilology,* **42,** 1092.

Lipedematous alopecia (References p. 530)

This rare condition has so far been reported only in Negroid women, was first described by Cornbleet in 1935, and was named lipedematous alopecia by Coskey *et al.* (1961). The cause is unknown. Hyperextensible joints were present in one case (Curtis & Heising 1964).

The epidermis shows some atrophy and some follicles are replaced by scar tissue. The subcutaneous fat was increased in thickness at the expense of the dermis. The latter showed some lymphocytic infiltration.

The patients, aged 28–75, complained of itching and soreness or tenderness of the scalp. The hair was sparse and short. The scalp was palpably thickened and was of spongy or boggy consistency.

References

Cornbleet, T. (1935) Cutis verticis gyrata? lipoma? *Archives of Dermatology and Syphilology*, **32**, 688.
Coskey, R.J., Fosnough, R.P. & Finn, G. (1961) Lipedematous alopecia. *Archives of Dermatology*, **84**, 619.
Curtis, J.W. & Heising, R.A. (1964) Lipedematous alopecia associated with skin hyperelasticity. *Archives of Dermatology*, **89**, 819.

Skin diseases in which lesions may occur in the scalp

Ichthyosis

The term ichthyosis is traditionally applied to a heterogeneous group of mainly hereditary disorders characterized in some degree by dryness and scaling of the skin. Ichthyosis vulgaris comprises two different diseases (Wells & Kerr 1965).

Autosomal dominant ichthyosis
In this, the commonest form of ichthyosis, dryness and scaling of the skin become apparent during the second year or later. The changes are most marked on the back and on the exterior aspects of the limbs, and the flexures are spread. The scales are small and white. Keratosis pilaris is frequent, and is often conspicuous. There may be some fine scaling of the scalp but there is no hair loss.

Sex-linked recessive ichthyosis
From early infancy large dark scales are present on the trunk and the side of the face, and tend to encroach on the flexures. The scalp is scaly and the hair is sometimes coarse and dry; there may be patches of cicatricial alopecia (Harris 1947).

References

Harris, H. (1947) A pedigree of sex-linked ichthyosis vulgaris. *Annals of Eugenics*, **14**, 10.
Wells, R.S. & Kerr, C.B. (1965) Genetic classification of ichthyosis. *Archives of Dermatology*, **92**, 1.

Darier's disease (References p. 532)

History and nomenclature
Jean Darier (1856–1938) of the Hôpital St Louis, Paris, described in 1889 the disease which now bears his name. Misinterpretation of the histological findings was responsible for the misleading term 'psorospermosis', which was soon abandoned. 'Keratosis follicularis', the term commonly applied, invites confusion with other forms of follicular keratosis, and the eponymous Darier's disease is therefore preferred.

Aetiology
Darier's disease is a hereditary defect of keratinization determined by an autosomal

dominant gene (Getzler & Flint 1966). Its prevalence in Denmark has been estimated as 1:100,000 (Svendsen & Albuchtron 1959); it has been reported from most countries.

The essential abnormality is a defect in the tonofilament–desmosome complex.

Pathology
Several lacunae appear above the basal cells and thence extend irregularly through the Malpighian layer. Cells around the lucunae undergo premature keratinization and become enlarged and separated from their neighbours; a dark nucleus is surrounded by clear cytoplasm. These cells are the so-called 'corps ronds', which give rise to the 'grains', shrunken cells seen in the upper layer of the epidermis.

Clinical features
The appearance of the first lesion is commonly in childhood, but may be developed until the fourth decade or later. The characteristic lesion is a brown, warty, rather greasy papule. These papules may coalesce to form warty, malodorous plaques (Fig. 17.13).

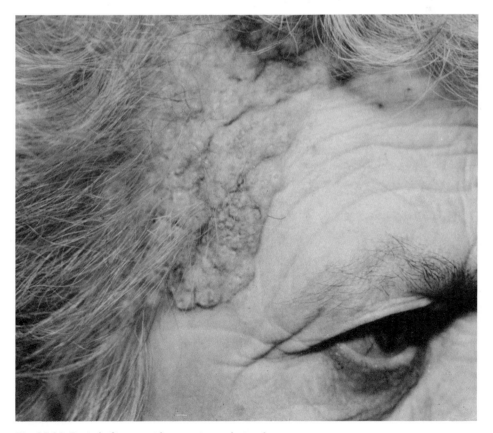

Fig. 17.13 Darier's disease with extensive scalp involvement.

The sites most commonly affected are the face, the flexures and the mid-chest and back. Some involvement of the scalp is frequent and may simulate seborrhoea. Less commonly, there are hypertrophic lesions of the scalp and behind the ears (Elsbach & Nater 1960). In such cases there may be some hair loss; exceptionally there may be extensive cicatricial alopecia (Kuske & Krebs 1965).

Whilst physical development may be normal, some affected individuals are of short stature, and in many intellectual development also is retarded. Distinct changes in the nails, longitudinal white and red bands associated with terminal V-shaped splits, may support the diagnosis, which can usually be made with confidence on clinical grounds, and is readily confirmed histologically.

Treatment

Treatment is on the whole disappointing, but the topical application of retinoic acid (Hesbacher 1970) causes temporary regression of the lesions, and can be repeated as necessary.

Good suppression of disease activity is possible with oral etretinate (Tigason UK; Tegison, USA)—0.5–1 mg/kg body weight per day).

References

Darier, J. (1889) De la psorospermie folliculaire végétante. *Annales de Dermatologie et de Syphiligraphie*, 10, 597.

Elsbach, E.M. & Nater, J.P. (1960) La forme hypertrophique de la maladie de Darier. *Dermatologica*, 120, 93.

Getzler, N.A. & Flint, A. (1966) Keratosis follicularis. *Archives of Dermatology*, **93**, 545.

Hesbacher, E.N. (1970) Zosteriform keratosis follicularis treated topically with tretinoin. *Archives of Dermatology*, **102**, 209.

Kuske, H. & Krebs, A. (1965) Morbus Darier mit subtotaler Alopecie. *Dermatologica*, **131**, 108.

Svendsen, I.B. & Albuchtron, B. (1959) The prevalence of dyskeratosis follicularis (Darier's disease) in Denmark. *Acta Dermato-Venereologica*, **39**, 256.

Dermatitis herpetiformis (References p. 534)

History and nomenclature

The bullous erythemas have suffered to an unusual extent from international confusion in nomenclature but dermatitis herpetiformis is now accepted. The history of the disease was reviewed by Alexander (1975) and Holubar (1990).

Aetiology

The disease affects all ages, but onset between 10 and 50 is usual. The pathogenesis is not fully understood; a gluten-sensitive enteropathy is commonly associated and immunofluorescence studies of the apparently normal skin show granular deposits of IgA in the tips of dermal papillae, or a band-like deposit of the same immunoglobulin (Fry 1990).

Pathology
The bullae are sub-epidermal. The initial lesion is a small collection of poly-morphonuclear and eosinophil leucocytes which invade a papilla, accumulate at its summit, and separate epidermis from dermis (Piérard & Whimster 1961). These lesions are the site of IgA deposition (Fry 1990).

Clinical features
A chronic, more or less symmetrical, papulovesicular eruption is present in variable severity for many years (Fig. 17.14). The sites of predilection are the elbows, buttocks, shoulders, knees, scalp and forearms. The neck, thigh, sacral area, temples and face are not uncommonly involved. In the early stages the scalp, or the scalp and face, may be the only sites affected (Björnberg & Hellgren 1962) and the scalp is involved at some stage in some 30% of cases (Alexander 1975).

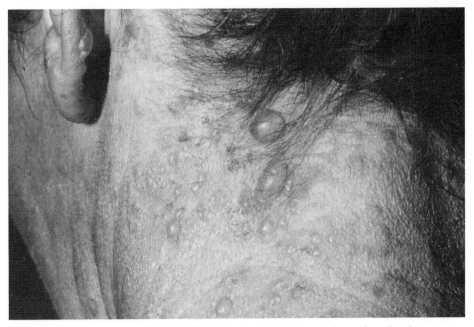

Fig. 17.14 Dermatitis herpetiformis with unusually florid lesions of the neck and scalp.

The presence of unexplained intensely irritable papules in the scalp should lead to a search for similar lesions elsewhere. Only in the rarer cases in which the scalp alone is involved initially or at some stage, will differentiation arise, and this can be resolved by biopsy.

Treatment
Thorough examination, investigation and evaluation should precede treatment with dapsone and perhaps a gluten-free diet.

References

Alexander, J. O'D. (1975) *Dermatitis Herpetiformis*, p. 22. Saunders, London.
Björnberg, A. & Hellgren, L. (1962) Dermatitis herpetiformis. *Dermatologica*, **125**, 205.
Fry, L. (1990) Dermatitis herpetiformis. In *Management of Blistering Diseases*, 1st edn., p. 139, eds. F. Wojnarowska & R. Briggaman. Chapman & Hall, London.
Holubar, K. (1990) Historical background. In *Management of Blistering Diseases*, 1st edn., p.1, eds. F. Wojnarowska & R. Briggaman. Chapman & Hall, London.
Piérard, J. & Whimster, I. (1961) The histological diagnosis of dermatitis herpetiformis, bullous pemphigoid and erythema multiforme. *British Journal of Dermatology*, **73**, 253.
Seah, P.P. & Fry, L. (1975) Immunoglobulins in the skin in dermatitis herpetiformis and their relevance in diagnosis. *British Journal of Dermatology*, **92**, 157.

Cicatricial pemphigoid (Brunsting–Perry variant of bullous pemphigoid)

This scarring bullous eruption of middle or old age may present with only a few lesions at one anatomical site (Fine 1990; Leenutaphong *et al.* 1989)—not infrequently the head or scalp (Brunsting–Perry variant). Mucous membranes, including the conjunctival sac (with blindness), may be affected during the slow spread of the disease.

References

Fine, J.-D. (1990) Cicatricial pemphigoid. In *Management of Blistering Diseases*, 1st edn., p. 83, eds. F. Wojnarowska & R. Briggaman, Chapman & Hall, London.
Leenutaphong, V., von Kries, R. & Plewig, G. (1989) Localized cicatricial pemphigoid. *Journal of the American Academy of Dermatology*, **21**, 1089.

Follicular mucinosis (References p. 537)

History and nomenclature
Descriptions of this distinctive clinico-pathological entity were published by Kreibich in 1926 and by Gougerot and Blum in 1932 (Degos *et al.* 1962). The clinical and histological features were clearly defined by Pinkus (1957). He proposed the term alopecia mucinosa, but most subsequent authors have preferred 'follicular mucinosis', since alopecia is clinically evident only when sites bearing terminal hairs are involved.

Aetiology
The cause of follicular mucinosis is unknown (Gibson *et al.* 1989). Most of the reported cases of this uncommon, but far from rare, disorder fall into one of three groups (Coskey & Mehregan 1970; Emmerson 1969; Gibson *et al.* 1989). The largest group consists of patients with solitary or few lesions, often on the face and scalp, clearing spontaneously in 2 months to 2 years. In a second group, also benign, the lesions are more extensive and persistent, or continue to develop at intervals for years without any evidence of associated disease. These benign forms occur at any age from early childhood onwards, but are most frequent between 10 and 40 years. In a third group of patients, somewhat older on average,

the mucinosis is associated with a reticulosis, histological evidence of which is present from the onset. Gibson *et al.* (1989) concluded that no single clinical or histopathological observation predicts which patients will have a benign or malignant course, suggesting that prolonged vigilance is required, including repeat biopsies.

Pathology
The outer root sheath and sebaceous gland become oedematous and develop cystic spaces in which mucin accumulates. These changes may extend to the full depth of the follicle, which may then be converted into a cystic cavity containing mucin and degenerate root sheath cells. Variable inflammatory changes in the dermis range from a sparse lymphocytic infiltrate to a granulomatous reaction. Unless the follicle is destroyed complete or almost complete reversion to normal usually occurs. Any cellular infiltrate should be carefully studied for evidence of a reticulosis (Gibson *et al.* 1989).

With the electron microscope (Orfanos & Gahlen 1964) the epidermis has been shown to be involved. Mainly in the stratum malpighii and the granular layer organelles in the perinuclear cytoplasm disappear and the nucleus shrinks.

Clinical features (Kim & Winkelmann 1962; Emmerson 1969; Gibson *et al.* 1989)
The acute benign form commonly affects the face, scalp, neck and shoulders. Skin-coloured papules or plaques of erythema show some fine scaling and patulous prominent follicles. If the scalp or eyebrows or male beard are involved the patient seeks advice on account of the loss of hair from the affected follicles. In sites covered by vellus hair the loss is less conspicuous. The plaques tend to be 2–5 cm in diameter and change little until they resolve, usually without trace after a few months, or sometimes rather longer. There may be a single plaque, or multiple plaques developing more or less simultaneously or at intervals.

Variations in the clinical picture have been reported, and may not be as rare as the paucity of recorded cases suggests, for they are easily misdiagnosed. A general-ized eruption of papules with horny plugs, not grouped into plaques, was associated with redness and scaling of the scalp and small patches of alopecia in the eyebrows (Fig. 17.15) (Bazex *et al.* 1962). In a boy aged 11, groups of papules on the neck, popliteal flexures, one knee and one buttock were followed by the appearance of a single patch of alopecia of the scalp (Fig. 17.16) (Zackheim 1958). The hairs remaining in this patch were distorted telogen hairs. A man aged 36 had suffered for 3 months from an eruption of pink papules of the face and scalp, with branny scaling and patchy alopecia. The dilated follicles contained horny plugs (Goldschlag & Jablonska 1960).

In the chronic benign form lesions are more numerous, more widely distributed and more diverse in their morphology. There may be red scaly patches or soft gelatinous plaques or nodules. The lesions may persist unchanged for years and the destruction of some follicles may lead to patches of permanent alopecia, sometimes

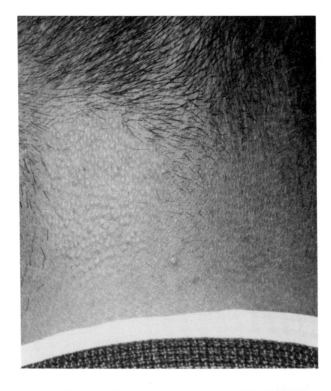

Fig. 17.15 Follicular mucinosis of the nape: typical appearance.

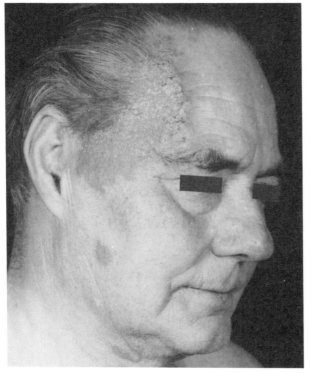

Fig. 17.16 Follicular mucinosis; more extensive erythema and scaling.

studded with horny plugs. A characteristic case of this form of follicular mucinosis was a man aged 38 in whom multiple plaques of the scalp, arms and buttocks were unchanged after 3 years (Stevanovic 1964).

In some 15–20% of all chronic cases a reticulosis is associated (Plotnich & Abrecht 1965). The skin lesions, which do not differ from those of the chronic benign form, may develop when the reticulosis is well advanced, or the latter may first be diagnosed in a biopsy of the mucinosis (Emmerson 1969; Pinkus 1964).

In all forms pruritus is an inconstant symptom. Occasionally it may be troublesome in the chronic forms.

Differential diagnosis
Problems in diagnosis occur when only the scalp is involved or when the lesions elsewhere are disseminated or otherwise atypical. A circumscribed plaque of erythema and scaling with total or partial loss of hair, especially in a child, may easily be confused with tinea; if examination under Wood's light is negative, and so is microscopy of epilated hairs, the diagnosis of follicular mucinosis should be considered. In all cases of unexplained patchy hair loss the whole skin surface should be examined. The diagnosis is confirmed by biopsy. Biopsy is advisable even in clinically obvious cases in adults, to exclude a reticulosis.

Treatment
None has been proved to be effective.

References
Bazex, A., Dupré, A., Parant, M. & Christol, B. (1962) Mucinose folliculaire; forme spinulosique généralisée. *Bulletin de la Société française de Dermatologie et de Syphiligraphie*, **67**, 484.
Coskey, R.J. & Mehregan, A.H. (1970) Alopecia mucinosa. *Archives of Dermatology*, **102**, 193.
Degos, R., Civatte, J. & Baptista, A.P. (1962) Mucinose folliculaire: La 'dermatose innominée alopéciante' de H. Gougerot et P. Blum (1932) en est-elle le premier cas? *Bulletin de la Société française de Dermatologie et de Syphiligraphie*, **69**, 228.
Emmerson, R.W. (1969) Follicular mucinosis. *British Journal of Dermatology*, **81**, 35.
Gibson, L.E., Muller, S.A., Leiferman, K.M. & Peters, M.S. (1989) Follicular mucinosis: clinical and histopathologic study. *Journal of the American Academy of Dermatology*, **20**, 441.
Goldschlag, F. & Jablonska, S. (1960) Mucinosis follicularis. *Australian Journal of Dermatology*, **5**, 173.
Kim, R. & Winkelmann, R.K. (1962) Follicular mucinosis (alopecia mucinosa). *Archives of Dermatology*, **85**, 490.
Kreibich, C. (1926) Mucin bei Hauterkrankung. *Archiv für Dermatologie und Syphilologie*, **150**, 243.
Orfanos, C. & Gahlen, W. (1964) Elektronmikroskopische Befunde bei der Mucinosis follicularis. *Archiv für klinische und experimentelle Dermatologie*, **218**, 435.
Pinkus, H. (1957) Alopecia mucinosa. *AMA Archives of Dermatology*, **76**, 419.
Pinkus, H. (1964) The relationship of alopecia mucinosa to malignant lymphomas. *Dermatologica*, **129**, 266.
Plotnich, H. & Abrecht, M. (1965) Alopecia mucinosa and lymphoma. *Archives of Dermatology*, **92**, 137.
Stevanovic, D.V. (1964) Mucinosis follicularis diffusa idiopathica. *Dermatologische Wochenschrift*, **149**, 352.
Zackheim, H. (1958) Alopecia mucinosa. *AMA Archives of Dermatology*, **78**, 715.

Granuloma annulare

Granuloma annulare rarely affects the scalp, but subcutaneous nodules in the scalp have accompanied typical lesions in other parts of the body (Grauer 1934).

Reference

Grauer, F.H. (1934) Granuloma annulare. *Archiv für Dermatologie und Syphilologie*, **30**, 785.

Elastosis perforans serpiginosa (Reference p. 539)

This unusual condition occurs particularly in persons with inherited abnormalities of connective tissue, but also in Down's syndrome, in patients receiving penicillamine, and in some apparently normal subjects.

The lesions occur most often on the face and neck, and in the latter site they extend some distance into the scalp (see Fig. 17.17).

The papules, which appear to be hyperkeratotic, are classically but not invariably grouped in circles or segments of circles.

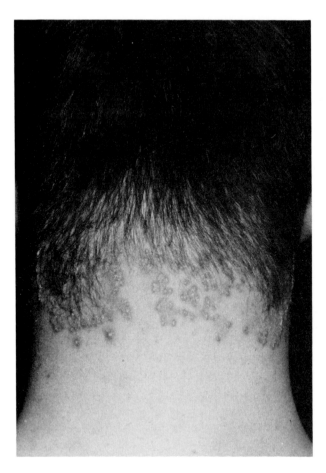

Fig. 17.17 Elastosis perforans serpiginosa in an 18-year-old male with Down's syndrome.

The diagnosis is confirmed by the histological appearance of a focal increase of large elastic fibres, which, in a necrotic state, are seen to be extruded through the overlying epidermis.

Reference

Uitto, J., Santa Cruz, D.J. & Eisen, A.Z. (1980) Connective tissue naevi of the skin. *Journal of the American Academy of Dermatology*, **3**, 441.

Eosinophilic cellulitis

History and nomenclature
Wells (1971) described as recurring granulomatous dermatitis with eosinophilia a distinct clinical entity, the cause of which remains unknown. Subsequently several similar cases have been recorded, the majority in adults but three in boys aged 11 and 12 (Wells & Smith 1979). In one of the children scalp lesions were present (Nielsen *et al.* 1981).

Pathology
During the acute stage there is dermal oedema with eosinophilic infiltration. This is followed by granulomatous changes with focal masses of disintegrating eosinophils and necrobiotic collagen fibres. These 'flame figures' are surrounded by histiocytes and foreign body giant cells.

Clinical features
Large infiltrated erythematous, oedematous, pruritic plaques develop with fever and marked peripheral eosinophilia. They resolve after a few weeks to leave slight atrophy. They may be associated with bullae which are sometimes haemorrhagic. Recurrences at irregular intervals are usual but not invariable.

In the only case in which the scalp has been involved by indurated plaques (Nielsen *et al.* 1981), these left large patches of permanent cicatricial alopecia.

Treatment
Systemic treatment with corticosteroids may shorten the course of the individual attack although these are eventually self-limiting without treatment. There may be only a single attack but more often the condition ends after one or more recurrences.

References

Nielsen, T., Schmidt, H. & Søgaard, H. (1981) Eosinophilic cellulitis (Wells' syndrome) in a child. *Archives of Dermatology*, **117**, 427.
Wells, G.C. (1971) Recurring granulomatous dermatitis with eosinophilia. *Transactions of St John's Hospital Dermatological Society*, **57**, 44.
Wells, G.C. & Smith, N.P. (1979) Eosinophilic cellulitis. *British Journal of Dermatology*, **100**, 101.

Chapter 18
Naevi, Tumours and Cysts of the Scalp

Superficial benign epidermal tumours
  Epidermal naevi
  Seborrhoeic keratoses
  Solar keratosis
  Cutaneous horn
Hair follicle tumours
  Keratoacanthoma
  Multiple self-healing epithelioma
  Pilomatrixoma
  Pilomatrix carcinoma
Other appendage tumours with hair differentiation
  Trichofolliculoma
  Trichoepithelioma
  Follicular infundibulum tumour
  Trichoadenoma
Sebaceous gland tumours
  Sebaceous adenoma
  Sebaceous carcinoma
  Microcystic adnexal carcinoma
Sweat gland tumours
  Dermal eccrine cylindroma
  Syringoma
  Primary adenoid cystic carcinoma
Basal cell carcinoma
Bowen's disease
Squamous cell carcinoma
Melanocytic tumours
  Melanocytic naevi
  Congenital pigmented naevi
  Juvenile melanoma
  Blue naevus
  Naevus of Ota
  Malignant melanoma
Perifollicular connective tissue tumours
Tumours of dermis and subcutis
  Dermatofibrosarcoma protuberans
  Gingival fibromatosis and multiple hyaline fibromas
  Neurofibromatosis
  Encephalocraniocutaneous lipomatosis
  Mastocytosis
Tumours of vessels
  Granuloma telangiectaticum
  Angiolymphoid hyperplasia with eosinophilia
  Vascular naevi
  Malignant angioendothelioma
  Cutaneous meningioma
Carcinoma metastatic to the scalp
Cysts of the scalp

Trichilemmal cysts
Cock's peculiar tumour
Epidermoid cysts
Congenital inclusion dermoid cysts
Heterotropic brain tissue cyst of scalp
Eruptive vellus hair cyst

Superficial benign epidermal tumours
(Reference p. 544)

Of the very large number of different tumours of the skin now recognised as distinct entities, the majority have at some time or another been reported as occurring in the scalp. The role of light exposure is such an important factor in increasing the incidence of many common tumours that they are rarely found in the scalp of those who retain a good protective covering of hair in old age. In the many who develop frontovertical baldness in early adult life however, the scalp, so conspicuously exposed to light, becomes very vulnerable.

The dense population of large pilosebaceous follicles in the scalp results in a relatively higher incidence of tumours derived from that source than the surface area would lead one to expect. The special anatomical peculiarities of the scalp modify the morphology and course of other tumours or demand special procedures in treating them.

In this account of tumours of the scalp only a brief description is given of tumours which are uncommon in this site, with no mention of those that have rarely if ever been reported in the scalp. Tumours which are common in the scalp and elsewhere receive greater attention, with emphasis on differential diagnosis. For more detailed information on skin tumours and on the general problem of carcinogenesis the reader is referred to standard textbooks of dermatopathology (McKee 1989). A relatively longer account is given in this chapter of tumours which are particularly characteristic of the scalp, as the dermal eccrine cylindroma.

Epidermal naevi (References p. 544)

The epidermal naevi are circumscribed developmental defects. They are classified according to their predominant component. Although many naevi contain other epidermal structures, this classification remains useful for the different types show differences in distribution, morphology and course. On clinical grounds they are often subdivided into three sub-types: verrucous naevus, naevus unius lateralis and ichthyosis hystrix. Rarely, basal and squamous carcinoma may complicate these entities (Horn *et al.* 1981).

Verrucous naevi

These naevi, warty and often linear, are not common in the scalp. In two patients with extensive verrucous naevi the scalp appeared normal but there were patches of hair abnormal in colour and texture (Bassas Grau *et al.* 1969).

Sebaceous naevi (Robinson 1932; Conner & Bryan 1967)

Sebaceous naevi are present at birth or in early infancy but may first appear later in childhood (Fig. 18.1). The majority are in the scalp or on the face (Wilson Jones & Heyl 1970). In infancy the naevus, which may be 1–2 cm in diameter,

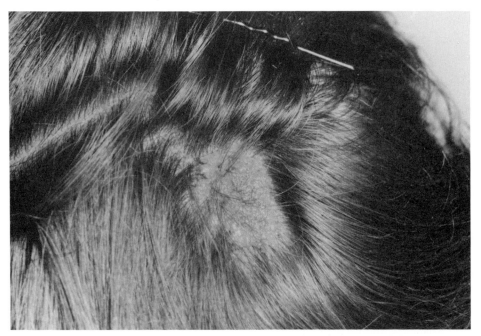

Fig. 18.1 Naevus sebaceous in the scalp of a man aged 19 years. It had enlarged during the previous 3–4 years. The granular texture of the surface can be seen.

or may cover a large area, is a flat or slightly elevated plaque with a velvet-like surface composed of numerous small elevations. It may be yellow or yellow-brown in colour. It is often more evident in infancy than in childhood for the sebaceous gland component regresses (Mehregan & Pinkus 1965; Steigleder & Cortes 1971). However, sebaceous naevi enlarge again with the approach of puberty. It is this enlargement which frequently induces the child's parents to seek medical advice.

Basal-cell carcinoma may develop in these naevi (Zugerman 1961; Castellain & Spitalier 1962; Fergin *et al.* 1981) and enlargement, induration or ulceration in one part of the naevus is an indication for biopsy.

Surgical removal of sebaceous naevi is the treatment of choice.

Naevus syringocystadenomatosus papilliferus (Helwig & Hackney 1955)
In this clumsily named naevus the apocrine sweat gland component predominates. The essential histological changes are villous papillary projections into the lumen of dilated sweat ducts, and cystic dilatation of the associated gland. The epidermis may be normal but may be grossly acanthotic and hyperkeratotic.

The typical lesion is a pink, domed, umbilicated nodule 2–10 mm in diameter. There may be a cluster of discrete nodules or they may be grouped to form a plaque with a warty surface (Fig. 18.2). Some 50% occur in the scalp. In about 30% of cases a sebaceous naevus is associated.

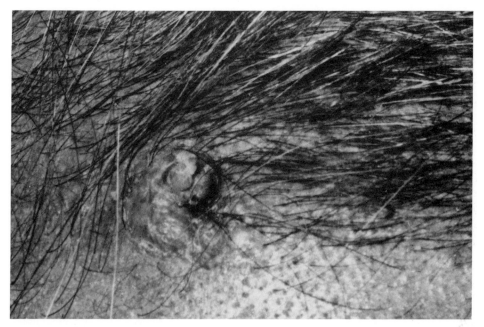

Fig. 18.2 Naevus syringocystadenomatosus.

This naevus is present at birth or develops in infancy. It may enlarge at puberty and become more verrucous (Pinkus 1954). Malignant change may eventually develop in about 10%.

Treatment is by excision.

Comedo naevus
The comedo naevus is perhaps not a single entity but a group of conditions characterized by dilated and plugged follicles (Leppard & Marks 1973). This naevus may be present at birth or may appear during childhood; exceptionally it may develop in old age (Nabai & Mehregan 1973). It may occur in any part of the body but in most cases on the neck, face or trunk. It is rare in the scalp but this was involved in a patient with extensive bilateral lesions (Paige & Mendelson

1967). In two cases (Leppard & Marks 1973; Peyri *et al.* 1978) lesions of the scalp were associated with palmoplantar lesions.

Histologically there are large horny plugs in dilated follicles with small atrophic sebaceous glands (Beerman & Harman 1959). Clinically the naevus presents as a circumscribed, often irregularly linear area in which dilated follicles contain large horny plugs. The intervening surface epidermis may appear normal or may be thickened.

Treatment is not entirely satisfactory. If the naevus is small excision may be considered but this is not appropriate in most cases. Retinoic acid 0.1% has been reported to be 'very effective' (Dechard *et al.* 1972). But we have not found it always to be so.

Epidermal naevus syndrome

An epidermal naevus of any of the four types described may be associated with other defects, skeletal and ocular, epilepsy and mental retardation. The syndrome was formerly linked principally to naevus sebaceous (Feuerstein & Mims 1962) but naevus syringocystoadenoma papilliferus (Jancar 1970) and naevus comedonicus (Rook 1953) may also form part of this somewhat variable syndrome (McKee 1989). In the presence of such naevi the other defects should be sought, though in many cases the epidermal naevus is an apparently isolated defect, but according to Solomon *et al.* (1968) some other developmental defects, although not the full syndrome, were found in some 60% of cases of epidermal naevus.

References

Bassas Grau, E., Capdevela, J., Castells, A. & Pinol Aguade, J. (1969) Naevus sistematizado con heterocromia areata del cabello. *Medicina Cutanea*, **3**, 1.

Beerman, H. & Harman, J.B. (1959) Naevus comedonicus. *Archiv für klinische und experimentelle Dermatologie*, **208**, 325.

Castellain, P.Y. & Spitalier, J.M. (1962) Epiteliome basocellulaire pigmentée sur naevus sebacée de Jadassohn. *Annales de Dermatologie et de Syphiligraphie*, **69**, 956.

Conner, A.E. & Bryan, H. (1967) Nevus sebaceus of Jadassohn. *American Journal of Diseases of Children*, **114**, 626.

Dechard, J.C., Mills, O. & Leyden, J.J. (1972) Naevus comedonicus—treatment with retinoic acid. *British Journal of Dermatology*, **86**, 528.

Fergin, P.E., Chu, A.C. & MacDonald, D.M. (1981) Basal cell carcinoma complicating naevus sebaceous. *Clinical and Experimental Dermatology*, **6**, 111.

Feuerstein, R.C. & Mims, L.C. (1962) Linear Nevus Sebaceus with convulsions and mental retardation. *American Journal of Diseases of Children*, **104**, 605.

Helwig, E.B. & Hackney, V.C. (1955) Syringadenoma papilliferum. Lesions with and without naevus sebaceus and basal cell carcinoma. *Archives of Dermatology and Syphilology (Chicago)*, **71**, 361.

Horn, M.S., Sausker, W.F. & Pierson, D.L. (1981) Basal cell epithelioma arising in a linear epidermal naevus. *Archives of Dermatology*, **117**, 247.

Jancar, J. (1970) Naevus syringocystadenomatosus papilliferus. *British Journal of Dermatology*, **82**, 402.

Leppard, B. & Marks, R. (1973) Comedone naevus. *Transactions of the St. John's Hospital Dermatological Society*, **59**, 45.

McKee, P.H. (1989) *Pathology of the Skin*, 1st edn. Gower Medical Publishing, London.

Mehregan, H. & Pinkus, H. (1965) Life history of organoid nevi. *Archives of Dermatology*, **91**, 574.

Nabai, H. & Mehregan, H. (1973) Naevus comedonicus. *Acta Dermato-Venereologica (Stockholm)*, **53**, 71.

Paige, T.M. & Mendelson, C.G. (1967) Bilateral nevus comedonicus. *Archives of Dermatology*, **96**, 172.

Peyri, J., Ferrandiz, C., Palou, J. & Mascaro, J.M. (1978) Naevus comedonicus palmoplantary y de cuero caballudo. *Medicina Cutanea I.L.A.* **6**, 227.

Pinkus, H. (1954) Life history of naevus syringocystadenomatosus papilliferus. *Archives of Dermatology and Syphilology*, **69**, 305.

Robinson, S.S. (1932) Nevus sebaceus (Jadassohn). *Archives of Dermatology and Syphilology*, **26**, 663.

Rook, A.J. (1953) Naevus comedonicus unilateralis with partial Sturge–Weber syndrome and extensive vascular naevi with haemangiomatous hypertrophy of leg. *Proceedings of Tenth International Congress of Dermatology*, p. 421, London.

Solomon, L.M., Fretzin, D.F. & De Wald, R.I. (1968) The epidermal nevus syndrome. *Archives of Dermatology*, **97**, 273.

Steigleder, G.K. & Cortes, A.C. (1971) Verhalten der Talgdrüsen in Talgdrüssenaevus während des Kindersalters. *Archiv für klinische und experimentelle Dermatologie*, **239**, 323.

Wilson Jones, E. & Heyl, T. (1970) Naevus sebaceous. *British Journal of Dermatology*, **82**, 97.

Zugerman, I. (1961) Basal-cell epithelioma in nevus syringocystadenomatosus papilliferus. *Archives of Dermatology (Chicago)*, **84**, 672.

Seborrhoeic keratoses (References p. 546)

Nomenclature

Numerous terms have been applied to these common lesions; Unna called them seborrhoeic verrucas but they are also known as senile warts and as basal-cell papillomas.

Aetiology

Seborrhoeic keratoses are benign neoplasms. They are so frequent that it is difficult to assess the role of genetic factors, but autosomal dominant inheritance seems probable in some families (Reiches 1953). They are extremely rare in childhood but have been reported as early as the age of 5 (Becker 1951). They become more frequent from the age of 30 onwards and are common in middle and old age.

Pathology (Becker 1951)

The epidermis is thickened and cells resembling basal cells form a solid epithelial mass, flat or irregularly serrated, or a retiform pattern with horn cysts or pseudocysts.

Clinical features

Typical seborrhoeic keratoses are sharply marginated flat papules, bright or dark brown in colour, with a velvet surface, greasy to the touch. They may become pedunculated with a smooth dull cerebriform surface. They can occur anywhere except on the palms and sole, but are most frequently seen on the face and scalp and on the trunk. There may be only one or two keratoses or very large numbers.

The rapid development of very numerous keratoses may be a manifestation of systemic malignant disease.

Differential diagnosis

The most important problem in differential diagnosis presented by seborrhoeic keratoses in the hairy scalp is that of distinguishing them from a melanocytic naevus or a malignant melanoma. The smooth dome-shaped seborrhoeic keratoses may be very deeply pigmented. If the diagnosis is in doubt the lesions should be excised if small, or submitted to biopsy if large. The typical flat seborrhoeic keratosis seen more often on the bald scalp must be differentiated from a solar keratosis and from a basal cell carcinoma. If the diagnosis is uncertain a biopsy is essential.

Treatment

These keratoses are premalignant and their removal is undertaken solely on cosmetic grounds. They are very easily curetted to leave less scarring than would follow excision. Cryosurgery using the cotton wool bud, liquid nitrogen method is now commonly employed, although liquid nitrogen spray gives higher success rates but may occasionally cause permanent hair loss with even short freeze times.

References

Becker, S.W. (1951) Seborrheic keratosis and verruca, with special reference to the melanotic variety. *Archives of Dermatology and Syphilology,* **63**, 358.
Reiches, A.J. (1953) Seborrheic keratoses. *Archives of Dermatology and Syphilology,* **65**, 600.

Solar keratosis (References p. 547)

Nomenclature

The synonym senile keratosis is not appropriate, for the incidence of these keratoses is related to age only in so far as the latter is a measure of cumulative exposure to solar radiation. Actinic keratosis is an acceptable synonym.

Aetiology

Solar keratoses are very common lesions of all exposed skin, including the bald or balding scalp. Their age of onset depends on the amount of light exposure in relation to the individual skin's capacity to tan. Given the same exposure to light, the fairer the skin, the earlier the onset of the keratoses.

Pathology (Pinkus 1958)

The parakeratotic epidermis has lost its granular layer. The prickle-cells are oedematous and vary in size and shape, and have lost their normal orderly stratified arrangement. The dermo-epidermal junction may be flat and the epidermis thin, or there may be acanthosis, but in either case the normal regular pattern of ridges and papillae is no longer apparent. The keratosis has sharp margins which slope upwards and inwards. The dermal collagen shows solar degenerative changes.

Clinical features

The patient complains initially of dry patches. Later, well-circumscribed, rough, adherent crusts develop. They are removed with difficulty and soon recur. In a simple keratosis the lesion feels superficial, and there is no underlying induration. If such is present the possibility of early squamous carcinoma must be considered. Some authors claim that solar keratoses frequently disappear spontaneously if careful observations are made.

Diagnosis

The sharply marginated rough patch on evidently light-damaged skin is not readily confused with seborrhoeic keratosis or with the red, often crusted appearance of Bowen's disease.

Treatment

If a single lesion is present it may be curetted under local anaesthesia, or destroyed with liquid nitrogen or trichloroacetic acid. If there are numerous lesions, as is often the case, 5-fluorouracil cream may be used (Almeida Gonçalves & de Noronia 1970); the latter is applied twice daily only until the lesion becomes red or sore. After this inflammatory phase most solar keratoses peel off spontaneously.

If the lesions are indurated, biopsy or excision-biopsy is essential.

References

Almeida Conçalves, J.C. & de Noronia, T. (1970) 5-Fluorouracil (5-FU) ointment in the treatment of skin tumours and keratoses. *Dermatologica*, **140** (Suppl.) 1, 97.
Pinkus, H. (1958) Keratosis senilis. *American Journal of Clinical Pathology*, **29**, 193.

Cutaneous horn

A cutaneous horn is a horny projection, a few millimetres or several centimetres in length, forming when conditions, such as protection from trauma, favour the accumulation of horn. It may arise on a wide variety of different lesions including virus warts, epidermal naevi, solar or seborrhoeic keratoses and squamous carcinoma.

When this purely clinical diagnosis is made, it must be regarded as the first stage of a two-stage diagnosis and the nature of the underlying lesion must be established clinically or, preferably, histologically.

Hair follicle tumours

Keratoacanthoma (Molluscum sebaceum) (References p. 549)

Aetiology
The keratoacanthoma (Fig. 18.3) is a common tumour of the skin occurring in the same populations as squamous carcinoma (Kern & McCray 1980) and in

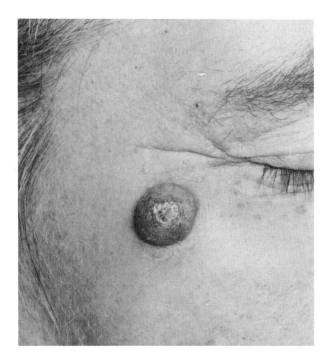

Fig. 18.3 Keratoacanthoma.

response to such carcinogenic environmental hazards as actinic radiation and tar, but at a significantly lower age than squamous carcinoma. In one large series of cases (Rook & Champion 1963) 24% of keratoacanthomas but only 6% of squamous carcinomas occurred in patients under 50 years of age, and only 9% of keratoacanthomas, but 18% of squamous carcinomas occurred in patients over 80 years of age. In this same series of cases of keratoacanthoma only 1% occurred on the scalp, 4% on the forehead, 5% on the thighs, 7% on the eyelids, 20% on the nose and 26% on the cheeks. Most of the remainder were on other areas of the face and neck or on the exposed skin of the back and forearms.

Pathology (Kopf 1976)
The keratoacanthoma is compact, circumscribed and superficial. A central mass of horn is surrounded by columns of hyperplastic epithelium, orderly and

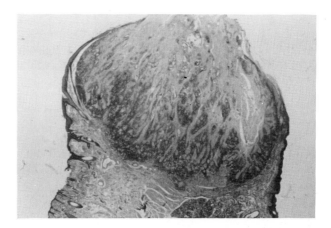

Fig. 18.4 Keratoacanthoma, showing the characteristic architecture.

symmetrical; mitoses are numerous. The general architecture of the lesion (Fig. 18.4) is usually characteristic.

Clinical features

A firm hemispherical papule enlarges rapidly to reach a diameter of 1–2 cm in 4–5 weeks, though further enlargement is unusual. The lesion is now a crateriform nodule of rubbery consistency, the central crater of which is filled by horn. After 6–8 weeks the lesion becomes softer and flatter and the plug of horn is shed. The rim slowly flattens and only a puckered scar remains.

Recurrence after removal is not unusual (Rook *et al.* 1967) but the recurrent lesion runs essentially the same course if left untreated.

Malignant change is possible and should be suspected in atypical lesions, particularly those on the lip or ear, and in elderly patients (Rook & Whimster 1979).

Diagnosis

The short history and the clinical appearance suggest the diagnosis which may be confirmed histologically from an adequate biopsy specimen. If the diagnosis is still in doubt, the lesion must be treated as a carcinoma.

Treatment

In the high proportion of cases in which the diagnosis is not in doubt the lesion can be curetted under local anaesthesia after a small elliptical biopsy has been taken for accurate histological diagnosis; the recurrence rates are longer after formal excision which may, however, be unnecessarily complicated in larger lesions.

References

Kern, W.H. & McCray, M.K. (1980) The histopathologic differentiation of keratoacanthoma and squamous cell carcinoma of the skin. *Journal of Cutaneous Pathology,* 7, 318.

Kopf, A.W. (1976) Keratoacanthoma. In *Carcinoma of the Skin*, p. 755, eds. R. Andrade, S.L. Gumport, G.L. Popkin & T.D. Rees. Philadelphia, Saunders.

Rook, A. & Champion, R.H. (1963) Keratoacanthoma. *National Cancer Institute Monograph*, 10, 257.

Rook, A. & Whimster, I. (1979) Keratoacanthoma—a thirty year retrospect. *British Journal of Dermatology*, 100, 41.

Rook, A., Kerdel-Vegas, F. & Young, J.A. (1967) Las recidivas en el queratoacantoma. *Medicina cutanea*, 2, 17.

Multiple self-healing epithelioma

In this uncommon syndrome, characterized by Ferguson Smith in 1934, the development of self-healing epitheliomas begins in the third or fourth decade, sometimes earlier (Sommerville & Milne 1950). There may be a family history of the disorder.

The tumours may be very widely distributed, but in most cases they have occurred predominantly in the scalp, on the face and ears, on the hands and in the anogenital region (Epstein *et al.* 1957). The presence of tumours in the scalp is a feature of almost all reported cases.

Clinically the tumours do not show the almost consistently crateriform structure of the keratoacanthoma. They are more deeply set irregular nodules.

Histologically the columns of squamous cells extend into the dermis and differentiation from an ordinary squamous cell carcinoma may be difficult. The history and presence of other lesions will suggest the diagnosis.

References

Epstein, N.M., Biskind, G.R. & Pollack, R.S. (1957) Multiple benign self-healing 'epitheliomas' of the skin. *Archives of Dermatology and Syphilology*, 75, 210.

Ferguson Smith, J. (1934) A case of multiple primary squamous celled carcinoma of the skin in a young man, with spontaneous healing. *British Journal of Dermatology*, 46, 267.

Sommerville, J. & Milne, J.A. (1950) Familial primary self-healing epithelioma of the skin (Ferguson Smith type). *British Journal of Dermatology*, 62, 485.

Pilomatrixoma (benign calcifying epithelioma of Malherbe) (References p. 551)

History and nomenclature

This distinctive tumour was named by Malherbe in 1880, 'calcified epithelioma of the sebaceous glands'. It had first been described in 1858 by Wilckens in his thesis at the University of Göttingen (Geiser 1959). The origin of the tumour was disputed for many years, but it is now accepted that it arises from the primitive epidermal germ cells differentiating towards hair matrix cells (Forbès & Helwig 1961) and the term pilomatrixoma is generally favoured.

Pathology (Forbès & Helwig 1961)

Pilomatrixoma is a circumscribed tumour situated in the lower dermis, and consisting of lobulated masses of cells. The small outer cells have large round basophilic nuclei. The central cells are large with eosinophilic cytoplasm, but no nuclear staining—the so-called shadow cells. Calcification may be seen in these cells and also sometimes in the abnormal connective tissue stroma. There is no reliable evidence that the tumour is inherited, but more than one case in a family has been reported on several occasions (Geiser 1960).

Clinical features

The tumours, which are usually solitary, though rarely up to four may be present, are often first observed in childhood and have been observed in early infancy; some 40% have been found in patients under 40. The majority are on the upper half of the body: scalp 6%, face 21%, neck 13%, arms 35% in one series of cases (Forbès & Helwig 1961); and scalp 12%, face 36.5%, arms 24.2% in another (Martins 1956). Perforating lesions may occur (Lo *et al.* 1989).

The lesion presents as a slowly enlarging dermal or subcutaneous lobular nodule up to 3 cm in diameter and of firm or hard consistency (Taafe *et al.* 1988).

Some lesions show melanocytic hyperplasia (Zaim 1987).

Treatment

Excision is the only effective treatment. Malignant change is thought to occur only rarely (Van der Walt & Rohlova 1984), but recurrences have followed incomplete excision.

References

Forbès, R. & Helwig, E.B. (1961) Pilomatrixoma. *Archives of Dermatology*, **83**, 601.

Geiser, J.D. (1959) l'Epithéliome calcifié de Malherbe. *Annales de Dermatologie et de Syphiligraphie*, **86**, 259, 583.

Geiser, J.D. (1960) Forme familiale de l'epithéliome (calcifié) de Malherbe. *Dermatologica*, **130**, 361.

Lo, J.S., Guitart, J., Bergfeld, W.F. *et al.* (1989) Perforating pilomatrixoma. *Cutis*, **44**, 130.

Martins, A.G. (1956) Tumor numificado de Malherbe. *Arquivo de Patologia*, **28**, 123.

Taaffe, A., Wyatt, E.H. & Bury, H.P.R. (1988) Pilomatrixoma. *International Journal of Dermatology*, **27**, 477.

Van der Walt, J.D. & Rohlova, B. (1984) Carcinomatous transformation in a pilomatrixoma. *American Journal of Dermatopathology*, **6**, 63.

Zaim, M.T. (1987) Pilomatrixoma with melanocytic hyperplasia. *Archives of Dermatology*, **123**, 865.

Pilomatrix carcinoma (Reference p. 552)

Green *et al.* (1987) reported a single case of this entity presenting as a large ulcerated mass in the axilla, and reviewed the findings of 16 cases in the world literature. Histology showed irregular nests of basaloid matrix cells with cystic centres containing necrotic debris and 'shadow cells'; the tumour invaded adjacent structures and was characterized by areas of cellular pleomorphism, crowding of cells and numerous mitotic figures.

Reference

Green, D.E., Sanusi, I.D. & Fowler, M.R. (1987) Pilomatrix carcinoma. *Journal of the American Academy of Dermatology*, **17**, 264.

Other appendage tumours with hair differentiation

Many of these are only firmly diagnosable histologically; details of the most common and esoteric forms are well described by McKee (1989). Only the clearly delineated types are considered here.

Reference

McKee, P.H. (1989) *Pathology of the Skin*, 1st edn. Gower Medical Publishing, London.

Trichofolliculoma (of Miescher)

This not uncommon hamartoma usually arises as a single dome-shaped lesion with a central pore—on the face, neck or scalp. Most characteristic is the presence of one or more silky-white thread-like hairs (trichoids) growing out of the central pore (Pinkus & Sutton 1965).

Reference

Pinkus, H. & Sutton, R.L. Jr. (1965) Trichofolliculoma. *Archives of Dermatology*, **91**, 46.

Trichoepithelioma (References p. 553)

This is a hamartomatous condition with less follicular differentiation than a trichofolliculoma (Gray & Helwig 1963). It may occur as a solitary nodule, multiple mainly centrifacial lesions and in a familial form (Gaul 1953). The type inherited as an autosomal dominant form is known as Epithelioma adenoides cysticum of Brooke.

Lesions begin to appear at puberty, increasing in number; they are skin-coloured or slightly pink. In contrast to basal cell carcinomas they do not usually ulcerate. Generalized trichoepitheliomas have been described with alopecia and myasthenia gravis (Miyakawa *et al.* 1988).

Histologically horn cysts are seen with a fully keratinized inner shell and outer shell of flattened basaloid cells; it has recently been suggested that papillary mesenchymal bodies are the pathological signs to look for in trichoepithelioma if basal cell carcinoma is difficult to differentiate (Brooke *et al.* 1989). Occasionally primitive hair papillae or hair shafts may occur within them.

As the tumours of trichoepithelioma are asymptomatic, treatment is mostly sought for cosmetic reasons. Excision, curettage, dermabrasion and X-irradiation all have advocates. Duhra and Paul (1988) obtained good results using cryosurgery.

References

Brooke, J.D., Fitzpatrick, J.E. & Golitz, L.E. (1989) Papillary mesenchymal bodies: differentiation of trichoepithelioma from basal cell carcinoma. *Journal of the American Academy of Dermatology*, **21**, 523.

Duhra, P. & Paul, J.C. (1988) Cryotherapy for multiple trichoepithelioma. *Journal of Dermatologic Surgery and Oncology*, **14**, 1413.

Gaul, L.E. (1953) Heredity of multiple benign, cystic epithelioma. *Archives of Dermatology*, **68**, 517.

Gray, H.R. & Helwig, E.B. (1963) Epithelioma adenoides cysticum and solitary trichoepithelioma. *Archives of Dermatology*, **87**, 102.

Miyakawa, S., Araki, Y. & Sugawara M. (1988) Generalized trichoepitheliomas with alopecia and myasthenia gravis. *Journal of the American Academy of Dermatology*, **19**(2), 361.

Follicular infundibulum tumour

This entity was clearly described by Mehregan and Butler (1961). Two distinctive terms have recently been delineated.

1 Eruptive infundibulomas in which there are hundreds of asymptomatic erythematous lesions 2–15 mm diameter with complex angular shapes in a mantle distribution over the upper portion of the chest, back and shoulders. Microscopy showed infundibular tumours with benign platelike proliferations of the external root sheath outlined by a prominent brushlike elastic network (Kossard *et al.* 1989).

2 Multiple lesions occurring on the sun-exposed areas of the head and neck of middle-aged men. These lesions often heal leaving discoid lupus erythematous-like scars (Findlay 1989).

References

Findlay, G.H. (1989) Multiple infundibular tumours of the head and neck. *British Journal of Dermatology*, **120**, 633.

Kossard, S., Finley, A.G., Poyzer, K. & Kossard, E. (1989) Eruptive infundibulomas. *Journal of the American Academy of Dermatology*, **21**, 361.

Mehregan, A.H. & Butler, J.D. (1961) A tumour of the follicular infundibulum. *Archives of Dermatology*, **142**, 177.

Trichoadenoma (of Nikolowski)

A benign hair follicle tumour, this yellowish nodular lesion typically on the head or neck, may be difficult to differentiate on clinical grounds from tri-chofolliculoma or trichoepithelioma, and histologically from basal cell carcinoma.

References

Bonvalet, D., Duterque, M. & Ducret, J.-P. (1988) Tricho-adénome de Nikolowski. *Annales de Dermatologie et de Vénéréologie*, **115**, 1186.

Rahbari, H., Mehregan, A. & Pinkus, H. (1977) Trichoadenoma of Nikolowski. *Journal of Cutaneous Pathology*, **4**, 90.

Sebaceous gland tumours

Sebaceous adenoma

These benign tumours are uncommon. They occur most frequently in men, usually over the age of 40. Histologically the tumours have a well-defined sebaceous structure. The peripheral cells of the lobules are small and eosinophilic; the more central cells contain lipid globules.

Clinically sebaceous adenomas are small nodules, skin coloured or yellow, and may have a keratotic surface. They are most common on the nose, cheeks or scalp. Multiple sebaceous adenomas should suggest the possibility of Torre's syndrome and a search for associated visceral cancer (Rulon & Helwig 1973).

The adenomas should be excised.

Reference

Rulon, D.B. & Helwig, E.B. (1973) Multiple sebaceous adenomas of the skin. *American Journal of Clinical Pathology*, 60, 745.

Sebaceous carcinoma (References p. 555)

History and nomenclature

Lever (1948) distinguished between the sebaceous carcinoma derived from the cells of the sebaceous gland and the basal cell or squamous epithelioma with sebaceous differentiation. Relatively few cases of sebaceous carcinoma of the skin have been reported; these tumours arise rather more frequently in the Meibomian glands but extra-ocular ones are well described. The peri-ocular variety is often aggressive and may metastasize widely. The confusion of these sebaceous carcinomas with basal cell epithelioma with sebaceous differentiation (Urban & Winkelmann 1961) accounts for the conflicting opinions as to its degree of malignancy (Graham *et al.* 1984).

Pathology (Civatte & Tsoitis 1976)

The tumour consists of lobules of sebaceous cells in various stages of differentiation. Atypical cells and mitoses are frequent. The eosinophilic cytoplasm is foamy or finely granular. Lipid may be demonstrable, particularly in the better differentiated cells. The stroma which may be dense and fibrous contains lymphocytes and plasma cells. Histological distinction from basal cell epithelioma or squamous cell epithelioma with sebaceous differentiation must be made.

Clinical features (Warren & Warvi 1943)

The tumour occurs most often on the face or scalp mainly over the age of 50. The clinical appearance is not diagnostic; there is a solid or ulcerated nodule which enlarges slowly. It may be yellow in colour but is not invariably so. Local invasion and metastasis may occur. The diagnosis must be confirmed histologically.

Treatment

Wide excision is advisable in an attempt to reduce the risk of recurrence (Beach & Serurann 1942).

References

Beach, A. & Serurann, A.D. (1942) Sebaceous gland carcinoma. *Annals of Surgery,* **115**, 258.

Civatte, J. & Tsoitis, G. (1976) Adnexal skin carcinomas. In *Cancer of the Skin,* vol. 2, p. 1045, eds. R. Andrade, S.L. Gumporte, G.L. Popkin & T.D. Rees. Saunders, Philadelphia.

Graham, R.H., McKee, P.H. & McGibbon, D.H. (1984) Sebaceous carcinoma. *Clinical and Experimental Dermatology,* **9**, 466.

Lever, W.F. (1948) Pathogenesis of benign tumours and cutaneous appendages and basal cell epithelioma. *Archiv für Dermatologie und Syphilologie Berlin),* **57**, 679.

Urban, F.H. & Winkelmann, R.K. (1961) Sebaceous malignancy. *Archives of Dermatology,* **84**, 63.

Warren, S. & Warvi W.N. (1943) Tumors of sebaceous glands. *American Journal of Pathology,* **19**, 441.

Microcystic adnexal carcinoma

Microcystic adnexal carcinoma is a rare, recently-described tumour showing benign features histologically but locally aggressive behaviour. Only one case has been described specifically affecting the scalp.

Reference

Chow, W.C., Cockerell, C.J. & Geronemus, R.G. (1989) Microcystic adnexal carcinoma of the scalp. *Journal of Dermatologic Surgery and Oncology,* **15**, 768.

Sweat gland tumours

Dermal eccrine cylindroma (turban tumour; Spiegler's tumour)
(References p. 557)

History and nomenclature

The earliest account of the scalp tumours that later acquired the name of cylindromas was given by Ancell in 1842. Many accounts were published, under almost as many different names, but the terms most widely adopted have been cylindroma, turban tumours and Spiegler's tumours. The term dermal eccrine cylindroma is preferred; it is more precise. Not all 'turban tumours' are eccrine cylindromas (Parker 1958) and the latter tumour does not always present in 'turban' distribution.

Trichoepitheliomas of the face may be present in association with cylindromas of the scalp and the two tumours form part of a single genetic entity (Welch *et al.* 1968). Inheritance is determined by an autosomal dominant gene with variable expression; either tumour may predominate. Penetrance probably approaches 100% in adult life.

Pathology (Sutherland 1956; Crain and Helwig 1961; Nödl 1965)
The cylindroma is of eccrine sweat gland origin. Closely packed masses of darkly staining cells are invested by condensed hyaline strands in variable mucinoid infiltration. Histological changes transitional between cylindroma and tricho-epithelioma may occur.

Clinical features
The cylindroma is a firm or hard raised nodule, pink or bluish-red in colour, domed or mushroom-shaped, and enlarging very slowly (Fig. 18.5). It may ultimately reach a diameter of several centimetres, or remain no more than pea-sized for several years. The first tumours have appeared in childhood, but the greatest number begin between the ages of 10 and 40.

Solitary lesions may occur in any part of the body, but both solitary and multiple lesions favour the forehead and scalp where, if present in great numbers, they may justify the clinical diagnosis 'turban tumour'. They normally

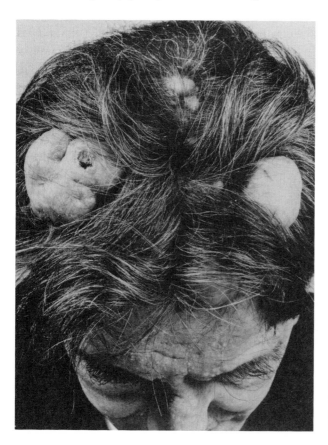

Fig. 18.5 Cylindromata (turban tumours) of the scalp (Dr C. Darley, London Hospital).

run an entirely benign course, but as they increase in number and size, may constitute a serious cosmetic disability.

Rarely local invasion and malignant degeneration (Urbanski *et al.* 1985) with fatal metastasis may overtake in middle-life lesions present since childhood (Luger 1949). In one woman in whom dedifferentiation and metastasis occurred at the age of 67 in an epithelioma present for 3 years, brachydactyly and racquet nails were also present (Greither & Rehrmann 1980). The authors suggest that this may represent an unrecognized syndrome.

Vernon *et al.* (1988) described a case associated with a solitary lung lesion.

Cylindromas formed part of a syndrome with milia in addition to trichoepitheliomas (Rasmussen 1975). The milia developed in the fourth decade.

Diagnosis

The confident clinical diagnosis of the solitary cylindroma may be impossible and biopsy is always advisable. Where multiple cylindromas of the scalp are present, epidermoid cysts must be excluded. Very rarely familial turban tumours have proved to have a modified squamous structure (Parker 1958).

Treatment

Excision, followed if necessary by grafting, is usually the treatment of choice, but local recurrence is frequent (Crain & Helwig 1961). Radiosensitivity is low, but the skilled application of contact therapy in high dosage can give excellent results (Graul 1954). Carbon dioxide laser therapy may be successful in selected cases (Stoner & Hobbs 1988).

References

Ancell, H. (1842) History of a remarkable case of tumour development on the head and face. *Medicochirurgical Transactions*, **25**, 227.

Crain, R.C. & Helwig, E.B. (1961) Dermal cylindroma (dermal eccrine cylindroma). *American Journal of Clinical Pathology*, **35**, 504.

Graul, E.H. (1954) Strahlenbiologische und strahlentherapeutische Untersuchungen an Spieglerschen Zylindromen, *Strahlentherapie*, **93**, 549.

Greither, A. & Rehrmann, A. (1980) Spiegler-Karzinome mit associerten Symptome, *Dermatologica*, **160**, 361.

Luger, A. (1949) Das Cylindrom der Haut und seine maligne Degeneration. *Archiv für Dermatologie und Syphilologie*, **188**, 155.

Nödl, F. (1965) Zur Histogenese der dermaler ekkriner Cylindroma. *Archiv für klinische und experimentelle Dermatologie*, **222**, 171.

Parker, R.A. (1958) Familial multiple cutaneous tumours of the head with a modified squamous structure. *Journal of Pathology and Bacteriology*, **75**, 435.

Rasmussen, J.E. (1975) A syndrome of trichoepitheliomas milia and cylindromas. *Archives of Dermatology*, **111**, 610.

Stoner, M.F. & Hobbs, E.R. (1988) Treatment of multiple dermal cylindromas with the CO_2 laser. *Journal of Dermatologic Surgery and Oncology*, **14**, 1263.

Sutherland, T.W. (1956) Non-papillary hyalinising hidradenoma, sometimes forming turban tumours. *Journal of Pathology and Bacteriology*, **72**, 663.

Urbanski, S.J., From, L., Asramowicz, A. *et al.* (1985) Metamorphosis of dermal cylindroma: possible relation to malignant transformation. *Journal of the American Academy of Dermatology,* **12**, 188.

Vernon, H.J., Olsen, E.A. & Vollmer, R.T. (1988) Autosomal dominant multiple cylindromas associated with solitary lung cylindromas. *Journal of the American Academy of Dermatology,* **19**, 397.

Welch, J.P., Wells, R.S. & Kerr, C.B. (1968) Ancell–Spiegler cylindromas (turban tumours) and Brooke–Fordyce trichoepitheliomas: evidence for a single genetic entity. *Journal of Medical Genetics,* **5**, 29.

Syringoma

Aetiology
This benign tumour, apparently not hereditary, is a malformation of the eccrine sweat ducts.

Pathology
In the upper part of the dermis are convoluted and cystic sweat ducts. On one side of the lesion a tail-like projection extends into the fibrous stroma, like the tail of a tadpole.

Clinical features
Syringomas, which are usually but not invariably multiple, develop from adolescence in crops or singly on the eyelids and the orbital skin, on the chest and on the abdomen. They are small, skin-coloured or pale yellowish-brown papules (Yung *et al.* 1981).

One patient, a man aged 47, had a plaque of cicatricial alopecia with a papular surface. He also had syringomas of the eyelids and cutis laxa (Dupré *et al.* 1981). The bald cicatricial area showed the pathological changes of syringoma.

A women aged 57 with progressive, irregular cicatricial alopecia of 20 years' duration, with no other skin changes was found histologically to have multiple syringomas of the scalp, replacing the hair follicles (Shelley & Wood 1980).

Diagnosis
In retrospect, knowing that syringoma can give rise to cicatricial alopecia, the diagnosis could have been suspected in the first case. The second case merely underlines the importance of taking a biopsy in unexplained cicatricial alopecia for there were no clinical grounds on which a diagnosis of syringoma could have been considered. Many papules occurring in flexures may mimic pseudo-xanthoma elasticum.

References
Dupré, A., Bonafe, J.L. & Christoe, B. (1981) Syringoma as a causative factor for cicatricial alopecia. *Archives of Dermatology,* **117**, 315.

Shelley, W.B. & Wood, M.G. (1980) Occult syringoma of the scalp associated with progressive hair loss. *Archives of Dermatology,* **116**, 843.

Yung, C.W., Saltani, K., Bernstein, J.E. *et al.* (1981) Unilateral linear naevoid syringoma. *Journal of the American Academy of Dermatology,* **4**, 412.

Primary adenoid cystic carcinoma

A malignant carcinoma which may occur in salivary glands, lacrimal and ceruminous glands and many other sites; Meyrick Thomas *et al.* (1987) described a case in the scalp—a smooth swelling with overlying alopecia.

Reference

Meyrick Thomas, R.H., Lowe, D.G. & Munro, D.D. (1987) Primary adenoid cystic carcinoma of the skin. *Clinical and Experimental Dermatology*, **12**, 378.

Basal cell carcinoma (basal cell epithelioma; rodent ulcer)
(References p. 561)

Aetiology

Basal cell carcinoma is not a rare tumour in the scalp; this was the site in some 5% of tumours in one series (Battle & Patterson 1960).

Tumours on the bald scalp do not differ from those in other light-exposed areas. Those in the hairy scalp may develop in scars, but many arise in previously normal skin for no known reason. X-ray overdosage for epilation in childhood ringworm may leave persistent radiodermatitis and cicatricial alopecia, but a somewhat smaller dose may be followed by a reasonable regrowth of hair, and atropy and the progressive reduction in follicle density may not be clinically apparent until age changes have added to those induced by the X-rays. The development of one or more basal cell carcinomas in the scalp in middle age should lead to a careful enquiry concerning ringworm in childhood. Binstock *et al.* (1981) described a very aggressive form occurring particularly in the hairy scalp of young adults.

Pathology

The pathology of these lesions in the scalp shows no features which distinguish it from that of basal cell carcinomas in other sites, other than those imposed by the anatomy of the scalp and by the greater tendency of patients to neglect lesions concealed by hair. Thus lesions tend to be larger and more advanced with destructive invasion of the periosteum, and even of bone (Howell & Riddell 1954). The depth of invasion may not be the same in all parts of a large tumour, and extension may occur along nerve sheaths as well as blood vessels and lymphatics.

Clinical features (Geiser 1980)

The typical smooth, translucent nodule, very slowly enlarging, with a few telangiectatic vessels crossing its surface occurs in the scalp as elsewhere (Figs 18.6 & 18.7). The nodule may be slightly or even deeply pigmented. Ulceration is frequent. The duration of the lesion when the patient seeks advice is measured in months or years; if a lesion of more than trivial size is reliably known to have been present only a few weeks, serious doubt should be thrown on the diagnosis.

The multicentric basal cell carcinoma is particularly characteristic of the scalp.

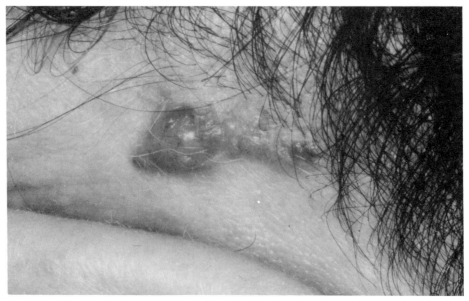

Fig. 18.6 Basal cell epithelioma arising at the age of 66 years in a congenital epidermal naevus of the scalp.

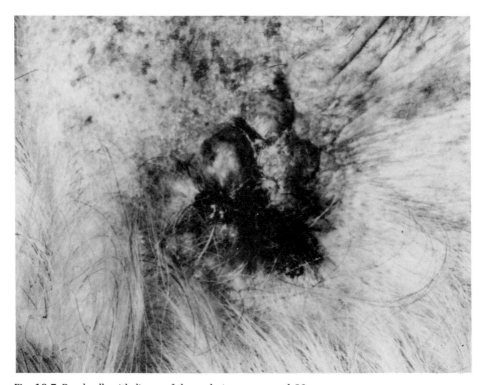

Fig. 18.7 Basal cell epithelioma of the scalp in a man aged 82 years.

It presents a rolled mother-of-pearl margin; its surface is moist and crusted and atrophic or ulcerated. Throughout the lesion some hair follicles are present in patches. Such lesions can be alarmingly destructive, involving even the meninges if they are neglected (James *et al.* 1950).

The uncommon morphoeic type of basal cell carcinoma also occurs in the scalp (Howell and Riddell 1954). The indurated, thickened plaque is not readily recognized as a tumour.

Haber *et al.* (1989) described an unusual case of basal cell carcinoma of the hairy scalp of a negroid individual with no preceding risk factors.

Diagnosis

A biopsy should be taken as soon as the diagnosis is suspected. If the lesion is large biopsies should be taken from two or more sites, to give some indication of the depth of invasion of dermis or periosteum.

Treatment

Very small carcinomas may be effectively treated by curettage, provided the patient can be kept under supervision, but wide excision is advisable. Whether excision or radiotherapy is preferred it is of the greatest importance to ensure that the initial treatment is adequate, for the treatment of recurrences presents even greater difficulties than in other parts of the body; modern surgical methods certainly give the best cosmetic results, particularly with large lesions. Some authors suggest that MOHS micrographic surgery should be used for all but the smallest lesions.

References

Battle, R.J.V. & Patterson, T.J.S. (1960) The surgical treatment of basal-celled carcinoma. *British Journal of Plastic Surgery*, **12**, 118.

Binstock, J.H., Stigman, S.J. & Tromovitch, T.A. (1981) Large aggressive basal cell carcinoma of the scalp. *Journal of Dermatologic Surgery and Oncology*, **7**, 565.

Geiser, T.D. (1980) Les tumeurs cutanées malignes du cuir chevelu. *Revue de Thérapeutique*, **37**, 578.

Haber, R.S., Beltrani, V.P., Yunakov, M.J. & Held, J.L. (1989) Basal cell carcinoma of the scalp in a black patient. *Cutis*, **44**, 59.

Howell, J.B. & Riddell, J.M. (1954) Cancer of forehead and scalp. *Journal of the American Medical Association*, **154**, 13.

James, A.G., Anderson, R.G., Scholl, J.A. & Martin, B.C. (1950) Cancer of the scalp. *American Journal of Surgery*, **80**, 441.

Bowen's disease
(Reference p. 562)

This intra-epidermal carcinoma may occur in any part of the skin. In the scalp it occurs most frequently in areas long exposed to solar damage by balding but multicentric Bowen's disease has occurred in the hairy scalp (Mora *et al.* 1980).

The lesion is a crusted, sharply marginated plaque which has been mistaken for psoriasis. It enlarges very slowly. An invasive squamous carcinoma may eventually develop.

The diagnosis should be confirmed histologically. Lesions on hairy sites should be excised; those on exposed, bald areas respond well to liquid nitrogen cryosurgery.

Reference

Mora, R.G., Jolly, H.W. & Vaughn, G.E. (1980) Localised multicentric Bowen's disease of the scalp. *Archives of Dermatology*, **116**, 841.

Squamous cell carcinoma
(References p. 563)

Squamous cell carcinoma in the scalp is uncommon, but early diagnosis is of such importance in prognosis that a knowledge of its precursors is essential.

The most frequent precursor of squamous carcinoma of the scalp is a solar keratosis. Such lesions occur in scalp which has long been bald and the lack of hair ensures that changes in the appearance of the keratosis should be rapidly detected.

The scalp is not infrequently the site of burns or scalds in childhood. Squamous carcinoma may develop after an interval of many years in long-forgotten scar tissue (Lawrence 1952; Cruickshank *et al.* 1963).

Skin damaged by X-ray epilation in the treatment of ringworm may later be the site of squamous carcinoma. Lupus vulgaris was at one time treated with X-rays and such lesions too may develop squamous carcinoma as may also chronic lupus erythematosus (Ratzer & Strong 1967). Routine therapeutic doses of Grenz rays, i.e. no more than 20 Gy/year or 100 Gy/lifetime may give rise to carcinomatous changes in the treated area—latency time up to 18 years (Frentz 1989). Most cases have resulted from the use of Grenz rays for scalp psoriasis and other benign dermatoses.

Clinical features

The development of induration around the base of a solar keratosis should raise the suspicion of malignant change. Ulceration of a long-standing scar does not necessarily imply a diagnosis of squamous carcinoma but it too is an indication for urgent biopsy. Any change in size or any ulceration of a chronic skin lesion of the scalp should be submitted to biopsy with the minimum of delay.

Treatment

If histological examination establishes the diagnosis of squamous carcinoma the management of the patient should be surgical though which dermatological surgery technique is applied will depend on the pathological type, the site and the size.

References

Cruickshank, A.H., McConnell, E.M. & Miller, D.G. (1963) Malignancy in scars, chronic ulcers and sinuses. *Journal of Clinical Pathology*, **16**, 573.

Frentz, G. (1989) Grenz ray induced nonmelanoma skin cancer. *Journal of the American Academy of Dermatology*, **21**, 475.

Lawrence, E.A. (1952) Carcinoma arising in the scars of thermal burns. *Surgery, Gynaecology and Obstetrics*, **95**, 579.

Ratzer, E.R. & Strong, E.W. (1967) Squamous cell carcinoma of the scalp. *American Journal of Surgery*, **114**, 570.

Melanocytic tumours

Melanocytic naevi

Melanocytic naevi (pigmented naevi) are formed by the proliferation of melano-cytes at the dermo-epidermal junction. Some naevi are present at birth but the majority appear during childhood or adult life. Relatively few new naevi develop after middle age and fewer are present in old age. If the activity at the dermo-epidermal junction ceases the naevus gradually becomes intra-dermal. If junctional activity persists after the intra-dermal naevus has formed then this is said to be of the compound type (Fig. 18.8).

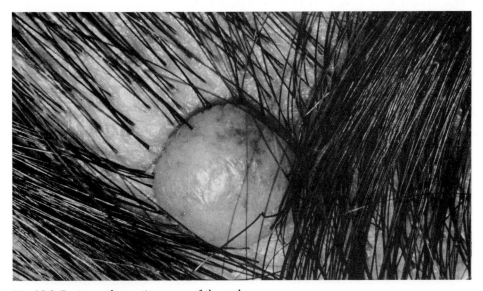

Fig. 18.8 Benign melanocytic naevus of the scalp.

Junctional naevi are flat brown macules. At a rate which varies with the site and with the individual, junctional naevi form compound naevi and become raised to a variable degree. At puberty the enlargement of some naevi and the growth of coarse hair in some, often brings them to the notice of parents. Each naevus may reach its maximum size in childhood or during adult life. Pigmented naevi may ultimately become pedunculated and be shed. It is important to think of the pigmented naevi in any individual as a changing population. Some new ones appear from time to time; the existing naevi mature at varying rates.

Pigmented naevi of the ordinary types are not uncommon in the scalp. Medical advice is often sought because of enlargement or because the comb catches in the naevus or because of a change in the appearance of the naevus.

An increase in size or in the depth of pigmentation, ulceration, bleeding or pain are indications for immediate excision and histological examination. The risk of melanoma developing in any individual naevus is slight, but this tumour is of such importance that early diagnosis is essential.

A naevus, usually on the neck in women, or in male adolescents may suddenly become swollen and tender. On careful examination it is often evident that the inflammatory swelling is situated beneath rather than within the naevus. The lesion is in fact a foreign body granuloma which will resolve or may recur. Excision is desirable both for this reason and because it allows histological confirmation of the diagnosis. We have seen these granulomas on the nape of the neck but not in other regions of the scalp.

The patient's attention may first be drawn to a previously unnoticed naevus of the scalp by the development of a mesh of white hairs which, on closer examination, can be shown to arise in a halo of leucoderma surrounding the naevus.

The dysplastic naevus (B-K mole) syndrome is of great importance because it sheds some light on the evolution of malignant melanoma and helps one to recognize 'at-risk' members of the population. It was originally described as a familial connection but sporadic examples do occur. The disease consists essentially of the tendency of affected individuals to develop large numbers of atypical naevi with melanocytic dysplasia with an increased incidence of malignant melanoma.

Treatment

In almost every case in which treatment is considered necessary or desirable, excision is to be preferred; if malignancy cannot be excluded or if the diagnosis is in any doubt, excision is mandatory. If malignancy is thought probable, plans must be made for further surgery to be undertaken without delay, should malignancy be proven. If the naevus is certainly benign the probable cosmetic benefits of excision should be carefully evaluated and unnecessary surgery should be avoided.

Congenital pigmented naevi (References p. 565)

Pigmented naevi present at birth differ in their morphology and natural history from the commoner pigmented naevi appearing during childhood or during adult life.

Histologically they are similar to compound naevi but the naevus cells extend more deeply.

Clinically they may be quite small with a surface which is warty or hairy, or both, but they may be very extensive, with a dermatomal distribution. If on the lower back they tend to involve the buttocks and thighs in a 'bathing trunk' pattern; if on the upper back they infest the shoulders and arms, and if in the cervical region, the scalp. There may be associated melanocytic infiltration of the meninges; this is associated particularly with cranial and cervical naevi but may occur with giant congenital naevi in any site (Reed *et al.* 1965).

Congenital naevi are dark brown with an irregularly thickened, sometimes verrucous, surface. The naevus becomes thicker and darker and the coarse hairs which are usually present become more conspicuous with the approach of puberty. Dark brown or black nodules may also be present.

Malignant melanoma develops in infancy, childhood, or less commonly in adult life in at least 10% of cases. In one series of giant naevi the incidence of malignancy was 17.5% (Pack & Davis 1961). Neurocutaneous melanosis is frequently fatal (Netherton 1936).

Another still rarer form of congenital naevus of the scalp is the cerebriform naevus (Gibson 1960). This irregularly convoluted naevus is melanocytic but is not clinically pigmented. Malignant change is rare in such naevi but does occur (Gross & Carter 1967).

Treatment

The high incidence of malignant melanoma even in infancy in congenital naevi, together with the serious cosmetic disfigurement they inflict, make excision the treatment of choice. A plastic surgeon should be consulted as soon as possible and excision in stages should be planned as soon as the child is old enough. Sometimes with very large naevi only very limited surgery can safely be undertaken in infancy. In such cases priority should be given to excising those areas in which the naevus appears to be most active. Techniques of excision which preserve the follicles may be applicable in some cases (Cronin 1953).

References

Cronin, T.D. (1953) Extensive pigmented naevi in the hair-bearing areas; resection of pigmented layer whilst preserving the follicles. *Plastic and Reconstructive Surgery,* **11**, 94.

Gibson, A.A.M. (1960) A giant benign naevus of the scalp. *Journal of Pathology and Bacteriology,* **80**, 185.

Gross, P.R. & Carter, D.M. (1967) Malignant melanoma arising in a giant cerebriform naevus. *Archives of Dermatology,* **96**, 536.

Netherton, E.W. (1936) Extensive pigmented nevus associated with primary melanoblastosis of leptomeninges of brain and spinal cord. *Archives of Dermatology and Syphilology (Chicago),* **33**, 238.

Pack, G.T. & Davis, J. (1961) Naevus giganticus pigmentosus with malignant transformation, *Surgery (St. Louis),* **89**, 347.

Reed, W.B., Beck, S.Q. & Nickel, W.R. (1965) Giant pigmented nevi, melanoma and leptomeningeal melanocytosis. *Archives of Dermatology,* **91**, 100.

Juvenile melanoma (Spitz naevus; spindle and epithelioid cell naevus)
(References p. 567)

This tumour is generally considered to be a special form of benign compound
naevus. Before it was characterized by Spitz in 1948 many such tumours were
misdiagnosed as melanomas and unnecessary radical treatment was carried out
(Kernen & Ackerman 1960).

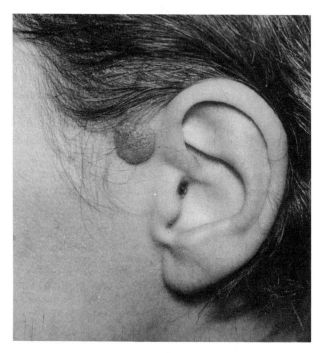

Fig. 18.9 Benign melanocytic
naevus.

Aetiology
The peak incidence of juvenile melanoma is between 3 and 15, but onset in infancy
or adult life may occur and persistence of lesions into adult life is not unusual. They
are most frequently seen on the face, particularly the cheeks, or on the arms or legs.
They are less common on the trunk. They have been reported in the scalp
(Gartmann 1959).

Pathology
The cells of the juvenile melanoma are larger than ordinary naevus cells, polygonal
or spindle-shaped, with abundant eosinophilic cytoplasm, and are arranged in
nests or cords in the upper or mid dermis. There are few or no mitoses.
Characteristic but inconstant are large giant cells, usually with three of four nuclei.
Pigment is absent or scanty. There may be an abundant lymphocytic infiltrate.
Telangiectases may be conspicuous in the oedematous subepidermal zone.

Clinical features

The juvenile melanoma commonly presents as a firm elevated nodule, pink, red, or red brown, with a smooth or slightly warty surface. It is commonly said to have developed very slowly. Bleeding with slight trauma is often noted, and the vascularity may suggest the diagnosis. The lesion persists but remains benign.

Differential diagnosis

Pyogenic granuloma, melanocytic naevus, malignant melanoma and lupus vulgaris are the main diagnostic problems.

Treatment

Simple excision is adequate.

References

Gartmann, H. (1959) Probleme des sogenannten Juvenilen Melanom. *Medizinische Kosmetik*, **8**, 301.

Kernen, J.A. & Ackerman, L.V. (1960) Spindle cell nevi and epithelioid cell nevi (so-called juvenile melanomas) in children and adults, *Cancer*, **13**, 612.

Blue naevus (References p. 568)

Aetiology

Blue naevi are circumscribed developmental defects in which persisting melanocytes are situated in the dermis.

Pathology

The common type of blue naevus consists of groups of melanocytes in the lower dermis. In the so-called cellular type there are also larger cells arranged in a neuroid pattern (Rodriguez & Ackerman 1986).

Clinical features

The common type of blue naevus is a flat or slightly elevated blue-black papule, usually small (Fig. 18.10). The cellular type is sometimes larger and more raised. The lesions occur most frequently on the face and the extremities but have occurred in most sites, including the scalp (Gartmann & Lischka 1972; Dawber 1972). They may be present at birth or may first appear at any age. Malignant change is uncommon.

Treatment

If the naevus is over 1 cm in diameter, or if it is enlarging, it should be excised with an adequate margin of normal tissue.

If it is small, flat and unchanging it may be removed on cosmetic grounds if the patient so wishes.

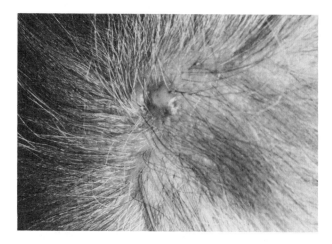

Fig. 18.10 Blue naevus. This patient also has ringed hair.

References

Dawber, R. (1972) Investigation of a family with pili annulati associated with blue naevus. *Transactions of St. Johns' Hospital Dermatological Society*, **58**, 51.

Gartmann, H. and Lischka, G. (1972) Maligner blauer Naevus. *Hautarzt*. **23**, 175.

Rodriguez, H.A. & Ackerman, L.V. (1986) Cellular blue naevus; clinicopathologic study of 45 cases. *Cancer*, **21**, 393.

Naevus of Ota (References p. 569)

The naevus of Ota is a developmental defect, not proved to be of hereditary origin, which consists of dermal melanocytosis in the distribution of the first two divisions of the trigeminal nerve. It is apparently considerably more frequent among the Japanese than in other races, but it is not confined to Mongoloids. About 80% of patients have been females (Fig. 18.11). Bluish black pigmentation may be present at birth and it appears before the end of the first year in about 50%; onset after the third decade has not been reported (Kopf & Weidman 1962; Hidano *et al.* 1967).

At its maximum the pigmentation extends, particularly during early life, to orbital and zygomatic skin but it may cover a wide area and exceptionally may be bilateral (Hidano *et al.* 1967). The pigmentation may spread from the forehead some 2 cm or more into the scalp margin (Pariser & Beerman 1949; Findlay 1951).

Melanocytosis may affect ocular structures such as the sclera, cornea, iris and fundus, and also the oropharyngeal mucous membrane.

Ota's naevus is essentially a cosmetic disability, and no more can be done to relieve it than to obtain for the patient expert advice on the use of covering creams. Malignant change is exceedingly rare but a fatal orbital melanoma has been reported in a woman age 64 (Jay 1965).

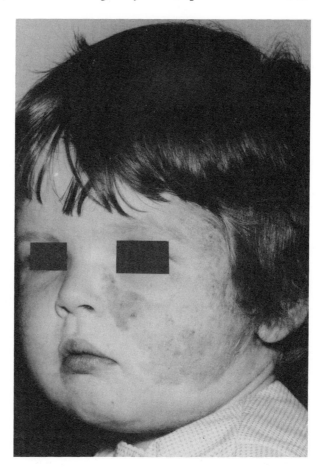

Fig. 18.11 Naevus of Ota
in a girl aged 2 years.

References

Findlay, G.H. (1951) Mesodermal abnormalities of the face and sclera. *South African Journal of Clinical Science*, **2**, 281.

Hidano, A., Kajima, H., Ikeda, S., Mizutani, H., Miyasata, H. & Miimura, M. (1967) Natural history of Nevus of Ota. *Archives of Dermatology*, **95**, 157.

Jay, B. (1965) Malignant melanoma of the orbit in a case of oculodermal melanosis. *British Journal of Ophthalmology*, **49**, 359.

Kopf, A.W. & Weidman, A.I. (1962) Nevus of Ota. *Archives of Dermatology*, **85**, 195.

Pariser, H. & Beerman, H. (1949) Extensive blue patch-like pigmentation. *Archives of Dermatology and Syphilology*, **59**, 396.

Malignant melanoma (References p. 571)

Aetiology

In most countries for which adequate statistics are available the incidence of malignant melanoma is increasing, as is the mortality from it. This increase may be due in part to increased exposure to sunlight of those who are susceptible by virtue of their fair skins. The capacity to form protective pigment is of course itself genetically determined, but there is also a more specific hereditary tendency to develop melanoma; in such families the age of onset of the melanoma is early, multiple primary tumours are not unusual, and the survival rate is higher than in patients with non-familial melanomas (Anderson 1971).

Some 30–50% of melanomas arise in benign pigmented naevi; the remainder develop in apparently normal skin. Melanomas in the scalp are largely of the nodular type arising in congenital naevi and occurring mainly in children and young adults, or of the lentigo malignant melanoma type, in sun-damaged bald scalp in the elderly.

In most series of cases all tumours of the head and neck are grouped together. When the scalp is separately classified the incidence of tumours in this site varies from less than 1% (Daland & Holmes 1939) to 3% (Farrell 1932). The latter series, like many from the Mayo Clinic, may include an unduly high proportion of cases which presented special treatment problems. A series of 48 cutaneous melanomas in Algeria (Merssini-Montpellier & Striet 1952) included seven in the scalp, of which five were in Europeans, one in a Negroid and one in an Asiatic. In three of 15 consecutive cases of disseminated melanomatosis, the primary tumour had been in the scalp (Tullis 1958). The early metastasis and poor prognosis of melanoma of the scalp is emphasized by a number of case reports (Russo 1947; Dionisi *et al.* 1951). In a French series of 623 melanomas (Maillard 1971) the 5-year survival rate for tumours of the forearm (70%) and face (50%) contrasted grimly with the 0% 5-year survival rate of melanomas of the scalp.

Pathology
The neoplastic melanocytes may invade the dermis laterally or vertically and the extent and direction of this invasion determines the indications for treatment and the prognosis (McGovern 1976). Scalp malignant melanomas, apart from in bald areas, more commonly present in a bad prognostic form as judged by the Clarke and Breslow histological criteria.

Clinical features
Any change in a congenital naevus should be regarded with suspicion; in particular localized increases in pigmentation, bleeding from an area of erosion, or complaints of itching or discomfort in the lesion.

The nodular form of melanoma, usually in middle-aged or elderly men, presents as a rather vascular reddish-brown nodule, raised or even pedunculated.

The melanomas in congenital naevi and the nodular melanoma may develop in hairy scalp and this delays their diagnosis, which in part accounts for their poor prognosis.

In contrast the lentigo maligna melanoma usually develops in bald scalp as a flat brown patch; as this slowly extends the pigmentation becomes more intensely black in some areas and redder in others. Eventually a nodule may form at a point within the pigmented area and may first present as localized crusting and ulceration.

Diagnosis

This involves a high level of suspicion of any pigmented lesion in the scalp or of any reddish-brown vascular nodule. If melanoma is considered to be a possible diagnosis excisional biopsy is desirable. If, however, the lesion is very large and excision would be a mutilating procedure incisional biopsy may be justifiable.

Treatment

This should be entrusted to an experienced plastic surgeon. The result of the surgical procedure will be determined by careful assessment of the clinical and histological features.

References

Anderson, D.E. (1971) Clinical characteristics of the genetic variety of cutaneous melanoma in man. *Cancer*, **28**, 721.

Daland, E.M. & Holmes, J.A. (1939) Malignant melanomas. *New England Journal of Medicine*, **220**, 651.

Dionisi, P., Orcel, L. & Kahn, J. (1951) Évolution aiguë d'un melanocarcinome du cuir chevelu. *Bulletin de L'Association française de Cancer*, **38**, 449.

Farrell, H.J. (1932) Cutaneous melanomas. *Archives of Dermatology and Syphilology*, **26**, 110.

Maillard, G.-F. (1971) Étude statistique de 623 mélanomes malins cutanés. *Annales de Dermatologie et de Syphiligraphie*, **98**, 5.

McGovern, V.J. (1976) *Malignant Melanomas. Clinical and Histological Diagnosis*. Wiley Medical, Sydney.

Merssini-Montpellier, J. & Striet, R. (1952) Le mélanoblastome malin. Quelques aspects Algériens. *Bulletin Algérien de Carcinologie*, **5**, 19.

Russo, P.E. (1947) Malignant melanoma in infancy. *Pediology*, **48**, 15.

Tullis, J.L. (1958) Triethylenephosphoramide in the treatment of disseminated melanoma. *Journal of the American Medical Association*, **166**, 37.

Perifollicular connective tissue tumours

These comprise three types of tumour: fibrofolliculoma of solitary and multiple types, trichodiscoma and perifollicular fibroma (Starink & Brownstein 1987). Multiple lesions may be inherited. The syndrome of Birt–Hogg–Dubé constitutes the occurrence together of hereditary multiple fibrofolliculomas, trichodiscomas and acrochordons (Birt *et al.* 1977; Rongioletti *et al.* 1988).

For further details of these uncommon tumours the reader is referred to more detailed textbooks of dermatology and dermatopathology.

References

Birt, A.R., Hogg, G.R. & Dubé, W.J. (1977) Hereditary multiple fibrofolliculomas with trichodiscomas and acrochordons. *Archives of Dermatology*, **113**, 1674.

Rongioletti, F., Hazini, R., Gianotti, G. & Regora, A. (1988) Birt–Hogg–Dubé syndrome associated
    with intestinal polyposis. *Clinical and Experimental Dermatology*, **14**, 72.
Starink, T.M. & Brownstein, M.H. (1987) Fibrofolliculoma: solitary and multiple types. *Journal of the
    American Academy of Dermatology*, **17**, 493.

Tumours of dermis and subcutis

Dermatofibrosarcoma protuberans (Darier and Ferrand's tumour)

This rare tumour usually begins in early adult life, but the diagnosis is often made
only after a considerable delay. It occurs most frequently on the trunk but is on the
head or neck in over 10% of cases (Shapiro & Brownstein 1976) and has been
reported in the scalp (Micoli *et al.* 1968).

Histologically the tumour consists of spindle-shaped cells in a closely woven
pattern.

Clinically there are protuberant firm nodules arising on a diffusely thickened
dermal plaque. Rockley *et al.* (1989) described three cases on the scalp of young
women and stressed that such lesions may directly invade the skull and
brain.

Excision must be wide as the risk of recurrence is considerable.

References

Micoli, G., Leofreddi, L. & Italia F. (1968) Dermatofibroma di Darier e Ferrand: Discussione di un
    caso a localizzazione al cuoio capelluto. *Gazzetta Istituto Medicinale Cuoio*, **73**, 2154.
Rockley, P.F., Robinson, J.K., Magid, M. & Goldblatt, D. (1989) Dermatofibrosarcoma of the scalp.
    Journal of the American Academy of Dermatology, **21**, 278.
Shapiro, L. & Brownstein, M.H. (1976) Dermatofibrosarcoma protuberans. In *Cancer of the Skin*, vol.
    2, p. 1069, eds. R. Andrade, S.L. Gumport, G.L. Popkin & T.D. Rees. Saunders, Philadelphia.

Gingival fibromatosis and multiple hyaline fibromas

Aetiology
The inheritance of this very rare disease is determined by an autosomal recessive
gene.

Clinical features
Gingival fibromatosis begins in infancy or early childhood. Soon numerous
subcutaneous nodules appear on the scalp, face, shoulders and digits. Later they
appear on the trunk and limbs. In the scalp they resemble cylindromas.
Histologically they consist of amorphous, PAS-positive ground substance in which
are embedded blood vessel and spindle-shaped cells.

There is no associated hypertrichosis.

Reference

Kitano, W. (1976) Juvenile hyaline fibromatosis. *Archives of Dermatology*, **112**, 86.

Neurofibromatosis (Von Recklinghausen's disease)

Aetiology
Neurofibromatosis is a neuro-ectodermal disorder, the inheritance of which is determined by an autosomal dominant gene. It is relatively common and occurs in 1 in 2500–3000 births (Crowe *et al.* (1956).

Pathology
Neurofibromas are derived from peripheral nerves and their supporting structures and consist of Schwann cells in collagenous interstitial tissue. Pigmented macules may contain macromelanosomes (Jimbow *et al.* 1974).

Clinical features
Neurofibromata can occur anywhere in the skin including the scalp where they are not uncommon. They are seen in several distinct clinical forms. The small, soft, lilac-pink molluscum fibrosum resembling a grape pip, contrasts with the diffuse elongated plexiform neuroma along the course of a nerve, and the diffuse overgrowth of skin and subcutaneous tissue producing the severely disfiguring pendulous folds of elephantiasis neuromatosa. Two types of pigmented lesion are characteristic of the disease: small freckles in the axillae and perineum are present in about 20% of cases and are pathognomonic (Crowe 1964); light-brown, more or less oval, café-au-lait spots are present in over 90% of cases. One or more such spots are present in 10% of normal subjects but the presence of six or more is highly suggestive of neurofibromatosis (Crowe *et al.* 1956).

The scalp may be involved with the face in neurofibromatous elephantiasis as in Treves' 'Elephant Man' (Howell & Ford 1980) but the commonest scalp lesions are single or multiple soft nodules, often appearing during the second or the third decade and sometimes becoming quite large. The soft consistency suggests the diagnosis and should lead to an investigation of the entire skin for other evidence of the disease. If this is found the patient should be kept under long-term supervision so that the involvement of other organ systems by the disease, should it occur, may be diagnosed early (Canale & Bebin 1972; Brasfield & Das Gupta 1972). The severity of neurofibromatosis is extremely variable and ranges from pigmentary changes with a few small mollusca to grossly disfiguring and disabling diseae with involvement of multiple systems.

Treatment
Excision is the only possible treatment and should be carried out if the scalp lesion is enlarging or is otherwise troublesome. Malignant change occurs in a significant proportion of lesions in deeper structures but is very unusual in superficial lesions.

References
Brasfield, R.D. & Das Gupta, T.K. (1972) Von Recklinghausen's disease—a clinicopathological study. *Annals of Surgery*, **175**, 86.

Canale, D.J. & Bebin, J. (1972) Von Recklinghausen's disease of the nervous system. In *Handbook of Clinical Neurology*, vol. 14, p. 132, eds. P.J. Vinken & G.W. Bruyn. North-Holland, Amsterdam.

Crowe, F.W. (1964) Axillary freckling as physical sign of neurofibromatosis. *Annals of Internal Medicine*, **66**, 1142.

Crowe, F.W., Schull, W.J. & Neel, J.V. (1956) *A Clinical, Pathological and Genetic Study of Multiple Neurofibromatosis*,Thomas, Springfield.

Howell M. & Ford P. (1980) *The True History of the Elephant Man*. Allison & Busby, London.

Jimbow, K., Szabo, G. & Fitzpatrick, T.B. (1974) Ultrastructure of giant pigment granules (macro-melanosomes) in the cutaneous pigmented macules of neurofibromatosis. *Journal of Investigative Dermatology*, **61**, 300.

Encephalocraniocutaneous lipomatosis

This syndrome, of which only four examples have been reported, cannot yet be too rigidly defined, as further cases may lead to some broadening of the clinical spectrum.

From birth soft papules and nodules are present in the scalp and on the face and neck; they have been unilateral in three cases and bilateral in one. Over the larger lesions in the scalp are patches of alopecia. Histologically the lesions are fibrolipomata or angiofibromata. Naevus lipomatosus cutaneous superficialis limited to the scalp and causing alopecia must be differentiated (Chanoki *et al.* 1989).

References

Chanoki, M., Sugamoto, I., Suzuki, S. & Hamada, T. (1989) Nevus lipomatosus cutaneous superficialis of the scalp. *Cutis*, **43**, 143.

Sanchez, N.P., Rhodes, A.R., Mandell, F. & Mihm, M.C. (1981) Encephalocraniocutaneous lipomatosis: a new neurocutaneous syndrome. *British Journal of Dermatology*, **104**, 89.

Mastocytosis (References p. 575)

The term mastocytosis is applied to a group of disorders in which mast cells are present in the tissues in excessive numbers.

In localized cutaneous mastocytosis one or sometimes two or three pigmented nodules are present at birth or appear in the first month of life. They may occur in any part of the body, including the scalp (Fig. 18.12). The urtication of the nodules when they are rubbed is a diagnostic feature. Sometimes blisters form on the nodules. Spontaneous resolution occurs during childhood.

Generalized cutaneous mastocytosis beginning in early childhood consists of light brown macules or nodular lesions, which urticate when rubbed. If the lesions are numerous the quantity of histamine released rubbing them may be sufficient to cause flushing. One boy aged 9 developed an attack of flushing when he visited his hairdresser (Marten 1957). Bullae may form on the lesions in early childhood; they have been sufficiently numerous to give rise to crusting of the scalp (Tavs 1947). This childhood form of the disease usually regresses before puberty. Rarely the

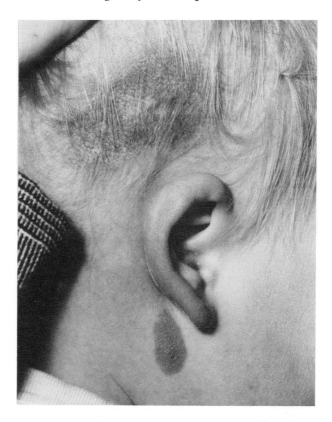

Fig. 18.12 Mast cell naevus in a child's scalp.

lesions are followed by conspicuous atrophy which, in the scalp, may give the appearance of scarring alopecia (Thivolet *et al.* 1981).

Involvement of the scalp is not a typical feature of the other forms of mastocytosis.

References

Marten, R.H. (1957) Urticaria pigmentation. *British Journal of Dermatology*, **69**, 151.

Tavs, L.E. (1947) Urticaria pigmentosa with bullae. *Archives of Dermatology and Syphilology*, **55**, 558.

Thivolet, J., Pierini, A.M., Cambazaud, F. *et al.* (1981) Mastocytose cutanée avec anétodermie secondaire et alopécie cicatricielle. *Annales de Dermatologie et de Vénéréologie* (*Paris*), **108**, 269.

Tumours of vessels

Granuloma telangiectaticum (granuloma pyogenicum; pseudobotryomycoma) (References p. 576)

Aetiology

The granuloma telangiectaticum, as the commonly employed synonym implies, was believed to be an abnormal tissue response to pyogenic infection of a minor abrasion but infection is probably secondary (Kerr 1951). The role of a virus has not been excluded. The lesion is seen in both sexes and at all ages, but is more common in childhood. The sexes are equally affected.

Pathology (Martens & McPherson 1956)
The granuloma consists of a mass of thin-walled newly formed capillaries in a connective tissue stroma, mucoid or fibrous, with an inconstant mixed cellular infiltrate.

Clinical features
It is a bright red, soft and highly vascular papule or nodule ranging in size from 2–3 mm to several centimetres in diameter, globular and pedunculated, mushroom-shaped or sessile. It enlarges for several weeks and then persists more or less indefinitely. It may be eroded or covered with a dried crust of foul-smelling seropurulent exudate. The base may be surrounded by a collar of thickened epidermis. Haemorrhage is often troublesome. The majority occur on the exposed parts, usually on the face in infancy and the face, hands, arms and upper trunk in older children and in adults. About 3% of those on the skin occur in the scalp (Kerr 1951). The mucous membranes of the oral cavity and nares are frequently affected. Lymphangitis is an occasional complication.

Diagnosis
Juvenile melanoma, malignant melanoma, and angiomatous naevi are most commonly confused. The history and the extreme friability of the lesion should serve to differentiate it from the angiomatous naevi. The juvenile melanoma may not be clinically distinguishable.

Treatment
Curettage and cautery or cryosurgery is usually satisfactory, but since the clinical diagnosis may be incorrect in about one case in three (McGeoch 1961), excision should be performed if there is any doubt in the clinician's mind. The lesion should always be examined histologically to exclude a serious diagnostic error, such as amelanotic malignant melanoma. Recurrences are occasionally seen, and excision is then advisable.

References
Kerr, D.A. (1951) Granuloma pyogenicum. *Oral Surgery*, **4**, 153.
Martens, V.E. & McPherson, D.J. (1956) Fibroangioma. *Archives of Pathology*, **61**, 120.
McGeoch, A.H. (1961) Pyogenic granuloma. *Australian Journal of Dermatology*, **6**, 33.

Angiolymphoid hyperplasia with eosinophilia (epithelioid haemangioma; Kimura's diseae) (References p. 577)

This angiomatous disorder occurs usually between the years of 25 and 45, in women more often than in men, and affects the scalp, the ears and occasionally the face. The lesions, which may be multiple, present as dome-shaped vascular nodules which may bleed easily.

Histologically the lesions show abnormal hypertrophic capillaries with swollen endothelial cells and an infiltrate of lymphocytes, histiocytes and eosinophils (Fig. 18.13).

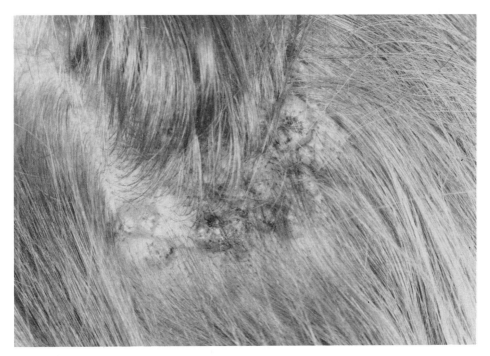

Fig. 18.13 Angiolymphoid hyperplasia.

The condition is benign, although recurrence may follow excision, which is the treatment of choice.

References

Berretty, P.J.M. & Faber, W.R. (1980) Angiolymphoid hyperplasia with eosinophils. *British Journal of Dermatology,* **103**, 578.

Vasques Botet, M. & Sanchez, J.L. (1978) Angiolymphoid hyperplasia with eosinophilia: report of a case and review of the literature. *Journal of Dermatologic Surgery and Oncology,* **4**, 931.

Wilson Jones, E. & Bleehen, S.S. (1969) Inflammatory angiomatous nodules with abnormal blood vessels occurring about the ears and scalp (pseudo or atypical pyogenic granuloma). *British Journal of Dermatology,* **81**, 804.

Vascular naevi (References p. 580)

The vascular naevi of the skin are circumscribed developmental defects of the dermal or subcutaneous vasculature. A simple classification of these naevi is:

1 Flat vascular naevi—telangiectatic naevi
      naevus flammeus—port-wine naevus
      (may also form part of complex syndromes)
2 Raised vascular naevi—cavernous
      superficial—strawberry mark
      deep

Flat vascular naevi

Nuchal naevus. The commonest flat naevus occurs on the nape of the neck and is
known as Unna's naevus. It was found in 20–30% of newborn babies in Malaya
(Tan 1972). A study of 2171 Danish schoolchildren aged 6–17 showed a nuchal
naevus in 46.2% of girls and 35.1% of boys (Oster & Nielsen 1970). The
reported incidence of the naevus in other population groups has ranged from 12
to 57%. The incidence in any population is the same in infancy and in middle
age. The naevus shows no tendency to disappear (Zumkeller 1957).
      The nuchal naevus is not a cosmetic problem, and is usually no more than an
incidental finding when the scalp is being examined.

Sturge–Weber syndrome. In this syndrome a port-wine naevus involves part of the
whole of the trigeminal distribution on the face and the front of the scalp. The
cutaneous naevus is associated with ocular and intra-cranial angiomatosis.
There is no constant relationship between the extent of skin involved and the
extent of intra-cranial lesions (Fig. 18.14).

Raised vascular naevi
Superficial raised naevi (strawberry mark) are present at birth or develop during
the first month after birth in some 90–95% of cases; in 5–10% they develop
from the second to the fifth month (Schnyder 1957; Simpson 1959). Subcutaneous cavernous naevi are essentially similar in their natural history. Both
superficial and subcutaneous types are about twice as common in girls as in
boys, and, although they may occur anywhere, are found predominantly on the
head and trunk (Fig. 18.15). In many reports the distribution of the naevi on the
head is not recorded in great detail, but 14% of Simpson's cases involved the
scalp.
      For the first 6–12 months the naevi continue to enlarge; indeed in a few
cases enlargement, but at a decreasing rate, may continue for 3 or 4 years. After
a year, but sometimes much earlier, greyish-blue patches mottle the previously
bright red surface, and the naevus begins to flatten. About 50% have involuted
without trace by the age of 5 and the process of involution continues in the
remainder. The residual changes when spontaneous involution has ceased
depend on the original size of the lesion and range from a few telangiectases to
redundant folds of atrophic skin. Superficial ulceration of naevi is not unusual in
infancy; it is not a serious complication and does not result in significant

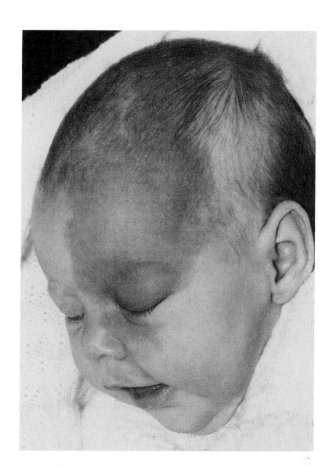

Fig. 18.14 Capillary naevus in the first two divisions of the left trigeminal nerve. This patient had Sturge–Weber syndrome.

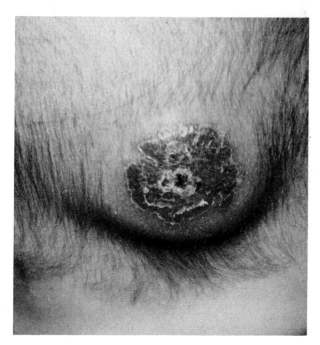

Fig. 18.15 Cavernous vascular naevus.

haemorrhage, but it may lead to some increase in scar formation. However, even in the scalp at least 50% of normal hair growth was preserved at the site of such a naevus (Simpson 1959).

Wallace (1953) had reported similar findings. Of 290 strawberry naevi, 120 disappeared without trace and a further 157 left slight atrophy which was no cosmetic disability. Of 121 deeper cavernous naevi 93 gave equally satisfactory results, though a slightly higher proportion had detectable atrophy. Bowers *et al.* (1960) made similar observations; they showed that spontaneous involution left only 6% with any ultimate cosmetic handicap.

Treatment. It is evident that in the majority of raised vascular naevi any form of treatment is unnecessary. Many potentially harmful measures, such as radiotherapy, have been used in the past, and the reluctance of the medical profession to accept the self-evident fact that most of the naevi involute spontaneously is now difficult to understand. Radiotherapy, even when it produced no local cutaneous damage, was associated with an increased incidence of thyroid carcinoma in childhood or adolescence (Brunner 1961).

A child's parents apprehensively watching the enlargement of a naevus on the face or scalp may put considerable pressure on their physician to provide some active treatment. Since such treatment is not in the best interests of the child it should never be given. If the parents can be shown serial photographs of the spontaneous involution of similar naevi, they will accept the advice that patience gives the best cosmetic results.

Where there are residual changes which require plastic surgery, this should be postponed until the comparison with photographs shows no further improvement over a year. Unnecessary surgery can then be avoided.

There are cases, however, in which active treatment is desirable or even essential. Treatment with systemic corticosteroids will hasten involution (Edgerton 1976) and is indicated when the naevus is obstructing orifices, or involves a vital organ or is causing cardiovascular decompensation (Lasser & Stein 1973).

Aggressive cryosurgery may cause large lesions to regress prematurely, but permanent alopecia is inevitable after such treatment.

References

Bowers, R.E., Graham, E.A. & Tomlinson, K.M. (1960) The natural history of the strawberry nevus. *Archives of Dermatology*, **82**, 167.
Brunner, K. (1961) Schilddrüsenkarzinom in Kinderalter nach Röntgenbestrahlen einer Nevus vascularis cutaneous von 12 Jahren. *Schweiz medizinische Wochenschrift*, **91**, 389.
Edgerton, M.T. (1976) The treatment of haemangioma. *Annals of Surgery*, **183**, 517.
Lasser, A.E. & Stein, A.F. (1973) Steroid treatment of hemangiomas in children. *Archives of Dermatology*, **108**, 565.
Oster, J. & Nielsen, A. (1970) Nuchal naevi and interscapular telangiectases. *Acta paediatrica Scandinavica*, **59**, 416.
Schnyder, U.W. (1957) Zur Klinik und Histologie der Angiome. IV. Die plano-tuberösen und tuberonodösen Angiome des Kleinkindes. *Archiv für klinische und experimentelle Dermatologie*, **204**, 457.

Simpson, J.R. (1959) Natural history of cavernous haemangiomata. *Lancet*, ii, 1057.

Tan, K.L. (1972) Nevus flammeus of the nape, glabella and eyelids. A clinical study of frequency, racial distribution, and association with congenital anomalies. *Clinical Pediatrics*, **11**, 112.

Wallace, H.J. (1953) The conservative treatment of haemangiomatous naevi. *British Journal of Plastic Surgery*, **6**, 78.

Zumkeller, R. (1957) A propos de la fréquence et de l'hérédité de 'Naevus vascularis uchae—Unna'. *Journal de Génétique Humaine*, **6**, 1.

Malignant angioendothelioma (angiosarcoma; haemangioendothelioma; haemangioblastoma)

Aetiology

Malignant angioendothelioma of the face and scalp has been characterized as a distinct clinicopathological entity (Wilson Jones 1964). Very rarely it may occur as early as the fourth decade but the average age of onset is between 70 and 80 with men more frequently affected than women (Hodgkinson *et al.* 1979; Knight *et al.* 1980; Drobacheff *et al.* 1989).

Pathology

The tumour consists of anastomosing irregular vascular channels and spaces which infiltrate but do not destroy the dermis. The channels are lined by atypical swollen endothelial cells which show a tendency to intra-luminal budding to form cords and islands of cells in syncytial arrangement.

Clinical features

The commonest presentation is with single or grouped bluish red nodules of the face and scalp. There may be some thinning of the hair over the tumours (Suurmond 1958) but alopecia is not a conspicuous feature of this form of the disease. Less well differentiated tumours appear as diffuse indurated plaques over which much hair is lost. Exceptionally there may be an extensive cicatricial alopecia (Knight *et al.* 1980). One morphological type is known to clinicians as the 'malignant bruise'.

Eventually a large area of face, neck and scalp may be involved, with gross oedema of the eyelids. The skin may ulcerate. Involvement of the cranial bones may occur and distant metastases are frequent (Kitawaga *et al.* 1987). The average duration of survival after onset is under 2 years.

Treatment

Palliative radiotherapy is the best that can be offered.

References

Drobacheff, C., Blanc, D. & Zultak, M. (1989) Malignant angioendotheliomas. *International Journal of Dermatology*, **28**, 454.

Hodgkinson, D.J., Soule, E.H. & Woods, J.E. (1979) Cutaneous angiosarcoma of the head and neck. *Cancer*, **44**, 1106.

Kitagawa, M., Tanaka, I., Takemura, T. *et al.* (1987) Angiosarcoma of the scalp. *Virchows Archives*, **412** (1), 83.

Knight, T.E., Robinson, H.M. & Sina, B. (1980) Angiosarcoma (angioendothelioma) of the scalp. *Archives of Dermatology*, **116**, 183.

Suurmond, D. (1958) Haemangioendothelioma (angioplastic sarcoma). *British Journal of Dermatology*, **70**, 132.

Wilson Jones, E. (1964) Malignant angioendothelioma of the skin. *British Journal of Dermatology*, **76**, 21.

Cutaneous meningioma

This is an extremely rare tumour which may occur in the scalp. A solitary nodule, usually in the midline of the occiput, is present from birth. The consistency of the tumour has been soft or rubbery. The overlying skin may be atrophic but has more often been thickened and sometimes hypertrophic. Some have enlarged slowly but others have remained unchanged. The ultimate size has ranged from 2 to 10 cm in diameter.

The diagnosis is suggested by the site and must be confirmed histologically. Treatment is by surgical excision.

Reference

Bain, G.O. & Schnitka, T.A. (1956) Cutaneous meningioma (psammoma). *Archives of Dermatology*, **74**, 590.

Carcinoma metastatic to the scalp
(References p. 584)

Aetiology and nomenclature

Carcinoma of an internal organ may involve the skin directly from an underlying organ or by extension through lymphatics, by lymphatic or bloodstream embolic dissemination, or by accidental implantation of tumour cells during the course of a surgical procedure (Mehregan 1961).

The incidence of metastatic carcinoma in the skin in any population reflects to some extent the efficiency with which malignant disease is sought, detected and treated. However, a cutaneous metastasis may be the presenting manifestation of an otherwise asymptomatic carcinoma; and indeed, even when the patient is fully investigated, the primary growth may not be discovered. In some cases, notably of carcinoma of the breast, a metastasis has appeared as long as 30 years after surgical removal of the original tumour (Michel *et al.* 1971).

In reported series the total incidence of cutaneous metastasis in patients with internal carcinoma has ranged from 2 to over 4%. The scalp is the site of such metastasis, particularly in hypernephroma (Rosenthal & Lever 1957), and carcinoma of the breast (Michel *et al.* 1971), but scalp metastasis also occurs from primary growth in bronchus, stomach, colon, rectum, ovary and prostate, and, more uncommonly, pancreas, liver, uterus and bone (Gómez Orbaneja *et al.*

1967; Cueto *et al.* 1970; Hernanez *et al.* 1979). Meningiomas may reach the scalp by direct extension, through operative defects in the skull or by metastasis (Waterson & Shapiro 1970).

Pathology
The cells in metastatic malignant deposits may retain recognizable characteristics of the primary tumour but may be too anaplastic for identification. Their metastatic origin is betrayed by their lack of any connection with cutaneous epithelial structures, but occasionally involvement of the epidermis by the cells of the metastasis may make diagnosis more difficult (Miescher 1955). Columns of cells may be seen within dilated lymphatics. Vascular dilatation is a variable feature.

The presence of mucin suggests that the primary tumour is in the digestive tract (Mehregan 1961). In metastasis from hypernephroma (Rosenthal & Lever 1957) the acinose arrangement of the cells of the original tumour may not be obvious, but vascular proliferation is often conspicuous.

Clinical features
Single or multiple firm non-tender nodules enlarging quite rapidly are the most frequent manifestation of metastatic carcinoma in the scalp. Sometimes when the patient's tissue reaction to the metastasis has been more effective there may be some oedema and inflammatory changes. In other changes dermal sclerosis around the deposit leads to destruction of hair follicles and the metastasis presents clinically as single or multiple areas of cicatricial alopecia (Fig. 18.16)—

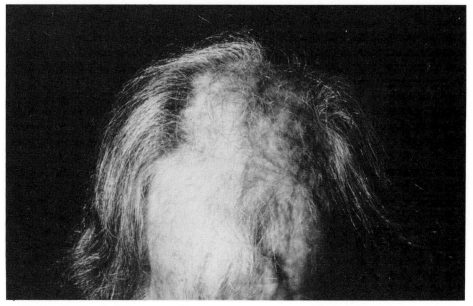

Fig. 18.16 Cicatricial alopecia caused by metastatic carcinoma of the breast.

scleroderma-like plaques of a few weeks' or months' duration (Delacrétaz & Chapuis 1958; Baran 1969; Baum *et al.* 1981).

Multiple nodules may simulate turban tumours (Ronchese 1940), but the latter develop slowly over many years.

Treatment

A biopsy should always be taken, and every attempt should be made to detect and treat the primary tumour. Usually the prognosis is very poor but, particularly in hypernephroma in which a solitary metastasis to the scalp may be the first evidence of the presence of the tumour, excision of both the affected kidney and the secondary may give a permanent cure.

Excision of the metastasis is always advisable unless of course it proves to be only one manifestation of generalized carcinomatosis. Even the long-delayed metastasis developing years after mastectomy should be excised (Michel *et al.* 1971) and the practicability of chemotherapy should be discussed. The patient's response to skin tests of delayed hypersensitivity may be of assistance in planning treatment (Anthony *et al.* 1974).

References

Anthony, H.M., Templeman, G.H., Madren, K.E. & Mason, M.K. (1974) The prognostic significance of DHS skin tests in patients with carcinoma of the bronchus. *Cancer*, **34**, 1901.
Baran, R. (1969) Les métastases alopéciantes scleroatrophiques des cancers mammaires. *Dermatologica*, **138**, 169.
Baum, E.M., Omura, E.F., Payne, P.P. & Little, W.P. (1981) Alopecia neoplastica—a rare form of cutaneous metastasis. *Journal of the American Academy of Dermatology*, **4**, 688.
Cueto, J.J., Rotman, J.-C., Castellato, R.H. & Veron, C.W. (1970) Metastasis alopeciante escleruoatrofica. *Archivos Argentinos de Dermatologia*, **20**, 167.
Delacrétaz, J. & Chapuis, H. (1958) Métastases cutanées alopéciantes. *Dermatologica*, **116**, 372.
Gómez Orbaneja, J., Ledo Pozueta, A. & de Castro Torres, A. (1967) Metastatic carcinomas to the skin. *Dermatologia Ibero Latino-Americana* (English edn.), **2**, 13.
Hernanez, J.M., Vives, P., Garcia Almazno, D. & Jacqueti, G. (1979) Alopecia neoplàsica. *Actas Dermosifilograficas*, **20**, 507.
Mehregan, A.H. (1961) Metastatic carcinoma to the skin. *Dermatologica*, **123**, 311.
Michel, P.-J., Cretin, J. & Grimaud, P.-S. (1971) A propos de certaines métastases cutanées isolées et tardives des cancers du sein. *Annales de Dermatologie et de Syphiligraphie*, **98**, 73.
Miescher, G. (1955) Über metastatische Invasio der Epidermis durch Tumorzellen (Melanom, Mammocarcinom). *Oncologia*, **8**, 203.
Ronchese, F. (1940) Metastasis of the scalp simulating turban tumours. *Archives of Dermatology and Syphilology*, **41**, 439.
Rosenthal, A.L. & Lever, W.F. (1957) Involvement of the skin in renal carcinoma. *AMA Archives of Dermatology*, **76**, 96.
Waterson, K.W. & Shapiro, L. (1970) Meningioma cutis. Report of a case. *International Journal of Dermatology*, **9**, 125.

Cysts of the scalp

The term sebaceous cyst is still widely used and is applied indiscriminately to epidermal cysts or trichilemmal cysts. It is best abandoned (Leppard & Sanderson 1976).

Trichilemmal cysts

Aetiology
This relatively common cyst occurs mainly in middle age, and more frequently in women than in men. The tendency to form such cysts is inherited, and it is determined by an autosomal dominant gene (Ingram & Oldfield 1937; Stephens 1959).

Pathology
The cysts are derived from the external root sheath, the trichilemma (Pinkus 1969). The wall consists of epidermis and the cyst contains keratin, but no granular layer is formed.

Clinical features
The cysts occur most frequently in the scalp, as single, or more often multiple, firm rounded nodules. If the cysts are large hair growth in the overlying scalp may be impaired.

Treatment
Treatment may be required on cosmetic grounds. The cysts can usually be dissected out without difficulty; occasionally excision may be necessary.

References
Ingram, J.T. & Oldfield, M.C. (1937) Hereditary sebaceous cysts. *British Medical Journal*, **i**, 960.
Leppard, B.J. & Sanderson, K.V. (1976) The natural history of trichilemmal cysts. *British Journal of Dermatology*, **94**, 379.
Pinkus, H. (1969) 'Sebaceous cysts' are trichilemmal cysts. *Archives of Dermatology*, **99**, 544.
Stephens, F.E. (1959) Hereditary multiple sebaceous cysts. *Journal of Heredity*, **50**, 299.

Cock's peculiar tumour

The case described by Bunker *et al.* (1989) clearly shows this expanding proliferative lesion of the scalp to be a giant pilar or trichilemmal cyst. They occur most commonly on the scalp of middle- to old-aged women and may mimic squamous cell carcinoma (Brownstein & Arluk 1981).

References
Brownstein, M.H. & Arluk, D.J. (1981) Proliferating trichilemmal cyst: a simulant of squamous cell carcinoma. *Cancer*, **48**, 1207.
Bunker, C.B., Smith, N.P., Russell, R.C.G. & Dowd, P.M. (1989) Cock's peculiar tumour. *Clinical and Experimental Dermatology*, **14**, 237.

Epidermoid cysts

Aetiology

Epidermoid cysts are common in adolescence and in adult life. They may occur as a complication of acne vulgaris.

They occur also in Gardner's syndrome.

Pathology

The wall of the cyst shows the normal layering of epidermis, but may be flattened by pressure. It contains lamellated keratin in which there may be cholesterol clefts.

Clinical features

Epidermoid cysts are firm and rounded nodules situated in the dermis and attached to the epidermis; there may be a central punctum.

They vary greatly in size, the largest cysts sometimes exceeding 50 mm in diameter. Recurrent episodes of inflammation are common, particularly in cysts associated with acne. The cysts occur most frequently on the face, neck and trunk, but are not uncommon in the scalp. They first appear in later childhood, and are frequently multiple.

Epidermoid cysts beginning in adolescence are a feature, often the earliest, of Gardner's syndrome, in which they are associated with fibromas, desmomas and lipomata of the skin and polyposis of the colon.

Treatment

Many cysts can be dissected out but cysts which have been inflamed may require excision, although some may be drained and pulverized.

Congenital inclusion dermoid cysts (Reference p. 587)

Aetiology

Most dermoid cysts develop from sequestrated epithelial cells along lines of embryonic fusion. In the scalp groups of epidermal cells are cut off from the surface epithelium at the suture lines as the cranial bones grow together (Colcock *et al.* 1955).

Pathology

The cysts are lined by stratified squamous epithelium and contain greasy material, keratinized debris and hair.

Clinical features

About 40% are present at birth and 60% by the fifth year. They slowly enlarge to reach a diameter of up to 5 cm. The skin is freely movable over them and they usually give rise to no symptoms.

Whilst the majority of cutaneous dermoids occur on the head and neck only a small proportion of them are in the scalp. In one series of cases the three cysts in the scalp were situated over the right parieto-occipital suture lines, the bregma and the anterior fontanelle respectively.

Treatment
Simple excision is usually adequate.

Reference
Colcock, B.P., Sass, R.D. & Standinger, L. (1955) Dermoid cysts. *New England Journal of Medicine*, **252**, 373.

Heterotropic brain tissue cyst of scalp

Commens *et al.* (1989) described two children who were noted at birth to have a single bald compressible nodule on the scalp surrounded by a collar of hypertrophic hair. Histology showed the lesions to be heterotropic brain tissue.

Reference
Commens, C., Rogers, M. & Kan, A. (1989) Heterotropic brain tissue presenting as bald cyst with a collar of hair. *Archives of Dermatology*, **125**, 1253.

Eruptive vellus hair cyst

This represents a relatively new entity of which only a few cases have so far been described (Benoldi & Allegra 1989). Small firm, sometimes keratotic papules develop in older children and young adults, the lesions particularly affecting the anterior chest and the flexor and extensor surface of the extremities (Lee *et al.* 1984).

Concurrent steatocystoma multiflex has been described (Jerasutus *et al.* 1989). Lesions may resemble keratosis pilaris, folliculitis or perforating dermatoses. Histologically thin-walled cysts are noted lined with a layer of squamous epithelium and containing multiple vellus hair.

References
Benoldi, D. & Allegra, F. (1989) Congenital eruptive vellus hair cysts. *International Journal of Dermatology*, **28**, 340.
Jerasutus, S., Suvanprakorn, P. & Sombatworapat, W. (1989) Eruptive vellus hair cyst and steatocystoma multiplex. *Journal of the American Academy of Dermatology*, **20**, 292.
Lee, S., Kim, J.G. & Kang, J.S. (1984) Eruptive vellus hair cysts. *Archives of Dermatology*, **120**, 1191.

Chapter 19
Investigation of Hair,
Hair Growth and the
Hair Follicle

Introduction

On being presented with a patient complaining, for example, of pruritus or a blistering eruption, most clinicians are fully competent to carry out a careful clinical examination and to use appropriate histological, biochemical and other laboratory investigations if required. The details of specific techniques for studying the pathogenesis of hair diseases seem for many clinicians and pathologists to be shrouded in mystery, mainly because the methods concerned are not within the province of any one speciality.

Many of the techniques required for studying hair and hair follicle abnormalities will be found in the chapter relating to the diseases in question. In this section are considered the clinical methods required for studying hair growth and also critical microscopic methods for detailed examination of hair shafts and hair follicles.

History-taking is of fundamental importance in assessing hair loss. A patient complaining of balding or hair loss may in fact have an increased shedding rate or a decrease in hairs per unit area. The complaint of thinning of hair may be due to a decrease in the number of hairs per unit area or a decrease in hair diameter; sometimes this may be worsened by a decrease in hair pigmentation. By careful questioning it is possible to assess these factors which guide one into particular lines of investigation and differential diagnosis. It is important that these factors should be quantified in order to assess accurately the progress (and prognosis) of hair disease and also to assess the changes induced by treatment. For example, in androgenetic alopecia and hirsutism, changes in the telogen count, linear growth rate, diameter of hair and pigmentation are detectable before the affected individual is able to subjectively observe the changes.

Hair growth may be measured by several easy clinical investigations. Daily hair growth may be measured with a graduated rule after shaving the skin. The length of the growth cycle (anagen) may be calculated by dividing the overall length of an uncut hair by the daily growth rate. In some circumstances it is only necessary to know the relative proportion of telogen/anagen hairs; this may be assessed by plucking hairs to examine the roots or by scalp biopsy. It should be noted that only telogen hairs are removed by combing or washing—anagen scalp hairs are bound too firmly to be removed in this manner.

Length of the hair cycle—examination of hair roots
(References p. 592)

The length of the hair cycle can be studied by observation (Pinkus 1947; Saitoh *et al.* 1970). This method relies on long periods of observations and accurate identification of individual hairs. It is more convenient to assess overall growth using hair length, daily linear growth (see below), in conjunction with an assessment of hair root status. This gives information on the length of the growth cycle (anagen = total length/daily growth) and the percentage of growing roots.

Hair roots are examined by plucking hairs (Fig. 19.1). The shafts should be

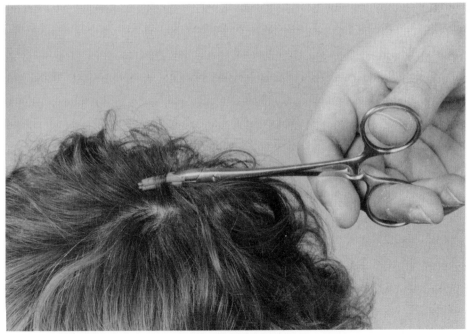

Fig. 19.1 Technique for plucking hairs. The hairs are grasped at a uniform point above the scalp and the forceps are rotated to ensure a firm grasp. The hairs are extracted with a firm pull.

grasped firmly and extracted briskly in the direction of their insertion. This ensures that the roots are not deformed (Van Scott *et al.*1957; Maguire & Kligman 1964). Surgical needle holders are used with the blades covered with fine rubber tubing or cellophane tape to ensure a firm grasp. Approximately 50 hairs should be extracted in order to reduce sampling errors. The roots are examined under a low-power microscope. The root morphology is stable and hairs can be kept for many weeks in dry packaging before analysis. Normal telogen counts are 13–15% on the vertex (Kligman 1961; Van Scott *et al.* 1957), but this figure will vary from site to site, with age, physiological androgen influences and many other factors. The appearance of the root is also important; shrivelled and atrophic roots are a feature of protein–calorie malnutrition (Bradfield *et al.* 1969, 1971, 1972).

Histological techniques
It is not always possible to obtain representative samples of hairs by plucking, particularly when examining the balding scalp or when assessing regrowth whilst the shafts are too short to grasp. In order to circumvent this problem several investigators have devised histological techniques. Uno *et al.* (1969) studied the stump-tailed macaque which, like *Homo sapiens*, also develops androgenic alopecia. They measured serial horizontal sections of skin along the length of the follicle and constructed a trichogram to compare different areas of the scalp, using follicle length and developmental stage as indices (see Fig.19.2). As the roots convert from terminal to vellus, their length decreases. Schreck-Purola *et al.* (1981) produced a similar histogram to display the different patterns and change of growth with therapy.

Kligman (1961) originally studied telogen effluvium by scalp histology demonstrating increased telogen roots in combination with a standardized combing technique and counting the shed hairs. This control data revealed that 90% of the normal population shed fewer than 75 hairs/day.

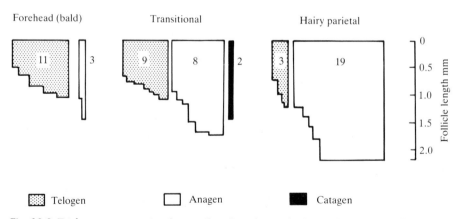

Fig. 19.2 Trichogram comparing density, length and growth phase of follicles at different sites on the scalp (adapted from Uno *et al.* 1969).

Headington (1984) has made detailed studies of hair roots by means of horizontal sections of scalp taken with 4–6 mm punch biopsies. He has defined the transverse appearance of the root in its different growth phase. Vellus hairs, which he defines as having a diameter less than 0.03 mm, are not seen below the entry of the sebaceous duct. Anagen hairs are recognized by the inner root sheath and absence of keratinocyte necrosis in the tricholemma. Catagen hair have a distinctive thickening of the basement membrane in the lower external root sheath. Telogen follicles have a bulbous configuration and have lost their inner root sheath. With this technique, a 6 mm punch biopsy will yield 22–30 follicular units or 60–80 terminal hairs. Once the orientation of this technique has been mastered, considerable data can be gleaned about the total number and density of follicular units, follicular structures and their developmental stage and hair shaft diameters.

Root volumes were first calculated by Van Scott and Ekel (1958), also using horizontal sections of skin. They assumed that the volume between sections approximated to truncated cones and that the total volume comprised the sum of the slices. The volume of the matrix was calculated by subtracting the volume of the papilla from the total root. They estimated that in normal hair the papilla was $338 \times 10^3 \ \mu m^3$ and contained 1220 cells, and that the matrix was $3370 \times 10^3 \ \mu m^3$ with 139 cells in mitosis. In a further series of experiments, Van Scott *et al.* (1963) found that the volume of the matrix was proportional to the height of the papilla. Ibrahim and Wright (1982) have found a constant relationship between the volume of the dermal papilla and the volume of the fully grown hair in rats and mice. An earlier method was employed by Crounse *et al.* (1970) who estimated root volumes by linear displacement of water in a calibrated capillary micropipette under a low-power microscope. The estimation of root volume may be of more general use than the measurement of hair growth as the root volume and protein content are directly proportional and correlate well with reduction in body weight (Crounse *et al.* 1970).

Follicle kinetics
Hair growth is the result of holocrine secretion by the hair follicle. This occurs in bursts of activity. Therefore, the ultimate measure of growth is by examination of the kinetics of the matrix cells. There are two methods of estimating mitotic activity: proliferative indices and metaphase arrest. The former is a count of the number of cells actively dividing at a given time and the latter is a count of the number of cells entering mitosis during a given period. The proliferative indices are the simplest and measure the proportion of cells at a particular phase within the cell cycle. The synthetic (S phase) and mitotic (M phase) are the most easily detected and are measured by the labelling index (S phase) and the mitotic index (M phase).

Mitotic index. Mitotic figures can be counted on wax-embedded sections. The mitotic index is the number of mitotic figures observed, divided by the total number of cells counted. There are four phases of mitosis; prophase, metaphase, anaphase and telophase. The early and late stages are difficult to identify and criteria for distinction must be defined early (Macdonald 1971). Van Scott *et al.* (1963) examined 84 anagen roots from 11 biopsies. The skin was fixed in Cajal's uranium nitrate–alcohol–formalin and wax-embedded. Horizontal sections were used to count the density and position of the mitotic figures within the matrix and they estimated the replacement time of the entire germinative matrix as 23 hours.

Labelling index. Cells synthesizing DNA (S phase) will incorporate [³H]thymidine which can then be visualized by autoradiography. After autoradiographic development the label appears as silver grains over the nucleus due to the emission of β-particles. Unfortunately, even after the subtraction of background radiographic interference, there are still many pitfalls in this technique (Maurer 1981). These studies can be performed *in vitro* by incubating skin slices in medium containing [³H]thymidine (92 MBq/ml) for 2.5 hours (Shahrad & Marks 1976), or *in vivo* using intra-dermal injections of 184 MBq [³H]thymidine and carrying out biopsies after fixed intervals (Weinstein & Mooney 1980). Unincorporated thymidine is rapidly cleared and only cells in the S phase will incorporate the injected thymidine (Cleaver 1967). For dynamic studies (Weinstein & Mooney 1980) results must be extrapolated from several individuals as multiple injections of [³H]thymidine are very toxic. The labelling index is the ratio of labelled cells counted.

Metaphase arrest. Cells can be arrested in metaphase by the administration of a stathmokinetic agent. Early studies on sheep performed using systemic Colcemid were sampled after 6 hours to study growth in different seasons (Fraser 1965). Cells with metaphase nuclei are counted and expressed as a ratio of the whole (metaphase index). Vincristine, which inhibits production of the mitotic spindle, is probably the best agent; it has been used to examine hair growth in pig skin (Dover 1985, personal communication) but not in human hair. A dose–response curve would need to be calculated prior to its use and this has only been performed for squamous epithelia (Duffill *et al.* 1977). The rate of increase of the metaphase index is proportional to the number of cells entering mitosis and therefore the birth rate of cells in the time between injection and sampling the tissue. The metaphase index, therefore, differs from the labelling index which only gives a state measurement with no information concerning cell production. The metaphase arrest technique offers the rate of cell production. It is a more accurate and enlightening method and should be used to study hair follicles.

References

Bradfield, R.B. (1971) Protein deprivation colon; comparative response of hair roots, serum protein and urinary nitrogen. *American Journal of Clinical Nutrition*, **24**, 405.
Bradfield, R.B. (1972) A rapid tissue technique for the field assessment of protein–calorie malnutrition. *American Journal of Clinical Nutrition*, **25**, 720.

Bradfield, R.B., Cordano, A. & Graham, G.G. (1969) Hair root adaptation to marasmus in Andean Indian children. *Lancet*, **ii**, 1395.

Cleaver, J.E. (1967) *Thymidine Metabolism and Cell Kinetics. Frontiers of Biology* ,vol. 6, p. 57. North Holland Publishing, Amsterdam.

Crounse, R.G., Bollet, A.J. & Owens, S. (1970) Quantitative tissue of human hair malnutrition using scalp hair roots. *Nature*, **228**, 465.

Dufill, M.B., Appleton, D.R., Dyson, P., Shuster, S., & Wright, N.A., (1977) The measurement of the cell cycle time in squamous epithelium using the metaphase arrest technique with vincristine. *British Journal of Dermatology*, **96**, 493.

Fraser, I.E.B. (1965) Cell proliferation in the wool follicle bulb. In *Biology of the Skin and Hair Growth*, p. 427, eds. A.G. Lyne & B.F. Short. Angus and Robertson, Sydney.

Headington, J.T. (1984) Transverse microscopic anatomy of the human scalp: a basis for a morphometric approach to disorders of the hair follicle. *Archives of Dermatology*, **120**, 449.

Ibrahim, L. & Wright, E.A. (1982) A quantitative study of hair growth using mouse and rat vibrissal follicles. 1. Dermal papilla volume determines hair volume. *Journal of Embryology and Experimental Morphology*, **73**, 209.

Kligman, A.M. (1961) Pathologic dynamics of human hair loss. *Archives of Dermatology*, **83**, 175.

Macdonald, D.G. (1971) Cell renewal in the oral epithelium. In *Current Concepts of the Oral Mucosa*, p.61, eds. C.A. Squirer & J. Meyer. C.C. Thomas, Springfield.

Maguire, H.C. & Kligman, A.M. (1964) Hair plucking as a diagnostic tool. *Journal of Investigative Dermatology*, **43**, 77.

Maurer, H.R. (1981) Potential pitfalls of [³H]thymidine techniques to a measure cell proliferation. *Cell Tissue Kinetics*, **14**, 111.

Pinkus, F. (1947) The story of a hair root. *Journal of Investigative Dermatology*, **9**, 91.

Saitoh, M., Uzaka, M. & Sakamoto, M. (1970) Human hair cycle. *Journal of Investigative Dermatology*, **54**, 65.

Schreck-Purola, I., Lindroos, B., Nystrom, R.E.A. & Sekala, K. (1981) Hair neogenesis in man: a histoquantitative study based on 1000 scalp biopsies. In *Hair Research*, p. 334, eds. C.E. Orfanos, W. Montagna & G. Stuttgen. Springer-Verlag, Berlin.

Shahrad, P. & Marks, R. (1976) Hair follicle kinetics in psoriasis. *Journal of Investigative Dermatology*, **94**, 7.

Uno, H., Adachi, K. & Montagna, W. (1969) Morphological and biochemical studies of hair follicle in common baldness of stump tailed macaque (*Macaca speciosa*). In *Advances in Biology of the Skin*, vol. IX, *Hair Growth*, p. 221, eds. W. Montagna & R.L. Dobson. Pergamon Press, Oxford.

Van Scott, E.J., Ekel, T.M. & Auerbach, R. (1963) Determinants of rate and kinetics of cell division in scalp hair. *Journal of Investigative Dermatology*,**41**, 269.

Van Scott, E.J. & Ekel, T.M. (1958) Geometric relationships between the matrix of the hair bulb and its dermal papilla in normal and alopecic scalp. *Journal of Investigative Dermatology*, **31**, 281.

Van Scott, E.J., Reinertson, R.P. & Steinmuller, R. (1957) The growing hair roots of human scalp and morphological changes therein following amethopterin therapy. *Journal of Investigative Dermatology*, **29**, 197.

Weinstein, G.D. & Mooney, K.M. (1980) Cell proliferation kinetics in the human hair root. *Journal of Investigative Dermatology*, **74**, 43.

Hair shaft length and diameter measurements
(References p. 596)

The hair shaft is measured using the parameters of length and diameter, and with these measurements the volume can be calculated from the formula $\pi r^2 l$, where r is the radius and l the length. The weight of hair is a comparable measure to volume but must be carefully standardized for shaving technique, washing and removal of epithelial débris. The easiest method to measure length is to bleach or shave the hair and measure the subsequent growth of undyed hair or stubble. Shaving does have the advantage of removing telogen hairs. Plucking hairs is not a useful manoeuvre as it introduces a variable lag in growth until the shaft has grown through the skin (Ibrahim & Wright 1978), and animal experiments suggest that plucking may alter linear growth (Dolnich 1969).

There are two widely used methods for measurement of linear growth; calibrated capillary tubes (Fig. 19.3) and macrophotography. Both of these

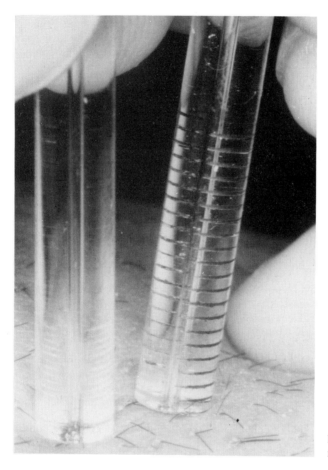

Fig. 19.3 Capillary tube measurement of hair growth.

methods are used after shaving, are repeatable and offer good correlation between observers. The capillary tube technique is easy and cheap, requiring only an accurately graduated tube. Macrophotography requires apparatus to ensure that magnification and orientation (Jones *et al.* 1981) are kept constant and that processing does not introduce any alterations in magnification. It does offer the advantage of clinical speed. The hairs are pressed flat against the skin with a microscope slide to ensure that the entire length is visualized (Burgess & Edwards 1978; Saitoh *et al.* 1969, 1970).

Reference points on the hair shaft can also be made by autoradiography after incorporation of radioisotopes. This technique was initially used in sheep (Downes & Syne 1959) with parenteral administration. Uptake of the isotope is rapid and [^{14}C]glucose can be detected in the hair bulb after 1 hour (Ryder 1956). [^{35}S]-Cystine is not taken up by the bulb but seems to enter the keratogenous zone directly. In the mouse, using [^{35}S]cystine, appreciable radioactivity can be seen after 2 minutes, but detectable activity is measurable as soon as 30 seconds which suggests immediate uptake (Ryder 1958). After 2 days the majority of the radioactivity is in the hair shaft above the keratogenous zone and after 6 days it is above the surface of the skin. No radioactivity within the follicle could be measured after 16 days (Harkness & Bern 1957). Edwards (1954), using the guinea-pig, administered [^{35}S]methionine intravenously, orally and by inunction to a defined area on the dorsum of the animal. He found identical patterns of shaft labelling with each form of administration, including labelling of the belly hair after inunction; incorporation into the hair with the intravenous route was 5% of the administered dose and only 1% with the topical route.

Munro (1966) developed the technique further for human use, using intra-dermal injections of [^{35}S]cystine. He initially demonstrated that the radioactivity which remains in rats' skin after intra-dermal injections of [^{35}S]cystine was only 30% after 10 minutes and had disappeared after 30 minutes. In view of these findings he felt that the risks of future carcinogenesis were negligible. He injected 185 Bq L-cystine in 0.05 ml saline intra-dermally, to form wheals approximately 6 mm in diameter, and repeated the injections after 3–4 weeks. The incorporated radioactivity was visualized in bands across the hair shaft on autoradiographs. In the three women investigated, scalp hair grew at 0.37 mm/day, forearm hair at 0.18 mm/day and thigh hair at 0.30 mm/day. Comaish used the identical technique to examine hair growth in uninvolved skin of patients with dermatoses (1969b) and monilethrix (1969a). He found no significant difference between these subjects or controls and no circadian growth rhythm. There was, however considerable variation in growth rates within each hair fibre. This information was discovered by injecting [^{35}S]cystine as frequently as every 3 days, and by careful alteration of the timing of each injection the data could be analysed to give growth rates for specific parts of the day.

Hair clippings can be used to determine length or diameter and may be measured using a graduated eye-piece graticule mounted on a low-power microscope. Micrometers cannot be used as hair is too soft and will yield to low compression forces. The hairs should be mounted on a glass microscope slide using a drop of water or more firmly fixed with cellophane tape (Barth *et al.* 1989), Canada balsam (Ebling *et al.* 1977), or Depex—a high viscosity plastic which sets as hard as glass on exposure to air (Peereboom-Wynia 1981). Bradfield (1972) floated the hairs on water in a Petri dish and Sims (1967) mounted the individual hairs in a syringe needle to measure the diameter in two dimensions. This may be important since a diameter variation between 77 and 39 μm (mean maximum and minimum dimensions) was found in normal hairs (Sims 1967). This observation of the oval cross-section of hair shafts has been confirmed by Rushton *et al.* (1983). Peereboom-Wynia (1981) measured hair diameters at several sites from the bulb to the shaft and found that if measurements were made above the outer root sheath the hair diameter was constant throughout the shaft, though greater in anagen than in telogen. Measurements of scalp hair show a constancy in diameter over the proximal 40 mm (Sims & Knollmeyer 1970). It should be noted that telogen hairs taper towards the bulb (Jackson *et al.* 1972).

Measurement of the diameter of hair may be complicated by swelling due to humidity and variations in the diameter due to the oral cross-section of hair shafts. Although we have not found these to introduce errors when a mean diameter of several hairs is required (Barth *et al.* 1989), several devices have been constructed to overcome these problems. Individual cells have been used which hold individual hairs with glue and hooks and allow rotation under a microscope (Barnard & White 1954; White & Stam 1949). White and Stam (1949) noted that the shaft diameter was not uniform along its length but that a representative number of major and minor diameters could be determined along a 20 mm fibre. A more sophisticated method relies on the relationship between vibration resonance and diameter (Dart & Peterson 1949). Laser beam diffraction has been used to measure diameter with very accurate results (Brancik & Datyner 1977).

Hair weight has been measured as an index of both human and animal hair growth (Marston 1955; Hamilton *et al.* 1969). The weight will be affected by oils and epidermis, and standardized methods must be established. This method appears to be suitable for measuring the small reductions in hair growth obtained with weak anti-androgen therapy (Casey *et al.* 1966).

References

Barnard, W.S. & White, H.J. (1954). The swelling of hair and a viscose rayon monofil in aqueous solutions. *Textile Research Journal*, **24**, 695.

Barth, J.H., Cherry, C.A., Wojnarowska F. & Dawber R.P.R. (1989) Spironolactone is an effective and well tolerated antiandrogen therapy for hirsute women. *Journal of Clinical Endocrinology and Metabolism*, **68**, 966.

Bradfield, R.B. (1972) A rapid tissue technique for the field assessment of protein–calorie malnutrition. *American Journal of Clinical Nutrition*, **25**, 720.

Brancik, J.V. & Datyner, A. (1977) The measurement of swelling of wool fibres in solvents by laser beam diffraction. *Textiles Research Journal*, **47**, 662.

Burgess, C.A. & Edwards, C.R.W. (1978) Hirsutography. *British Journal of Photography*, **36**, 770.

Casey, J.H., Burger, H.G., Kent, J.R. *et al.* (1966) Treatment of hirsutism by adrenal and ovarian suppression. *Journal of Clinical Endocrinology*, **26**, 1370.

Comaish, S. (1969a) Autoradiographic studies of hair growth and rhythm in monilethrix. *British Journal of Dermatology*, **81**, 443.

Comaish, S. (1969b) Autoradiographic studies of hair growth in various dermatoses: investigation of a possible circadian rhythm in human hair growth. *British Journal of Dermatology*, **81**, 283.

Dart, S.L. & Peterson, L.E. (1949) A strain-gage system for fibre testing. *Textiles Research Journal*, **19**, 89.

Dolnich, E.H. (1969) Variability in hair growth in *Macaca mulatta*. In *Advances in Biology of the Skin*, vol. IX, *Hair Growth*, p. 121, eds. W. Montagna & R.L. Dobson. Pergamon Press, Oxford.

Downes, A.M. & Syne, A.G. (1959) Measurement of the rate of growth of wool using cystine labelled with sulphur. *Nature*, **184**, 1884.

Ebling, F.J., Thomas, A.K., Cooke, L.D., Randall, V.A., Skinner, J. & Cawood, M. (1977) Effect of cyproterone acetate on hair growth, sebum excretion and endocrine parameters in an hirsute subject. *British Journal of Dermatology*, **97**, 371.

Edwards, L.J. (1954) The absorption of methionine by the skin of the guinea pig. *Biochemistry*, **57**, 542.

Hamilton, J.B., Terada, H., Mestler, G.E. & Tirman, W. (1969) I. Coarse sternal hairs, a male characteristic that can be measured quantitatively: the influence of sex, age and genetic factors. II. Other sex differentiating characters: relationship to age, to one another and to coarse sternal hairs. In *Advances in Biology of the Skin*, vol. IX, *Hair Growth*, p. 129, eds. W. Montagna & R.L. Dobson. Pergamon Press, Oxford.

Harkness, D.R. & Bern, H.A. (1957) Radioautographic studies of hair growth in the mouse. *Acta Anatomica*, **31**, 35.

Ibrahim, L. & Wright, E.A. (1978) The effect of a single plucking at different times in the hair cycle on the growth of individual mouse vibriassae. *British Journal of Dermatology*, **99**, 365.

Jackson, D., Church, R.E. & Ebling, F.J. (1972) Hair diameter in female baldness. *British Journal of Dermatology*, **87**, 361.

Jones, K.R., Katz, M., Keyzer, C. & Gordon, W. (1981) Effect of cyproterone acetate on rate of hair growth in hirsute females. *British Journal of Dermatology*, **105**, 685.

Marston, H.R. (1955) Wool growth. In *Progress in the Physiology of Farm Animals*, vol. 2, p. 543, ed. J. Hammond. Butterworths, London.

Munro, D.D. (1966) Hair growth measurement using intradermal sulphur-35 cystine. *Archives of Dermatology*, **933**, 119.

Peereboom-Wynia, J.D.R. (1981) Comparative studies of the diameters of hairshafts in anagen and in telogen phases in male adults without alopecia and in male adults with androgenic alopecia. In *Hair Research*, p. 294, eds. C.F. Orphanos, W. Montagna & G. Stuttgen. Springer Verlag, Berlin.

Rushton, H., James, K.C. & Mortimer, C.H. (1983) The unit area trichogram in the assessment of androgen dependent alopecia. *British Journal of Dermatology*, **109**, 429.

Ryder, M.L. (1956) Use of radioisotopes in the study of wool growth and fibre composition. *Nature*, **178**, 1409.

Ryder, M.L. (1958) Nutritional factors influencing hair and wool growth. In *The Biology of the Skin*, vol. IX, *Hair Growth*, p. 320, eds. W. Montagna & R.A. Ellis. Academic Press, London.

Saitoh, M., Uzuka, M., Sakomoto, M. & Kobori, T. (1969) Rate of hair growth. In *Advances in Biology of the Skin*, vol. IX, *Hair Growth*, p. 183, eds. W. Montagna & R.L. Dobson. Pergamon Press, Oxford.

Saitoh, M., Uzaka, M. & Sakamoto, M. (1970) Human hair cycle. *Journal of Investigative Dermatology*, **54**, 65.

Sims, R.T. (1967) Hair growth in kwashiorkor. *Archives of Diseases of Children*, **42**, 397.

Sims, R.T. & Knollmeyer, H.H.F. (1970) Multivariate normal frequency distributions for the analysis of scalp hair measurements. *British Journal of Dermatology*, **83**, 200.

White, H.J. & Stam, P.B. (1949) An experimental and theoretical study of the absorption and swelling isotherms of human hair in water vapour. *Textiles Research Journal*, **19**, 136.

Hair shaft morphology—vellus hair index
(Reference p. 600)

Androgenic stimulation of hair roots mediates the conversion of vellus into terminal and vice versa. Madanes and Novothy (1987) have suggested using the ratio of vellus/terminal hair as an index for hair growth in hirsuties. The skin is shaved (approximately 5×7.5 cm but there is no need to accurately define the field) and the hair shafts are examined microscopically and the number of vellus and terminal hairs counted. The ratio significantly differs between males, hirsute women and non-hirsute women, but it is unknown at present whether it is adequately sensitive to detect alterations with anti-androgen therapy.

Compound measurements
(References p. 600)

The trichogram is a composite measurement of several growth parameters. It was developed in order to formulate a more dynamic expression of growth. The term has been used by several authors to describe their different concepts. Uno *et al.* (1969), Schreck-Purola *et al.* (1981) and Headington (1984) have used solely histological features as described above.

Barman *et al.* (1964) have described a less invasive means of multiple measurement which collates the number of hairs per unit area and shaft diameter, growth, and root-cycle stage. A specifically designed microscope was used with $60 \times$ magnification. This is placed on the skin surface which acts as the stage; two eye-pieces are used, one with a micrometer scale calibrated down to $1/40$ mm and the other containing a reticulum defining an area of 4 mm^2. This area was then shaved and re-examined for length of growth after 5–10 days. Root status was measured, as before, by plucking. Using this technique they have collected data on the normal pattern of growth in the newborn child (Pecoraro *et al.* 1964a), prepubertal children (Pecoraro *et al.* 1964b), adults (Barman *et al.* 1965), pregnant women (Pecoraro *et al.* 1969), pubic hair (Astore *et al.* 1979) and axillary hair (Pecoraro *et al.* 1971). Stencils have been used to delineate the area for repeatability (Melick & Taft 1959; Rushton *et al.* 1983). Rushton *et al.* (1983) modified this trichogram by means of an intense washing and combing programme for 3 days, including the sample day, prior to plucking the hairs individually from a larger area of 35–45 mm^2. They also measured shaft diameter in two planes.

Hair pluckability

During studies of children suffering from protein–calorie malnutrition (PCM), it was noticed that the hair was not fully pigmented, was thin, sparse, straight and easily plucked (Jelliffe 1966). Therefore, hair has been suggested as an easily obtained tissue source for assessment of PCM using anagen/telogen ratios, shaft diameter and bulb morphology (Bradfield & Jelliffe 1970; Bradfield 1971). Chase *et al.* (1981) have developed a trichotillometer; this is a plucking device which comprises a spring dynamometer with a clamp to hold individual hairs, and a scale graduated at 1.4 g intervals from 0–62 g. The mean epilation force required to pluck 10 hairs has been assessed in normal and malnourished children and was found to correlate well with the serum albumin. The normal epilation force is > 36 g whereas in kwashiorkor it is < 19 g. This measure correlates well with shaft diameter which is also a good index of hair growth. They encourage the use of this technique which requires little training and no laboratory facilities. Regional epilation forces have been measured for hair from the scalp (Tsuda 1957), eyebrows and cilia (Sato 1960) and axillary and pubic hairs (Bessho & Okamoto 1960). However, this technique still needs to be rigorously evaluated on normal hair to determine variations with growth status (anagen or telogen) and with diameter.

Growth pattern analysis

Most mammals have synchronized hair growth which permits seasonal moulting. Hair growth in rats which spreads in a cephalo-caudal direction may be observed by administering a dye that colours the hair shaft (Johnson 1958). This would clearly be unacceptable in man and in any case would probably be inappropriate as man does not appear to moult. In a human clinical setting it is more useful to measure the changing pattern of hair growth. The patterns of androgenic hair growth on the body (hirsutism) and on the scalp (androgenic alopecia) have been formally defined, and grading systems formulated for the varying degrees of severity (Ferriman & Gallwey 1961; Hamilton 1951; Ludwig 1977) (see Chapter 5). These scores are easy to perform but are subject to considerable observer bias as is demonstrated in Fig. 19.4. This illustration compares the hirsutism score of

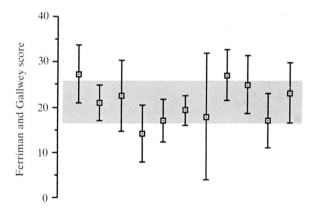

Fig. 19.4 This illustration compares 11 studies which have used the Ferriman and Gallwey (1961) scale to measure hirsutism: each study is represented as mean ± SD. The wide variation in scores of hirsute women (who may be assumed to be a homogeneous population) clearly states that no valid comparison may be made between these groups.

11 studies, all of which used the Ferriman and Gallwey system (1961); the mean and standard deviation of each study is drawn. It is reasonable to assume that the population of hirsute women presenting to any physician is similar and therefore no valid comparison can be made between these studies which have a wide scatter of values. This indicates that multicentre comparisons of therapies for androgenic alopecia or hirsuties cannot rely on subjective grading and must be supplemented with objective criteria.

References

Astore, I.P., Pecoraro, V. & Pecoraro, E.G. (1979) The normal trichogram of pubic hair. *British Journal of Dermatology*, **101**, 441.

Barman, J.M., Astore, I. & Pecoraro, V. (1965) The normal trichogram of the adult. *Journal of Investigative Dermatology*, **44**, 233.

Barman, J.M., Pecoraro, V. & Astore, I. (1964) Method, technique and computations in the study of the trophic state of human scalp hair. *Journal of Investigative Dermatology*, **42**, 421.

Bessho, I. & Okamoto, S. (1960) The extractive strength of human axillary and pubic hairs. *Journal of Kyoto Preferential Medical University*, **68**, 1325.

Bradfield, R.B. (1971) Protein deprivation colon; comparative response of hair roots, serum protein and urinary nitrogen. *American Journal of Clinical Nutrition*, **24**, 405.

Bradfield, R.B. & Jelliffe, E.F.P. (1970) Early assessment of nutrition. *Nature*, **225**, 283.

Chase, E.S., Weinsier, R.L., Laven, G.T. & Krumdieck, C.L. (1981) Trichotillometry: the quantitation of hair pluckability as a method of nutritional assessment. *American Journal of Clinical Nutrition*, **34**, 2280.

Ferriman, D. & Gallwey, J.D. (1961) Clinical assessment of body hair growth in women. *Journal of Clinical Endocrinology*, **21**, 1440.

Hamilton, J.B. (1951) Patterned loss of hair in man: types and incidence. *Annals of the New York Academy of Science*, **53**, 708.

Headington, J.T. (1984) Transverse microscopic anatomy of the human scalp: a basis for a morphometric approach to disorders of the hair follicle. *Archives of Dermatology*, **120**, 449.

Jackson, E. (1958) Quantitative studies of hair growth in the albino rat. I. Normal males and females. *Journal of Endocrinology*, **16**, 337.

Jelliffe, D.B. (1966) The assessment of the nutritional status of the community. *WHO Monograph Series* No. 53 (Geneva).

Ludwig, E. (1977) Classification of the types of androgenic alopecia (common baldness) occurring in the female sex. *British Journal of Dermatology*, **97**, 247.

Madanes, A.E. & Novotny, M.N. (1987) The vellus index: a new method of assessing hair growth. *Fertility and Sterility*, **48**, 1064.

Melick, R. & Taft, H.P. (1959) Observations on body hair in old people. *Journal of Clinical Endocrinology and Metabolism*, **19**, 1597.

Pecoraro, V., Astore, I. & Barman, J.M. (1964a) Cycle of the scalp hair of new born children. *Journal of Investigative Dermatology*, **43**, 145.

Pecoraro, V., Astore, I., Barman, J.M. & Araujo, C.I. (1964b) The normal trichogram in the child before the age of puberty. *Journal of Investigative Dermatology*, **42**, 427.

Pecoraro, V., Astore, I., & Barman, J.M. (1969) Growth rate and hair density of the human axilla. *Journal of Investigative Dermatology*, **56**, 362.

Pecoraro, V., Barman, J.M. & Astore, I. (1967) The normal trichogram of pregnant women. In *Advances in Biology of the Skin*, Vol. IX, *Hair Growth*, p. 203, eds. W. Montagna & R.L. Dobson. Pergamon Press, Oxford.

Rushton, H., James, K.C. & Mortimer, C.H. (1983) The unit area trichogram in the assessment of androgen dependent alopecia. *British Journal of Dermatology*, **109**, 429.

Sato, M. (1960) The extractive strength of human eyebrows and cilia. *Journal of Kyoto Preferential Medical University*, **67**, 1405.

Schreck-Purola, I., Lindroos, B., Nystrom, R.E.A. & Sekala, K. (1981) Hair neogenesis in man: a histoquantitative study based on 1000 scalp biopsies. In *Hair Research*, p. 344, eds. C.E. Orfanos, W. Montagna & G. Stuttgen. Springer-Verlag, Berlin.

Tsuda, K. (1957) Study on the extractive strength of human head hairs. *Journal of Kyoto Preferential Medical University*, **61**, 936.

Uno, H., Adachi, K. & Montagna, W. (1969) Morphological and biochemical studies of hair follicle in common baldness of stump tailed macaque (*Macaca speciosa*). In *Advances in Biology of the Skin*, vol. IX, *Hair Growth*, p. 221, eds W. Montagna & R.L. Dobson. Pergamon Press, Oxford.

Hair and hair follicle microscopy
(References p. 605)

Hair shaft microscopy is essential for the diagnosis of many abnormalities, particularly fungal disease, congenital and hereditary hair shaft disorders and to
assess hair weathering (Caserio 1987a,b).

In the diagnosis of fungal diseases of hair (Rebell & Taplin 1976) plucked hairs
are mounted in 20% potassium hydroxide solution; if the microscopy is to be
carried out within 30 minutes then dimethylsulphoxide (DMSO) may speed the
clearing time. DMSO may cause false negative results beyond this time since hyphal
destruction occurs. The kerion type of infection may show only arthrospores on the
proximal part of the plucked hair shaft despite massive inflammatory changes in
the skin.

Optical microscopy

Routine light microscopy of hair shafts is essential for the diagnosis of diseases such
as hereditary and congenital shaft abnormalities. To assess intrinsic shaft changes
only the proximal 1–2 cm of plucked hairs should be examined since more distal
changes may be extrinsic and due to weathering (Dawber 1980). Hairs may be
mounted dry if they are required for further studies; however, in routine
transmitted light microscopic examination the surface of dry-mounted hairs will
scatter light. More detail is seen and higher magnification will be possible if
a standard mounting medium is used; potassium hydroxide and water are not
satisfactory. 'Colour' changes seen by routine light microscopy may be due to
pigment alterations, or structural changes not transmitting light and thus giving
dark areas. If reflected light is used then the dark areas in structural diseases such as
pili annulati (Chapter 7) become light (Dawber 1972); pigmentation changes are
not altered by this technique. Careful examination using routine light microscopy
provides most of the information required in clinical practice. Polarization
microscopy may provide extra information regarding the biochemical make-up of
the hair and fine structural changes may become more obvious. Using this method
it is possible to determine refractive index and the birefringence of fibres (the
numerical difference between the refractive indexes parallel and perpendicular to
the hair axis), a physical phenomenon that reflects the orientation of internal
structures in the hair. In the examination of hair from patients with a neuroectodermal symptom complex (Price *et al.* 1980), polarizing microscopy revealed
striking bright and dark regions on viewing the hair between cross polarizers.
Turning the microscopic stage approximately 10° (5° on each side of the position of
maximum extinction) reversed the bright and dark areas; between cross polarizers
with the hair axis parallel to the vibration direction of the polarizer (maximum
extinction or 0°), the hair revealed transverse lines. This abnormality was

associated with sulphur, and high sulphur (matrix) protein deficiency. Dupré and Bonafe (1978) and Price (1979) have used polarization microscopy in many structural abnormalities of hair and have shown that the colour changes of polarization show up the abnormalities seen under transmitted light with greater clarity. The subtlety of optical microscopic methods can be enhanced by various specialized techniques (Swift 1977). The scale pattern can be examined in detail by examining a hair cast or impression of the hair in a suitable plastic material; an impression made by rolling the hair in the medium enables the whole circumference to be viewed. Interference microscopy, using monochromatic sodium light, greatly facilitates the examination of minute surface changes (Tolansky 1948).

Electron microscopy

Optical microscopy is limited in resolution to approximately 0.2 μm and has a narrow depth of focus. Transmission electron microscopy is capable of very high resolution (down to 2 nm for biological materials) and has a depth-of-image focus that is greater than the normal specimen thickness (approximately 100 nm). Routine electron microscopic preparation may be suitable for examination of hair follicles, but the presence of keratinized hair within the follicle and the nature of hair structure, make it necessary to modify routine procedure to get the best resolution and meaningful results. Glass knives give poor sectioning; a diamond

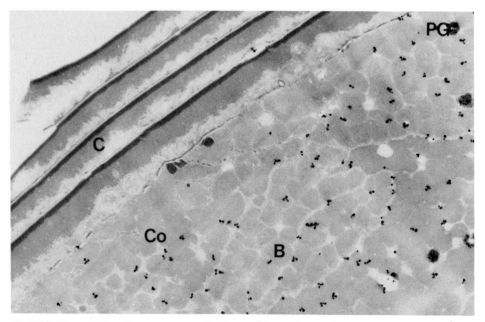

Fig. 19.5 Transmission electron micrograph of normal hair: silver methenamine stain (reduced from × 27,000). The cortex has four layers with the most dense stain (due to sulphur control) outermost. The inner cortex is composed of longitudinal fibres which are seen cut transversely. Cortex (Co); cuticle (C); pigment granule (PG); bundle of longitudinal fibres (B).

knife is necessary for cutting ultra-thin sections of hair without distortion. Needless to say this is a very skilful procedure not always available in electron microscope laboratories. Hair is a rather amorphous structure and must be stained with a heavy metal to show anatomical detail. Uranyl acetate and lead citrate enable the overall structure to be seen; dodecatungstophoric acid gives added detail of cortex matrix proteins and cortical cell membranes. For transverse sections of hair fibres, ammoniacal silver or the silver methenamine stain (Swift 1968) which specifically stain cystine, give more contrast to cuticular and cortical structure (Fig. 19.5) by highlighting the cystine-rich exocuticle and cortical matrix protein (Leonard *et al.* 1980). Other electron histochemical techniques already usefully applied to tissue from many other organs have not yet been fully exploited in hair follicle disease; these include the identification and localization of enzyme systems and antigen–antibody reactions (Swift 1977).

Scanning electron microscopy is very diverse in its modes of operation and gives a wealth of information about surface architecture (Dawber & Comaish 1970; Brown & Swift 1975), elemental composition (if an X-ray microanalytical attachment is available), crystalline make-up and electrical and magnetic properties of specimens. It is a research tool and it cannot be stressed too greatly that all the detail needed by the clinician regarding hair microstructure can be obtained by optical microscopic methods.

Follicular microscopy

Biopsy technique must be considered carefully if useful histological results are to be obtained. The level of the biopsy must extend deep into subcutaneous fat to avoid cutting off hair bulbs. The epidermal surface of the excised tissue should be opposed to a rigid piece of paper, to avoid curling of the tissue, and immediately placed in fixative; if necessary it can be glued or pinned to the paper if longitudinal follicular cutting is desired (Fig. 19.6), since follicles have a great propensity for bending prior to hardening, leading to cross-cutting in the dermis. Punch biopsies (6 mm) and horizontal sectioning at various levels gives more dynamic information about the hair cycle status at the site from which the tissue was taken (Headington 1984). After processing, the embedded tissue requires careful orientation prior to cutting to maximize the chance of obtaining longitudinal follicular sections. Routine paraffin-embedded tissue has never been entirely satisfactory for visualizing cytological detail within the follicle; where possible, tissue should be fixed and embedded as for routine electron microscopy and 1 µm sections cut (Fig. 19.6) to give greater cytological clarity. Haematoxylin and eosin staining reveals the general detail of the various cell layers in the follicle. Other histochemical stains may specifically enhance the appearance of various cell layers (Pinkus 1980). The lower border of the internal root sheath takes up the Giemsa stain; this stains the keratinized internal root sheath specifically dark blue. The intra-follicular hair cuticle stains with toluidine blue and rhodamine B, first becoming visible as a thin

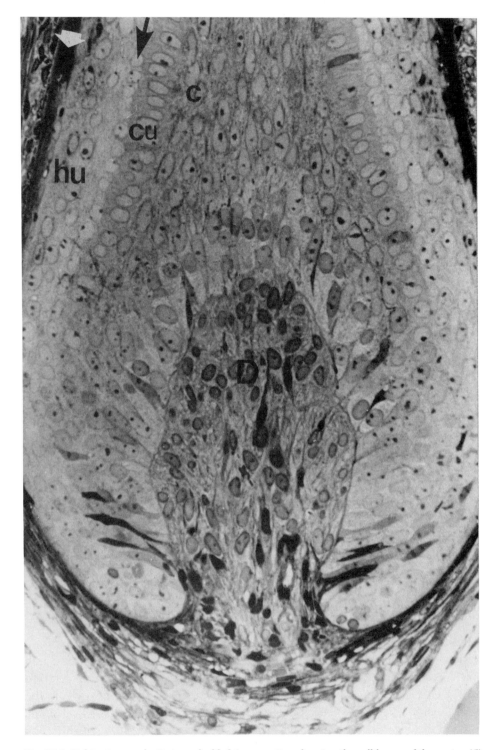

Fig. 19.6 Light micrograph. Resin-embedded 1 μm section showing the cell layers of the cortex (C), cuticle of hair (Cu), the internal root sheath cuticle (black arrow), Huxley layer (Hu), Henle layer (white arrow) and the dermal papilla.

blue layer surrounding the presumptive hair. The Van Gieson stain gives a yellow colour to the hair and the club in telogen roots; the tissue surrounding the club is brownish-red with PASHPA stain whilst rhodamine B stains the cuticle a faint blue colour and the surrounding tricholemmal layer brilliant red. Useful screening techniques for abnormal hair keratins are the fluorescence methods using either acridine orange or thioflavine T; normal hair keratin fluoresces blue with dilute acridine orange, whereas altered keratins such as the tip of hairs in trichorrhexis nodosa, dystrophic hairs in kwashiorkor, or weathered fibres, fluoresce red or orange. The peracetic oxidation and thioflavine T fluorescent method (Jarrett 1958) stain the disulphide bonds in cystine, enabling sites of mature keratin to be detected in the exocuticle or cortex. —SH bonds can be specifically stained by a fluorogenic maleimide, N(7-dimethyl-amino-methyl coumarinyl) maleimide (DACM). This substance only fluoresces on combining with —SH bonds (Taneda *et al.* 1980). This method requires frozen tissue; it has the advantage that the emission maximum of DACM does not overlap with any of the aromatic residues of proteins such as tryptophan.

References

Brown, A.C. & Swift, J.A. (1975) Hair breakage: the scanning electron microscope as a diagnostic tool. *Journal of the Society of Cosmetic Chemists,* **26**, 289.

Caserio, R.J. (1987a) Diagnostic techniques for hair disorders. Part I: microscopic examination of the hair shaft. *Cutis,* **40**, 265.

Caserio, R.J. (1987b) Diagnostic techniques for hair disorders. Part II: microscopic examination of hair bulbs, tips and casts. *Cutis,* **40**, 321.

Dawber, R.P.R. (1972) Investigations of a family with pili annulati associated with blue naevi. *Transactions of the St John's Hospital Dermatological Society,* **58**, 51.

Dawber, R.P.R. (1980) Weathering of hair in some genetic hair dystrophies. In *Hair, Trace Elements and Human Illness,* p. 273, eds. A.C. Brown & R.G. Crounse. Praeger, New York.

Dawber, R.P.R. & Comaish, S. (1970) Scanning electron microscopy of normal and abnormal hair shafts. *Archives of Dermatology,* **101**, 316.

Dupré, A. & Bonafe, J.L. (1978) Pilar dystrophies studied by polarised light. *Annales de Dermatologie et de Vénéréologie,* **105**, 921.

Headington, J.T. (1984) Transverse microscopic anatomy of the human scalp: a basis for a morphometric approach to disorders of the hair follicle. *Archives of Dermatology,* **120**, 449.

Jarrett, A. (1958) Chemistry of inner root sheath and hair keratins. *British Journal of Dermatology,* **70**, 271.

Leonard, J.L., Gummer, C.L. & Dawber, R.P.R. (1980) Generalised trichorrhexis nodosa. *British Journal of Dermatology,* **103**, 85.

Pinkus, H. (1980) Factors in the formation of club hairs. In *Hair, Trace Elements and Human Illness,* p. 147, eds. A.C. Brown & R.G. Crounse. Praeger, New York.

Price, V.H. (1979) Strukturanomalien des Haarschaftes. In *Haar und Haarkrankheiten,* p. 387, ed. C.E. Orfanos. Fischer, Stuttgart.

Price, V.H., Odom, R.B., Ward, W.H. & Jones, F.T. (1980) Trichothiodystrophy: sulphur-deficient brittle hair as a marker for a neuroectodermal symptom complex. *Archives of Dermatology,* **116**, 1375.

Rebell, G. & Taplin, D. (1976) *Dermatophytes: Their Recognition and Identification,* 2nd edn. University of Miami Press, Florida.

Swift, J.A. (1968) Electron histochemistry of cystine-containing proteins in thin transverse sections of human hair. *Journal of the Royal Microscopy Society,* **88**, 449.

Swift, J.A. (1977) The histology of keratin fibres. In *The Chemistry of Natural Protein Fibres*, p. 81, ed. R.S. Asquith. Wiley, London.

Taneda, A., Ogawa, H. & Hashimoto, K. (1980) The histochemical demonstration of protein-bound sulphydryl groups and disulphide bonds in human hair by a new staining method (DACM staining). *journal of Investigative Dermatology*, **75**, 365.

Tolansky, S. (1948) *Multiple Beam Interferometry*. Clarendon Press, Oxford.

Index

Note: Page numbers in *italic* refer to figures.